Exercise and Sport Sciences Reviews

Volume 26, 1998

EXERCISE AND SPORT SCIENCES REVIEWS

Volume 26, 1998

Editor

JOHN O. HOLLOSZY, M.D.

Professor of Medicine
Department of Internal Medicine
Washington University School of Medicine
St. Louis, Missouri

American College of Sports Medicine Series

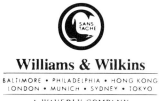

Williams & Wilkins

BALTIMORE • PHILADELPHIA • HONG KONG
LONDON • MUNICH • SYDNEY • TOKYO

A WAVERLY COMPANY

Accurate indications, adverse reactions, and dosage schedules for drugs are provided in this book, but it is possible that they may change. The reader is urged to review the package information data of the manufacturers of the medications mentioned.

Printed in the United States of America
(ISBN 0-683-18346-x)

98 99 00 01 02
1 2 3 4 5 6 7 8 9 10

Preface

Exercise and Sport Sciences Reviews, an annual publication sponsored by the American College of Sports Medicine, reviews current research concerning behavioral, biochemical, biomechanical, clinical, physiological, and rehabilitational topics involving exercise science. The Editorial Board for this series currently consists of 13 recognized authorities who have assumed responsibility for one of the following general topics: athletic medicine, biochemistry, biomechanics, environmental physiology, epidemiology, exercise physiology, gerontology, growth and development, metabolism, molecular biology, physical fitness, psychology, and rehabilitation. The organization of the Editorial Board should help foster the commitment of the American College of Sports Medicine to publish timely reviews in areas of broad interest to clinicians, educators, exercise scientists, and students. The goal for this Editorial Board is to provide reviews in each of these 13 areas whenever sufficient new information becomes available on topics that are likely to be of interest to the readership of *Exercise and Sport Sciences Reviews.* Further, the Editor selects additional topics to be developed into chapters based on current interest, timeliness, and importance to the above audience. The contributors for each volume are selected by the Editorial Board members and the Editor.

John O. Holloszy, M.D.
Editor

Contributors

Gregory R. Adams, Ph.D.
Department of Physiology and Biophysics
University of California, Irvine
Irvine, California

Carl J. Caspersen, Ph.D., M.P.H.
Physical Activity Epidemiologist
Physical Activity and Health Branch
Division of Nutrition and Physical Activity
National Center for Chronic Disease
    Prevention and Health Promotion
Centers for Disease Control and Prevention
Atlanta, Georgia

George N. DeMartino, Ph.D.
University of Texas
Southwestern Medical Center
Dallas, Texas

Robert H. DuRant, Ph.D.
Department of Pediatrics
Brenner Children's Hospital
Wake Forest University School of Medicine
Winston-Salem, North Carolina

Claire T. Farley, Ph.D.
Department of Integrative Biology
University of California, Berkeley
Berkeley, California

Daniel P. Ferris, M.S, Ed.
Department of Integrative Biology
University of California, Berkeley
Berkeley, California

Charles S. Fulco, Sc.D.
Thermal and Mountain Medicine Division
U.S. Army Research Institute of Environmental Medicine
Natick, Massachusetts

Paul L. Greenhaff, Ph.D.
Department of Physiology and Pharmacology
School of Biomedical Sciences
University Medical School
Queen's Medical Centre
Nottingham, United Kingdom

James M. Hagberg, Ph.D.
Department of Kinesiology
University of Maryland
College Park, Maryland

Ben F. Hurley, Ph.D.
Department of Kinesiology
University of Maryland
College Park, Maryland

Steven F. Lewis, Ph.D.
Department of Health Sciences
Boston University
Boston, Massachusetts

Patricia A. Nixon, Ph.D.
Department of Pediatrics
University of Pittsburgh
Pittsburgh, Pennsylvania

George A. Ordway, Ph.D.
Department of Physiology
University of Texas
Southwestern Medical Center
Dallas, Texas

Richard L. Seip, Ph.D.
Health, Physical Education, and Recreation Department
University of Nebraska
Kearney, Nebraska

Clay F. Semenkovich, M.D.
Departments of Medicine and
   Cell Biology and Physiology
Washington University School of Medicine
St. Louis, Missouri

Robert J. Sonstroem, Ph.D.
University of Rhode Island
Kingston, Rhode Island

Donald B. Thomason, Ph.D.
Department of Physiology and Biophysics
University of Tennessee
Memphis, Tennessee

James A. Timmons, B.Sc., Ph.D.
Department of Physiology and Pharmacology
School of Biomedical Sciences
University Medical School
Queen's Medical Centre
Nottingham, United Kingdom

Charles M. Tipton, Ph.D.
Department of Physiology
University of Arizona
Tucson, Arizona

Anton J.M. Wagenmakers, Ph.D.
Department of Human Biology &
   Stable Isotope Research Centre
Maastricht University
Maastricht, The Netherlands

William W. Winder, Ph.D.
Department of Zoology
Brigham Young University
Provo, Utah

Contents

Preface | *v*

Contributors | *vii*

1 INTERACTION BETWEEN AEROBIC AND ANAEROBIC
   METABOLISM DURING INTENSE MUSCLE
   CONTRACTION | 1
   Paul L. Greenhaff, Ph.D., James A. Timmons, Ph.D.

2 ROLE OF INSULIN-LIKE GROWTH FACTOR-I IN THE
   REGULATION OF SKELETAL MUSCLE ADAPTATION TO
   INCREASED LOADING | 31
   Gregory R. Adams, Ph.D.

3 OPTIMIZING HEALTH IN OLDER PERSONS: AEROBIC OR
   STRENGTH TRAINING? | 61
   Ben F. Hurley, Ph.D., James M. Hagberg, Ph.D.

4 A NEW APPROACH TO STUDYING MUSCLE FATIGUE AND
   FACTORS AFFECTING PERFORMANCE DURING DYNAMIC
   EXERCISE IN HUMANS | 91
   Steven F. Lewis, Ph.D., Chalres S. Fulco, Sc.D.

5 MALONYL-CoA—REGULATOR OF FATTY ACID OXIDATION IN
   MUSCLE DURING EXERCISE | 117
   William W. Winder, Ph.D.

6 PHYSICAL SELF-CONCEPT: ASSESSMENT AND EXTERNAL
   VALIDITY | 133
   Robert J. Sonstroem, Ph.D., FACSM

7 TRANSLATIONAL CONTROL OF GENE EXPRESSION IN
   MUSCLE | 165
   Donald B. Thomason, Ph.D.

8 SKELETAL MUSCLE LIPOPROTEIN LIPASE: MOLECULAR
   REGULATION AND PHYSIOLOGICAL EFFECTS IN RELATION
   TO EXERCISE | 191
   Richard L. Seip, Ph.D., Clay F. Semenkovich, M.D.

9 UBIQUITIN-PROTEASOME PATHWAY OF INTRACELLULAR
   PROTEIN DEGRADATION: IMPLICATIONS FOR MUSCLE
   ATROPHY DURING UNLOADING | 219
   George N. DeMartino, Ph.D., George A. Ordway, Ph.D.

10 BIOMECHANICS OF WALKING AND RUNNING: CENTER OF
    MASS MOVEMENTS TO MUSCLE ACTION | 253
    Claire T. Farley, Ph.D., Daniel P. Ferris, M.S.

11 MUSCLE AMINO ACID METABOLISM AT REST AND DURING
    EXERCISE: ROLE IN HUMAN PHYSIOLOGY AND
    METABOLISM | 287
    Anton J. M. Wagenmakers, Ph.D.

12 CONTEMPORARY EXERCISE PHYSIOLOGY: FIFTY YEARS AFTER
    THE CLOSURE OF HARVARD FATIGUE LABORATORY | 315
    Charles M. Tipton, Ph.D.

13 PHYSICAL ACTIVITY EPIDEMIOLOGY APPLIED TO CHILDREN
    AND ADOLESCENTS | 341
    Carl J. Caspersen, Ph.D., M.P.H., Patricia A. Nixon, Ph.D.,
    Robert H. DuRant, Ph.D.

Index | *405*

1
Interaction Between Aerobic and Anaerobic Metabolism During Intense Muscle Contraction

PAUL L. GREENHAFF, PH.D.
JAMES A. TIMMONS, PH.D.

Adenosine tri-phosphate (ATP) is the only fuel available for maintenance of skeletal muscle homeostasis and contractile function. Exercise rapidly increases the energy demand of skeletal muscle, and since the store of ATP in skeletal muscle is limited (~24 mmol/kg dry muscle, or dm), this means that an equivalent increase in the rate of ATP resynthesis must occur for exercise to continue. At the onset of submaximal exercise, phosphocreatine (PCr) degradation and glycogen hydrolysis to lactate provide a significant proportion of ATP resynthesis until steady-state metabolic regulation is once again achieved. This is commonly referred to as anaerobic ATP resynthesis, or more correctly, as ATP resynthesis derived from substrate level phosphorylation. Having achieved a steady state, oxidative phosphorylation becomes the major contributor to ATP resynthesis. During maximal exercise, when a steady-state situation is never achieved, the ATP demand of contraction is very high (e.g., 11 mmol ATP/kg dm/s), and muscle fatigue occurs rapidly. Under these circumstances, ATP resynthesis derived from substrate level phosphorylation normally makes the largest contribution to total ATP resynthesis. By way of example, Bangsbo et al. [3] reported that during 192 seconds (sec) of exercise at a workload equivalent to 130% of maximal oxygen consumption (VO_2 max.), anaerobic ATP resynthesis during the initial 30 sec of exercise contributed approximately 80% of the total ATP turnover. Anaerobic ATP resynthesis then declined to 45% during 60 to 90 sec, and declined to 30% after 120 sec of exercise, and appeared to be accompanied by an increase in oxidative phosphorylation. Therefore, it is apparent that during intense muscular contraction, the contribution made by anaerobic and aerobic ATP resynthesis will vary with exercise duration, and that the time constant for recruitment of the various ATP resynthesis pathways will differ greatly [79].

This chapter will concern itself with the physiological and biochemical regulation of these ATP regenerating pathways, and which identified factors, if any, determine their interaction during contraction. In particular,

1

we will highlight some of the recent information concerning individual human skeletal muscle fiber type responses to intense contraction. We will also consider some of the factors that determine ATP resynthesis during repeated periods of exercise. This exercise will then be used as a model to help explain the interaction between anaerobic and aerobic metabolism. Finally, the factors that are thought to determine the rate of onset of oxygen consumption, and hence the contribution made by oxidative ATP regeneration during intense muscle contraction, will be evaluated.

METABOLIC RESPONSES TO MAXIMAL EXERCISE

In the 1960s, Margaria et al. [76] reported that during maximal exercise of 10–5 sec duration, the total energy demand of contraction could be met solely by hydrolysis of muscle ATP and PCr stores. The authors concluded that only when the muscle PCr stores were depleted would ATP resynthesis occur via glycolysis (with the reduced nicotinamide adenine dinucleotide—NADH—produced being oxidized via the formation of lactate). This was a popular belief since PCr is stored in the cytosol in close proximity to the sites of energy utilization, and because PCr hydrolysis is rapidly activated by ADP accumulation and does not necessitate the completion of several metabolic reactions before energy is transferred to fuel ATP resynthesis. It is now accepted, however, that PCr hydrolysis and lactate production do not occur in isolation, and that both are initiated rather rapidly at the onset of contraction [6, 11, 68, 69]. For example, in a study by Bergström et al. [6], muscle PCr concentration declined by ~16 mmol/kg dm and the lactate concentration increased by ~15 mmol/kg dm, all within 6.6 sec of isometric contraction.

With the introduction of percutaneous electrical stimulation for use in human physiology [65], it became possible to investigate *in vivo* muscle metabolism and fatigue independent of subject motivation. These investigations were performed under conditions where metabolite efflux from the muscle could be minimized by occluding blood flow, thus creating a metabolically closed compartment. The use of electrical stimulation also enabled muscle biopsy samples to be obtained during contraction, a procedure that is not possible during dynamic exercise. Using this technique, it was demonstrated that as little as 1.3 sec of intense electrical stimulation was sufficient to degrade PCr by 11 mmol/kg dm, and increase lactate accumulation by 2 mmol/kg dm [64]. This study confirmed the earlier findings of Bergström et al., where PCr and lactate production appeared to occur simultaneously at the onset of intense muscle contraction [6].

While it is accepted that degradation of glycogen to lactate makes a significant contribution to ATP resynthesis during the initial period of intense exercise, the importance of PCr hydrolysis lies in the extremely rapid rates at which the creatine kinase (CK) reaction can resynthesis ATP. This is

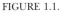

FIGURE 1.1.
Rates of anaerobic ATP production from phosphocreatine (PCr) and glycolysis during intense electrically evoked muscle contraction in man.

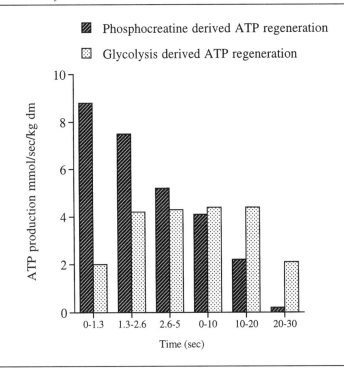

especially important during maximal short-duration exercise. For example, Figure 1.1 shows the rate of muscle ATP resynthesis from PCr hydrolysis during 30 sec of maximal electrically-evoked isometric contraction [62]. It should be noted that PCr hydrolysis was at its highest within 2 sec of the initiation of contraction. It is expected, through our understanding of the CK reaction, that a momentary rise in ADP concentration at the onset of contraction would be the primary stimulus for this rapid hydrolysis. However, after 2.6 sec of contraction, the rate of ATP production from PCr declined by about 15%, and following 10 sec of contraction, was reduced by more than 50%. The contribution of PCr to ATP resynthesis in the last 10 sec of 30 sec contraction was very small, amounting to only 2% of the initial rate. The mechanisms responsible for the rapid decline in the rate of PCr utilization during maximal contraction are presently unknown. These mechanisms may be related to a local myofibrillar decline in PCr availability, since the rate of creatine (Cr) rephosphorylation by the mitochondrial CK may not be able to operate sufficiently fast enough to regenerate PCr. It should be emphasized that PCr resynthesis, whether it be during each duty cycle or at the end of exercise, is entirely dependent on oxidative phosphorylation [85]. It is also apparent that there is a decline in muscle force production associated with the rapid decline in PCr stores [62], and, as a consequence, there is also a decline in the flux of ADP from the myofibrils to the mitochondria.

From the rapid decline in the rate of ATP resynthesis arising from PCr hydrolysis shown in Figure 1.1, it is clear that for maximal exercise to continue beyond only a few seconds, glycolysis must proceed at a very rapid rate following the initiation of contraction. The activation of muscle contraction by calcium (Ca^{2+}) and the accumulation of the products of ATP and PCr hydrolysis—adenosine diphosphate (ADP), adenosine monophosphate (AMP), inosine monophosphate (IMP), ammonia (NH_3) and inorganic phosphate (Pi)—all act as stimulators of glycogenolysis and glycolysis. In this way, they stimulate glycolytic ATP production, at least in the short term. A seminal study by Hultman et al., which delineated much of what we know about human skeletal muscle PCr metabolism during exercise, demonstrated that ATP regeneration from PCr degradation and substrate level phosphorylation from glycolysis interact [61]. Some of the factors that may bring about this interaction will be discussed below.

Interaction of Adenine Nucleotide, PCr, and Glycogen Metabolism

Glycogenolysis is the hydrolysis of muscle glycogen to glucose-1-phosphate. Glucose-1-phosphate, together with glucose derived from the circulation, form glucose-6-phosphate, with glycolysis being the sequence of events from glucose-6-phosphate to pyruvate formation. Control of muscle glycogenolysis is a highly complex process that can no longer be considered to simply center around the degree of transformation of less active glycogen phosphorylase *b* to the more active *a* form [26]. For example, researchers know that glycogenolysis can proceed at a negligible rate in resting skeletal muscle, despite almost total transformation of phosphorylase to the *a* form [18]. Conversely, an increase in glycogenolytic rate has been observed during resting circulatory occlusion, despite a relatively low mole fraction of the phosphorylase *a* form [26]. From this and other related work, it was concluded that Pi accumulation arising from ATP, and more importantly, PCr hydrolysis during muscle contraction, played a key role in the regulation of the glycogenolytic activity of phosphorylase *a*. These responses then served as a link between the ATP turnover associated with contraction and the rate of substrate mobilization. This interpretation is further supported by the observation that the reduction in skeletal muscle PCr degradation during fatiguing contraction following dichloroacetate administration (a known pyruvate dehydrogenase complex—PDC—activator) is associated with a substantial reduction in the rate of glycogenolysis [108].

That glycogenolysis occurs within 2 sec of the onset of muscle contraction without any measurable increase in Pi [63], and that glycogenolysis can proceed at a low rate despite a high phosphorylase *a* form and Pi concentration [89], suggests that factors other than simply the degree of phosphorylase transformation and Pi availability are involved in the regulation of glycogenolysis *in vivo*. For example, there is substantial evidence to suggest that both IMP and AMP are important regulators of glycogenolysis during exercise [90, 93]. IMP is thought to exert its effect by increasing the activity of phosphorylase *b* during contraction (apparent Km of phosphorylase *b* for IMP ~1.2 mmol/l intracellular water) [25, 75]. Indeed, IMP accumulation is thought to be one of the best indicators of the imbalance between ATP utilization and resynthesis pathways [52], and a teleologically efficient way of regulating glycogenolysis during contraction. AMP has also been shown to increase the activity of phosphorylase *b*, but is thought to require a non-physiological accumulation of free AMP to do so (apparent Km of phosphorylase *b* for AMP ~1.0 mmol/l intracellular water) [25, 75]. For this reason, most researchers believe that the principal function of AMP accumulation is to act as a positive modulator of phosphorylase *a* activity. However, because 90% or more of the total cell content of AMP is thought to be bound to cell proteins *in vivo* [99], researchers have questioned whether the increase in free AMP during contraction is of sufficient magnitude to affect the kinetics of phosphorylase *a* [90]. In contrast, it has been demonstrated that a small increase in AMP concentration (10 umol/l) can markedly increase the *in vitro* activity of phosphorylase *a* [90]. *In vivo* evidence that demonstrates a close relationship between muscle ATP turnover and glycogen utilization suggests that exercise-induced increases in free AMP and Pi concentrations may be the key regulators of glycogen degradation during muscle contraction [90, 93].

Glycolysis involves several more steps than PCr hydrolysis; however, compared with the rate of onset of oxidative phosphorylation (half-time of ~1 sec vs. half-time of 15–20 sec), glycolysis is still a very rapid method of maintaining ATP availability. As shown in Figure 1.1, ATP resynthesis from glycolysis during 30 sec of maximal electrically-evoked contraction occurs almost immediately at the onset of contraction. Furthermore, unlike PCr hydrolysis, ATP production from glycolysis does not reach its maximal rate until after 5 sec of contraction. Since ATP production from glycolysis is maintained at this high rate for several seconds, after more than 30 sec of intense contraction, the total contribution from glycolysis to ATP resynthesis is nearly double that from PCr. This high rate of flux through glycolysis is reflected by the very high muscle lactate concentrations (>100 mmol/kg dm) that are achieved during maximal exercise lasting 30 sec or more. It should be noted, however, that lactic acid production per se does not result in ATP regeneration, but functions as a mechanism for the regeneration of cytosolic nicotinamide adenine dinucleotide (NAD^+), thus allowing flux through glycolysis to be maintained.

ATP resynthesis derived from glycolysis during maximal exercise can be maintained only for relatively short periods of time (as demonstrated in Figure 1.1). The mechanisms responsible for this decline in glycolysis are unclear, but are unlikely to be related to a depletion (local or otherwise) of muscle glycogen stores, as levels are still high at the end of maximal exercise [88, 105]. Indeed, unlike prolonged submaximal exercise, it is unlikely that glycogen availability will limit glycolysis, and hence maximal exercise performance, until the pre-exercise concentration falls below 100 mmol/kg dm in human skeletal muscle [4, 14, 67]. A pH-mediated decrease in the activity of phosphorylase and phosphofructokinase (PFK) is suggested as a possible mechanism that may be responsible for the fall in the rate of glycolysis. However, it is now generally accepted that any potential for a pH-mediated inhibition of glycolysis is overcome *in vivo* by the accumulation of the activators of PFK, such as AMP and NH_3^+ [101].

As stated earlier, both AMP and IMP are associated with the regulation of glycogen degradation during exercise. It is thought that once the rate of glycogen utilization has reached a peak, a decrease in the sarcoplasmic concentration of free AMP will result in a diminished activation of phosphorylase *a*. The decrease in the sarcoplmasmic concentration of free AMP is believed to be a consequence of a decrease in the rate of ADP formation and/or a pH-induced increase in the activity of AMP deaminase, the enzyme which catalyses the deamination of AMP to IMP. This decrease may be responsible for the decline in the rate of glycogenolysis and glycolysis during maximal exercise [62] It is also clear that metabolites that accumulate during maximal exercise will inevitably result in inhibition of excitation-contraction coupling, and hence, muscle force production [34]. It is possible, therefore, that the decline in the flux through glycolysis results from the overall decline in the demand for ATP by the fatiguing muscle.

Based on the prior discussion, it could be inferred that the regulation of ATP resynthesis from substrate level phosphorylation is more closely related to the turnover of ATP than the actual concentration of any of the punitive modulators of glycogenolysis or glycolysis listed previously. This discussion highlights the first level at which aerobic metabolism can, theoretically, interact with anaerobic ATP regeneration, since mitochondrial function, the CK reaction, and glycogenolysis will all be sensitive, directly or indirectly, to the availability or turnover of ATP (or ADP) within the muscle. Skeletal muscle, however, is often composed of various different fiber types that demonstrate very different biological properties, thus making it difficult to directly relate whole-muscle metabolic changes to the regulation of cellular metabolism. This difficulty will be discussed in more detail later in this review.

Cr Supplementation and Exercise Metabolism

The importance of PCr as a substrate during intense exercise was confirmed by recent experiments that demonstrated that dietary Cr supplementation can markedly increase muscle Cr content and subsequent maximal exercise performance in man. Using the muscle biopsy technique, it is apparent that the ingestion of 20 g of Cr each day in solution for 5 days (4×5 g doses) can lead to an average increase in muscle total Cr concentration of about 20%, of which approximately 30% is in the form of PCr. However, the variation between subjects is quite large [40, 47]. Furthermore, it appears that the majority of muscle Cr retention occurs during the initial days of supplementation [47], and that the time-course for the return of muscle Cr concentration to its pre-supplementation value takes several weeks rather than days [66].

Ingestion of 4×5 g of Cr/day for 5 days was shown to significantly increase exercise performance by ~5–7% in healthy male volunteers, during repeated bouts of fatiguing, short-lasting maximal exercise (e.g., maximal isokinetic knee extensor exercise, maximal dynamic cycling exercise, maximal isokinetic cycling exercise, and controlled "track" running experiments [2, 8, 42, 48]. Some studies also reported an increase in maximal strength or torque at the onset of contraction [8]. However, the effects of Cr supplementation on maximal exercise performance are equivocal, and there is some evidence that Cr has no effect on performance [33]. More recently, however, results from our laboratory indicated that approximately 30% of subjects who ingested Cr in an attempt to increase muscle Cr concentration failed to retain substantial quantities of Cr [15, 40], possibly explaining the observed variation in efficacy. Indeed, our results showed that improvements in exercise performance using Cr supplementation were clearly associated with the extent of muscle Cr retention during supplementation. In other words, those individuals who experienced the highest muscle Cr accumulation during supplementation were those that demonstrated the better improvements in exercise performance (Figure 1.2) [15]). In support of this interpretation, we further demonstrated that those individuals who experienced more than a 25% increase in muscle total Cr concentration following 5 days of Cr ingestion also demonstrated an accelerated rate of PCr resynthesis during 2 min of recovery from intense fatiguing muscular contraction. Conversely, those individuals who experienced no or little Cr accumulation during ingestion (on average, an 8% increase) showed no measurable change in PCr resynthesis during recovery [40].

The exact mechanism by which Cr ingestion improves performance during maximal exercise is not yet clear. The available data indicate that this improvement may be related to the stimulatory effect that Cr has upon pre-exercise PCr availability [15] and on PCr resynthesis during recovery [40]. By maintaining ATP regeneration during maximal exercise, PCr availability could be expected to be an important determinant of performance during maximal exercise. This suggestion is supported by reports that indicate that the accumulation of plasma ammonia and hypoxanthine (accepted markers of skeletal muscle adenine nucleotide loss) are reduced during maximal

FIGURE 1.2.

Individual increases in muscle total creatine (Cr) concentration before and after 5 days of Cr ingestion (20 g/day), plotted against the change in work production during 2 × 30 sec bouts of maximal isokinetic cycling after Cr ingestion. Values on the y-axis were calculated by subtracting total work output during exercise before Cr ingestion from the corresponding value after Cr ingestion.

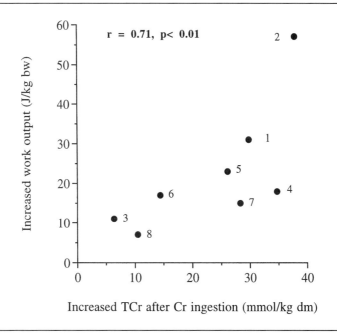

exercise following Cr ingestion, despite achieving a higher work output [2, 8, 41]. More convincing evidence comes from a recent study that showed that Cr supplementation can reduce the extent of muscle ATP degradation by 25% during maximal isokinetic cycling exercise, while at the same time, increasing work output [15] (Figure 1.3). The latter study also demonstrated that the increase in resting PCr in type II muscle fibers following Cr supplementation was positively correlated with PCr degradation in this fiber type during subsequent exercise ($r = 0.78$, $n = 8$, $p < 0.01$), as well as with the increase in work production observed during exercise ($r = 0.66$, $n = 8$, $p < 0.05$). No corresponding correlation was observed with respect to type I muscle fibers. These observations suggested that the improvements in exercise performance resulted from the increase in pre-exercise PCr concentration in type II muscle fibers maintaining ATP resynthesis during exercise following Cr ingestion.

FIGURE 1.3.

*The decline in muscle ATP concentration during 2 bouts of 30 sec maximal intensity, isokinetic cycling exercise. Each bout of exercise was performed at 80 rev/min and separated by 4 min of passive recovery. Total decline in ATP refers to the sum of the decline during bouts 1 and 2. Significant difference pre and post Cr supplementation is donated by * (p<0.05).*

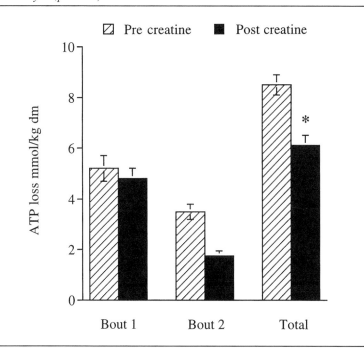

It is important to note at this point that the roles of free Cr, PCr, and the CK reaction in maintaining ATP resynthesis during contraction will differ between skeletal muscle fiber types. This makes it difficult to demonstrate the precise mechanisms of action of Cr supplementation from the current body of literature. For example, in type I skeletal muscle fibers, the K_m of the adenine nucleotide translocase for ADP is relatively high when assessed *in vitro* (~200 μM). However, the high activity of the mitochondrial isoform of CK (mi-CK), coupled with adequate Cr availability, reduces the effective K_m of the adenine nucleotide translocase for ADP by ~50% [112]. This results in a steeper relationship between mitochondrial ADP concentration and VO$_2$, and hence tighter coupling between changes in ADP concentration and mitochondrial respiration. In contrast to type I fibers, the K_m of the adenine nucleotide translocase for ADP in type II fibers is very low (~10μM), such that PCr and the CK reaction primarily behave as an "energy buffering" mechanism in this fiber type [112]. This interpretation is in agreement with the hypothesis of Wallimann et al. [114], and our own recent findings (based on single human fibers) [15], that showed that PCr acts mainly as a temporal buffer of cytosolic ADP accumulation in type II fibers during exercise. Therefore, it is unlikely that in terms of mitochondrial ATP production, Cr has an important role in type II muscle fibers during contraction. Indeed, it has been shown that Cr does not stimulate mitochondrial respiration in type II muscle fibers taken from the gastrocnemius muscle group in mice [112].

Single Muscle Fiber Glycogenolysis and PCr Metabolism

The quadriceps muscle group of man is composed of at least two main fiber types. Both are very divergent in their metabolic and physiological characteristics [5, 12, 32, 51]. Type I fibers are characterized as being highly oxidative and fatigue resistant. Conversely, type II fibers are highly glycolytic and fatigue rapidly. As might be expected from this description, the two fiber types differ in their maximal rates of ATP utilization (reflecting the different isoforms of myosin ATPase present) and their abilities to generate and sustain power output [38]. It should be noted, however, that a natural biochemical and physiological continuum probably exists between both type I and II fibers, such that the present classification system exists mainly for convenience. The majority of studies aimed at investigating the biochemical and physiological differences between muscle fiber types have been performed using animal skeletal muscle predominantly composed of a single fiber type [5, 12, 32, 51]. These studies demonstrated that fast-contracting muscle has a relatively high initial power output that is accompanied by a high rate of anaerobic ATP utilization, but which cannot be sustained for more than several seconds. Conversely, muscle composed of predominantly type I fibers has a relatively low initial power output and ATP utilization rate, both of which can be maintained during prolonged contraction [5, 12, 32, 51]. As previously stated, the quadriceps muscle group in man is not homogeneous with respect to fiber type. Therefore, it is reasonable to suggest that the analysis of mixed-fiber muscle biopsy samples will not accurately reflect the metabolic and physiological responses that occur in human skeletal muscle during exercise. In turn, this limits our ability to interpret and establish the mechanisms responsible for regulating ATP turnover during contraction.

We have studied, in a quantitative manner, the metabolic responses of type I and II human muscle fibers during exercise, and have attempted to relate the biochemical changes observed to the development of fatigue during contraction. In one particular study [98], muscle biopsy samples were obtained from the vastus lateralis at rest and after 10 and 20 sec of intermittent electrical stimulation (1.6 sec stimulation, 1.6 sec rest, at a frequency of 50 Hz) with muscle blood flow intact. The concentrations of ATP and PCr were measured in type I and II muscle fibers dissected from

FIGURE 1.4.

Muscle isometric force production (□) and ATP (O) and PCr (△) concentrations in type I (open symbols) and type II (closed symbols) muscle fibers during 20 sec of intense electrical stimulation (1.6 sec stimulation, 1.6 sec rest; 50 Hz) in man.

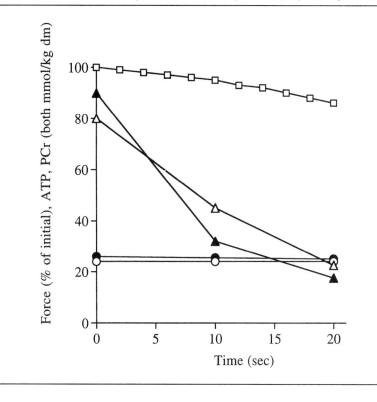

each biopsy sample, as depicted in Figure 1.4. During the initial 10 sec of contraction, the rate of PCr degradation was 60% greater in type II fibers. However, during the remaining 10 sec of contraction, PCr degradation declined in type II fibers by 60%, such that there was no difference in the rate of PCr degradation between fiber types during this period. These findings indicate that the decline in type II fiber PCr concentration, during the initial period of maximal exercise, will constitute the greatest proportion of the observed decline in a mixed muscle fiber biopsy.

We also investigated glycogenolysis in different muscle fiber types during maximal contraction in man. This was done under a variety of experimental conditions that included electrical stimulation (1.6. sec stimulation, 1.6 sec rest for 64 sec) with open circulation [43], electrical stimulation with open circulation and adrenaline infusion [43], electrical stimulation with occluded circulation, [44] and maximal sprint exercise [42]. The results are

FIGURE 1.5.

Glycogenolytic rates in type I (hatched bars) and type II (open bars) fibers during 30 sec of intermittent electrical stimulation at 50 Hz with open circulation (circ.), open circulation with adrenaline infusion, occluded circulation, and during 30 sec of maximal sprint running in man.

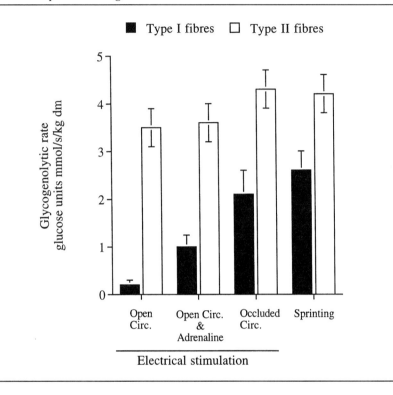

depicted in Figure 1.5. They show that during intense contraction with circulation intact, glycogenolysis proceeds maximally in type II fibers, such that when attempts were made to stimulate glycogenolysis further using adrenaline infusion and circulatory occlusion (to increase positive modulators of glycogenolysis), no further increase in glycogenolysis was observed. The suggestion that glycogenolysis is maximally activated in type II fibers under these conditions is supported by Harris et al. who found that the rates of glycogenolysis observed were close to the Vmax of phosphorylase measured in type II fibers dissected from human muscle biopsy samples [46].

Unexpectedly, glycogenolysis was negligible in type I fibers during maximal electrically-evoked contraction with limb blood flow intact. This was probably attributable to the comparatively low anaerobic ATP turnover rate of this fiber type during contraction, and the oxidative resynthesis of ATP during the 1.6 sec of recovery between each contraction. This latter suggestion has recently been confirmed by an experiment in which the interval between each contraction was reduced from 1.6 sec to 0.8 sec, which resulted in a rapid increase in type I fiber glycogenolysis (i.e., the oxidative rephosphorylation of ADP between each contraction was not sufficient to prevent AMP accumulation and the activation of glycogen phosphorylase) (Greenhaff et al. unpublished observation). Similarly, during ischemic or sprint exercise, the rate of glycogenolysis was dramatically increased in type I fibers to close to the Vmax of phosphorylase found in this fiber type (Figure 1.5), presumably by the same mechanism. The failure of oxidative phosphorylation to match the demand for ATP regeneration under these conditions is illustrated by the dramatic decline in type I fiber ATP concentration [44, 42]. This emphasizes the importance of what is known as the "duty cycle" in defining the metabolic response to contraction (i.e., the metabolic response to a fixed amount of work can be dramatically altered by varying the recovery period between successive contractions). The increase in glycogenolysis in type I fibers during contraction following adrenaline infusion (Figure 1.5) probably occurred as a direct result of a cyclic AMP mediated activation of phosphorylase [43], and highlights the fact that extra-muscular factors can also alter the metabolic response of skeletal muscle during contraction.

Repeated Bouts of Muscle Contraction as a Model for Studying the Interaction of Anaerobic and Aerobic Metabolism

When repeated bouts of exercise are performed, there are apparent dissociations between the maintenance of contractile function and the magnitude of the changes in PCr hydrolysis and glycogen utilization [10, 16, 35, 77]. For example, during 4 bouts of 30 sec maximal isokinetic cycling, with 4 min of recovery after each bout, the rate of muscle glycogen utilization was markedly diminished by the third bout (~20% of the rate during the first bout), even though the total work done was still maintained at the level of ~60% of the first bout [77]. A possible explanation for this observation is that a greater oxidative and much more efficient utilization of glycogen stores occurred (~16 time greater ATP yield per glucosyl unit from glycogen oxidation compared with the net ATP yield from glycolysis alone). It was also demonstrated that the extent of PCr hydrolysis remained similar during each bout of exercise, such that PCr hydrolysis and glycogenolysis did not appear related [77], which is in contrast to what we described previously.

When looking more closely at the two main fiber types, the picture becomes more complex. For example, we demonstrated that during two bouts of 30 sec maximal isokinetic cycling with 4 min of recovery, there was a significant reduction in the extent of type II fiber ATP and PCr hydrolysis during the second exercise bout. This we believe was a direct consequence of incomplete resynthesis of ATP and PCr in this fiber type during the recovery period [16]. However, the metabolic responses of type I fibers were not altered from bout one to bout two. Once again, these observations highlight the importance of differentiating between muscle fiber types when attempting to investigate the metabolic responses of human skeletal muscle to intense contraction.

It is apparent that the metabolic profile of sequential bouts of exercise will be partly dependent on the length of the recovery interval between exercise bouts, as well as the actual duration of the exercise bout itself. For instance, during ten bouts of 6 sec maximal sprint cycling with 30 sec recovery between each bout, work performed during the final five bouts decreased by ~20% when compared to the first five bouts [35]. However, in the case of PCr, the extent of degradation was reduced by ~40% during the final bout, when compared with the first bout. This indicates that similar to the conclusion outlined previously, the reduction in PCr degradation was a reflection of the fact that PCr concentration did not return to its resting values during the 30 sec recovery period. It also indicates that other mechanisms for ATP regeneration must have occurred to partly compensate for the reduction in PCr hydrolysis in order for function to be maintained proportionately better. It is important to note that the reduction in glycogenolysis observed in previous studies [9, 77] also occurred in this study [35], suggesting that factors that can also influence contractile efficiency (e.g., lactate anion accumulation) have to be taken into account when considering the balance between ATP utilization, provision, and exercise performance.

Based on the above discussion, it can be concluded that an imbalance between the rate of ATP demand and provision also can be partly responsible for the development of fatigue under maximal exercise conditions. Indeed, studies have shown that a significant relationship exists between the extent of PCr resynthesis between exercise bouts and subsequent exercise performance [9, 16]. For example, we recently demonstrated that when two bouts of 30 sec maximal isokinetic cycling exercise were performed, separated by 4 min of recovery, the extent of PCr resynthesis during recovery was positively correlated with work output during the second bout of exercise ($r = 0.8$, $n = 9$, $p < 0.05$) [16]. Furthermore, it was demonstrated that the rate of PCr hydrolysis during the first bout of exercise was 35% greater in type II fibers, as compared to type I fibers. This result agrees with the suggestion that the depletion of PCr specifically in type II muscle fibers may be primarily responsible for fatigue. However, during the second bout of exercise, the rate of PCr hydrolysis declined by 33% in type II fibers (Figure 1.6), which was attributable to incomplete resynthesis of PCr in this fiber type during recovery. In type I fibers, however, PCr resynthesis was almost complete following recovery from exercise bout one, making PCr utilization unchanged in this fiber type during exercise bout two (Figure 1.6). We concluded that the reduction in work output during the sec-

FIGURE 1.6.

*Changes in PCr in type I and type II muscle fibers during 2 bouts of 30 sec maximal intensity, isokinetic cycling exercise in man. Each bout of exercise was performed at 80 rev/min and separated by 4 min of passive recovery. * indicates significant differences between fiber types (p<0.05) and †† indicates significantly different from exercise bout 1 (p<0.01).*

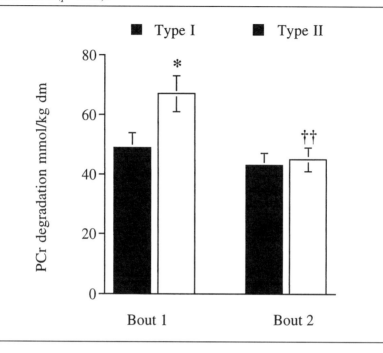

ond bout of exercise may have been related to a slower resynthesis, and consequently a reduced availability of PCr in type II muscle fibers [16].

In general, it would appear that during repeated bouts of high intensity exercise, the reduction in glycogenolysis and PCr degradation (in type II fibers), and hence anaerobic ATP resynthesis, can be partly compensated for by an increased contribution from aerobic ATP resynthesis. This hypothesis is confirmed by the decline in muscle lactate accumulation with successive exercise bouts. It appears that in the past the contribution from oxidative ATP resynthesis during this type of exercise has not been fully acknowledged. Indeed, in a recent study [111], oxidative ATP resynthesis appeared to provide the majority of the calculated ATP resynthesis in the later stages of a 30 sec bout of maximal exercise. However, regardless of whether assessed during a single bout or following repeated bouts of high intensity exercise, PCr hydrolysis provides the majority of ATP regeneration during the initial ~10 sec of exercise [10, 77, 111].

Some of the factors that undoubtedly limit the contribution made by oxidative ATP regeneration during intense contraction will be discussed later in this review. However, it is important to consider first those factors that regulate muscle oxygen consumption (VO_2) in order to highlight the important intracellular factors that may link the pathways of aerobic and anaerobic ATP regeneration.

REGULATORS OF MUSCLE OXYGEN CONSUMPTION DURING CONTRACTION

As mentioned previously, as the duration of exercise increases, aerobic ATP resynthesis becomes the predominant pathway for maintaining energy provision during intense muscle contraction. The integration of the factors that regulate skeletal muscle VO_2 and function during exercise are, however, extremely complex. It is also apparent that the important regulators of muscle VO_2 will also regulate contractile function, such that establishing the primary function of any one component is rather difficult. In addition, several factors interact to regulate VO_2 and glycolysis. These factors include the oxygen partial pressure at the level of the mitochondria (PO_{2mito}), the cell phosphorylation state, the cellular redox state, and the metabolic demand or the required rate of ADP rephosphorylation [36, 52]. One example of how VO_2 and glycolysis appear to interact is as follows: The PO_{2mito} is determined primarily by the oxygen gradient between the red blood cell (RBC) and the mitochondria. This, in turn, reflects muscle blood flow and oxygen content. However, the PO_{2mito} is also affected by the metabolic rate within the contracting muscle, where H^+ efflux will augment the unloading of oxygen from the RBC (the Bohr effect) by shifting the oxyhemoglobin curve to the right [115]. In fact, the Bohr effect may account for up to ~30% of VO_2 max. *in vivo* [97]. Whether this is an evolutionary development or simply a physiological correlate is unclear.

Calcium as a Regulator of Muscle Oxygen Consumption During Contraction

One of the most favored mechanisms for the integration of skeletal muscle VO_2 and contractile function centers on the role of changes in intracellular Ca^{2+} concentration [28, 45]. Not only is Ca^{2+} involved with the activation of glycolysis and several mitochondrial enzymes, but it also has a primary role in the coordination of skeletal muscle cross-bridge formation. Ca^{2+} mediated activation of the intramitochondrial dehydrogenases (pyruvate dehydrogenase, NAD^+-isocitrate dehydrogenase, and 2-oxoglutarate dehydrogenase) is thought to be a fundamental step in the regulation of mitochondrial respiration [28]. In turn, the electron transport chain uses the NADH generated from the intramitochondrial dehydrogenases, so that the activity of these enzymes can influence the overall process of oxidative phosphorylation [81]. Ca^{2+} is transported into mitochondria by the membrane potential component of the proton gradient that is also responsible for driving ATP production at the respiratory chain. It also has been demonstrated that not only do changes in intracellular Ca^{2+} effect mitochondrial function, mitochondria themselves can independently alter intracellular Ca^{2+} handling, thus highlighting the degree of interaction between intracellular and intramitochondrial events [70].

A word of caution is necessary, since all of the data presented in support of a role for intracellular Ca^{2+} as the regulator of muscle energy metabolism originates from *in vitro* data. In fact, it was demonstrated *ex vivo,* under conditions where mitochondrial Ca^{2+} uptake was blocked, that both mitochondrial respiration and muscle contractile function can continue as normal [106]. In addition, it is recognized that in large muscle groups, such as the quadriceps, increased force production, and hence oxygen consumption, is achieved by additional muscle fiber recruitment rather than increased frequency of stimulation [73]. As a result, intracellular Ca^{2+} may not actually differ in individual active fibers as whole muscle force production increases. Since it is the fluctuations (so called waves) in Ca^{2+} concentration that would be considered the primary regulatory factor, it would appear that the role for Ca^{2+} in the coordination of skeletal muscle metabolism during contraction is far from established.

Adenine Nucleotides as a Regulator of Muscle Oxygen Consumption During Contraction

A more convincing mechanism for controlling muscle VO_2 during contraction involves changes in cell phosphorylation state, and in particular, temporal changes in ADP flux. It was established *in vivo* that as the rate of oxygen consumption increased, a reduction in the cell phosphorylation state occurred (i.e., an increase in free ADP and AMP and a decrease in ATP and PCr). These biochemical changes were thought to be essential for driving the increase in oxygen consumption. In skeletal muscle, the maximal rate of aerobic ATP regeneration that can be achieved for a given oxygen presentation will reflect the extent to which changes in the cell phosphorylation state can adjust to maintain the stimulus to mitochondrial respiration. Ultimately, however, a reduction in the cellular phosphorylation state will result in the inhibition of excitation-contraction coupling force production, and so a reduction in the requirement for both ADP rephosphorylation and VO_2 [55, 102].

As the cell phosphorylation state is reduced during contraction, greater contributions from PCr hydrolysis, glycogenolysis, and glycolysis also occur. In this way, the biochemical alterations that are required for increasing mitochondrial function also result in an increase in ATP production from substrate level phosphorylation. It is clear, therefore, that during intense muscle contraction, both systems for ATP resynthesis will be "recruited" rapidly. Nevertheless, the factors that determine the proportionate contribution from each are unclear. It is commonly perceived that a lag in the rate of delivery of oxygen is a major determinant of this response during intense contraction [96]. In order to gain a better understanding of the integration of substrate level phosphorylation and VO_2 during intense contraction, discussed below are some of the factors that determine the lag in and limits to VO_2. The importance of oxygen delivery to the contracting muscle will also be discussed.

Limits to Muscle Oxygen Consumption During Intense Contraction

No one single determinate exists to explain the maximum possible contribution from oxidative phosphorylation to ATP regeneration in contracting skeletal muscle *in situ,* or during whole body exercise [55, 91, 113], since it is well known that both oxygen availability and blood flow can independently influence VO_2 [1, 55]. Further, it appears that *in vivo,* a reduction in the stimulus to mitochondria respiration occurs before the theoretical maximal rate of oxygen consumption is achieved. This observation reflects both the pattern of muscle blood flow [27, 30] and the inherent biochemical characteristics of the muscle [29, 58, 59]. In this sense, when considering the limit to VO_2, it has not been possible to dissociate the effects of metabolic inhibition of contractile function from a failure in the ADP mediated drive to mitochondrial respiration [113]. However, recent work suggests that under conditions of maximal blood flow, mitochondrial oxygen consumption is limited at the level of the tricarboxylic acid (TCA) cycle [9].

In particular, it has been stated that the maximum activity of the enzyme oxoglutarate dehydrogenase (5.1 μmol/min/g wet muscle) was similar to the flux through the TCA cycle calculated from muscle oxygen consumption during maximal single leg exercise (4.6 μmol/min/g wet muscle). This interpretation is, however, limited by the fact the maximal activity of PDC, and hence the maximal rate of carbohydrate oxidation, is approximately 3 μmol/min/g wet muscle in humans [84]. This suggests that the calculated flux through the TCA cycle has been overestimated [9], such that *in vivo,* mitochondrial function may be limited under these conditions by maximal PDC activity.

During submaximal, steady-state force production, a given rate of ATP regeneration is required to maintain contractile function, and it appears that within certain limits, ATP demand and supply are coregulated in such a way that ATP concentration is maintained relatively constant at the expense of muscle PCr stores [1, 23, 60, 92]. In this respect, the utilization of PCr during the transition from rest to exercise is approximately proportional to the final steady-state work load, and, therefore, explains the majority of the shift in cellular phosphorylation state [1, 60, 96, 117]. It is clear, however, that there is a critical steady-state workload for a given oxygen presentation whereby aerobic ATP regeneration can no longer meet the rate of ATP utilization; at that time, a progressive contribution from anaerobic ATP regeneration occurs [21, 72]. In this sense, the metabolic responses to intense contraction can be mimicked simply by reducing the availability of oxygen to the mitochondria through a reduction in skeletal muscle blood flow [44, 110].

It should be pointed out that although lactate production is dependent on the prevailing PO_{2mito}, lactate production does not indicate that oxygen presentation is limiting mitochondrial respiration. In fact, lactate production is partly a consequence of maintaining mitochondrial respiration in the face of a falling PO_{2mito} [23, 94]. When the partial pressure of oxygen in arterial blood is reduced (hypoxia) during skeletal muscle contraction, the reduction in oxygen presentation is accompanied by a further reduction in the phosphorylation state of the muscle to compensate for the reduced PO_{2mito}. It is this biochemical change that also stimulates glycolysis and hence muscle lactate production [53]. Hypoxia has been often used in this manner to manipulate muscle metabolism during contraction, as well as being used to establish a relationship between arterial oxygen content and arterial lactate concentration, or the rate of muscle lactate production [54, 71, 74, 103]. However, it is accepted that the function of blood flow is not simply to present oxygen and substrates to the muscle, but also to remove metabolites such as lactate and H^+. In this way, the potential inhibition of excitation-contraction coupling, cross bridge cycling, and glycogenolytic flux are also reduced. It should also be remembered that the free energy yield from ATP hydrolysis ($\Delta G'_o$) is not constant, but varies according to the prevailing biochemical environment (e.g., changes in the concentration of Pi and ADP). This also has implications for skeletal muscle contractile efficiency, and hence, estimates of ATP consumption from external work done.

Most agree that the aforementioned physiological regulators of mitochondrial respiration interact, as described above, to stimulate VO_2 as the demand for ATP regeneration increases. However, debate continues in regards to the precise order of events by which this regulation is achieved, particularly during the transition from rest to steady-state contraction. The biochemical alterations that are required to maintain the electron transport chain function are also a function of the mitochondrial density (in particular, the number of adenine nucleotide translocases), such that mitochondrial density is one example of an intracellular limitation to the adaptability of skeletal muscle oxidative metabolism as the demand for ATP increases [29, 36].

Regulation of Muscle Oxygen Consumption During the Rest Steady-State Transition Period

As previously discussed, at the onset of intense exercise, the principal mechanism for ATP regeneration is the rapid utilization of PCr mediated by the CK reaction [22, 60, 80]. There is also rapid accumulation of muscle lactate during this period, which reflects the proportion of the ATP regeneration being derived from glycolysis [63]. In terms of the integration of aerobic and anaerobic pathways during the rest-to-steady-state period, it has been hypothesized that NADH derived from glycolysis (in addition to that derived from the intramitochondrial dehydrogenases) is an essential stimulus for the increased rate of mitochondrial respiration during this period [22, 58]. Connett et al. suggested that the rapid increase in glycolytic flux, and the associated accumulation of cytosolic NADH, was an essential part of the regulatory mechanism by which greater mitochondrial respiration occurs, implying that the biochemical changes that occur at the onset of contraction are highly regulated.

The metabolic responses during the rest-to-steady-state period also appear to be sensitive to alterations in training status and hence mitochondrial function. For example, a reduction in muscle lactate accumulation and PCr degradation was observed after short-term exercise training, when subjects exercised at identical works loads before and after training [13, 39]. Under these conditions, it would be expected that muscle mitochondrial density would increase only modestly, and therefore, would not be entirely responsible for the observed changes [19, 100]. These changes could also reflect a reduction in motor unit recruitment (i.e., an improvement in motor control). This would result in a reduction of PCr degradation and lactate accumulation when assessed in a biopsy containing a mixture of active and inactive muscle fibers. In addition, it was demonstrated that the oxygen deficit, which represents PCr degradation and lactate production during the rest-to-work transition period, was not dependent on the rate of transition, but rather the final steady-state workload. This, then, suggests that these alterations are likely to be relatively independent of any changes in blood flow [87, 95]. It is also possible that the faster rate of onset of VO_2 during the rest-to-work transition following endurance training [50, 56, 57] partly reflects an alteration in mitochondrial regulation, rather than simply an increase in the mitochondrial density or the concentration of oxidative enzymes. In this context, mitochondrial substrate availability was recently shown to partly determine the metabolic responses during the rest-to-steady-state transition [107, 109, 110]

PDC AS A SITE FOR THE INTERACTION BETWEEN AEROBIC AND ANAEROBIC METABOLISM

It appears that lactate accumulation can occur in contracting skeletal muscle even when oxygen availability is high [23]. This suggests that lactate formation may be a consequence of the failure to utilize the presented oxygen. Or lactate formation may simply reflect the reduction in cellular phosphorylation state, and hence accumulation of positive modulators of glycogenolysis, that is required to support the increased rate of oxidative

ATP regeneration [23, 101]. Indeed, recent data from our laboratory demonstrated that a large proportion of muscle lactate accumulation is unrelated to oxygen availability under conditions where the maximal intrinsic capacity of the mitochondria is not exceeded [107, 108,110]. Specifically, this work centered on alterations in PDC activation status, and provided evidence that PDC may be an important site for the interaction of aerobic and anaerobic ATP regeneration during intense muscle contraction.

PDC is a multiple enzyme complex composed of three enzyme components (pyruvate dehydrogenase, dihydrolipoyl transacetylase, and dihydrolipoyl dehydrogenase) which are thought to regulate carbohydrate entry into the TCA cycle [86]. PDC is situated in the inner mitochondrial membrane and catalyses the irreversible reaction whereby pyruvate undergoes decarboxylation to acetyl-CoA (requiring NAD^+ and CoA). Regulation of the rate of formation of acetyl-CoA by PDC (i.e., flux through the enzyme complex) is achieved by two strategies. First, 0 the amount of PDC that exists in its active, dephosphorylated form is altered. This is achieved by the covalent modification of PDC either from its inactive to its active, dephosphorylated form, catalyzed by PDC phosphatase, or vice versa, catalyzed by PDC kinase [24]. In turn, the PDC kinase and phosphatase are sensitive to muscle ATP requirements and oxidative substrate accumulation. Second, the rate of pyruvate oxidation by PDC is regulated by end product inhibition of flux through the enzyme complex by NADH and acetyl-CoA, which reflect both substrate availability and the availability of oxygen [49].

Flux through the enzyme complex during muscle contraction (at least at the onset of contraction) is thought to be related to both the availability of free carnitine, as well as the rate of oxidative phosphorylation [7, 20]. A high rate of acetyl group formation by the PDC reaction results in the transfer of the acetyl group from Co-A to carnitine via the carnitine acetyltransferase reaction, thus maintaining the availability of Co-A for TCA cycle function. It has been proposed that lactate production may be a function of a mismatch between glycogenolysis, glycolysis, and the activation of PDC, which has been termed the "mass effect" [102]. Recent evidence implies that PDC may play an important role in determining the amount of muscle lactate accumulation during repeated bouts of high intensity exercise [84].

As described previously, at the onset of contraction, the principal substrates for ATP regeneration are PCr hydrolysis and glycogenolysis. There are many debates as to whether the extent of this so-called anaerobic ATP regeneration is due to a lag in oxygen delivery to the contracting muscle, or whether it is due to a lag in the rate of onset of oxygen utilization [37, 74]. In support of the lag in oxygen delivery hypothesis, it has been shown that compared to normoxia, exercise during hypoxic conditions results in greater PCr degradation during exercise, [71] (although this result has not been observed in all studies) [74]. Furthermore, during ischemic conditions at the same absolute submaximal workload and oxygen consumption,

PCr degradation is substantially greater [104]. However, this observation of increased reliance on PCr also reflects the greater muscle recruitment, and hence more active fibers within a muscle biopsy sample [104]. Therefore, we cannot say that the reduction in muscle oxygen availability reduces the PCr concentration in each muscle cell.

At the onset of skeletal muscle contraction, the kinetics of PCr degradation follow a similar pattern to that of muscle VO_2 kinetics [78]. Furthermore, during low and high intensity muscle contraction occurring in hypoxia, the time constant for pulmonary VO_2 slows and the oxygen deficit increases [31, 82]. These data have been interpreted to mean that the kinetics of oxygen delivery or diffusion to the muscle determines the extent of PCr degradation during the early stages of exercise. However, it has been demonstrated when using lower body positive pressure, that a reduction in leg blood flow during exercise does not alter the VO_2 kinetics at the onset of exercise [116]. Further, if the kinetics of PCr degradation were determined by oxygen delivery, one would expect that a slower transition from rest to exercise would result in a reduced reliance on PCr stores. When this hypothesis was directly tested, the rate of transition from rest to steady-state did not alter the extent of PCr degradation [95]. It does not appear, therefore, that PCr degradation during the transition from rest to exercise reflects a limitation in oxygen delivery.

We recently established in a canine model that activation of PDC and accumulation of oxidative substrate, in the form of acetylcarnitine, substantially reduces muscle PCr degradation during intense muscle contraction under conditions of controlled blood flow and arterial oxygen content [108, 109]. These data provided direct evidence that a large proportion of the PCr degradation during skeletal muscle contraction is unrelated to oxygen availability, but rather reflects an inherent lag in intracellular oxidative metabolism even during conditions of low blood flow. This latter point is in agreement with the conclusion reached by Grassi et al. [37], whereby the early lag in VO_2 kinetics was not determined by the bulk delivery of O_2 to the contracting limb. It was also demonstrated that at the onset of skeletal muscle contraction, NADH concentration transiently fell, which further suggested that a substrate limitation, probably at the level of the TCA cycle, occurred during this period [83]. In a recent study, we demonstrated that PDC activation reduced the reliance on PCr stores by ~50% during 3 min of human muscle contraction [107]. If the proportionality between oxygen consumption and PCr hydrolysis holds [80], then a faster onset of oxidative phosphorylation must have occurred during the initial 3 min of contraction following PDC activation.

As demonstrated *in vitro*, activation of the intramitochondrial dehydrogenases, and PDC in particular, can play an important role in the overall regulation of oxidative phosphorylation [81]. In particular, it was shown that when the concentration of NAD-linked substrates was low, dehydrogenase activity was a major limit to flux through oxidative phosphorylation. This limitation (or regulatory feature) is lost when substrates, such as pyruvate and 2-oxoglutarate, are in excess [81]. It could be argued, therefore, that the high accumulation of acetylcarnitine (~10 mmol/kg dm) following PDC activation, a substrate store for the TCA cycle dehydrogenases, was the mechanism for the more rapid onset of mitochondrial respiration (reflected by the sparing of PCr). If this interpretation is correct, then these studies [107–110] would be consistent with observations in isolated mitochondrial preparations that demonstrated that a certain degree of the metabolic control of oxidative phosphorylation resides at the level of the intramitochondrial dehydrogenases [17, 81]. It was also noted in our *in vivo* studies that early during contraction, there was a net decline in acetylcarnitine concentration following PDC activation, and a greater rate of accumulation of NADH. This, then, could account for the reduction in ATP derived from substrate level phosphorylation [109]. These findings also indicate that at least some of the "stock pile" of oxidative substrate was indeed utilized early during contraction, and suggests that flux through PDC is a site of limitation to mitochondrial substrate availability and hence respiration.

These discoveries also have important implications for our understanding of *in vivo* mitochondrial regulation during skeletal muscle contraction. During conditions of adequate blood flow in resting skeletal muscle, regulation of mitochondrial respiration is thought to be analogous to that of state 4 in isolated mitochondria (i.e., saturated with both reduced substrate—NADH—and oxygen) [17]. Once contraction is initiated, an increased rate of ADP rephosphorylation occurs, and it has been suggested that this process may be limited by the availability of ADP at the mitochondrial level. This has led to the suggestion that the increase in VO_2 at the onset of contraction may reflect a diffusion-limited process between the myofibrils and the mitochondria, or more likely across the mitochondrial membrane [80]. One piece of evidence for an ADP-limited process is that the greater mitochondrial density following endurance training is associated with a faster onset of oxygen consumption [36]. It is thought that the greater number of adenine-nucleotide translocators post-training increases the transport of ADP; consequently, a faster onset of respiration occurs [36]. Another theory suggested that intracellular "energy" fluxes might be mediated by the PCr shuttle [17]. When this occurs, CK isoforms mediate a process whereby ADP is rephosphorylated at the myofibrils by PCr, and the free Cr then diffuses across to the mitochondria interacting with the mitochondrial pool of ADP, reforming PCr, which then diffuses back to the myofibrils. However, it has now been established that during the transition from rest to work, the reliance on PCr stores can be reduced by 50%, while force production and hence ADP turnover is constant [108, 107]. It would appear therefore, that *in vivo* oxidative rephosphorylation of ADP during the transition from rest to exercise is not limited by the availability of ADP.

SUMMARY: METABOLIC CHANGES WITH CONTRACTION: INTERACTION OR CORRELATION?

The previous findings suggest that during intense muscular contraction, ATP is supplied at near maximal rates by PCr degradation and glycolysis. As exercise duration progresses, it would appear that anaerobic ATP turnover is reduced due to the depletion of PCr and a reduction in the rate of glycogenolysis. This, in turn, results in a reduction in muscle force and power output. The precise reasons for the reduction in glycogenolysis are not yet established but may relate to the reduction in ADP production.

More recent studies implicated the depletion of PCr specifically in type II muscle fibers with the development of fatigue during intense exercise. The importance of PCr availability to ATP resynthesis has been confirmed by studies demonstrating that Cr supplementation can increase muscle PCr concentration at rest, improve exercise performance, and facilitate PCr resynthesis during recovery from exercise. Finally, recent studies also demonstrated that the reduction in work production during repeated bouts of maximal exercise is less than the reduction observed in anaerobic energy provision. This led to the suggestion that the contribution of oxidative phosphorylation to total ATP production during intense muscle contraction may have been underestimated. This increased contribution from oxidative phosphorylation, particularly during repeated bouts of maximal exercise, may reflect greater oxidative substrate availability prior to the onset of contraction. This conclusion is supported by recent studies that demonstrated that mitochondrial acetyl group availability partly determines the aerobic, and hence anaerobic, contribution to ATP regeneration during skeletal muscle contraction. Finally, the relative contribution made by aerobic and anaerobic metabolism during exercise is likely to be determined primarily by the demand for ADP rephosphorylation, which can clearly influence glycogenolysis, PCr metabolism, and mitochondrial function. Whether the changes in metabolite concentration described above are actually responsible for the overall integration of substrate level phosphorylation and oxidative phosphorylation during skeletal muscle contraction remains to be established.

ACKNOWLEDGEMENTS

The authors would like to acknowledge the substantial contributions made by Kristina Bodin, Anna Casey, Eric Hultman, Simon Poucher, Karin Söderlund, and Tim Constantin-Teodosiu in the work described in this review. We would also like to acknowledge the support of The Wellcome Trust,

The DERA Centre for Human Sciences, Smithkline Beecham (UK), Zeneca Pharmaceuticals (UK), and The Gatorade Sport Science Institute.

REFERENCES

1. Arthur, P.G., M.C. Hogan, D.E. Bebout, P.D. Wagner, and P.W. Hochachka. Modelling the effects of hypoxia on ATP turnover in exercising muscle. *J. Appl. Physiol.* 73:737–742, 1992.
2. Balsom, P.D., B. Ekblom, K. Söderlund, B. Sjödin, and E. Hultman. Creatine supplementation and dynamic high-intensity intermittent exercise. *Scand. J. Med. Sci. Sports* 3: 143–149, 1993.
3. Bangsbo, J., P.D. Gollnick, T.E. Graham, et al. Anaerobic energy production and O_2 deficit–debt relationship during exhaustive exercise in humans. *J. Physiol.* 422:539–559, 1990.
4. Bangsbo, J., T.E. Graham, B. Kiens, and B. Saltin. Elevated muscle glycogen and anaerobic energy production during exhaustive exercise in man. *J. Physiol.* 451:205–227, 1992.
5. Barany, M. ATPase activity of myosin correlated with speed of muscle shortening. *J. Gen. Physiol.* 50:197–218, 1967.
6. Bergstrom, J., R.C. Harris, E. Hultman, and L.O. Nordesjo. Energy rich phosphagens in dynamic and static work. *Adv. Exp. Med. Biol.* 11:341–355, 1971.
7. Bieber, L.L., R. Emaus, K. Valkner, and S. Farrell. Possible functions of short–chain and medium–chain carnitine acyltransferases. *Fed. Proc.* 41:2858–2862, 1982.
8. Birch, R., D. Noble, and P.L. Greenhaff. The influence of dietary creatine supplementation on performance during repeated bouts of maximal isokinetic cycling in man. *Eur. J. Appl. Physiol.* 69:268–270, 1994.
9. Blomstrand, E., G. Rådegran, and B. Saltin. Maximum rate of oxygen uptake by human skeletal muscle in relation to maximal activities of enzymes in the Krebs cycle. *J. Physiol.* 501.2:455–460, 1997.
10. Bogdanis, G.C., M.E. Nevill, L.H. Boobis, and H.K.A. Lakomy. Contribution of phosphocreatine and aerobic metabolism to energy supply during repeated sprint exercise. *J. Appl. Physiol.* 80:876–884, 1996.
11. Boobis, L., C. Williams, and S.A. Wootton. Human muscle metabolism during brief maximal exercise. *J. Physiol.* 338:21–22P, 1982.
12. Burke, R.E., D.N. Levine, F.E. Zajac III, et al. Mammalian motor units: physiological-histochemical correlation in three types of cat gastrocnemius. *Science* 174:709–712, 1971.
13. Cadefau, J., H.J. Green, R. Cuss, M. Ball-Burnett, and G. Jamieson. Coupling of muscle phosphorylation potential to glycolysis during work after short term training. *J. Appl. Physiol.* 76:2586–2593, 1994
14. Casey, A., A.H. Short, S. Curtis, and P.L. Greenhaff. The effect of glycogen availability on power output and the metabolic response to repeated bouts of maximal isokinetic exercise in man. *Eur. J. Appl. Physiol.* 72:249–255, 1996.
15. Casey, A., D. Constantin-Teodosiu, S. Howell, E. Hultman, and P.L. Greenhaff. Creatine supplementation favourably affects performance and muscle metabolism during maximal intensity exercise in humans. *Am. J. Physiol.* 271:E31–E37, 1996.
16. Casey, A., D. Constantin-Teodosiu, S. Howell, E. Hultman, and P.L. Greenhaff. The metabolic response of type I and II muscle fibers during repeated bouts of maximal exercise in humans. *Am. J. Physiol.* 271:E38–E43, 1996.
17. Chance, B., and G.R. Williams. The respiratory chain and oxidative phosphorylation. *Adv. Enzymol.* 17:65–134, 1956.
18. Chasiotis, D., K. Sahlin, and E. Hultman. Regulation of glycogenolysis in human muscle in response to epinephrine infusion. *J. Appl. Physiol.* 54:45–50, 1983.

19. Chesley, A., G.J.F. Heigenhauser, and L.L. Spriet. Regulation of muscle glycogen phosphorylase activity following short-term endurance training. *Am. J. Physiol.* 270:E328–E335, 1996.

20. Childress, C.C., B. Sacktor, and D.R. Traynor. Function of carnitine in the fatty acid oxidase-deficient insect flight muscle. *J. Biol. Chem.* 242:754–760, 1966.

21. Connett, R.J., T.E.J. Gayeski, and C.R. Honig. Lactate accumulation in fully aerobic, working dog gracilis muscle. *Am. J. Physiol.* 246:H120–H128, 1984.

22. Connett, R.J., T.E.J. Gayeski, and C.R. Honig. Energy sources in fully aerobic rest-work transitions: a new role for glycolysis. *Am. J. Physiol.* 248:H922–H929, 1985.

23. Connett, R.J., and C.R. Honig. Regulation of VO2 in red muscle: do current biochemical hypotheses fit *in vivo* data? *Am. J. Physiol.* 256:R898–R906, 1989.

24. Cooper, R.H., P.J. Randle, and R.M. Denton. Stimulation of phosphorylation and inactivation of pyruvate dehydrogenase by physiological inhibitors of the pyruvate dehydrogenase reaction. *Nature* 257:808–809, 1975.

25. Cori, G.T. The effect of stimulation and recovery on the phosphorylase a content of muscle. *J. Biol. Chem.* 158:333–339, 1945.

26. Cori, G.T., S.P. Colowick, and C.F. Cori. The action of nucleotides in the disruptive phosphorylation of glycogen. *J. Biol. Chem.* 123:381–389, 1938.

27. Damon, D.H., and B.R. Duling. Evidence that capillary perfusion heterogeneity is not controlled in striated muscle. *Am. J. Physiol.* 248:H386–H392, 1986.

28. Denton, R.M., J.G. McCormack, and N.J. Edgell. Role of calcium ions in the regulation of intramitochondrial metabolism. *Biochem. J.* 190:107–118, 1980.

29. Dudley, G.A., P.C. Tullson, and R.L. Terjung. Influence of mitochondrial content on the sensitivity of respiratory control. *J. Biol. Chem.* 262:9109–9114, 1987.

30. Duling, B.R., and D.H. Damon. An examination of the measurement of flow heterogeneity in striated muscle. *Circ. Res.* 60:1–13, 1986.

31. Engelen, M.J., Porszasz, M. Riley, K. Wasserman, K. Maehara, and T.J. Barstow. Effects of hypoxic hypoxia on O2 uptake and heart rate kinetics during heavy exercise. *J. Appl. Physiol.* 81:2500–2508, 1996.

32. Faulkner, J.A., D.R. Claflin, and K.K. McCully. Power output of fast and slow fibers from human skeletal muscles. N.L. Jones, N. McCartney, A.J. McComas, (eds.). *Human Muscle Power.* Champaign, IL: Human Kinetics, 1986, pp. 81–89.

33. Febbraio, M.A., T.R. Flanagan, R.J. Snow, S. Zhao, and M.F. Carey. Effect of creatine supplementation on intramuscular TCr, metabolism and performance during intermittent, supramaximal exercise in humans. *Acta. Physiol. Scand.* 155:387–395, 1995.

34. Fitts, R. H. Cellular mechanisms of fatigue. *Physiol. Rev.* 74:49–94, 1994.

35. Gaitanos, G.C., C. Williams, L.H. Boobis, and S. Brooks. Human muscle metabolism during intermittent maximal exercise. *J. Appl. Physiol.* 75:712–719, 1993.

36. Gollnick, P.D., M. Riedy, J.J. Quintinskie, and L.A. Bertocci. Differences in metabolic potential of skeletal muscle fibres and their significance for metabolic control. *J. Exp. Biol.* 115:191–199, 1985.

37. Grassi, B., D.C. Poole, R.S. Richardson, D.R. Knight, B.K. Erickson, and P.D. Wagner. Muscle O2 uptake kinetics in humans: implications for metabolic control. *J. Appl. Physiol.* 80:988–998, 1996.

38. Green, H.J. Muscle power: fiber type recruitment, metabolism and fatigue. N.L. Jones, N. McCartney, A.J. McComas, (eds.). *Human Muscle Power.* Champaign, IL: Human Kinetics, 1986, pp. 65–79.

39. Green, H.J., S. Jones, M. Ball-Burnett, D. Smith, J. Livesey, and B. Farrance. Early muscular and metabolic adaptations to prolonged exercise training in humans. *J. Appl. Physiol.* 70: 2032–2038, 1991.

40. Greenhaff, P.L., K. Bodin, K. Söderlund, and E. Hultman. The effect of oral creatine supplementation on skeletal muscle phosphocreatine resynthesis. *Am. J. Physiol.* 266: E725–E730, 1994.

41. Greenhaff, P.L., A. Casey, A.H. Short, R.C. Harris, K. Söderlund, and E. Hultman. Influence of oral creatine supplementation on muscle torque during repeated bouts of maximal voluntary exercise in man. *Clin. Sci.* 84:565–570, 1993.

42. Greenhaff, P.L., M.E. Nevill, K. Söderlund, et al. The metabolic responses of human type I and II muscle fibers during maximal treadmill sprinting. *J. Physiol.* 478:149–155, 1994.

43. Greenhaff, P.L., J.M. Ren, K. Söderlund, and E. Hultman. Energy metabolism in single human muscle fibers during contraction without and with epinephrine infusion. *Am. J. Physiol.* 260:E713–E718, 1991.

44. Greenhaff, P.L., K. Söderlund, J.M. Ren, and E. Hultman. Energy metabolism in single human muscle fibers during intermittent contraction with occluded circulation. *J Physiol.* 460:443–453, 1993.

45. Hansford, R.G. Role of calcium in respiratory control. *Med. Sci. Sports Exerc.* 26:44–51, 1994.

46. Harris, R.C., B. Essen, and E. Hultman. Glycogen phosphorylase in biopsy samples and single muscle fibers of musculus quadriceps femoris of man at rest. *Scand. J. Clin. Lab. Invest.* 36:521–526, 1976.

47. Harris, R.C., K. Söderlund, and E. Hultman. Elevation of creatine in resting and exercised muscle of normal subjects by creatine supplementation. *Clin. Sci.* 83:367–374, 1992.

48. Harris, R.C., M. Viru, P.L. Greenhaff, and E. Hultman. The effect of oral creatine supplementation on running performance during maximal short term exercise in man. *J. Physiol.* 467:74, 1993.

49. Hennig, G., G. Loffler, and O.H. Wieland. Active and inactive forms of pyruvate dehydrogenase in skeletal muscle as related to the metabolic and functional state of the cell. *FEBS* 59:142–145, 1975.

50. Hickson, R.C., H.A. Bomze, and J.O. Holloszy. Faster adjustment of O_2 uptake to the energy requirement of exercise in the trained state. *J. Appl. Physiol.* 44:877–881, 1978.

51. Hintz, C.S., M.M.Y. Chi, R.D. Fell, et al. Metabolite changes in individual rat muscle fibers during stimulation. *Am. J. Physiol.* 242:C218–C228, 1982.

52. Hochachka, P.W., and G.O. Matheson. Regulating ATP turnover rates over broad dynamic work ranges in skeletal muscles. *J. Appl. Physiol.* 73:1697–1703, 1992.

53. Hogan, M.C., P.G. Arthur, D.E. Bebout, P.W. Hochachka, and P.D. Wagner. Role of O_2 in regulating tissue respiration in dog muscle working in situ. *J. Appl. Physiol.* 73:728–736, 1992.

54. Hogan, M.C., R.S. Richardson, and S. Kurdak. Initial fall in skeletal muscle force development during ischemia is related to oxygen availability. *J. Appl. Physiol.* 77:2380–2384, 1994.

55. Hogan, M.C., J. Roca, J.B. West, and P.D Wagner. Dissociation of maximal O_2 uptake from O_2 delivery in canine gastrocnemius in situ. *J. Appl. Physiol.* 66:1219–1226, 1989.

56. Holloszy, J.O. Adaptations of skeletal muscle to endurance exercise. *Med. Sci. Sports Exerc.* 7:155–164, 1975.

57. Holloszy, J.O., and E.F. Coyle. Adaptations of skeletal muscle to endurance exercise and their metabolic consequences. *J. Appl. Physiol.* 56:831–838, 1984.

58. Honig, C.R., R.J. Connett, and T.E.J. Gayeski. O_2 transport and its interaction with metabolism: a systems view of aerobic capacity. *Med. Sci. Sports Exerc.* 24:47–53, 1992.

59. Horstman, D.H., M. Gleser, and J. Delehunt. Effects of altering O_2 delivery on VO_2 of isolated, working muscle. *Am. J. Physiol.* 230:327–334, 1976.

60. Hultman, E. Studies on muscle metabolism of glycogen and active phosphate in man with special reference to exercise and diet. *Scan. J. Clin. Lab. Invest.* 19:1–63, 1967.

61. Hultman, E., J. Bergstrom, and N. McLennan Anderson. Breakdown and resynthesis of phosphocreatine and adenosine triphosphate in connection with muscular work in man. *Scan. J. Clin. Lab. Invest.* 19:56–66, 1967.

62. Hultman, E., P.L. Greenhaff, J.M. Ren, and K. Söderlund. Energy metabolism and fatigue during intense muscle contraction. *Biochem. Soc. Trans.* 19:347–353, 1991.

63. Hultman, E., and H. Sjöholm. Energy metabolism and contraction force of human skeletal muscle in situ during electrical stimulation. *J. Physiol.* 345:525–532, 1983.

64. Hultman, E., and H. Sjoholm. Substrate availability. H.G. Knuttgen, H.G. Vogel, J.A.-Poortmans, (eds.). *Biochemistry of Exercise.* Champaign: Human Kinetics, 1983, pp. 63–75.

65. Hultman, E., I. Sjoholm, E.K. Jaderholm, and J. Krynicki. Evaluation of methods for electrical stimulation of human muscle in situ. *Pfluegers Arch.* 398:139–141, 1983.

66. Hultman, E., K. Söderlund, J.A. Timmons, G. Cederblad, and P.L Greenhaff. Muscle creatine loading in man. *J. Appl. Physiol.* 81:232–237, 1996.

67. Jacobs, I., P. Kaijser, and P. Tesch. Muscle strength and fatigue after selective glycogen depletion in human skeletal muscle fibers. *Eur. J. Appl. Physiol.* 46:47–53, 1981.

68. Jacobs, I., P. Tesch, O. Bar-Or, et al. Lactate in human skeletal muscle after 10 and 30 sec of supramaximal exercise. *J. Appl. Physiol.* 55:365–367, 1983.

69. Jones, N.L., N. McCartney, T. Graham, et al. Muscle performance and metabolism in maximal isokinetic cycling at slow and fast speeds. *J. Appl. Physiol.* 59:132–136, 1985.

70. Jouaville, L.S., F.I. Ekhson, L. Holmuhamedov, P. Camacho, and J.D. Lechleiter. Synchronisation of calcium waves by mitochondrial substrates in Xenopus laevis oocytes. *Nature* 377:438—441, 1995.

71. Katz, A., and K. Sahlin. Effect of decreased oxygen availability on NADH and lactate contents in human skeletal muscle during exercise. *Acta. Physiol. Scand.* 131:119–127, 1987.

72. Katz, A., and K. Sahlin. Regulation of lactic acid production during exercise. *J. Appl. Physiol.* 65:509–518, 1988.

73. Laframboise, J., and E. Cafarelli. Differential effects of voluntary and involuntary activation on contractile characteristics of two human muscles. *J. Appl. Physiol.* 76:1400–1402, 1994.

74. Linnarsson, D., J. Karlsson, L. Fagraeus, and B. Saltin. Muscle metabolites and oxygen deficit during exercise with hypoxia and hyperoxia. *J. Appl. Physiol.* 36:399–402, 1974.

75. Lowry, O.H., D.W. Schulz, and J.V. Passoneau. Effects of adenylic acid on the kinetics of muscle phosphorylase a. *J. Biol. Chem.* 239:1947–1953, 1964.

76. Margaria, R., D. Oliva, P.E. Di Prampero, and P. Cerretelli. Energy utilisation in intermittant exercise of supramaximal intensity. *J. Appl. Physiol.* 26:752–756, 1969.

77. McCartney, N., L.L. Spreit, G.J.F. Heigenhauser, J.M. Kowalchuk, J.R. Sutton, and N.L. Jones. Muscle power and metabolism in maximal intermittent exercise. *J Appl. Physiol.* 60:1164–1169, 1986.

78. McCreary, C.R., P.D. Chilibeck, G.D. Marsh, D.H. Paterson, D.A. Cunningham and R.T. Thompson. Kinetics of pulmonary oxygen uptake and muscle phosphates during moderate-intensity calf exercise. *J. Appl. Physiol.* 81(3):1331–1338, 1996.

79. Medbo, J.I., and I. Tabata. Relative importance of aerobic and anaerobic energy release during short-lasting exhausting bicycle exercise. *J. Appl. Physiol.* 67:1881–1886, 1989.

80. Meyer, R.A., H.L. Sweeney, and M.J. Kushmerick. A simple analysis of the "phosphocreatine shuttle." *Am. J. Physiol.* 246:C365–C377, 1984.

81. Moreno-Sanchez, R., B.A. Hogue, and R.G. Hansford. Influence of NAD-linked dehydrogenase activity on flux through oxidative phosphorylation. *Biochem. J.* 268:421–428, 1990.

82. Murphy, P.C., L.A. Cuervo, and R.L. Hughson. A study of cardiorespiratory dynamics with step and ramp exercise tests in normoxia and hypoxia. *Cardiovasc. Res.* 23:825–832, 1989.

83. Olgin, J., R.J. Connett, and B. Chance. Mitochondrial redox changes rest-work transition in dog gracilis muscle. *Adv. Exp. Med. Biol.* 191:855–862, 1985.

84. Putman, C.T., N.L. Jones, L.C. Lands, T.M. Bragg, M.G. Hollidge-Horvat, and G.J.F. Heigenhauser. Skeletal muscle pyruvate dehydrogenase activity during maximal exercise in humans. *Am. J. Physiol.* 269:E458–E468, 1995.

85. Quistorff, B., L. Johansen, and K. Sahlin. Absence of phosphocreatine resynthesis in human calf muscle during ischemic recovery. *Biochem. J.* 291:681–686, 1992.

86. Randle, P.J., P.B. Garland, C.N. Hales, and E.A. Newsholme. The glucose fatty-acid cycle: its role in insulin sensitivity and the metabolic disturbances of diabetes mellitus. *Lancet* 1:785–789, 1963.

87. Ren, J.M., S. Broberg, and K. Sahlin. Oxygen deficit is not affected by the rate of transition from rest to submaximal exercise. *Acta. Physiol. Scand.* 135:545–548, 1989.

88. Ren, J.M., S. Broberg, K. Sahlin, and E. Hultman. Influence of reduced glycogen level on glycogenolysis during short term stimulation in man. *Acta Physiol. Scand.* 139:427–474, 1990.

89. Ren, J.M., and E. Hultman. Regulation of glycogenolysis in human skeletal muscle. *J. Appl. Physiol.* 67:2243–2248, 1989.

90. Ren, J.M., and E. Hultman. Regulation of phosphorylase a activity in human skeletal muscle. *J. Appl. Physiol.* 69:919–923, 1990.

91. Richardson, R.S., B. Kennedy, D.R. Knight, and P.D. Wagner. High muscle blood flows are not attenuated by recruitment of additional muscle mass. *Am. J. Physiol.* 269: H1545–H1552, 1995.

92. Sahlin, K. Metabolic changes in limiting muscle performance. B. Saltin (ed.). *Biochemistry of Exercise VI.* Champaign, IL: Human Kinetics, 1986, pp. 323–343.

93. Sahlin, K., J. Gorski, and L. Edstrom. Influence of ATP turnover and metabolite changes on IMP formation and glycolysis in rat skeletal muscle. *Am. J. Physiol.* 259:C409–C412, 1990.

94. Sahlin, K., and A. Katz. Lactate formulation during submaximal exercise is oxygen dependent. Taylor, Grollnick, Green, et al. (eds.). *Biochemistry of Exercise VII.* Champaign, IL: Human Kinetics, 1990, pp. 79–82.

95. Sahlin, K., J.M. Ren, and S. Broberg. Oxygen deficit at the onset of submaximal exercise is not due to a delayed oxygen transport. *Acta Physiol. Scand.* 134:175–180, 1988.

96. Saltin, B. Anaerobic capacity: past, present and prospective. A.W. Taylor, P.D. Gollnick, H.J. Green, C.D. Ianuzzo, E.G. Noble, G. Métivier, and J.R. Sutton (eds.). *International Series on Sport Science, Vol. 21:Biochemistry of Exercise VII.* Champaign, IL: Human Kinetics, 1990, pp. 387–421.

97. Severinghaus, J.W. Exercise O_2 transport model assuming zero cytochrome PO_2 at VO_2max. *J. Appl. Physiol.* 77:671–678, 1994.

98. Söderlund, K., P.L Greenhaff, and E. Hultman. Energy metabolism in type I and type II human muscle fibers during short term electrical stimulation at different frequencies. *Acta Physiol. Scand.* 144:15–22, 1992.

99. Sols, A., and R. Marco. Concentrations of metabolites and binding sites: implications in metabolic regulation. *Curr. Topics Cell Reg.* 2:227–273, 1970.

100. Spina, R.J., M.M.Y. Chi, M.G. Hopkins, P.M. Nemeth, O.H. Lowry, and J.O. Holloszy. Mitochondrial enzymes increase in muscle in response to 7–10 days of cycle exercise. *J. Appl. Physiol.* 80:2250–2254, 1996.

101. Spriet, L.L., K. Söderlund, M. Bergstrom, and E. Hultman. Anaerobic energy release in skeletal muscle during electrical stimulation in men. *J. Appl. Physiol.* 62:611–615, 1987.

102. Stainsby, W.N., W.F. Brechue, D.M. O'Drobinak, and J.K. Barclay. Oxidation/reduction state of cytochrome oxidase during repetitive contractions. *J. Appl. Physiol.* 67:2158–2162, 1989.

103. Stainsby, W.N., W.F. Brechue, D.M. O'Drobinak, and J.K. Barclay. Effects of ischemic and hypoxic hypoxia on VO_2 and lactic acid output during tetanic contraction. *J. Appl. Physiol.* 68:574–579, 1990.

104. Sundberg, C.J. Exercise and training during graded leg ischemia in healthy man. *Acta Physiol. Scand.* 150(S615):2–50, 1994.

105. Symons J.D., and I. Jacobs. High intensity exercise performance is not impaired by low intramuscular glycogen. *Med. Sci. Sports Exerc.* 21:550–557, 1989.

106. Tan, Z.T. Ruthenium red, ribose, and adenine enhance recovery of reperfused rat heart. *Coronary Artery Disease* 4:305–309, 1993.

107. Timmons, J.A., T. Gustavsson, C.J. Sundberg, et al. Substrate availability limits human skeletal muscle oxidative APT regeneration at the onset of exercise. *J. Clin. Invest.* (In Press).

108. Timmons, J.A., S.M. Poucher, D. Constantin-Teodosiu, I.A. Macdonald, and P.L. Greenhaff. The metabolic responses from rest to steady state determine contractile function in ischemic skeletal muscle. *Am. J. Physiol.* 273:E001–E007, 1997.

109. Timmons, J.A., S.M. Poucher, D. Constantin-Teodosiu, V. Worrall, I.A. Macdonald and P.L. Greenhaff. The metabolic responses of canine gracilis muscle during contraction with partial ischemia. *Am. J. Physiol.* 270:E400–E406, 1996.

110. Timmons, J.A., S.M. Poucher, D. Constantin-Teodosiu, V. Worrall, I.A. Macdonald, and P.L. Greenhaff. Increased acetyl group availability enhances contractile function of canine skeletal muscle during ischemia. *J. Clin. Invest.* 97:879–883, 1996.

111. Trump, M.E., G.J.F. Heigenhauser, C.T. Putman, and L.L. Spriet. Importance of muscle phosphocreatine during intermittent maximal cycling. *J. Appl. Physiol.* 80:1574–1580, 1996.

112. Veksler, V.I., A.V. Kuznetsov, K. Anflous, et al. Muscle creatine kinase-deficient mice. *J. Biol. Chem.* 270:19921–19929, 1995.

113. Wagner, P.D. Gas exchange and peripheral diffusion limitation. *Med. Sci. Sports Exerc.* 24:54–58, 1989.

114. Wallimann, T., M. Wyss, D. Brdiczka, K. Nicolay, and H.M. Eppenberger. Intracellular compartmentation, structure and function of creatine kinase isoenzymes in tissues with high and fluctuating energy demands: the "phosphocreatine circuit" for cellular energy homeostasis. *Bioch. J.* 281:21–40, 1992.

115. Wasserman, K., J.E. Hansen, and D.Y. Sue. Facilitation of oxygen consumption by lactic acidosis during exercise. *News Physiol. Sci.* 6:29–34, 1991.

116. Williamson, J.W., P.B. Raven, and B.J. Whipp. Unaltered oxygen uptake kinetics at exercise onset with lower-body positive pressure in humans. *Exp. Physiol.* 81:695–705, 1996

117. Wilson, D.F., M. Erecinska, C. Brown, and I.A. Silver. Effect of oxygen tension on cellular energetics. *Am. J. Physiol.* 233:C135–C140, 1977.

2
Role of Insulin-Like Growth Factor-I in the Regulation of Skeletal Muscle Adaptation to Increased Loading

GREGORY R. ADAMS, PH.D.

Mammalian skeletal muscle is a dynamic tissue that is capable of substantial remodeling in response to alterations in functional demand [15]. While the causes and effects of skeletal muscle adaptation have been extensively reported, the mechanisms that mediate these changes at the cellular level are less well documented. This review represents an attempt to present and to some extent interpret the role of one putative mediator of the skeletal muscle adaptational process, insulin-like growth factor (IGF)-I.

IGF-I has been studied extensively at the molecular, cellular, and organismal level. As a result, many of the important concepts related to this growth factor have been worked out in great detail. Consequently, the bulk of this review focuses on information that is germane to the topic of skeletal muscle adaptation in adult mammalian systems. The more global IGF-I-related information is summarized primarily from recent reviews [9, 11, 71]. The abridged presentations included herein are intended to provide a context for the specific points raised and should not be considered a comprehensive treatment. The general format of each section is to present background information and then address the proposed involvement of IGF-I based on recent experimental results.

This review provides: (1) the rationale for focusing on IGF-I; (2) a brief description of the components of the IGF-I signaling system; (3) the generally accepted effects of IGF-I on skeletal muscle; (4) a survey of the effects of manipulation of circulating IGF-I levels in human and animal models in the context of muscle adaptation; (5) a discussion of the evidence for and importance of autocrine/paracrine IGF-I systems in skeletal muscle; (6) an introduction to the concept of myogenesis as a key component of hypertrophic adaptation; (7) a brief presentation of potential processes that could be impacted via altered IGF-I homeostasis during muscle atrophy; and (8) a discussion of potential interactions between IGF-I and a second hormonal system (thyroid hormone) known to have extensive and profound effects on muscle phenotype.

The express purpose of this review is to examine the role of IGF-I in the adaptation of skeletal muscle; however, only a sparse amount of literature exists which directly addresses this topic. More accurately, the primary thrust of this review is a presentation of the background information from related fields which has been used to generate working hypotheses regarding the function of IGF-I in skeletal muscle. The few studies that examined the role of IGF-I at the level of intact skeletal muscle functioning *in vivo* have generally involved increased loading leading to muscle hypertrophy. As a result, the content of this review will, of necessity, be heavily weighted toward discussion of this aspect of muscle adaptation.

Definitions

A variety of relatively common terms take on specific meanings within various branches of science. To avoid any confusion in this review, the following definitions specific to the topics covered are provided: **Proliferation** is the process of entering and completing the cell cycle to produce cellular progeny. Agents (e.g., growth factors, cell surface components, hormones, etc.) that stimulate cells to proliferate are called mitogens. **Differentiation** is the process by which cells committed to a particular functional fate begin to express specific proteins indicative of that fate. Myogenesis is the process by which cells differentiate into myofibers. **Development** relates to the processes by which cells transition from relatively undifferentiated states toward the attainment of the morphology and phenotype indicative of that found in the adult organism. **Primary cell culture** is the process of removing a particular cell type intact from living tissue and maintaining and possibly propagating these cells *in vitro*. This process does not include the fusion of the wild-type cell with a transformed cell to produce an "immortal" cell line. The phrase **muscle cell lines** is used to distinguish between primary muscle cell cultures and any of a number of immortal cell culture[1] lines that express some subset of characteristics found in muscle cells *in vivo*. Such cell lines may be derived from: (a) wild-type cell fusion with a transformed cell type; (b) a naturally occurring transformed cell type that expresses some muscle-specific proteins (e.g., myogenin, creatine kinase, α-actin, myosin, etc.); or (c) a transformed cell type that has been transfected with gene elements which force the expression of a muscle-specific phenotype. **Myoblasts** are differentiated cells found in developing muscle tissue that proceed to fuse and form multinucleated myotubes which subsequently mature into functional muscle cells (myofibers). The term myoblast is often applied to cells derived from muscle cell culture lines as well as to recently

---

[1] Much of the information related to IGF-I in skeletal muscle has been derived from studies conducted *in vitro*. While muscle cell lines have various attributes that render them muscle-like in nature, the reader should bear in mind that none of these cell lines or for that matter primary muscle cell culture systems represent high-fidelity analogues of mature skeletal muscles functioning *in vivo*.

differentiated stem cells found in hypertrophying and/or regenerating skeletal muscles. **Satellite cells** are mononucleated, quiescent stem cells found between the sarcolemma and basal lamina of myofibers. These cells are capable of proliferating and then differentiating into myoblasts.

OVERVIEW: ADAPTATION AND IGF-I

Alterations in the loading state chronically imposed on skeletal muscles are known to result in remodeling processes which can be measured as changes in muscle mass and can also be detected at the cellular and molecular levels in the myofibers of affected muscles. Manifestations of these adaptations are seen when muscles are exposed either to increased loading, as with resistance training, or unloading, exemplified by bed rest or chronic exposure to microgravity. Despite the extensive body of knowledge associated with skeletal muscle biochemistry and physiology at the present time there is relatively little information concerning the cellular, subcellular, and molecular factors that mediate the alteration in myofiber size.

Some key elements of the hypertrophy response involve processes such as altered protein synthesis and degradation, which are part of the basic "housekeeping" activities of muscle cells. However, the results of recent studies suggest that the hypertrophy response also includes an obligatory component that is "myogenic" in nature [89, 92, 93]. This component is myogenic, not in the sense that new muscle fibers are formed, but rather in regard to the fact that quiescent undifferentiated cells (i.e., satellite cells) are stimulated successively to proliferate and then begin expressing muscle-specific proteins in a process that resembles developmental myogenic events [19]. This suggests that the mechanisms that mediate the hypertrophy response must coordinate both increased protein production within existing myofibers and the initiation of myogenic processes in populations of satellite cells.

The interest in IGF-I as a potential mediator of hypertrophic adaptations is driven at least in part by reports that this growth factor appears to stimulate anabolic, mitogenic, and myogenic processes in various *in vitro* and *in vivo* systems employed in the study of muscle cell biology [40]. In particular, the ability to stimulate both proliferation and differentiation in myogenic cells appears to be unique to IGF-I within the ranks of growth factors. Recent emperical findings indicate that IGF-I expression in skeletal muscle appears to be increased during the process of compensatory hypertrophy in response to increased loading [2, 27, 30, 117]. These various findings have suggested that IGF-I is an attractive candidate for involvement in the control of muscle adaptation to changes in muscle loading.

In traditional endocrinology, IGF-I (originally called somatomedin C) appears as a component of the somatic growth and development system

FIGURE 2.1.

IGF-I can be viewed in two different contexts: (A) IGF-I as an intermediary in GH-regulated control of growth as described by the "somatomedin hypothesis," or (B) IGF-I acting as an autocrine and/or paracrine growth factor mediating localized processes.

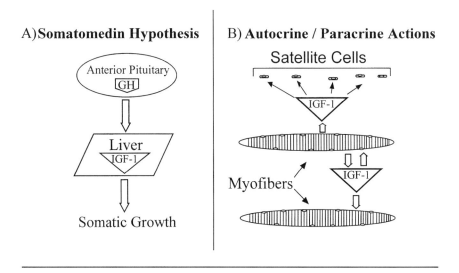

A) **Somatomedin Hypothesis**

B) **Autocrine / Paracrine Actions**

(Figure 2.1A) mediated by growth hormone (GH) (originally somatotrophin). Much of the literature concerning the role of IGF-I in relation to skeletal muscle appears in two major contexts: (1) IGF-I as a component of the GH control axis [125], and (2) the role of IGF-I in myogenesis during the process of development [40]. In the GH context, much of the emphasis has been on the insulin-like metabolic and anabolic effects of IGF-I. In developmental scenarios, the role of IGF-I in stimulating both mitogenic and myogenic processes has been the major point of emphasis. In contrast to these established theories, the concept of a major role for GH-independent, autocrine/paracrine function of IGF-I (Figure 2.1B) was developed relatively recently.

COMPONENTS OF THE IGF-I SYSTEM

IGF-I Expression

IGF-I is a 70-amino acid peptide similar in structure to proinsulin [71]. Circulating levels of IGF-I are generally thought to reflect GH-mediated production by the liver [38]. However, at the molecular level there is evidence that suggests tissue-specific GH-independent regulation of IGF-I expression in non-hepatic tissues that probably does not represent a primary endocrine function [66, 110]. To illustrate this point, significant increases in skeletal muscle IGF-I expression ($\approx$50 fold) are not reflected by an increase in plasma IGF-I concentration [24].

A key component of the theory of tissue-specific regulation of IGF-I involves the structure of the IGF-I gene. Two of the six exons of the IGF-I gene contain multiple transcription initiation sequences, which in conjunction with alternative splicing, can result in a large number of IGF-I mRNAs. Of particular interest are two primary classes of transcripts associated with promoter regions that code for alternative leader sequences [66, 110]. Exon 2 gives rise to class II IGF-I transcripts found primarily in the liver, whereas expression of exon I results in the production of a class I IGF-I transcript that is found in most other tissues, including skeletal muscle. In addition, Yang et al. recently reported the presence of a specific IGF-I transcript that is only expressed following mechanical stretching in skeletal muscles [124]. The identification of a specific, apparently load-sensitive, skeletal muscle IGF-I transcript would clearly support a hypothesis that autocrine/paracrine muscle IGF-I production may be a significant player in muscle adaptational processes.

IGF-I Receptors and Signaling Processes

The IGF-I receptor binds both IGF-I and IGF-II [2] with high affinity. As a result, it has been proposed that the IGF-I receptor is more appropriately termed the type 1 IGF receptor (IGFR1) [83]. The IGFR1 and insulin receptor (IR) are closely related members of the large growth factor receptor family [105]. Insulin also binds to the IGFR1 but with 100- to 1000-fold lower affinity than IGF-I [9, 40]. IGFR1 knockout experiments result in mice that have extreme growth retardation and animals that die at birth due to the lack of sufficient respiratory muscle development [40].

Structurally, the IGFR1 is a multimeric transmembrane glycoprotein consisting of two α and two β subunits [105]. The α subunits are found located on the extracellular face of the plasma membrane and contain the ligand binding sites while the β subunits span the membrane and exhibit the tyrosine kinase activity required for signal transduction [60]. Hybrid receptors containing $\alpha\beta$ dimers from both the IR and IGFR1 have been identified in cells that normally express both receptors, including skeletal muscle [9, 40, 105]. Two different IGFR1 mRNAs resulting from alternative splicing have been detected in some tissues [105]. In addition, a structural and functional IGFR1 variant is found in fetal muscle [40]. Hence, there is the potential for significant heterogeneity in IGFR1 populations, which may be physiologically relevant in some tissues.

---

[2] IGF-II appears to promote many of the same responses attributed to IGF-I in skeletal muscle-related systems [40].

The structure of the IGF-II receptor appears to be unrelated to that of the IR/IGFR1 family. In striated muscle it is generally thought that the IGFR1 mediates the actions of both IGF-I and IGF-II. [40].

As with other members of the growth factor receptor family, IGFR1-ligand interactions stimulate the intrinsic tyrosine kinase activity of the β subunit to catalyze autophosphorylation at multiple sites on that subunit [9, 105]. Subsequently, the activated IGFR1 phosphorylates intracellular signaling proteins, such as insulin receptor substrate (IRS)-1 (IRS-1) (or IRS-2 /4PS) and Src homology-containing proteins (Shc) [9, 40, 86]. IRS-1 has multiple sites for its phosphorylation which, when phosphorylated, allow for the interaction with various other cytoplasmic signaling molecules, such as Grb2 and c-Crk [8, 40, 78]. In muscle, a well-characterized target of phosphory-lated IRS-1 is the regulatory (p85) subunit of phosphatidyl-inositol-3-kinase (PI3-kinase). IRS-1 (or 2) binding to p85 increases PI3-kinase activity [9, 86]. Downstream events attributed to PI3-kinase activity include activation of p70-s6 kinase, which phosphorylates the S6 protein component of ribo-somes, possibly modulating the rate of translation and thereby protein syn-thesis [40, 71, 75]. The IRS-1/Grb2 pathway has been shown to lead to the exchange of guanosine 5'-triphosphate (GTP) for guanosine 5'-diphos-phate (GDP) on RAS protein leading to RAS activation of the mitogen activated protein (MAP) kinase cascade [9, 78]. In some mammalian sys-tems, activation of the MAP kinase cascade is associated with mitogenic effects, such as the activation of c-*fos,* c-*jun,* and c-*myc* transcription factors [9, 71, 82].

These examples of the events that follow IGFR1 activation are similar to or the same as those described for insulin receptor activation, and IGF-I can in fact stimulate many of the same cellular responses as insulin [88, 105]. In addition, many cell types, including skeletal muscle, express both IR and IGFR1, raising the question of how a specificity of response is ob-tained. One possibility lies in the kinetics of receptor-ligand interactions and the fate of the different ligands. Following ligand binding, both IR and IGFR1 are internalized [46, 90, 109, 128]. In rat fibroblasts, Zapf et al. found that compared to insulin, the rate of internalization of IGF-I-IGFR1 was much slower, and that once internalized, IGF-I remains associated with its receptor much longer [128]. These authors also found that the intracel-lular fate of ligands was different; much of the internalized insulin was separated from its receptor and degraded. In contrast, a large proportion of the IGF-I remained attached to receptors, which were recycled to the plasma membrane where the IGF-I was released. This might suggest that the differences in internalization and degradation between the IR and IGFR1 are responsible for some of the divergent functional consequences of the activation of these two receptors. However, recent cell culture studies in which amino acid substitution reduced IGFR1 internalization suggest that IGF-I-specific effects, such as the stimulation of cell proliferation, were not affected [109].

Although internalization per se may not differentiate between insulin from IGF-I-mediated responses, differences in receptor-ligand kinetics may still play a role. DeMeyts et al. [29] recently reported that synthetic insulin analogues with unaltered metabolic effects were highly mitogenic compared to insulin. An interesting characteristic of the more mitogenic analogues was that they dissociated from the IR much more slowly than insulin, a characteristic reminiscent of IGF-I. DeMeyts et al. suggested that the kinetics of receptor occupation may function as a "timer" resulting in specificity of transduction. More recently, Shooter et al. [104] published results demonstrating alterations in potency for the stimulation of protein synthesis by synthetic IGF-I analogues that appear to support the concept of receptor occupation kinetics as a modulating factor.

Recent reports state that IGF-I, IGF-I-binding proteins, and IGFR1 can be localized in the nucleus of cells *in vivo* [20] and in cell culture [68]. Such results suggest that the effects of IGF-I might be mediated via nuclear transduction routes as well as the more extensively characterized cytoplasmic pathways.

As noted previously, many of the downstream events following IGF-IGFR1 binding have been elucidated. However, most of the steps in these pathways appear to be similar to those associated with insulin binding to IR. The data suggesting that receptor ligand kinetics or nuclear localization may distinguish IGF-I from insulin-mediated effects offer suggestions for further study but cannot be considered conclusive at this time.

IGF Binding Proteins

Most of the circulating IGF-I ($\approx 99\%$) in the plasma is bound to members of a family of IGF-I-specific transport proteins. There is a significant presence of IGF binding proteins (IGFBPs) in the extravascular spaces as well. The IGFBPs modulate the availability of IGF-I via a number of processes, including: (a) increasing the half-life of circulating IGF-I; (b) mediating IGF-I transport out of the circulation; and (c) localizing IGF-I in specific tissues [22, 25].

IGFBP-IGF-I binding has a higher affinity than that of IGF-I-IGFR1 interactions [22]. Several IGF-I analogues have high affinity for the IGFR1 but do not bind to IGFBPs, which indicates that separate portions of the IGF-I structure are responsible for receptor or IGFBP binding [22]. This suggests that IGF-I might not need to be released from IGFBPs in order to interact with IGFR1. For example, in cultured smooth muscle, the mitogenic responses to IGF-I are potentiated by addition of IGFBPs [22]. There is also evidence that the various IGFBPs have intrinsic biological activities separate from the modulation of IGF-I availability [25].

IGFBP-3 is the primary plasma transport binding protein and is maintained at relatively stable levels [25]. In contrast, circulating levels of IGFBP-1 and -2 tend to vary throughout the day and appear to be particularly responsive to a fasting metabolic state [25]. IGFBP-2 is present at relatively low levels in plasma, but is the major IGFBP present in cerebrospinal fluid (CSF) [25], and has also been found in cardiac tissue [21]. IGFBP-4 is detected mainly in extracellular fluid spaces [25]. IGFBP-2 and -4 have relatively low molecular weights and are postulated to be involved with the transport of IGF-I across the endothelial surface to specific cell types [14, 21]. IGFBP-5 is found at high levels in fetal tissues and in various tissues in adults [25]. IGFBP-5 mRNA has also been identified in rat muscle [42]. IGFBP-6 is found in serum and CSF and has a much higher affinity for IGF-II than IGF-I [25]. A seventh IGFBP was recently identified but is not well characterized at this time [120].

IGFBP actions are often described as being inhibitory, in relation to IGF-I-mediated processes, due to the fact that the addition of binding proteins to cell culture systems decreases the concentration of free IGF-I [25]. *In vivo*, increases in some of the more labile IGFBPs most certainly function to decrease IGF-I activity while others function to facilitate IGF-I effects via transport and localization.

Various processes may alter the affinity of IGFBPs for IGF-I [22, 25]. IGFBP-1 can be phosphorylated, thereby increasing its affinity for IGF-I. Both IGFBP-1 and -2 have amino acid sequences that suggest the capability to bind to integrins, a process that might alter their affinity for IGF-I [22, 25]. IGFBP-5 binds to extracellular matrix components (inhibited by heparin), a process that significantly lowers IGFBP-5 affinity for IGF-I [25].

Of particular recent interest is the involvement of IGFBP-specific proteases in the modulation of IGF-I activity [12, 23, 25, 64]. Proteolysis of IGFBP-3 in the plasma decreases its affinity for IGF-I, possibly causing the release of IGF-I or IGF-I bound to IGFBP-3 subunits for transendothelial transport. In the interstitial space, IGFBP proteolysis may serve a similar function by providing free IGF-I, which is then available to bind with the cell surface IGFR1. These various processes could provide a wide range of flexibility in both the temporal and spatial coordination of IGF-I function.

Various studies using muscle cell lines suggest a role for IGFBPs in the modulation of IGF-I effects in muscle. Some muscle cell lines [53, 73] produce IGFBP-4 and/or -5. James et al. reported that over-expression of IGFBP-5 in C2 cells prevents differentiation [53], while cytokines that block differentiation have also inhibited IGFBP-4 and -5 production *in vitro* [74].

Figure 2.2 presents an overview of some of the components of the IGF-I signaling system. As with all hormone-like systems, modulation of IGF-I actions can be accomplished via the control of cellular IGF-I production and secretion as well as the manipulation of cell surface IGFR1 populations and components of the intracellular signaling pathways. The presence of

FIGURE 2.2.
Schematic representation of some components of the IGF-I signaling system. (A) Extra-cellular modulation can be accomplished by controlling the amount of circulating (endocrine) or locally produced (autocrine /paracrine) IGF-I. Another level of extracel-lular modulation is provided by the presence of IGFBPs and associated proteases, which further regulate the bioavailability IGF-I. (B) IGF-I binding to cells will be a function of the concentration of free IGF-I and IGFR1 density on the cell membrane (C) IGF-I binding to IGFR1 results in autophosphorylation of the β subunit and subsequent phosphorylation of various intracellular messenger molecules that initiate signaling cascades.

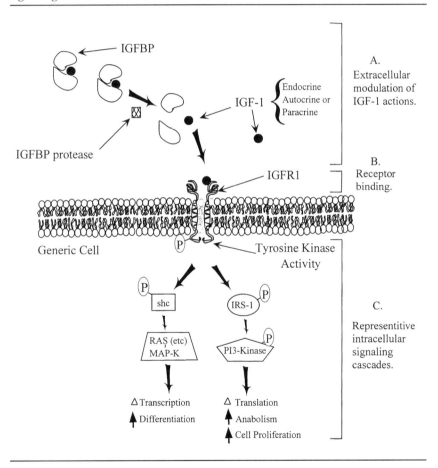

IGFBPs and IGFBP proteases provides another level of complexity in the control of IGF-I signaling.

THE EFFECT OF IGF-I ON SKELETAL MUSCLE

Anabolic Effects of IGF-I

Increased net protein production is an obvious requirement for muscle hypertrophy to occur. It is generally acknowledged that IGF-I exerts anabolic effects similar to those produced by insulin [40]. In rats, IGF-I injections have been shown to increase skeletal muscle protein synthesis rates when delivered in conjunction with insulin or amino acids [51]. In muscle cell culture studies, IGF-I has been shown to suppress protein degradation and increase amino acid uptake and stimulate protein synthesis [36, 40]. IGF-I-mediated depression of protein degradation may involve regulation of components of the ubiquitin degradation pathway [121]. In intact isolated skeletal muscles, IGF-I infusion or incubation has been shown to result in an increase in the uptake of amino acids and increased synthesis of RNA [36]. In keeping with one of the IGF-I-related signal transduction schemes outlined above, Dardevet et al. [28] found that IGF-I or insulin-stimulated protein synthesis can be blocked by PI3-kinase inhibitors in superfused rat muscles. The well-established ability of IGF-I to mediate anabolism represents one attribute of this growth factor that could clearly contribute to the hypertrophy process in skeletal muscle.IGF-I

IGF-I and Muscle Development

The literature relating to the effects of IGF-I in developmental systems provides much of the background which suggests the potential for the involvement of this growth factor in the mediation of muscle adaptation. IGF-I is a critical growth factor for the embryonic development of skeletal muscle [9, 40]. Ordered development of any tissue involves proliferation of progenitor cells and subsequent differentiation of the progeny which coalesce into the mature tissue. IGF-I has been shown to stimulate the proliferation of muscle cell lines and to promote the expression of muscle-specific proteins. In addition, in some cell lines, IGF-I can induce differentiated cells to fuse and form myotubes. The IGF-I-stimulated transition from proliferation to differentiation is inhibited by the presence of other proliferation promoting growth factors, particularly basic-fibroblast growth factor (bFGF) and transforming growth factor-β (TGFβ) [40]. In developmental and cell culture studies, IGF-I-mediated expression of muscle-specific proteins appear to be linked to expression of myogenic regulatory factors (MRF), which in mammals include myoD, myogenin, Myf-5, and MRF-4 [38, 39, 40, 97]. Members of the MRF family are known to bind to specific sites in the promoter region of several muscle-specific genes, thereby initiating the myogenic program in myoblasts. Interestingly, an IGF response element has been identified in the 5'-upstream region of the mouse myogenin gene promoter [39]. As an example of IGF-I-MRF interactions, Engert et al. [35] recently reported that IGF-I stimulation of L6E9 cells results initially in the decreased expression of myogenic factors such as myogenin, while markers of proliferation such as the cell cycle protein cyclin D1 were increased. This relationship was reversed over time (≈48 hours) and the IGF-I-stimulated cells subsequently formed myotubes. The expression of myoD and myogenin has also been detected in adult mammalian muscle [47].

In the context of developmental processes, there appear to be several distinct outcomes stimulated by IGF-I-IGFR1 binding, which suggests separate intracellular signaling pathways. Kaliman et al. [59] reported that PI3-kinase inhibitors block IGF-I-stimulated differentiation but not proliferation in L6E9 cells. Florini and Ewton [37] found that an antisense oligo-deoxy-ribonucleotide specific to myogenin mRNA eliminated the differentiation response of L6 cells to IGF-I, but it had no effect on the anabolic actions of this growth factor. In further dissection of distinct IGF-I-stimulated signaling pathways, Florini's group [26, 40] recently showed that inhibition of the MAP kinase signaling cascade prevents proliferation in L6 cells, while inhibition of the pathway, which includes PI3-kinase and/or $p70^{s6kinase}$, prevents IGF-I-stimulated differentiation.

In conclusion, there is an extensive body of literature, primarily representing *in vitro* experiments, indicating that IGF-I modulates both mitogenic and myogenic effects in developing muscle tissues. Further, these two IGF-I-stimulated processes, proliferation and differentiation, can be dissociated in muscle cell lines. As will be discussed, there is increasing evidence that the processes of proliferation and differentiation, which are traditionally associated with the development of skeletal muscle, may also be active during muscle adaptation to changes in loading state.

SYSTEMIC IGF-I AND MUSCLE

Increased Circulating IGF-I in Humans

A variety of studies in humans report that GH treatment, which increases systemic IGF-I levels, causes growth of both muscle and non-muscle tissues, resulting in increased lean body mass but no improvements in muscle-related parameters, such as strength or relative muscle mass [125]. The primary observation that prompted researchers to undertake these studies was that circulating levels of IGF-I are known to be depressed in elderly humans. In light of this observation, investigators postulated that IGF-I or GH therapy might improve the muscle mass and/or the response of elderly humans to resistance training. A number of studies had in fact reported increased nitrogen balance and/or skeletal muscle protein synthesis following administration of GH as well as relatively high doses of IGF-I. However, these studies did not include information such as measurements of muscle function, muscle mass, or in some cases, alterations in the nutritional state of the subjects, all of which would speak to the practica! applications for such treatments [17, 98, 125]. For example, Butterfield et al. [17] recently reported that daily injections of either GH or IGF-I (0.12 mg·kg^{-1}) for 28 days resulted in increased nitrogen balance and increased protein synthesis in the vastus lateralis muscles of four elderly women; however, no muscle strength or morphological measurements were obtained, so the functional impact of the observed increases in muscle protein synthesis could not be assessed. In studies where muscle function and/or mass was determined, the overall impact of experimentally increasing circulating IGF-I levels were negligible [112, 113, 126]. In one such study, investigators attempted to augment resistance training-induced strength gains in elderly men via exogenous GH treatment. The GH treatment doubled the circulating levels of IGF-I in these subjects, but it did not augment the strength gains elicited by the resistance training program [113]. Similarly, Yarasheski et al. found that GH administration doubled circulating IGF-I levels in elderly subjects, but it had no effect on the protein synthesis rate in the trained muscles nor did it augment the measured strength gains [126].

Increased Circulating IGF-I in Animal Models

IGF-I has only recently become available in quantities sufficient to allow systemic supplementation. However, there is a substantial body of literature where GH supplementation was provided and measures of muscle morphology and/or function were subsequently obtained. GH treatment results in significant increases in circulating IGF-I, thus, these studies can be viewed as manipulations of the levels of this growth factor as well.

Comparisons of human studies which have experimentally increased circulating GH and/or IGF-I levels with studies conducted in animal models are hampered by a tendency to use the hypophysectomized (Hypox) rat model. In addition to depressed GH levels, Hypox rats lack other pituitary hormones, such as thyroxine, that also have known effects in skeletal muscle. Further complication results from the fact that growth factor treatment of Hypox animals restores generalized body growth, making muscle-specific effects difficult to discern unless the data are normalized. For example, Bates et al. gave GH injections to Hypox rats and reported a restoration of growth such that normalized muscle weights (e.g., medial gastrocnemius, or MG) were similar to those of control animals [8]. In contrast, a study published about the same time reported that GH treatment of Hypox rats caused significant hypertrophy in several muscles, including the MG [43]. In the latter study [43], the absolute muscle weights were analyzed without consideration of the restoration of body growth. When corrected for body weight gains, the GH treatment in this study [43] did not appear to result in a functional hypertrophy (i.e., increased muscle to body weight ratio), which indicates agreement between the two studies. Similar results were seen in a different model where circulating GH levels were increased via the implantation of GH-secreting cells [116]. Using this model, the data of Turner et al. [116] indicate that GH induced a generalized somatic growth during which the muscle weights failed to keep pace with the overall increase in body mass. For example, the relative gastrocnemius muscle mass from the GH-treated animals was actually smaller than that of the controls. In contrast, there was a relative hypertrophy of the heart [116]. Since the gastrocnemius is a weight-bearing muscle, these results would suggest that despite an absolute increase in muscle mass, the GH treatment might have placed this muscle at a functional disadvantage. Although slightly out of context, it is interesting to note that *in vitro* studies indicate that high levels of IGF in the culture medium appear to suppress autocrine/paracrine production of IGF-I by many myoblast cell lines [40].

A variety of animal studies have combined exogenous GH treatment with exercise training [125]. For example, in an attempt to counter unloading-induced skeletal muscle atrophy, Linderman et al. [69] treated tail-suspended rats with GH and in a subgroup provided both GH supplementation and resistance training. These authors found that GH treatment alone did not prevent the atrophy process; however, resistance training in conjunction with GH treatment did result in a modest sparing of myofibrillar protein in unloaded gastrocnemius and soleus muscles. When carefully examined, the data from the majority of studies using animal models indicate a general failure of systemic GH or IGF-I treatment to produce a functionally significant enhancement (i.e., increased muscle to body weight ratio) of skeletal muscle [7, 43, 96, 116, 125]. Nonetheless, failure of GH treatment to produce a functional muscle hypertrophy in animals is not a universal finding. In a study that employed normal (non-Hypox) rats, GH treatment resulted in functional hypertrophy of the soleus muscle [12]. This result is in contrast to those reported from Hypox rats that found that the soleus muscle was refractory to GH treatment [7, 43]. In the study by Bates et al. cited above, GH did induce hypertrophy in MG muscles of rats that were calorically restricted to prevent total body mass increases [7]. While caloric restriction in and of itself represents an experimental intervention for the manipulation of muscle mass, these results do indicate that GH may be causing the selective delivery and uptake of nutrients to potentiate anabolic processes.

As a result of their survey of the literature, several reviewers conclude that circulating (endocrine) IGF-I at best plays a minor role in the modulation of the mass of specific skeletal muscles during adaptation to changes in loading [70, 125]. In the context of skeletal muscle adaptation to altered loading, and assuming that the primary relevant effect of GH treatment is to increase circulating IGF-I, these collective results raise questions as to the relative importance of circulating IGF-I in functional adaptations of skeletal muscle (i.e., functionally significant increases in strength or mass). Taken together, the majority of the literature from both human and animal studies suggests that circulating IGF-I levels are of minimal importance in the adaptation of specific muscles to changes in loading.

AUTOCRINE/PARACRINE IGF-I FUNCTION AND MUSCLE ADAPTATION

Teleologically, a local autocrine/paracrine system that mediates the adaptation of specific muscles to changes in loading state may be easier to envision than one that requires cells to respond to increases in levels of circulating factors which are normally present in relatively high concentrations (e.g., IGF-I, >200 ng•ml^{-1} in humans [103, 113, 126] and >400 ng•ml^{-1} in rodents [2, 24]). The suggestion that muscle adaptation, specifically muscle hypertrophy, occurring *in vivo* may be relatively independent of circulating levels of GH and IGF-I is also supported by several lines of evidence. First, there are substantial data indicating that muscle cells produce IGF-I as an autocrine and/or paracrine growth factor both: (a) *in vitro*, in studies using primary muscle cell culture or muscle cell lines that have demonstrated that IGF-I is expressed in these cell types [58, 87, 117]; and (b) *in vivo*, where an accumulating number of studies convincingly demonstrated that skeletal muscles express IGF-I [18, 40, 49, 55, 124] even when circulating GH and IGF-I levels are depressed [2, 30, 127]. Second, examination of the literature indicates that high circulating levels of IGF-I do not appear to be a necessary condition for muscles to grow [70] or to enlarge in response to increased loading [2]. Most notably, when the GH axis is interrupted via surgical hypophysectomy (Hypox), plasma levels of IGF-I in the rat are significantly depressed ($\approx$80%) [2, 7, 49]. Even so, the muscles of Hypox rats can respond to increased loading with substantial increases in muscle mass [2, 30, 41].

Muscle IGF-I and Regeneration

A number of studies report evidence of increased IGF-I expression (mRNA and/or peptide) in satellite cells, myotubes, or myofibers in both Hypox and normal rat muscles during skeletal muscle regeneration [34, 54–56, 108]. Using a muscle regeneration model, Jennische and Hansson [55] demonstrated that IGF-I immunoreactivity was detected in the cytoplasm and was probably associated with polyribosomes. In this study, the most intense immunoreactivity was seen within myoblasts and myotubes [55]. LeFaucheur and Sebille recently reported that antibodies that neutralized either IGF-I or bFGF activity reduced the number and size of regenerating fibers with the anti-IGF-I treatment demonstrating a higher potency [65].

The known *in vitro* myogenic effects of IGF-I, coupled with evidence of expression of this growth factor, lead to the common assumption that IGF-I is participating in the regenerative process [48]. The increased IGF-I seen in the regenerating muscles of Hypox rats further suggests that this response is occurring independent of GH stimulation [108].

Muscle IGF-I and Hypertrophy

Numerous studies employing *in vitro* models demonstrate that IGF-I stimulates anabolic, mitogenic, and myogenic processes in muscle cell lines and in primary muscle cell culture [40]. For example, Vandenburgh et al. [117] found that myoblasts, isolated from avian skeletal muscle and cultured under continuous tension in a collagen matrix, form myofibers and that these myofibers hypertrophied in response to the addition of IGF-I.

Studies employing *in vivo* models known to result in muscle hypertrophy demonstrate that muscle expression of IGF-I increases very early in the hypertrophy process. Several studies report that stretch-induced hypertrophy of mammalian skeletal muscle is accompanied by increased expression of IGF-I mRNA [27, 101, 124] and that some of this increased IGF-I mRNA was localized to the myofibers of the affected muscles [124]. In rat skeletal muscles which were functionally overloaded for 8 days via the removal of synergists, DeVol et al. [30] detected increased IGF-I mRNA. This particular study employed Hypox rats, which further suggests that the observed IGF-I mRNA expression was GH independent. In a time-course study using the functional overload model in both Hypox and normal rats, Adams and Haddad found that increased muscle IGF-I peptide and mRNA levels were detected prior to the attainment of significant muscle hypertrophy and remained elevated for up to 28 days during the hypertrophy process [2]. In a very different model, Zanconato et al. [127] suppressed circulating GH and IGF-I levels by using antibodies to GH-releasing hormone. Treadmill training of these GH-suppressed rats increased muscle IGF-I mRNA by 55% and IGF-I peptide by 250% [127].

Though descriptive in nature, these studies demonstrate that increased skeletal muscle IGF-expression is associated with adaptation to increased loading and strongly suggest that this growth factor is involved with some aspects of the hypertrophy process.

IGF-I Stimulated Hypertrophy

Recent studies provide strong support for a cause and effect relationship between increased skeletal muscle IGF-I expression and muscle hypertrophy using two very different approaches. In one study, Coleman et al. [24] constructed a transgene using the regulatory elements of the avian skeletal α-actin gene coupled to IGF-I cDNA and then used this construct to create a transgenic mouse line that overexpressed IGF-I only in muscle tissues. The overexpression of IGF-I peptide in muscle (≈50 fold) induced muscle hypertrophy (normalized mass) while other tissues were unaffected. It is interesting to note that this large increase in muscle IGF-I was not reflected by an increase in plasma IGF-I concentrations [24]. Using a different approach in adult rats, we recently found that IGF-I in and of itself can induce muscle hypertrophy in specifically targeted rat skeletal muscles *in vivo* [1]. This was accomplished via the implantation of osmotic pumps containing IGF-I and attached to catheters that were secured under the fascia of the tibialis anterior (TA) muscles in rats. Compared to the contralateral muscles or those of saline-infused control animals, infusion of non-systemic doses ($990 \eta g \cdot day^{-1}$) of IGF-I directly into the implanted TA muscles resulted in increased muscle mass and protein content in the absence of changes in the loading state of the muscle (Figure 2.3). Infusion of IGF-I had no effect on body weight, the weight of the heart, or of the extensor digitorum longus, a muscle that lies directly beneath the TA. After 2 weeks of IGF-I infusion, hypertrophy of the TA was accompanied by a 21% increase in muscle DNA ($\mu g \cdot mg \, protein^{-1}$) (Figure 2.3). These results clearly establish a link between IGF-I exposure, muscle enlargement, and DNA incorporation into the muscle. As discussed below, the process of DNA incorporation appears necessary to maintain DNA to protein ratios as the myofibers enlarge.

The various studies cited in the previous two sections clearly suggest a cause and effect relationship between the hypertrophy process and increased, GH-independent, autocrine/paracrine IGF-I expression in skeletal muscle. The maintenance of a "normalized" DNA to protein ratio in hypertrophied skeletal muscle points to a potential key role for IGF-I in this process that is separate from this growth factor's known anabolic effects.

FIGURE 2.3.
Effects of 2 and 3 weeks of IGF-I infusion (990 ηg/day) on the normalized muscle weight (left) and DNA concentration (right) of rat TA muscles. Contra, sham operated-contralateral TA.

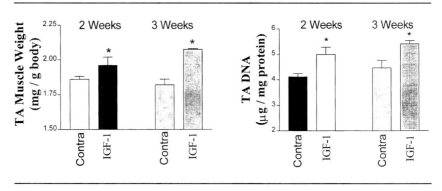

"MYOGENIC" ASPECTS OF HYPERTROPHY

Although increased protein production is an obvious requirement for muscle to hypertrophy, it is becoming increasingly evident that other processes, such as the acquisition of additional myonuclei, are also required to support this process.

Hypertrophy and Proliferation

As noted previously, IGF-I is acknowledged to have two primary effects on skeletal muscle that can impact the hypertrophy process: (1) a clearly established, insulin-like anabolic effect and (2) a critical role in embryonic developmental schemes that are in some ways analogous to processes that are activated during hypertrophy.

Skeletal muscle is a dynamic tissue capable of undergoing extensive remodeling that can include substantial increases in muscle size. An increasing body of evidence indicates that there is a relationship between skeletal muscle fibers size (e.g., cross-sectional area, cytoplasmic volume, etc.) and the number of myonuclei present on the myofiber [33, 114]. Nevertheless, shortly after birth, mammalian myofibers are permanently differentiated and thus cannot undergo mitotic division or directly increase their myonuclear number (i.e., myonuclear division) [19, 111]. Therefore, myofibers undergoing hypertrophy would need an external source of new nuclei in order to maintain or reestablish a relatively constant myonucleus to fiber size ratio. Recent studies suggest that mechanisms do exist which result in the maintenance of a consistent myonucleus to myofiber size ratio [3]. It has been proposed that any new myonuclei found in skeletal muscle are most likely of satellite cell origin [19, 118].

The Role of Satellite Cells in Muscle Adaptation

Satellite cells are small mononucleated skeletal muscle stem cells located between the basal lamina of the muscle and the sarcolemma of myofibers. Satellite cells appear to be mobilized in response to increased loading or after injury to muscle cells [3].

Initial events after satellite cell activation appear to be a proliferative response in which all the activated satellite cells undergo at least one mitotic cycle. Following this initial phase, some of the activated cells and/or their progeny differentiate into myoblast-like cells. In regenerating muscle, these myoblast-like cells can fuse with each other to form new myofibers or can be incorporated into damaged but viable existing myofibers [13, 72, 76]. In the case of the hypertrophy response, satellite cell derived myoblasts are thought to fuse with existing myofibers, thereby providing additional myonuclei (i.e., DNA) [19, 99, 100, 107]. In addition, several studies strongly suggest that satellite cell proliferation may be required to support the compensatory hypertrophy process [3, 89, 92, 93, 100]. For example,

Phelan and Gonyea [89] recently used γ-radiation to prevent satellite cell proliferation prior to initiating skeletal muscle functional overloading. These authors demonstrated that the irradiated overloaded muscles failed to hypertrophy [89].

The mechanisms underlying the recruitment of satellite cells for either regenerative or hypertrophy processes have not been established. Based on developmental models, such as those involving embryonic and muscle cell line studies, there appears to be a role for various growth factors in the mobilization of satellite cells. Several of the well-characterized growth factors, including fibroblast growth factors (FGF) and platelet-derived growth factors (PDGF), were shown to stimulate satellite cell proliferation *in vitro* [6, 39, 57, 91, 119]. While growth factors such as FGF may in fact be important in the initial activation of satellite cells, the presence of these growth factors has been shown to inhibit the second phase of satellite cell responses (i.e., differentiation and fusion) [40]. In contrast, IGF-I has been shown to stimulate proliferation, differentiation, and fusion of satellite cells in primary cultures [19, 31]. In the *in vivo* study of Phelan and Gonyea [89] cited above, irradiated, overloaded muscles increased IGF-I production, but the targeted muscle failed to hypertrophy [89]. Taken together, these findings suggest that skeletal muscle IGF-I is functioning in a paracrine mode and contributing to the hypertrophy process via the mobilization of satellite cells during muscle remodeling.

Using an avian muscle satellite primary cell culture preparation, Duclos et al. reported that DNA synthesis can be initiated via binding of IGF-I and IGF-II and, to a lesser extent, insulin, to the IGFR1 [32]. We also recently reported that the increase in IGF-I seen in rat skeletal muscles during compensatory hypertrophy was paralleled by an increase in muscle DNA content [2]. Our analysis indicated that there was a significant positive correlation between the increase in muscle DNA content and muscle IGF-I expression. These results also support the hypothesis that IGF-I might be mediating the hypertrophy response by stimulating the proliferation of satellite cells.

In an attempt to illustrate the role of cell proliferation in the hypertrophy process, we overloaded rat plantaris muscles by removing the synergistic soleus and gastrocnemius muscles. One week later, we implanted (intraperitoneally) mini-osmotic pumps (Alzet, Mountain View, CA) in order to dispense bromo-deoxyuridine (BRdU). BRdU is a nucleotide analogue that is incorporated into DNA during *de novo* synthesis and thus can be used as a marker of nuclear proliferation. The results indicated that the overloaded muscles contained a significant number of new nuclei compared to the contralateral control plantaris (Figure 2.4).

Satellite Cell Proliferation

As noted above, it is generally assumed that new myonuclei are provided by satellite cells that enter the cell cycle and then differentiate. The prolifer-

FIGURE 2.4.

BRdU-positive nuclei in overloaded and contralateral control plantaris muscles. Results expressed as BRdU-positive nuclei per myofiber counted on muscle cross-sections.

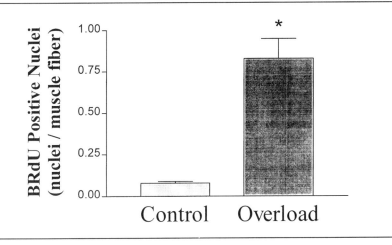

ative phase of activated satellite cells is characterized by progression through successive steps of the cell cycle [19]. Progression of quiescent cells from G_0 into G_1 and on through the mitotic process is shown to be under the control of cyclin proteins that are complexed with various cyclin-dependent kinases (cdk). In a given population of activated satellite cells, some are known to pass through one or more cell cycles and then subside into a quiescent state, while others will irreversibly exit the cell cycle and become differentiated myoblasts that produce muscle-specific proteins such as myogenin (and/or myoD), muscle creatine kinase, and various sacromeric proteins such as myosin heavy chain [19, 40, 94]. In satellite primary cell culture, myoD and myogenin are reported to be present in activated but not in quiescent cells [106, 122]. Also in satellite cell culture, Smith et al. found that myoD mRNA increased prior to proliferation, while the appearance of myogenin mRNA was found to coincide with differentiation [106].

IGF-I has been shown to stimulate proliferation in satellite cells in primary cultures and in a variety of muscle cell-related *in vitro* systems [5, 19, 31]. As part of this process, IGF-I appears to stimulate the expression of cyclins D1 and D2 [35]. FGF has also been shown to stimulate proliferative processes in developing skeletal muscles, satellite cells, and muscle-related *in vitro* systems, which further suggests that this growth factor is likely to be involved in the proliferative phase of the response to muscle injury or increased loading in mature muscles as well [44, 57, 85, 95, 119, 123].

Differentiation of Satellite Cells

If the hypothesis that activated satellite cells provide myonuclei during the hypertrophy process is correct, then satellite cell proliferation must be followed by differentiation in some members of the satellite cell population.

A number of well-characterized growth factors have the potential to stimulate cell proliferation in various muscle cell types associated with skeletal muscle [48]. However, the actions of growth factors other than IGF-I (and IGF-II) are generally antagonistic to differentiation [40, 50, 61, 84]. For example, transgenic chicken embryos over-expressing the FGF type 1 receptor (FGFR1) in somatic cells demonstrate appropriate cell migration to limb buds but a failure to differentiate into myotomal muscle [50]. These results prompted the authors to suggest that a down-regulation of the FGFR1 is necessary to allow differentiation to proceed. In a more generalized result, Lagord et al. [62, 63] demonstrated that inhibitors of cAMP-dependent protein kinase (PKA), which is often associated with the signaling pathways of non-IGF growth factors, such as FGF and TGF-β [84], will stimulate differentiation in primary cultures of rat satellite cells. In particular, the cAMP pathway and PKA have been shown to inhibit the activity of MRF proteins which are required for myogenesis and are putative targets for IGF-I stimulation [67].

These results highlight the unique contrast between IGF-I and other growth factors. To date, the IGFs are the only well-characterized growth factors that have been found to induce both the processes of proliferation and differentiation in satellite primary cell culture and muscle cell lines [94].

In summary, the literature suggests that skeletal muscle hypertrophy appears to involve both anabolic and myogenic events that provide for both the increase in muscle protein associated with increased myofiber size and the provision of new myonuclei via the incorporation of satellite cells into existing myofibers. A working model for further investigation is proposed in Figure 2.5. Based on the foregoing literature, this model proposes that IGF-I is a likely candidate in mediating anabolic and particularly myogenic events required to support skeletal muscle hypertrophy.

Myonuclei, Satellite Cells, and Muscle Atrophy

In further support of the concept of a relationship between myofiber size and myonuclear number, several studies link reductions in muscle loading with alterations in myonuclear number in skeletal muscles. In growing rats subjected to reduced muscle loading via hind-limb suspension, it was reported that soleus muscle growth retardation was accompanied by cessation of mitotic activity in muscle [102]. In another study, the soleus muscles from rats that were suspended from postpartum day 20 to day 30 had 45% fewer satellite cells and 42% fewer myonuclei than those of the control group. In denervated cat soleus muscles, Allen et al. reported a significant

FIGURE 2.5.

(A) Increased loading stimulates a myofiber to increase production and secretion of IGF-I. (B) Satellite cells lying beneath the basal lamina of the myofiber are stimulated by the increased local concentration of IGF-I to enter the cell cycle and begin to proliferate. (C) Continued exposure to elevated IGF-I levels induces expression of muscle-specific proteins in some adjacent satellite cells. (D) Differentiated satellite cells (myoblasts) fuse with the hypertrophying myofiber providing additional myonuclei.

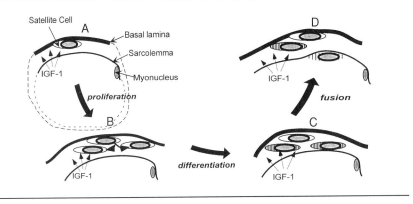

loss of myonuclei associated with fast myofibers [3]. Recent studies on rats exposed to microgravity indicate that the number of myonuclei skeletal in muscles decreased as a result of mechanical unloading [4, 45].

These studies suggest that the mitogenic and myogenic events associated with muscle hypertrophy are mirrored by antipodal processes during unloading-induced muscle atrophy. The decrease in satellite cell activation and in particular the finding that myofibers appear to lose myonuclei as a result of unloading strongly suggest that the coordinate regulation of the myonucleus to fiber size (or DNA to protein) ratio is a symmetrical process during muscle adaptation to both increased and decreased loading.

Thyroid Hormones and IGF-I

A number of agents other than IGF-I are reported to positively affect muscle cell differentiation [40]. Among these agents, thyroid hormone (T_3) has been shown to exert a powerful effect on skeletal muscle [15] and may impact some of the same processes as IGF-I [77]. For example, thyroid response elements (TRE) have been identified in the myoD and myogenin genes of myogenic cell lines [77]. Using the L6 cell line, Thelen et al. reported that T_3 and IGF-I act synergistically to increase SERCA1 levels [115]. In a series of papers [77], Muscat et al. reported findings that show that IGF-I, T_3, or retinoic acid can induce myogenic cell lines to exit the proliferation phase and fuse into myotubes.

FIGURE 2.6.

Proposed function for IGF-I in the skeletal muscle hypertrophy process. (A) Increased loading of muscle stimulates (B) increased myofiber IGF-I production and secretion. This IGF-I can act as an autocrine factor (C), possibly stimulating anabolic processes, and as a paracrine growth factor (D) impacting satellite cells and possibly other myofibers.

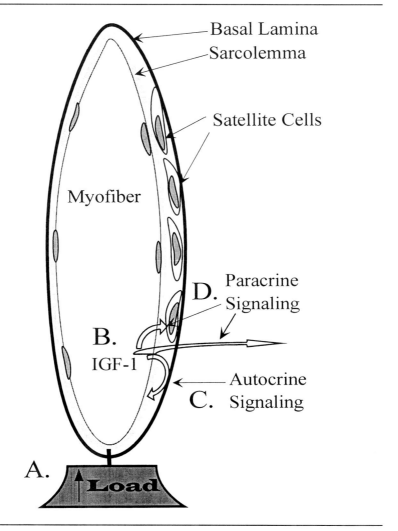

In addition to these similar effects on skeletal muscle, there is some evidence that the thyroid axis may be involved with the modulation of cellular responses to IGF-I. Based on both *in vivo* and *in vitro* studies involving satellite cells, Jacobs et al. [52] concluded that satellite cell ability to differentiate and fuse with existing myofibers was depressed under hypothyroid conditions. T_3 has also been shown to regulate several components of the IGF-I system *in vitro* and *in vivo*. Nanto-Salonen et al. found that hypothyroidism in rat neonates disrupts normal developmental patterns of IGF-I and -2 and IGFBP expression, and in adult rats depresses levels of IGFBP3 and -4 [79–81]. Also, GH administration alone in hypothyroid rats was found to be insufficient in normalizing circulating IGF-I levels [16].

Taken together, these various reports suggest the potential for complex interactions between the IGF-I and T_3 signaling pathways that mediate muscle adaptation in adult mammalian skeletal muscles.

SUMMARY

Adaptations in muscle mass stimulated by changes in muscle loading state entail alternations in the synthesis and degradation of myofiber proteins and the modulation of myonuclear number such that the ratio between the number of myonuclei and the size of the myofibers remains relatively constant.

As depicted schematically in Figure 2.6, the literature regarding the role of IGF-I in mediating muscle adaptation to alterations in loading state suggests the following conclusions: During periods of increased loading, myofibers upregulate the expression and secretion of IGF-I. Acting as an autocrine and/or paracrine growth factor, IGF-I stimulates myofiber anabolic processes. Acting as a paracrine growth factor, IGF-I also stimulates adjacent satellite cells to enter the cell cycle and proliferate. Continued myofiber production of IGF-I stimulates some satellite cells to differentiate and then fuse with myofibers, thus providing additional myonuclei in order to maintain or reestablish the myonucleus to myofiber size ratios of the enlarged myofibers.

REFERENCES

1. Adams, G.R. Muscle hypertrophy resulting from direct IGF-I infusion. *Med. Sci. Sports Exerc.* 29:S114, 1997.
2. Adams, G.R., and F. Haddad. The relationships between IGF-I, DNA content, and protein accumulation during skeletal muscle hypertrophy. *J. Appl. Physiol.* 81:2509–2516, 1996.
3. Allen, D.L., S.R. Monke, R.J. Talmadge, R.R. Roy, and V.R. Edgerton. Plasticity of myonuclear number in hypertrophied and atrophied mammalian skeletal muscle fibers. *J. Appl. Physiol.* 78(5):1969–1976, 1995.
4. Allen, D.L., W. Yasui, T. Tanaka, et al. Myonuclear number and myosin heavy chain expression in rat soleus single muscle fibers after space flight. *J. Appl. Physiol.* 81:145–151, 1996.

5. Allen, R.E., and L.K. Boxhorn. Regulation of skeletal muscle satellite cell proliferation and differentiation by transforming growth factor-beta, insulin-like growth factor 1, and fibroblast growth factor. *J. Cell. Physiol.* 138:311–315, 1989.

6. Allen, R.E., S.M. Sheehan, R.G. Taylor, T.L. Kendall, and G.M. Rice. Hepatocyte growth factor activates quiescent skeletal muscle satellite cells in vitro. *J. Cell. Physiol.* 165: 307–312, 1995.

7. Bates, P.C., P.T. Loughna, J.M. Pell, D. Schulster, and D.J. Millward. Interactions between growth hormone and nutrition in hypophysectomized rats: Body composition and production of insulin-like growth factors. *J. Endocrinol.* 139:117–126, 1993.

8. Beitner-Johnson, D., V.A. Blakesley, Z. Shen-Orr, et al. The proto-oncogene product c-Crk associates with insulin receptor substrate-1 and 4PS. *J. Biol. Chem.* 271:9287–9290, 1996.

9. Benito, M., A.M. Valverde, and M. Lorenzo. IGF-I: a mitogen also involved in differentiation processes in mammalian cells. *Int. J. Biochem. Cell Biol.* 28:499–510, 1996.

10. Bigard, A.X., F. Lienhard, D. Merino, B. Serrurier, and C.Y. Guezennec. Effects of growth hormone on rat skeletal muscle after hindlimb suspension. *Eur. J. Appl. Physiol.* 69: 337–343, 1994.

11. Binoux, M. The IGF system in metabolism regulation. *Diabete Metab.* 21:330–337, 1995.

12. Binoux, M., C. Lalou, C. Lassarre, C. Blat, and P. Hossenlopp. Limited proteolysis of insulin like growth factor binding protein-3 (IGFBP-3). *Ann. N.Y. Acad. Sci.* 343:293–300, 1993.

13. Bischoff, R. Analysis of muscle regeneration using single myofibers in culture. *Med. Sci. Sports Exerc.* 21:S164–S172, 1989.

14. Boes, M., B.B. Booth, A. Sandra, B.L. Dake, A. Bergold, and R.S. Bar. Insulin-like growth factor binding protein (IGFBP)4 accounts for the connective tissue distribution of endothelial cell IGFBPs. *Endocrinology* 131:327–330, 1992.

15. Booth, F.W., and K.M. Baldwin. Muscle plasticity: energy demand and supply processes. L.B. Rowell, J.T.Shepard (eds). *Handbook of Physiology* Section 12. Oxford Univ. Press, 1996, pp. 1074–1123.

16. Burstein, P.J., B. Draznin, C.J. Johnson, and D.S. Schalch. The effect of hypothyroidism on growth, serum growth hormone, the growth hormone dependent somatomedin, IGF and its carrier proteins. *Endocrinology* 104(4):1107–1111, 1979.

17. Butterfield, G.E., J. Thompson, M.J. Rennie, R. Marcus, R.L. Hintz, and A.R. Hoffman. Effect of rhGH and rhIGF-I treatment on protein utilization in elderly women. *Am. J. Physiol.* 272:E94–E99, 1997.

18. Caroni, P., and C. Schneider. Signaling by insulin-like growth factors in paralyzed skeletal muscle: rapid induction of IGF1 expression in muscle fibers and prevention of interstitial cell proliferation by IGF-BP5 and IGF-BP4. *J. Neurosci.* 14:3378–3388, 1994.

19. Chambers, R.L., and J.C. Mcdermott. Molecular basis of skeletal muscle regeneration. *Can. J. Appl. Physiol.* 21:155–184, 1996.

20. Chen, C., and D. Roy. Up-regulation of nuclear IGF-I receptor by short term exposure of stilbene estrogen, diethylstilbestrol. *Mol. Cell. Endocrinol.* 118:1–8, 1996.

21. Chen, Y., and H.J. Arnqvist. Differential regulation of insulin-like growth factor binding protein-2 and -4 mRNA in muscle tissues and liver by diabetes or fasting. *J. Endocrinol.* 143:235–242, 1994.

22. Clemmons, D.R. IGF binding proteins and their functions. *Mol. Reprod. Dev.* 35:368–375, 1993.

23. Clemmons, D.R., J.I. Jones, W.H. Busby, and G. Wright. Role of insulin like growth factor binding proteins in modifying IGF actions. *Ann. N.Y. Acad. Sci.* 692:10–21, 1993.

24. Coleman, M.E., F. DeMayo, K.C. Yin, H.M. Lee, R. Geske, C. Montgomery, and R.J. Schwartz. Myogenic vector expression of insulin like growth factor-1 stimulates muscle cell differentiation and myofiber hypertrophy in transgenic mice. *J. Biol. Chem.* 270(20): 12109–12116, 1995.

25. Collett-Solberg, P.F., and P. Cohen. The role of the insulin-like growth factor binding proteins and the IGFBP proteases in modulating IGF action. *Endocrinol. Metabol. Clin. North Am.* 25:591–614, 1996.

26. Coolican, S.A., D.S. Samuel, D.Z. Ewton, F.J. McWade, and J.R. Florini. The mitogenic and myogenic actions of insulin-like growth factors utilize distinct signaling pathways. *J. Biol. Chem.* 272:6653–6662, 1997.

27. Czerwinski, S.M., J.M. Martin, and P.J. Bechtel. Modulation of IGF-I mRNA abundance during stretch induced skeletal muscle hypertrophy and regression. *J. Appl. Physiol.* 76: 2026–2030, 1994.

28. Dardevet, D., C. Sornet, T. Vary, and J. Grizard. Phosphatidylinositol 3-kinase and p70 S6 kinase participate in the regulation of protein turnover in skeletal muscle by insulin and insulin-like growth factor 1. *Endocrinology* 137:4087–4994, 1996.

29. De Meyts, P., B. Urso, C.T. Christoffersen, and R.M. Shymko. Mechanism of insulin and IGF-I receptor activation and signal transduction specificity. *Ann. N.Y. Acad. Sci.* 766: 388–401, 1995.

30. DeVol, D.L., P. Rotwein, J. Levis Sadow, J. Novakofski, and P.J. Bechtel. Activation of insulin like growth factor gene expression during work induced skeletal muscle growth. *Am. J. Physiol.* 259:E89–E95, 1990.

31. Dodson, M.V., R.E. Allen, and K.L. Hossner. Ovine somatomedin, multiplication-stimulating activity, and insulin promote skeletal muscle satellite cell proliferation in vivo. *Endocrinology* 117:2357–2363, 1985.

32. Duclos, M.J., R.S. Wilkie, and C. Goddard. Stimulation of DNA synthesis in chicken muscle satellite cells by insulin and insulin-like growth factors: evidence for exclusive mediation by a type-I insulin-like growth factor receptor. *J. Endocrinol.* 128:35–42, 1991.

33. Edgerton, V.R., and R.R. Roy. Regulation of skeletal muscle fiber size, shape and function. *J. Biomechan..* 24(S1):23–133, 1991.

34. Edwall, D., M. Schalling, E. Jennische, and G. Norstedt. Induction of insulin like growth factor 1 messenger ribonucleic acid during regeneration of rat skeletal muscle. *Endocrinology* 124(2):820–825, 1989.

35. Engert, J.C., E.B. Berglund, and N. Rosenthal. Proliferation precedes differentiation in IGF-I stimulated myogenesis. *J. Cell Biol.* 135:431–440, 1996.

36. Florini, J.R. Hormonal control of muscle growth. *Muscle Nerve* 10:577–598, 1987.

37. Florini, J.R., and D.Z. Ewton. Highly specific inhibition of IGF-I-stimulated differentiation by an antisense oligodeoxyribonucleotide to myogenin mRNA. *J. Biol. Chem.* 265: 13435–13437, 1990.

38. Florini, J.R., and D.Z. Ewton. Induction of gene expression in muscle by the IGFs. *Growth Regul.* 2:23–29, 1992.

39. Florini, J.R., D.Z. Ewton, and K.A. Magri. Hormones, growth factors, and myogenic differentiation. *Ann. Rev. Physiol.* 53:201–216, 1991.

40. Florini, J.R., D.Z. Ewton, and S.A. Coolican. Growth hormone and insulin like growth factor system in myogenesis. *Endocr, Rev.* 17:481–517, 1996.

41. Goldberg, A.L. Work induced growth of skeletal muscle in normal and hypophsectomized rats. *Am. J. Physiol.* 213:1193–1198, 1967.

42. Gosteli-Peter, M.A., K.H. Winterhalter, C. Schmid, E.R. Froesch, and C. Zapf. Expression and regulation of IGF-I and IGF-binding protein mRNA levels in tissues of hypophysectomized rats infused with IGF-I IGF 1. *Endocrinology* 135(6):2558–2567, 1994.

43. Grindeland, R.E., R.R. Roy, V.R. Edgerton, et al. Interactive effects of growth hormone and exercise on muscle mass in suspended rats. *Am. J. Physiol.* 267:R316–R322, 1994.

44. Hannon, K., A.J. Kudla, M.J. McAvoy, K.L. Clase, and B.B. Olwin. Differentially expressed fibroblast growth factors regulate skeletal muscle development through autocrine and paracrine mechanisms. *J. Cell Biol.* 132:1151–1159, 1996.

45. Hikida, R.S., S. Van Nostran, J.D. Murray, R.S. Staron, S.E. Gordon, and W.J. Kraemer. Myonuclear loss in atrophied soleus muscle fibers. *Anat. Rec.* 247:350–354, 1997.

46. Hsu, D., P.E. Knudson, A. Zapf, G.C. Rolband, and J.M. Olefsky. NPXY motif in the insulin like growth factor 1 receptor is required for efficient ligand mediated receptor internalization. *Endocrinology* 134:744–750, 1994.

47. Hughes, S.M., J.M. Taylor, S.J. Tapscott, C.M. Gurley, W.J. Carter, and C.A. Peterson. Selective accumulation of myoD and myogenin mRNAs in fast and slow adult skeletal muscle is controlled by innervation and hormones. *Development* 118:1137–1147, 1993.

48. Husmann, I., L. Soulet, J. Gautron, I. Martelly, and D. Barritault. Growth factors in skeletal muscle regeneration. *Cytokine Gro. Fac. Rev.* 7:249–258, 1996.

49. Isgaard, J. Expression and regulation of IGF-I in cartilage and skeletal muscle. *Growth Regul.* 2:16–22, 1992.

50. Itoh, N., T. Mima, and T. Mikawa. Loss of fibroblast growth factor receptors is necessary for terminal differentiation of embryonic muscle. *Development.* 122:291–300, 1996.

51. Jacob, R., X. Hu, D. Neiderstock, S. Hasan, et al. IGF-I stimulation of muscle protein synthesis in the awake rat: permissive role of insulin and amino acids. *Am. J. Physiol.* 270: E60–E66, 1996.

52. Jacobs, S.C., P.R. Bar, and A.L. Bootsma. Effect of hypothyroidism on satellite cells and postnatal fiber development in the soleus muscle of rat. *Cell Tissue Res.* 286:137–144, 1996.

53. James, P.L., C.E.H. Stewart, and P. Rotwein. Insulin like growth factor binding protein-5 modulates muscle differentiation through an insulin-like growth factor-dependent mechanism. *J. Cell Biol.* 133:683–693, 1996.

54. Jennische, E. Sequential immunohistochemical expression of IGF-I and the transferrin receptor in regenerating rat muscle in vivo. *Acta Endocrinol.* 121:733–738, 1989.

55. Jennische, E., and H.A. Hansson. Regenerating skeletal muscle cells express insulin-like growth factor 1. *Acta Physiol. Scand.* 130:327–332, 1987.

56. Jennische, E., and G.L. Matejka. IGF-I binding and IGF-I expression in regenerating muscle of normal and hypophysectomized rats. *Acta Physiol. Scand.* 146:79–86, 1992.

57. Johnson, S.E., and R.E. Allen. Activation of skeletal muscle satellite cells and the role of fibroblast growth factor receptors. *Exp. Cell Res.* 219:449–453, 1995.

58. Kajstura, J., W. Cheng, K. Reiss, and P. Anversa. The IGF-I-IGF-I receptor system modulates myocyte proliferation but not myocyte cellular hypertrophy in vitro. *Exp. Cell Res.* 215:273–283, 1994.

59. Kaliman, P., F. Vinals, X. Testar, M. Palacin, and A. Zorzano. Phosphatidylinositol 3-kinase inhibitors block differentiation of skeletal muscle cells. *J. Biol. Chem.* 271: 19146–19151, 1996.

60. Kato, H., T.N. Faria, B. Stannard, C.T. Roberts, and D. LeRoith. Role of tyrosine kinase activity in signal transduction by the insulin like growth factor 1 (IGF-I) receptor. *J. Biol. Chem.* 268:2655–2661, 1993.

61. Kong, Y., S.E. Johnson, E.J. Taparowsky, and S.F. Konieczny. Ras p21val inhibits myogenesis without altering the DNA binding or transcriptional activities of the myogenic basic helix-loop-helix factors. *Mol. Cell. Biol.* 15:5205–5213, 1995.

62. Lagord, C., G. Carpentier, M. Leibovitch, J. Gautron, and I. Martelly. Stimulation of rat satellite cell myogenesis by inhibitors of ser/thr protein kinases. *Neuromuscul. Disord.* 3: 379–383, 1993.

63. Lagord, C., G. Carpentier, J. Moraczewski, G. Pons, F. Climent, and I. Martelly. Satellite cell myogenesis is highly stimulated by the kinase inhibitor iso-H7. *Biochem. Biophys. Res. Commun.* 191:928–936, 1993.

64. Lamson, G., L.C. Giudice, P. Cohen, et al. Proteolysis of IGFBP-3 may be a common regulatory mechanism of IGF action in vivo. *Growth Regul.* 3:91–95, 1993.

65. LeFaucheur, J.P., and A. Sebille. Muscle regeneration following injury can be modified in vivo by immune neutralization of fibroblast growth factor, transforming growth factor beta 1 or insulin-like growth factor I. *J. Neuroimmunol.* 57:85–91, 1995.

66. LeRoith, D., V.M. Kavsan, A.P. Koval, and C.T. Roberts. Phylogeny of the insulin like growth factors (IGFs) and receptors: a molecular approach. *Mol. Reprod. Dev.* 35:332–338, 1993.

67. Li, L., R. Heller-Harrison, M. Czech, and E.N. Olson. Cyclic AMP-dependent protein kinase inhibits the activity of myogeninc helix-loop-helix proteins. *Mol. Cell. Biol.* 12: 4478–4485, 1992.

68. Li, W., J. Fawcett, H.R. Widmer, P.J. Fielder, R. Rabkin, and G.A. Keller. Nuclear transport of insulin-like growth factor-1 and insulin-like growth factor binding protein-3 in opossum kidney cells. *Endocrinology* 138:1763–1766, 1997.

69. Linderman, J.K., K.L. Gosselink, F.W. Booth, V.R. Mukku, and R.E. Grindeland. Resistance exercise and growth hormone as countermeasures for skeletal muscle atrophy in hindlimb-suspended rats. *Am. J. Physiol.* 267:R365–R371, 1994.

70. Loughna, P.T., P. Mason, and P.C. Bates. Regulation of insulin like growth factor 1 gene expression in skeletal muscle. *Symp. Soc. Exp. Biol.* 46:319–330, 1992.

71. Lowe, W.L. Insulin-like growth factors. *Sci. Am. Sci. Med.* 3:62–71, 1996.

72. Luque, E., J. Pena, P. Salas, and J.D. Martin. Changes in satellite cell population associated with regenerating muscle fibers in rats. *J. Submicrosc. Cytol. Pathol.* 28:305–311, 1996.

73. McCusker, R.H., C. Camacho-Hubner, and D.R. Clemmons. Identification of the types of insulin-like growth factor-binding proteins that are secreted by muscle cells in vitro. *J. Biol. Chem.* 264:7795–7800, 1989.

74. McCusker, R.H., and D.R. Clemmons. Effects of cytokines on insulin-like growth factor binding protein secretion by muscle cells in vitro. *Endocrinology* 134:2095–2102, 1994.

75. Mendez, R., M.G. Meyers, M.F. White, and R.E. Rhoads. Stimulation of protein synthesis, eukaryotic translation initiation factor 4E phosphorylation, and PHAS-I phosphorylation. *Mol. Cell. Biol.* 16:2857–2864, 1996.

76. Molnar, G., M.L. Ho, and N.A. Schroedl. Evidence for multiple satellite cell populations and a non-myogenic cell type that is regulated differently in regenerating and growing skeletal muscle. *Tissue Cell.* 28:547–556, 1996.

77. Muscat, G.E.O., M. Downes, and D.H. Dowhan. Regulation of vertebrate muscle differentiation by thyroid hormone: the role of the myoD gene family. *Bioessays* 17:211–218, 1995.

78. Meyers, M.G., L. Wang, X.J. Sun, et al. Role of IRS-1-GRB-2 complexes in insulin signaling. *Mol. Cell. Biol.* 14:3577–3587, 1994.

79. Nanto-Salonen, K., G.F. Glasscock, and R.G. Rosenfeld. The effects of thyroid hormone on insulin-like growth factor (IGF) and IGF-binding protein (IGFBP) expression in the neonatal rat: prolonged high expression of IGFBP-2 in methimazole-induced congenital hypothyroidism. *Endocrinology* 129:2563–2570, 1991.

80. Nanto-Salonen, K., and R.G. Rosenfeld. Insulin-like growth factor binding protein expression in hyperthyroid rat is age dependent. *Endocrinology* 131:1489–1496, 1992.

81. Nanto-Salonen, K., H.L. Muller, A.R. Hoffman, T.H. Vu, and R.G. Rosenfeld. Mechanisms of thyroid hormone action on the insulin-like growth factor system. *Endocrinology* 132: 781–788, 1993.

82. Oemar, B.S., N.M. Law, and S.A. Rosenzweig. Insulin-like growth factor-1 induces tyrosyl phosphorylation of nuclear proteins. *J. Biol. Chem.* 266:24241–24244, 1991.

83. Oh, Y., H.L. Muller, E.K. Neely, G. Lamson, and R.G. Rosenfeld. New concepts in insulin like growth factor receptor physiology. *Growth Regul.* 3:113–123, 1993.

84. Olson, E.N. Interplay between proliferation and differentiation within the myogenic lineage. *Dev. Biol.* 154:261–272, 1992.

85. Olwin, B.B., K. Hannon, and A.J. Kudla. Are fibroblast growth factors regulators of myogenesis in vivo? *Prog. Growth Factor Res.* 5:145–158, 1994.

86. Patti, M.E., X.J. Sun, J.C. Bruening, E. Araki, M.A. Lipes, M.F. White, and C.R. Kahn. 4PS/Insulin receptor substrate (IRS-)-2 is the alternative substrate of the insulin receptor in IRS-1 deficient mice. *J. Biol. Chem.* 270:24670–24673, 1995.

87. Perrone, C.E., D. Fenwick-Smith, and H.V. Vandenburgh. Collagen and stretch modulate autocrine secretion of insulin like growth factor-1 and insulin like growth factor binding proteins from differentiated skeletal muscle cells. *J. Biol. Chem.* 270:2099–2106, 1995.

88. Pessin, J.E., and A.L. Frattali. Molecular dynamics of insulin/IGF-I receptor transmembrane signaling. *Mol. Reprod. Dev.* 35:339–345, 1993.

89. Phelan, J.N., and W.J. Gonyea. Effect of radiation on satellite cell activity and protein expression in overloaded mammalian skeletal muscle. *Anat. Rec.* 247:179–188, 1997.

90. Prager, D., H. Li, H. Yamasaki, and S. Melmed. Human insulin like growth factor 1 receptor internalization. *J. Biol. Chem.* 269:11934–11937, 1994.

91. Quinn, L.S., B. Steinmetz, A. Maas, L. Ong, and M. Kaleko. Type 1-insulin like growth factor receptor over-expression produces dual effects on myoblast proliferation and differentiation. *J. Cell. Physiol.* 159:387–398, 1994.

92. Rosenblatt, J.D., and D.J. Parry. Adaptation of rat extensor digitorum longus muscle to gamma irradiation and overload. *Pflugers Arch.* 423:255–264, 1993.

93. Rosenblatt, J.D., D. Yong, and D.J. Parry. Satellite cell activity is required for hypertrophy of overloaded adult rat muscle. *Muscle Nerve* 17:608–613, 1994.

94. Rosenthal, S.M., and Z. Cheng. Opposing early and late effects of IGF-I on differentiation and cell cycle regulatory retinoblastoma protein in skeletal myoblasts. *Proc. Natl. Acad. Sci. USA* 92:10307–10311, 1995.

95. Rotwein, P., P.L. James, and K. Kou. Rapid activation of insulin-like growth factor binding protein-5 gene transcription during myoblast differentiation. *Mol. Endocrinol.* 9:913–923, 1995.

96. Roy, R.R., C. Tri, E.J. Grossman, et al. IGF-I, growth hormone and/or exercise effects on non-weight-bearing soleus of hypophysectomized rats. *J. Appl. Physiol.* 81:302–311, 1996.

97. Rudnicki, M.A., and R. Jaenisch. The myoD family of transcription factors and skeletal myogenesis. *Bioessays* 17:203–209, 1995.

98. Russell-Jones, D.L., A.M. Umpleby, T.R. Hennessy, et al. Use of a leucine clamp to demonstrate that IGF-I actively stimulates protein synthesis in normal humans. *Am. J. Physiol.* 267:E591–E598, 1994.

99. Salleo, A., G. LaSpada, G. Falzea, M.G. Denaro, and R. Cicciarello. Response of satellite cells and muscle fibers to long-term compensatory hypertrophy. *J. Submicrosc. Cytol.* 15: 929–940, 1983.

100. Schiaffino, S., S. P. Bormioli, and M. Aloisi. The fate of newly formed satellite cells during compensatory muscle hypertrophy. *Virchows Arch.* B 21:113–118, 1976.

101. Schlechter, N.L., S.M. Russell, E.M. Spencer, and C.S. Nicoll. Evidence suggesting that the growth promoting effect of GH on cartilage in vivo is mediated by local production of somatomedin. *Proc. Natl. Acad. Sci. USA* 83:7923–7934, 1986.

102. Schultz, E. Satellite cell behavior during skeletal muscle growth and regeneration. *Med. Sci. Sports Exerc.* 21:S181–S186, 1989.

103. Schwarz, A.J., J.A. Brasel, R.L. Hintz, S. Mohan, and D.M. Cooper. Acute effect of brief low- and high-intensity exercise on circulating insulin-like growth factor (IGF) I, II, and IGF-binding protein-3 and its proteolysis in young healthy men. *J. Clin. Endocrinol. Metabol.* 81:3492–3497, 1996.

104. Shooter, G.K., B. Magee, M.A. Soos, G.L. Francis, K. Siddle, and J.C. Wallace. Insulin-like growth factor (IGF)-1 A- and B-domain analogues with altered type 1 IGF and insulin receptor binding specificities. *J. Mol. Endocrinol.* 17:237–246, 1996.

105. Siddle, K. The insulin receptor and type 1 IGF receptor: comparison of structure and function. *Prog. Growth Factor Res.* 4:304–320, 1992.

106. Smith, C.K., M.J. Janney, and R.E. Allen. Temporal expression of myogenic regulatory genes during activation, proliferation, and differentiation in rat skeletal muscle satellite cells. *J. Cell. Physiol.* 159:379–385, 1994.

107. Snow, M.H. Satellite cell response in rat soleus muscle undergoing hypertrophy due to surgical ablation of synergists. *Anat. Rec.* 227:437–446, 1990.

108. Sommerland, H., M. Ullman, E. Jennische, A. Skottner, and A. Oldfors. Muscle regeneration. *Acta Neuropatol.* 78:264–269, 1989.

109. Stannard, B., V. Blakesly, H. Kato, C.T. Roberts, and D. LeRoith. Single tyrosine substitution in the insulin like growth factor 1 receptor inhibits ligand induced receptor autophosphorylation. *Endocrinology* 136:4918–4924, 1995.

110. Steenbergh, P.H., E. Jansen, F.M.A. van Schiak, and J.S. Sussenbach. Functional analysis of the human IGF-I gene promotors. *Mol. Reprod. Dev.* 35:365–367, 1993.

111. Stockdale, F.E., and H. Holtzer. DNA synthesis and myogenesis. *Exp. Cell Res.* 24:508–520, 1961.

112. Taaffe, D.R., I.H. Jin, T.H. Vu, A.R. Hoffman, and R. Marcus. Lack of effect of recombinant human growth hormone (GH) on muscle morphology and GH-insulin-like growth factor expression in resistance-trained elderly men. *J. Clin. Endocrinol. Metabol.* 81: 421–425, 1996.

113. Taaffe, D.R., L. Pruitt, J. Reim, et al. Effect of recombinant human growth hormone on the muscle strength response to resistance exercise in elderly men. *J. Clin. Endocrinol. Metabol.* 79:1361–1366, 1994.

114. Talmadge, R.J., R.R. Roy, G.R. Chalmers, and V.R. Edgerton. MHC and sarcoplasmic reticulum protein isoforms in functionally overloaded cat plantaris muscle fibers. *J. Appl. Physiol.* 80:1296–1303, 1996.

115. Thelen, M.H., A. Muller, M.J. Zuidwijk, G.C. van der Linden, W.S. Simonides, and C. van Hardeveld. Differential regulation of the expression of fast type sarcoplasmic reticulum $Ca2+$-ATPase by thyroid hormone and insulin like growth factor-I in the L6 muscle cell line. *Biochem. J.* 303:467–474, 1994.

116. Turner, J.D., P. Rotwein, J. Novakofski, and P.J. Bechtel. Induction of mRNA for IGF-I and -II during growth hormone stimulated muscle hypertrophy. *Am. J. Physiol.* 255: E513–E517, 1988.

117. Vandenburgh, H.H., P. Karlisch, J. Shansky, and R. Feldstein. Insulin and IGF-I induce pronounced hypertrophy of skeletal myofibers in tissue culture. *Am. J. Physiol.* 260: C475–C484, 1991.

118. White, T.P., and K.A. Esser. Satellite cell and growth factor involvement in skeletal muscle growth. *Med. Sci. Sports Exerc.* 21:S158–S163, 1989.

119. Wilkie, R.S., I.E. O'Neil, S.C. Butterwith, M.J. Duclos, and C. Goddard. Regulation of chick muscle satellite cells by fibroblast growth factors: Interaction with insulin like growth factor-1 and heparin. *Growth Regul.* 5:18–27, 1995.

120. Wilson, E.M., Y. Oh, and R.G. Rosenfeld. Generation and characterization of an IGFBP-7 antibody: Identification of a 31kD IGFBP-7 in human biological fluids. *J. Clin. Endocrinol. Metabol.* 82:1301–1303, 1997.

121. Wing, S.S., and N. Bedard. Insulin-like growth factor 1 stimulates degradation of an mRNA transcript encoding the 14kDa ubiquitin-conjugating enzyme. *Biochem. J.* 319: 455–461, 1996.

122. Yablonka-Reuveni, Z., and A.J. Rivera. Temporal expression of regulatory and structural muscle proteins during myogenesis of satellite cells on isolated adult rat fibers. *Dev. Biol.* 164:588–603, 1994.

123. Yamada, S., N. Buffinger, J. Dimario, and R.C. Strohman. Fibroblast growth factor is stored in the fiber extracellular matrix and plays a role in regulating muscle hypertrophy. *Med. Sci. Sports Exerc.* 21:S173–S180, 1989.

124. Yang, S., M. Alnaqeeb, H. Simpson, and G. Goldspink. Cloning and characterization of an IGF-I isoform expressed in skeletal muscle subjected to stretch. *J. Muscle Res. Cell Motil.* 17:487–495, 1996.

125. Yarasheski, K.E. Growth hormone effects on metabolism, body composition, muscle mass, and strength. *Exerc. Sport Sci. Rev.* 22:285–312, 1994.

126. Yarasheski, K.E., J.J. Zachwieja, J.A. Campbell, and D.M. Bier. Effect of growth hormone and resistance exercise on muscle growth and strength in older men. *Am. J. Physiol.* 268: E268–E276, 1995.

127. Zanconato, S., D.Y. Moromisato, M.Y. Moromisato, et al. Effect of training and growth hormone suppression on insulin like growth factor 1 mRNA in young rats. *J. Appl. Physiol.* 76(5):2204–2209, 1994.

128. Zapf, A., D. Hsu, and J.M. Olefsky. Comparison of the intracellular itineraries of insulin like growth factor-I and insulin and their receptors in rat-1 fibroblasts. *Endocrinology* 134: 2445–2452, 1994.

3
Optimizing Health in Older Persons: Aerobic or Strength Training?

BEN F. HURLEY, PH.D.
JAMES M. HAGBERG, PH.D.

The average American now lives nearly twice as long as he/she did only one hundred years ago. As a result, by the year 2000, approximately 35 million, or one out of every eight Americans, will be over 65 yrs of age [17]. In addition, it is estimated that by the year 2000, 4.5 million people, or approximately 2% of the population, will be over 85 yrs of age [17]. Even more sobering, the number of Americans over 65 yrs of age is expected to double to 70 million by the year 2040. At that time, the elderly will represent nearly one out of every four Americans. Moreover, by the year 2040, the number of Americans over 85 yrs of age will increase to 12 million and will represent 4% of the United States population [17].

This "graying" of the American population, and of all industrialized countries around the world, has led to dramatic increases in health care costs—costs that cannot be sustained into the future without a severe impact on the economy of all countries. Most evidence indicates that the best method for optimizing health and reducing health care costs in the elderly is to prevent potential medical problems from reaching an overt clinical state [21]. Interventions designed to optimize health and reduce health care costs in older men and women must address cardiovascular (CV) diseases since they are the major cause of death and disability in the elderly [17]. These interventions must also address the numerous declines in the musculoskeletal system that occur with aging, and that are associated with deterioration in functional capacity and increased risk of falls and hip fractures. A number of interventions have been used in an effort to affect CV disease and musculoskeletal health in older adults, including diet and hormonal supplements, such as estrogen, testosterone, and growth hormone. Increased physical activity also is frequently proposed and used as a preventive measure for older men and women.

Though little evidence documenting the effects of increased physical activity in the elderly was available until the early 1980s, subsequently, an abundance of data have been published. Most studies initially investigated the effects of aerobic exercise training (AT) in the elderly; however, the increased recognition that musculoskeletal health is especially critical in

61

the elderly resulted in a large number of studies assessing the effects of strength training (ST) in the elderly. This chapter will review the evidence documenting the effects of AT and ST on CV and musculoskeletal health in the elderly.

CARDIOVASCULAR DISEASE AND AGING

More than any other medical disorder, CV disease is responsible for higher rates of morbidity and mortality in Americans over 65 yrs of age [52]. In 1986, there were almost 4 million patients with CV disease over the age of 65, [127] and ~60% of all patients who were hospitalized for acute myocardial infarction were in this age group [128]. It was anticipated that by 1996, 80% of all myocardial infarction patients would be over 65 yrs of age [50].

EFFECTS OF AT AND ST ON CV DISEASE RISK FACTORS

There are no long-term prospective primary prevention trials examining the effects of either AT or ST on CV disease morbidity or mortality. Furthermore, due to their immense cost, it is doubtful that such trials will be conducted in the future. At this time, therefore, the best option available as a surrogate for such trials is to assess the impact of these different forms of exercise training on the major modifiable CV disease risk factors predictive of a person's risk of developing CV disease. This approach is based on the assumption that improving a person's or population's CV disease risk factors should, in the long-term, result in decreased rates of CV morbidity and mortality. The major modifiable CV disease risk factors addressed here include low CV fitness levels, abnormal plasma lipoprotein-lipid profiles, glucose intolerance and insulin resistance, hypertension, left ventricular (LV) hypertrophy, and abdominal obesity.

Low CV Fitness Levels

Blair et al. documented that CV fitness, indexed as treadmill test duration as a surrogate for VO_2max, is an important risk factor for all-cause mortality in both men and women [11]. In fact, the relative risk associated with a lack of CV fitness is similar to the risk associated with high cholesterol levels, elevated fasting glucose levels, and a family history of CV disease. Furthermore, these data indicate that moving a person only from the lowest to the next quintile of CV fitness substantially reduces all-cause mortality. Aging is associated with a marked decrease in CV fitness, as indicated by a decline in VO_2max [67]. However, it appears that as much as half of this reduction may be due to secondary factors, such as increased body fat and decreased physical activity, rather than primary aging. [67].

A number of early studies indicated that older men and women did not increase their VO$_2$max with AT [8, 131]; however, these studies generally used very short or low-intensity AT programs. Later studies showed that prolonged and relatively intense AT elicits substantial increases in VO$_2$max in 60–80 yr old men and women [64, 65, 164]. Seals et al. reported a 12% increase in VO$_2$max in healthy 60–69 yr old men and women after 6 months of training at 50% of VO$_2$max, and a further increase of 18% after a subsequent 6 months of training at 75–85% of VO$_2$max, totaling to a 30% increase in VO$_2$max after a year of training [164]. Hagberg et al. reported a 28% increase in VO$_2$max in 60–69 yr old hypertensive men and women with 9 months of training at 70–75% of VO$_2$max [65]. Hagberg et al. also found a 22% increase in VO$_2$max in healthy 70–79 yr old men and women with 6 months of training at 70–75% of VO$_2$max [64]. Thus, it is clear that prolonged and relatively intense AT (>75% of VO$_2$max) results in substantial increases in VO$_2$max in older individuals, and that men and women increase VO$_2$max to a similar degree [94]. However, older women may increase their VO$_2$max via different mechanisms than older men, i.e., widening of the arteriovenous O$_2$ difference without an increase in maximal cardiac output [177].

According to some evidence, prolonged, low-intensity AT (40–60% of VO$_2$max) increases VO$_2$max in older men and women [164, 166], although these increases are less (<12%) than those resulting from higher-intensity AT [164, 166]. Furthermore, other studies have not found significant increases in VO$_2$max with prolonged low- to moderate-intensity AT in older men and women [65].

Studies that have compared the effects of AT and ST on changes in VO$_2$max in older persons indicate that AT increases VO$_2$max substantially, while ST does not. Hagberg et al. found that 6 months of moderate- to high-intensity AT in healthy 70–79 yr old men and women increased VO$_2$max by 22%, whereas 6 months of ST did not alter VO$_2$max [64]. In two studies, Smutok et al. found that 20 wks of AT increased VO$_2$max by 18% in middle-aged and older men, while 20 wks of ST resulted in a non-significant 5% increase in VO$_2$max [173, 175]. These studies all measured VO$_2$max during a progressive-inclined maximal treadmill exercise test.

Frontera et al. also reported a 5% increase in VO$_2$max after 12 wks of ST in healthy 60–72 yr old men; however, this change, measured during cycle ergometer exercise, was statistically significant [54]. Since non-cyclists are usually unable to achieve true VO$_2$max on a cycle ergometer, it is unlikely that a true VO$_2$max was measured on these subjects. It should be noted that in contrast to VO$_2$max on the treadmill, cycle ergometer performance appears to be limited by non-cardiovascular factors, such as leg strength or power[70, 112]. Supporting the possibility that true VO$_2$max did not change in the study of Frontera et al. [54] are the data of Hickson et al. [70]. They found that 10 wks of ST in young men resulted in a significant increase in VO$_2$peak on a cycle ergometer, but did not change true VO$_2$max measured during a progressive-inclined maximal treadmill exercise test [70]. Furthermore, most studies indicate that VO$_2$max in young persons does not increase appreciably with ST.

ST may, however, elicit other more generalized adaptations that might benefit the CV systems of older men and women. Ades et al. found that 12 wks of ST increased treadmill walking endurance at 80% of VO$_2$max by 38% in 65–79 yr old women, even though their VO$_2$max did not change [1]. Furthermore, the change in treadmill endurance time was significantly related to change in leg strength. Parker et al. reported that 16 wks of ST in 60–77 yr old women decreased heart rate, blood pressure, and rate pressure product (an index of myocardial VO$_2$) significantly during a weight-loaded submaximal treadmill walking test) [135]. Heart rate, blood pressure, and rate pressure product during an acute resistive exercise are also lower after ST [114].

Thus, it is clear from studies comparing AT and ST, and those assessing the effects of both training modes independently, that AT is the most effective intervention to improve CV fitness in older persons. Almost all previous results indicated that AT elicited substantial improvements in CV fitness, generally indexed as VO$_2$max. Conversely, virtually all evidence indicates that ST does not increase CV fitness appreciably; however, ST may elicit other adaptations that might benefit the CV systems of older persons.

Abnormal Plasma Lipoprotein-Lipid Profiles

Studies that have examined the relationship of age, lipoprotein-lipid profiles, and morbidity and mortality from CV disease in the elderly have produced mixed results. For example, in an 8 yr follow-up of ~4900 men and women 20–79 yrs of age, Wilson et al. [195] found that total blood cholesterol levels actually declined with age. Others have suggested that disease, rather than age, may cause age-associated decreases in blood cholesterol [158]. Although subjects with CV disease and cancer were excluded from the study of Wilson et al. [195], declines in high-density lipoprotein (HDL) cholesterol levels with age were still observed. The total cholesterol to HDL cholesterol ratios increased slightly from young to middle-aged men, and stayed about the same in middle-aged to elderly men, whereas this ratio continued to increase from young to middle-aged women, and from middle-aged to the oldest women.

Studies investigating the predictive value of lipid profiles in the elderly have also produced mixed results. Krumholtz et al. [100] concluded that neither high total cholesterol nor low HDL cholesterol levels predict all-cause mortality, mortality due to CV disease, or CV events in people >70 yrs of age. In contrast, Frost et al. [55] reported (from the Systolic Hypertension in the Elderly Program) that lipid profiles do predict CV events for people over the age of 60, while Schaeffer et al. [159] found that both low-density lipoprotein (LDL) and HDL cholesterol are important predictors of longevity. Thus, it appears that abnormal lipoprotein-lipid profiles confer increased CV disease risk in individuals at least until the age of 70 yrs.

Many investigators have studied the effects of AT on lipoprotein-lipid profiles in the elderly [23, 27, 71, 76, 130, 160]. Hill et al. [71] found a significant decline in total cholesterol with AT in older men, but not in older women, and a significant increase in HDL cholesterol in the women, but not in the men. There was a significant increase in the HDL cholesterol/total cholesterol ratio when all subjects were combined. Schwartz et al. [160] found that both young and older men increased HDL cholesterol levels significantly with AT, but only the older men had a significant increase in HDL cholesterol, and a significant decline in triglycerides (TG) and the LDL to HDL ratio. Therefore, the overall lipoprotein-lipid profile appeared to improve to a greater extent in the older than in the younger men. Another study reported increases in HDL cholesterol and decreases in the total cholesterol/HDL ratio with AT in both older men and women [122]. However, total cholesterol, LDL cholesterol, and TG levels did not change significantly in either group. After completing AT, these subjects stopped exercising for 4 wks, and experienced a significant decrease in HDL cholesterol and a significant increase in the total cholesterol/HDL ratio. In another study with postmenopausal women, training with or without estrogen therapy resulted in significant decreases in total cholesterol, LDL cholesterol, and TG, as well as an increase in the HDL/LDL cholesterol ratio [104]. Training-induced reductions in TG and elevations in HDL cholesterol were also reported in a number of other studies that involved middle-aged and older individuals [103, 163].

Not all studies with older persons show improved plasma lipoprotein-lipid profiles with AT. For example, Hughes et al. [76] reported that AT did not alter lipoprotein-lipid levels in middle-aged and older men and women, unless a low fat diet was added. A low fat diet alone, or combined with regular exercise, decreased total cholesterol, HDL cholesterol, and LDL cholesterol levels. Other investigators also observed no significant changes in plasma lipoprotein-lipid profiles with AT in the elderly [23, 27, 130].

Two epidemiological studies addressed the relationship among muscular strength, ST, and plasma lipoprotein-lipid profiles. Kohl et al. [93] examined the association between muscular strength and serum lipoprotein-lipid levels in 1,193 women and 5,460 men. They found no association in either men or women between strength, total cholesterol, or LDL cholesterol. However, there was a direct association between both upper and lower body strength and TG levels in men, and an inverse relationship between muscular strength and HDL cholesterol in men. In contrast, Tucker and Silvester [188] studied 8,499 male employees of more than 50 companies, and observed a reduced risk of hypercholesterolemia among subjects undergoing ST. However, only those who performed ST 4–7 hrs per week maintained this reduced risk, when other potentially confounding variables were controlled.

Published reports on the effects of ST on plasma lipoprotein-lipid profiles have been limited preponderantly to adolescent, young, and middle-aged subjects. Some of these studies showed improvements in lipid profiles with ST in young [15, 51] and middle-aged [80, 83] subjects, but most of these studies either did not control for normal variations in lipoproteins, used subjects who were not at risk for CV disease, lacked proper dietary controls, or did not control for other factors that influence lipid profiles [79, 97]. When an attempt is made to control for at least some of these factors, most studies show no improvements in lipid profiles with ST [14, 98, 110, 149, 173, 185]. Rhea et al. [149] recently found no significant improvements in lipoprotein-lipid values in postmenopausal women as a result of ST with or without weight loss. Manning et al. [110] and Treuth et al. [185] reported similar findings of no improvements in lipid profiles in older women with ST. Thus, we are not aware of any studies using elderly subjects that demonstrated improvements in lipid profiles with ST.

Considering that there are many more studies showing improved lipid profiles with AT than with ST in middle-aged and older subjects, it is quite surprising that none of the published reports comparing these training modalities show any differences. In fact, to date, only five published studies could be found that compared the effects of AT and ST on plasma lipoprotein-lipids. None of these studies showed that either training modality improved plasma lipoprotein-lipid profiles significantly [14, 69, 102, 173, 196].

Thus, some but not all data support the conclusion that AT improves plasma lipoprotein-lipid profiles in the elderly, specifically resulting in reduced TG levels, increased HDL cholesterol levels, and increased HDL cholesterol/total cholesterol ratios. On the other hand, virtually no evidence indicates that ST improves plasma lipoprotein-lipid profiles in the elderly.

Glucose Intolerance and Insulin Resistance

In addition to being important in the etiology of diabetes, glucose intolerance and insulin resistance are independent CV disease risk factors [6, 43, 180]. They are also associated with hypertension [142] and elevated and decreased levels of LDL and HDL cholesterol, respectively [200]. The prevalence of glucose intolerance increases with age [12, 66, 123, 154, 167] due to insulin resistance [154]. This leads to hyperinsulinemia, [22, 38, 123] and may be due to increased adiposity and/or decreased physical activity [18, 68, 134]. Pacini et al. [134] found no independent association between age and glucose tolerance when the effects of obesity and physical activity were eliminated from consideration. Broughton and Taylor [18] reached a similar conclusion based on their analysis of previous studies. Glucose intolerance is also associated with age-related losses of muscle mass [12].

However, age-associated deterioration in glucose tolerance and increase in hyperinsulinemia is not observed in older athletes who do not participate in the type of exercise that leads to muscular hypertrophy [162], whereas it is observed in older athletes who have substantially greater muscle mass [81]. Moreover, AT reduces plasma insulin responses to an oral glucose challenge in older individuals, even though it does not increase muscle mass [163]. Thus, there is little evidence to support the hypothesis that a reduced muscle mass with age is responsible for deterioration in glucose tolerance.

Most studies investigating the effects of AT on glucose tolerance report no significant changes in plasma glucose responses during an oral glucose tolerance test (OGTT) in older individuals [16, 40, 84, 91, 162, 184]. However, reductions in plasma insulin responses to an OGTT have been consistently reported, providing evidence of improved glucose homeostasis [16, 31, 40, 84, 91, 162, 184]. Glucose clamp studies indicate that this improvement is due to an increase in glucose disposal because of an improvement in insulin action, most likely due to an increase in insulin sensitivity [39, 40, 77, 84, 85, 90, 91]. The mechanism for this response appears to be increases in the GLUT-4 transporter [45, 48, 74, 77]. However, reduced insulin secretion [84], increased muscle capillary cross-sectional area and number [96], and increased insulin receptor-binding [176] have also been suggested as potential mechanisms.

It was commonly believed, based on the notion that improvements in glucose metabolism were dependent on reductions in body fat [4] and increases in VO$_2$max [96], that only AT should be recommended for improving glucose homeostasis [33]. However, ST has been observed to improve glucose metabolism in subjects with normal [80, 173] and abnormal glucose metabolism [174], even when body fat or VO$_2$max are not changed. Some subjects with impaired glucose tolerance become normalized following ST [173]. Glucose metabolism is improved in both young [46, 120] and older subjects [35] with ST, most often in the form of blunted plasma insulin responses to an OGTT; however, a blunted glucose response has also been demonstrated in middle-aged subjects [173, 174]. In contrast to these findings, Hersey et al. [69] found that ST did not improve glucose or insulin responses to an OGTT in healthy 70–79 yr old men and women. Others have observed a ST-induced increase in glucose uptake, as measured by the hyperinsulinemic euglycemic clamp procedure in older subjects [119, 156], or by the minimal model of labeled glucose disappearance [199]. In one study, 4 months of heavy resistance ST increased glucose uptake by 23% [119]. In another study, similar benefits were lost in six subjects when growth hormone administration was added to ST [199]. Ryan et al. [156] found that ST, with or without weight loss, in postmenopausal women increased insulin action and reduced hyperinsulinemia. In contrast to AT, no published data identified a potential mechanism as to how ST might improve glucose tolerance and/or insulin sensitivity.

Only three studies have compared the effects of AT and ST on glucose homeostasis in middle-aged to older men and women [69, 173, 174]. Hersey et al. [69] found that only AT blunted the plasma insulin responses to an OGTT, whereas Smutok et al. [173, 174] observed that both AT and ST reduced glucose and insulin responses to an OGTT. There are a number of potentially important differences between these studies. The subjects in Hersey et al. were older than the subjects in Smutok et al. (70–79 yr olds vs. 50–70 yr olds). Hersey et al. also studied both men and women, whereas Smutok et al. studied only men. The increases in both upper and lower body muscular strength were also much greater in the Smutok et al. study, as compared to those in the Hersey et al. study. Thus, it is possible that older individuals, and perhaps specifically older women, may not be able to improve their glucose and insulin responses to an OGTT with ST to the same degree as middle-aged men. However, it is also possible that heavier resistance ST than was used by Hersey et al. may be required to improve glucose and insulin responses to an OGTT in older men and women.

Therefore, substantial evidence exists to support the conclusion that in older persons, both AT and ST improve glucose homeostasis, indexed as improved glucose disposal and/or increased insulin sensitivity. The majority of the available data also indicate that AT and ST improve glucose homeostasis, to a similar degree and consistency.

Hypertension

In industrialized countries, blood pressure (BP) increases with age, so that by age 60–70, approximately 50% of men and women are hypertensive [87]. Elevated BP remains a major CV disease risk factor in the elderly, except for those over 85 yrs of age [87]. As noted earlier, hypertension is also often accompanied by a constellation of other CV disease risk factors, including obesity, insulin resistance, hyperinsulinemia, and abnormal plasma lipoprotein-lipid profiles. Optimal intervention programs in older hypertensives should address all of these risk factors, rather than focusing solely on BP.

In the only known study that compared the effects of AT and ST in older persons with essential hypertension, 70–79 yr old men and women with initially elevated BP reduced their systolic and diastolic BPs by 8 and 9 mmHg, respectively, with 6 months of AT [32]. These systolic and diastolic BP reductions are similar to the average BP reductions shown in a number of reviews based on all available AT studies of persons with essential hypertension, irrespective of age [20, 62, 63]. In the same study, 6 months of ST did not change BP in 70–79 yr old men and women with initially elevated BPs. Though this study had relatively small sample sizes, these results in older persons are consistent with the general conclusions in previous review articles. Furthermore, an American College of Sports Medicine Position Stand concluded that ST by itself does not consistently elicit significant reductions in BP in hypertensive individuals [63].

Additional studies provide further evidence that AT is effective in reducing BP in older persons with essential hypertension [65, 166]. Hagberg et al. [65] reported that in otherwise healthy 60–69 yr old men and women with essential hypertension, 9 months of low-intensity AT (50% VO$_2$max) resulted in 20 and 12 mmHg reductions in systolic and diastolic BP, respectively. Nine months of AT at 70% VO$_2$max decreased systolic and diastolic BPs by 8 and 11 mmHg, respectively, with only the change in diastolic BP being statistically significant. Seals and Reiling [166] found that 6 months of low-intensity AT (47% VO$_2$max) in 50–74 yr old men and women with essential hypertension resulted in significant reductions in both systolic and diastolic BP, but that 6 additional months of AT, at a somewhat higher intensity (57% VO$_2$max), resulted in slightly greater reductions in both systolic and diastolic BPs. No studies could be found that independently assessed the effect of ST on the BP of older adults with essential hypertension.

Thus, the available evidence supports the conclusion that AT is effective in reducing BP in older hypertensives, and that low- to moderate-intensity training may elicit the same or greater reductions in BP as higher intensity AT. Conversely, ST does not appear to reduce BP significantly in older hypertensives.

Left Ventricular Hypertrophy

Another important CV disease risk factor that often accompanies elevated BP, especially in the elderly, is left ventricular (LV) hypertrophy. One major negative consequence of pathological LV hypertrophy is delayed LV diastolic filling, which by itself, or in conjunction with reduced LV systolic function, can lead to congestive heart failure.

Kokkinos et al. [99] found that middle-aged and older African-American men with severe hypertension who were first treated with medications to reduce their BP, reduced LV mass by 13% (from an initial very high level) with 16 wks of AT. The reduced LV mass was primarily the result of decreased wall thicknesses. Baglivo et al. [5] reported that 16 months of AT in middle-aged hypertensive men and women decreased LV mass by 9% (P = 0.056). It may be important to note that the subjects in the Baglivo et al. study had initial LV mass indices that were substantially lower than the subjects in the Kokkinos et al. study (139 vs. 164 g/m^2). Kelemen et al. [89] found that LV mass actually increased by ~10 g/m^2 with combined AT and ST in middle-aged hypertensives, primarily as a result of increased LV internal dimensions. These subjects had the lowest initial LV mass indices of the three studies, with values averaging 129 g/m^2. Other studies showed that AT in older men with normal LV mass indices resulted in physiological increases in LV mass and increased LV internal dimensions [47, 165, 177]. However, other evidence indicates that these same adaptations may not occur in postmenopausal women, perhaps because of their estrogen deficiency [177, 178]. No known studies have compared the effects of AT and ST on LV hypertrophy in the elderly, or independently assessed the effects of ST on LV hypertrophy in the elderly.

Thus, it appears that AT may reduce LV mass in older hypertensives with marked LV hypertrophy, over and above the effect that simply lowering BP has on LV mass. On the other hand, AT appears to elicit increases in LV mass, at least in older men with initially normal LV mass indices. There are no data documenting the effects of ST on LV mass in older persons with either initially abnormal or normal LV mass.

Abdominal Obesity

Reducing a person's level of obesity must be considered as an important outcome of risk factor intervention programs, as it may have concomitant beneficial effects on other major CV disease risk factors. Both AT [64, 65, 164] and ST [187] can reduce total body fat stores in older men and women, even when subjects are not undergoing caloric restriction. However, since abdominal obesity is more consistently related to a metabolic profile predictive of CV disease risk than general obesity [42], a more important issue may be the effects of AT and ST on abdominal adipose tissue depots.

Aging is associated with a preferential deposition of fat in the abdominal region, especially in men [30]. Abdominal obesity may increase the risk for CV disease independent of other CV disease risk factors [44], but it is also closely associated with other risk factors [22, 41]. Abdominal obesity is thought to be the first step in a series of events that leads to insulin resistance, glucose intolerance, abnormal lipoprotein-lipid profiles, and hypertension [22, 41, 123]. This constellation of risk factors for CV disease, diabetes, and hypertension has been called many names, including syndrome X, the deadly quartet, the Reaven syndrome, the insulin resistance syndrome, the abdominal obesity syndrome, the atherothrombogenic syndrome [3], the plurimetabolic syndrome [42], and the metabolic syndrome [22, 41, 123]. Although there may be a genetic predisposition for abdominal obesity, increasing age, high fat diets, and a sedentary lifestyle are also thought to be important determinants [22, 41].

Several studies have shown that AT produces significant losses in abdominal adipose tissue. For example, Schwartz et al. [161] compared abdominal fat losses in older men vs. younger men in response to AT. Before training, the older men had twice as much intra-abdominal fat as the younger men. In the older men, AT resulted in significant reductions in body weight, the percentage of body fat, intra-abdominal fat mass, and waist:hip ratio, whereas only intra-abdominal fat mass changed significantly in the young men. Kohrt et al. [95] also reported reductions in central body fat stores with AT in both older men and women. Lehmann et al. [103] reported similar findings with AT in middle-aged and older diabetics. However, there is some evidence that the effects of AT on central fat may depend on how the measurements are taken. In this regard, Houmard et al. [75] found a significant reduction with AT in the waist:hip ratio in middle-aged men and older men when the umbilicus circumference was divided by the maximal hip circumference, and when the minimal waist was divided by maximal hip circumference. However, no significant change was found when the circumference at the umbilicus was divided by either the circumference at the anterior superior iliac spine or greater trochanter.

Very little information is available on the effects of ST on abdominal fat in older individuals. Using dual energy x-ray absorptiometry, Treuth et al. [187] observed reductions in truncal fat mass of older men after 16 weeks of total body ST. In a follow-up study that used computed tomography (CT), Treuth et al. [185] found significant ST-induced reductions in intra-abdominal fat in older women.

Diet cannot be ruled out as a factor that could have affected the results of AT and ST studies addressing the effects of training on intra-abdominal fat. Although no study that measured abdominal fat adequately controlled diet throughout the entire training program, Ross et al. performed some of the best-controlled studies that assessed the effects of diet and exercise training [152, 153]. In their studies, magnetic resonance imaging (MRI) was used to provide a direct measurement of fat tissue so that regional fat losses from diet combined with either AT or ST could be compared. In their first study, Ross et al. [152], found no differences between the two groups for losses in either whole body subcutaneous fat or visceral fat; however, within each group, there was a significantly greater visceral fat loss compared to subcutaneous fat loss. In a follow-up study Ross et al. [153] isolated the effects of AT and ST by comparing the responses to diet alone and diet combined with each training modality in 33 middle-aged obese men. All three groups lost a substantial amount of whole body subcutaneous and visceral fat, and all three groups experienced a significantly greater visceral fat loss compared to whole body subcutaneous fat loss. The changes amounted to a 39% reduction in visceral fat in the diet and AT group, a 40% reduction in the diet and ST group, and a 32% reduction in the diet-only group. These differences were not significant. We estimated that the low-volume ST program required less than one-third of the energy required for the AT. When comparing losses from the abdominal subcutaneous fat depot to those from the gluteal-femoral (leg) region, there was a preferential loss from the abdominal region in the two training and diet groups, but no preferential losses in the diet-only group. Both training and diet groups maintained whole body skeletal muscle tissue, whereas the diet-only group lost muscle tissue.

Therefore, it appears that both AT and ST are effective in reducing intra-abdominal fat stores in older persons. It is somewhat surprising that AT does not result in significantly greater fat losses compared to ST, since the caloric expenditure associated with ST is substantially less than that of AT. It is unclear exactly what accounts for this discrepancy in energy balance, but one possible explanation could be increases in resting metabolic rate (RMR) with ST.

Resting Metabolic Rate

Aging is associated with a loss of fat free mass (FFM) and an increase in fat mass [30]. Loss of FFM is accompanied by a decline in RMR, which can lead to obesity [140]. Although FFM is by far the major determinant of RMR, explaining ~60–70% of the interindividual variability [182], the age-related reduction in the Na-K pump activity [141] and VO_2 max [136] also contribute to the decline in RMR with age. RMR is not an independent CV disease risk factor; however, because of its mechanistic links with obesity, RMR should probably be considered when assessing the impact of AT and ST modalities on overall CV disease risk.

Poehlman et al. [139] observed a 9% increase in RMR after AT, despite no changes in body composition. A 22% increase in norepinephrine appearance and no change in norepinephrine clearance also occurred. Thus, one possible mechanism for training-induced increases in RMR may be increased sympathetic nervous system activity. In another study, this increased sympathetic activity was associated with an increase in fat oxidation [138]. Nevertheless, not all studies show increases in RMR with AT [117, 155, 194].

In a cross-sectional study, Poehlman et al. [137] found higher RMR values in ST athletes compared to untrained controls. Increases in RMR have also been reported with ST in longitudinal studies of older men and women [25, 144]. Pratley et al. [144] studied 50 to 65-yr-old men before and after 16 wks of heavy resistance ST, and observed a 2.6% increase in FFM, a 7.7% increase in RMR, and a 36% increase in resting plasma norepinephrine levels. They concluded that the increases in FFM and the increased activity of the sympathetic nervous system may be responsible for the training-induced increase in RMR [144]. Campbell et al. [25] also found increases in FFM and RMR in older men and women with ST. However, they concluded that the increase in RMR was due to an increase in the metabolic activity of lean tissue and not an increase in FFM. Although FFM increased with ST in the Campbell et al. study, they determined that the increase was due mainly to an increase in body water. Ryan et al. [155] observed a significant rise in RMR in postmenopausal women as a result of ST, with and without weight loss.

However, not all ST studies show increases in RMR. Taaffe et al. [181] reported that neither low- nor high-intensity ST altered RMR significantly. In addition, Treuth et al. [186] found that increases in RMR, as a result of

ST in postmenopausal women, were not significant when increases in FFM were taken into account. Similar findings were reported by Van Etten et al. [189] who observed no significant increases in metabolic rate during sleep as a result of ST. As was previously well established for AT, both Van Etten et al. [189] and Treuth et al. [186] reported that ST significantly increased fat oxidation. Thus, while there is evidence indicating that both AT and ST can increase RMR, other studies show that no changes in RMR occur with either training modality. Differences in training regimes and testing conditions may explain some of the discrepancies on this issue.

MUSCULOSKELETAL HEALTH AND AGING

Osteoporosis is one of the most prevalent conditions in postmenopausal women. The prevalence of osteoporosis also increases with age in men, though it is a much greater public health concern in women. The morbid events associated with osteoporosis consist of fractures, primarily occurring in the neck of the femur, the vertebrae, and the forearm in older men and women. In women, the loss of bone mineral density (BMD) after menopause results in a doubling of hip fracture risk for every 5 yrs of age past the age of 50 [36]. These fractures are so common that one-third of 80 yr old women will experience a hip fracture, and one-third of them will experience two hip fractures [36]. The overall result is that osteoporosis affects 25 million people, the majority of whom are women, and is the primary cause of 1.5 million fractures yearly [106].

The total costs each year associated with osteoporosis are estimated at nearly $18 billion, with hip fractures alone costing $7 billion [72]. Osteoporosis annually results in ~750,000 physician office visits and ~20 million restricted activity days [57]. Potentially more problematic are the facts that hip fractures result in 5–20% excess mortality, some long-term loss in function in 60% of fracture cases, and the need for long-term care in 30% of fracture cases [106]. Perhaps the most significant statistic regarding hip fractures is that only 20% of hip fracture cases return to their original functional status [106].

A second major component of musculoskeletal health is the loss of muscle mass and strength (sarcopenia) that occurs with aging. This decrease is associated with an increased risk for falls, low BMD, and hip fractures. Furthermore, decreased muscular strength is a major determinant of an older person's ability to maintain an active, high-quality lifestyle, and, perhaps, his/her ability to minimize increased adiposity with aging because of the reduction in muscle mass, a highly metabolically active component of body composition. Thus, when attempting to optimize health and function in the elderly, all aspects of musculoskeletal health, including bone and skeletal muscle, must be considered as a composite because of their close interactive relationships in the physiology of aging humans.

Bone Mineral Density

One major component of musculoskeletal health and a major risk factor for hip fracture is low BMD. BMD decreases markedly in women in the 2–5 yrs immediately after menopause and continues to decline at a slower rate thereafter [106]. As a result, maintenance or enhancement of BMD in older persons, especially older women, is a major public health concern. Determining whether various forms of physical activity enhance BMD at critical skeletal sites in postmenopausal women has been a major area of research over the past 15 yrs.

It appears that only one study has compared the effects of AT and ST on BMD at critical skeletal sites in postmenopausal women. Chow et al. found that 12 months of combined AT and ST increased BMD in the general area of the trunk and upper thigh by ~50% more than AT alone, but the difference was not statistically significant [29]. However, both training modalities increased BMD significantly more than the control group.

A number of other studies also indicate that AT increases BMD at critical skeletal sites in postmenopausal women. Other studies demonstrated that AT maintained BMD in older women, while BMD in the control group decreased over time, as would be expected [171, 172]. Such changes result in decreased hip fracture risk with training compared to the controls, but not an actual decrease in hip fracture risk in the exercise training group when compared to their initial risk.

Dalsky et al. showed that in postmenopausal women, AT combined with calcium supplements increased BMD significantly, as compared to women only given calcium supplements [37]. It is important to note that although most of the training these women completed was aerobic in nature, the training also included specific exercise training designed to load the axial skeleton. In addition, many of the early studies that assessed the effect of AT on BMD in postmenopausal women included some ST in the training program [171, 172]. This may also be relevant to the recent results of Bloomfield et al. who found that cycle ergometer AT increased BMD in postmenopausal women [13]. The training in this study consisted of cycling at 60 revolutions/min, which would result in substantial muscular forces at the hip and lumbar spine. However, it must also be kept in mind that a number of studies have not found significant increases in BMD with AT in postmenopausal women.

In a cross-sectional study, Bevier et al. reported that muscular strength was a better predictor of BMD in older men and women than VO_2max [10]. Other studies have also documented positive relationships between muscular strength and BMD in both young and older persons [24, 78]. Similarly, a number of studies have documented that strength-trained persons have markedly enhanced BMD, compared to their sedentary peers [61, 86, 88].

Nelson et al. [129] found that in 50–70 yr old women, heavy resistance ST essentially maintained BMD (0.9 and 1.0% increases at femoral neck and lumbar spine, respectively), whereas BMD decreased by 2.5% at the femoral neck and 1.8% in the lumbar spine in the control group. The changes in both femoral neck and the lumbar spine BMD were significantly greater in the ST intervention group compared to the control group. Notel-ovitz et al. [132] found that 1 yr of ST combined with estrogen replacement therapy, produced a greater increase in spine, radial midshaft, and total body BMD in surgically postmenopausal women than estrogen replacement therapy alone. Pruitt et al. reported that 9 months of ST in women with an average age of 54 yrs increased BMD at the lumbar spine, but not the femoral neck and distal wrist. [146]. Results from our laboratory indicate that men 50–70 yrs of age increase femoral neck BMD and tend to increase lumbar spine BMD with 16 wks of ST that results in substantial increases in both upper and lower body muscular strength [116, 157]. However, a number of other studies indicate that ST does not increase BMD in young and older women [150, 191].

To summarize, it appears that in older individuals, ST may have a more consistently beneficial effect than AT on BMD, especially in postmenopausal women. However, AT can also beneficially affect BMD in older persons. Furthermore, in most cases, it is probably more appropriate to conclude that the exercise intervention, be it AT or ST, may effectively maintain BMD in older persons compared to nonexercising control subjects who lose BMD over the same period of time. The magnitude of the change in BMD resulting from these interventions is, in general, not substantial enough to markedly reduce an older person's risk of suffering a fracture once a fall occurs [34].

Fall Prevention

Some researchers estimate that increases in BMD of greater than 20% would be required to provide adequate protection against bone fractures resulting from falls [34]. Given the fact that most studies report less than a 5% increase in BMD from any exercise training modality, it is more likely that exercise training could play a role in the prevention of falls rather than fractures once a fall occurs. Cognitive impairment, visual deficits, environmental conditions, and medication use may combine with physical activity-related risk factors, such as neuromuscular gait and balance impairments to increase the risk of falls [124]. Although many authors emphasize the importance of regular exercise for prevention of falls in the elderly, only very limited data are available on this topic, and the information available is not conclusive. Means et al. [115] observed no significant differences in falls or injuries from falls following a 6-wk exercise program, consisting of stretching, postural control, endurance walking, and coordination exercises designed to improve balance and mobility. In contrast, following a yearlong, low-intensity exercise program consisting of stand-ups from a sitting position and step-ups on a 6-inch stool, MacRae et al. [109] reported that 36% of the exercising subjects sustained a fall, compared to 45% of attention control subjects. Furthermore, none of the 10 fallers in the exercise group required medical attention, whereas three of the 14 fallers in the control group required medical attention. In a pre-planned meta-analysis of seven independent, randomized, controlled clinical trials that assessed intervention efficacy in reducing falls in elderly patients, it was concluded that interventions that included regular exercise reduced risk of falls [145]. However, the exercise interventions were very diverse and often included nonexercise components.

Good evidence exists to indicate that the use of ST reduces risk factors for falls [49], but we are unaware of any data showing a reduction in the number of falls with a ST intervention program. Lipsitz et al. [107] compared fall rates in residents of Japanese and American nursing homes, hypothesizing that Japanese nursing home residents would have lower fall rates due to greater quadriceps strength. Fall rates were, in fact, nearly 4-fold higher in American nursing home residents; however, these differences could not be attributed to differences in quadriceps strength, since American residents also had a greater number of medical diagnoses and a greater use of medications than the Japanese nursing home residents. Thus, the association between muscle weakness and falls was potentially confounded by differences in medical status between the groups. Messier et al. [118] compared the effects of AT, ST, and an attention control health education class on gait mechanics and knee pain in older adults with knee osteoarthritis. The AT group significantly improved temporal components of gait, as well as knee and joint kinematics, and the ST group significantly increased ankle plantar flexion velocity. Both training interventions improved walking mechanics and resulted in significantly less knee pain, as compared to the control group. No data on the effects of the training programs on fall rates were reported.

To summarize, due to the prolonged time period and expense required for studies on fall rates, most investigations into the effects of AT and ST have focused on risk factors for falls, rather than actual fall incidence rates. These studies provide evidence that both AT and ST can improve neuromuscular function, gait, and balance, which are all very important risk factors for falls in the elderly. The one study that compared the effects of AT to ST found that both modalities improved walking mechanics, AT improved gait and joint kinematics, and ST improved ankle plantar flexion velocity, suggesting a reduction in risk of falling.

Muscle Quality

It is well established that with age there is a loss of muscle strength and mass [101, 105], and that in older men and women, both can be increased relatively quickly with ST. [19, 25, 49, 53, 69, 82, 119, 143, 147, 151, 155, 156, 168, 169, 181, 185, 187, 199]. However, the effects of age and ST on muscle quality, the inherent strength of muscle independent of changes in mass, are less well understood. Many investigators have assessed strength in relation to muscle mass or cross-sectional area of muscle (specific tension) as an index of muscle quality. Young et al. [197] found no difference in muscle quality between 70–80 and 20–30 yr old women, whereas lower muscle quality was reported in older men compared to younger men [133, 148, 198]. Hortabagyi et al. [73] found no age-related changes in estimated muscle quality in either men or women in relation to eccentric strength, whereas Lindle et al. [105] observed losses in muscle quality for eccentric strength in men, but not women.

Castro et al. [26] reported higher torque per cross-sectional area of muscle (muscle quality) in strength-trained subjects compared to untrained subjects for both men and women. Narici et al. [126] reported a nonsignificant 11% increase in muscle quality following a ST program. In a more recent study, Narici et al. [125] found a similar 12% increase in muscle quality with ST, but this change was statistically significant. Welle et al. [192] compared muscle quality responses to ST in young and older men and women. Both the young and older groups increased their muscle quality with ST, and there was no difference in response to training between the age groups for most muscle groups tested, with the exception of the knee flexors, which increased to a greater extent in the older group.

Only one study appears to have compared the effects of AT and ST on muscle strength in older persons. Hagberg et al. found that 6 months of ST in healthy 70–79 yr old men and women increased lower and upper body strength by 9–18%, respectively, whereas 6 months of AT, that resulted in a 22% increase in VO$_2$max, did not significantly change either lower or upper body strength [64]. These results are consistent with the likelihood that muscle quality did not change with AT in these older men and women as they did not change lean body mass. Therefore, it is clear that ST is the only training method that effectively increases muscle mass and strength in older men and women. Most evidence also indicates that in older persons, ST reverses the losses in muscle quality—the strength per unit of muscle mass. There is no evidence that AT improves muscle strength or quality in older persons.

Flexibility

The loss of joint range of motion (flexibility) with age is well-documented [7, 59], and is related to dysfunction and a decline in health status [9, 58]. This loss in flexibility may be associated with difficulty in climbing stairs, getting up from a chair or bed, and the need for walking aids [9]. It is thought that much of this loss is due to inactivity, and that increasing muscular activity might at least delay losses in flexibility [28, 190]. Kligman and

Pepin [92] concluded that older adults who maintain high levels of muscular strength and flexibility are rarely candidates for long-term health care. Improving flexibility [2, 170] could alleviate several musculoskeletal disorders. However, there is minimal information available on the impact of either AT or ST on flexibility in older adults. Furthermore, most AT and ST studies that investigated the effects of training on flexibility used flexibility exercises in the training program. Thus, the independent effects of AT or ST on flexibility are not well established. In one of the few studies that did not include flexibility exercises, Taunton et al. [183] found no improvements in flexibility with either land- or water-based AT, and concluded that neither program was specific enough to improve flexibility.

It is often assumed that properly performed ST (i.e., going through the full range of motion, and exercising both the agonist and antagonist muscle groups) improves flexibility [108, 179]. However, published results do not support this assumption. Despite performing all exercises through the full range of motion, training both the agonist and antagonist muscle groups, and performing stretching exercises before and after every training session as is recommended for improving flexibility [108, 179], Girourard et al. [60] found no significant improvements in flexibility beyond those of an inactive control group. Moreover, there was a significantly greater improvement in shoulder abduction in a group who performed the identical stretching exercises without ST [60].

The few studies that assessed whether ST can improve flexibility either used only young subjects [56, 193], did not indicate if stretching exercises were incorporated [113], included aerobic exercise in the training program [111, 121, 147], used only low-resistance exercise [147], or did not control for other factors that can affect flexibility [113, 147]. These methodological differences may explain why investigators report increases [28, 121, 193], no changes [56, 113], and losses [113] in flexibility with ST. Thus, there is no definitive evidence that a total body ST program improves flexibility in older adults. Because of the limitations in previous studies, there is a great need for well-designed studies on the effects of heavy resistance ST on flexibility in older individuals. In the meantime, it should not be assumed that ST alone will increase range of motion, simply by exercising the agonist and antagonist muscle groups, and by going through the full range of motion with each exercise. Even brief warm-up and cool-down stretching may not be enough to improve flexibility significantly, particularly in the shoulder region [59, 60, 113, 147]. Therefore, prolonged stretching should be an integral part of any properly designed ST program.

In summary, it appears that exercise training programs, whether they are aerobic or resistive in nature, should specifically include flexibility exercises if increased flexibility is a desired outcome from a training program for older men and women. ST and AT programs alone do not improve joint flexibility in older adults, and it is possible that both modalities may actually inhibit joint range of motion if stretching exercises are not included in the training program.

CONCLUSIONS

A vast amount of research has been conducted in the past 15 yrs to quantify the impact of both AT and ST on older men and women. We have attempted to review the data concerning the effects of both training modalities on CV and musculoskeletal health in older adults. The available literature does not provide definitive answers relative to many critical aspects of CV and musculoskeletal health in older persons, as only a small number of studies have addressed some key parameters, and because data are often lacking for specific responses in women. Furthermore, there is a virtual lack of data assessing the interactions between both forms of training and hormonal replacement therapy in postmenopausal women.

However, the available data clearly indicate that both AT and ST offer a wide range of benefits to older adults. Some evidence indicates that both AT and ST may improve BMD, glucose homeostasis, and overall risk for falling. However, if older persons want to increase their CV fitness, decrease their elevated BP, improve their plasma lipoprotein-lipid profile, or ameliorate their LV hypertrophy to optimize their health status, AT would appear to be the most efficacious training mode. On the other hand, if older adults want to increase their muscle mass and strength, and possibly also their muscle quality, ST should clearly be their first choice. For other CV and musculoskeletal health variables, the optimal training mode is not known, often because not enough data are available relative to the variable in question. However, with the possible exception of flexibility, which may decrease with both AT and ST, neither form of training has been shown to result in worsening of any of the key CV and musculoskeletal health parameters. Perhaps the best concluding recommendation we can provide to older adults who want a program to optimize their current and future health, is to initiate a well-rounded physical activity program, one that includes both AT and ST and probably also incorporates specific flexibility and balance exercises.

REFERENCES

1. Ades, P., D. Ballor, T. Ashikaga, J. Utton, and K. Nair. Weight training improves walking endurance in healthy elderly persons. *Ann. Int. Med.* 124:568–572, 1996.
2. Amatuzzi, M., M. Frazzi, and M. Varella. Pathological synovial plica of the knee: results of conservative treatment. *Am. J. Sports Med.* 18:466–469, 1990.
3. Anderssen, S., Hjermann, I, P. Urdal, P. Torjesen, and I. Holme. Improved carbohydrate

metabolism after physical training and dietary intervention in individuals with the ather-othrombogenic syndrome. Oslo diet and exercise study(ODES). A randomized trial. *J. Int. Med.* 240:203–209, 1996.

4. Anonymous. National Institute of Health. Consensus Development Conference on diet and exercise in non-insulin-dependent diabetes mellitus. *Diabetes Care* 10:639–644, 1987.

5. Baglivo, H., H. Fabregues, R. Burrieza, R. Esper, M. Talarico, and R. Esper. Effect of moderate physical training on left ventricular mass in mild hypertensive persons. *Hypertension* 15:1153–1156, 1990.

6. Barret-Conner, E., D. Wingard, M. Criqui, and L. Suarez. Is borderline fasting hyperglycemia a risk factor for cardiovascular death? *J. Chron. Diseases* 37:773–779, 1984.

7. Bell, R., and T. Hoshizaki. Relationships of age and sex with joint range of motion of seventeen joint actions in humans. *Can. J. Appl. Sport Sciences* 6:202–206, 1981.

8. Benestad, A. Trainability of old men. *Acta Medica Scandinavica* 178:321–327, 1965.

9. Bergstrom, G., A. Aniansson, A. Bjelle, G. Grimby, B. Lundgren-Lidquist, and A. Svanborg. Functional consequences of joint impairment at age 79. *Scan. J. Rehab. Med.* 17: 183–190, 1985.

10. Bevier, W., R. Wiswell, G. Pyka, K. Kozak, K. Newhall, and R. Marcus. Relationship of body composition, muscle strength and aerobic capacity to bone mineral density in older men and women. *J. Bone Min. Research* 4:421–432, 1989.

11. Blair, S., H. Kohl III, R. Paffenbarger Jr., D. Clark, K. Cooper, and L. Gibbons. Physical fitness and all-cause mortality: a prospective study of healthy men and women. *JAMA* 262:2395–2401, 1989.

12. Bloesch, D., Y. Schultz, E. Breitenstein, E. Jequier, and J. Felber. Thermogenic response to an oral glucose load in man: comparison between young and elderly subjects. *J. Am. Col. Nutrition* 7:471–483, 1988.

13. Bloomfield, S., N. Williams, D. Lamb, and R. Jackson. Nonweightbearing exercise increases lumbar bone mineral density in healthy postmenoupausal women. *Am. J. Phys. Med. Rehab.* 72:204–209, 1993.

14. Blumenthal, J., K. Matthews, M. Fredrikson, et al. Effects of exercise training on cardiovascular function and plasma lipid, lipoprotein, and apolipoprotein concentrations in premenopausal and postmenopausal women. *Arterio.Thromb.* 11:912–917, 1991.

15. Boyden, T., R. Pamenter, S. Going, et al. Resistance exercise training is associated with decreases in serum low-density lipoprotein cholesterol levels in premenopausal women. *Arch. Int. Med.* 153:97–100, 1993.

16. Braun, B., M. Zimmermann, and N. Kretchmer. Effects of exercise intensity on insulin sensitivity in women with non-insulin-dependent diabetes mellitus. *J. Appl. Physiol.* 78: 300–306, 1995.

17. Brock, D., J. Guralnick, and J. Brody. Demography and epidemiology of aging in the US. E. Schneider and J. Rowe (eds.). *Handbook of the Biology of Aging.* San Diego: Academic Press, 1990, pp 3-23.

18. Broughton, D., and R. Taylor. Review: Deterioration of glucose tolerance with age: the role of insulin resistance. *Age Aging* 20:221–225, 1991.

19. Brown, A., N. McCartney, and D. Sale. Positive adaptation to weight-lifting in the elderly. *J. Appl. Physiol.* 69:1725–1733, 1990.

20. Brown, M., and J. Hagberg. Does exercise training play a role in the treatment of essential hypertension? *J. Card. Risk* 2:296–302, 1995.

21. Buchner, D., and E. Wagner. Preventing frail health. *Clin. Ger. Med.* 8:1–17, 1992.

22. Buemann, B., and A. Tremblay. Effects of exercise training on abdominal obesity and related metabolic complications. *Sports Med.* 3:191–212, 1996.

23. Busby, J., M. Notelovitz, K. Putney, and T. Grow. Exercise, high-density lipoprotein-cholesterol, and cardiorespiratory function in climacteric women. *South. Med. J.* 78: 769–773, 1995.

24. Calmels, P., L. Vico, C. Alexandre, and P. Minaire. Cross-sectional study of muscle strength and bone mineral density in a population of 106 women between the ages of 44 and 87 years: relationship with age and menopause. *Eur. J. Appl. Physiol.* 70:180–186, 1995.

25. Campbell, W., M. Crim, V. Young, and W. Evans. Increased energy requirements and changes in body composition with resistance training in older adults. *Am. J. Clin. Nutrition* 60:167–175, 1994.

26. Castro, M., D. McCann, J. Shaffrath, and W. Adams. Peak torque per unit cross-sectional area differs between strength-trained and untrained young adults. *Med. Sci. Sports Exerc.* 27:397–403, 1995.

27. Cauley, J., A. Kriska, R. LaPorte, R. Sandler, and G. Pambianco. A two year randomized exercise trial in older women: effects on HDL-cholesterol. *Atherosclerosis* 66:247–258, 1987.

28. Chapman, E., H. deVries, and R. Swezey. Joint stiffness: effects of exercise on young and old men. *J. Gerontol.* 27:218–221, 1972.

29. Chow, R., J. Harrison, and C. Notarius. Effect of two randomised exercise programmes on bone mass of healthy postmenopausal women. *Brit. Med. J.* 295:1441–1444, 1987.

30. Cohn, S., A. Vaswani, I. Zanzid, and J. Aloia. Changes in body chemical composition with age measured by total-body neutron activation. *Am. J. Physiol.* 25:85–95, 1976.

31. Cononie, C., A. Goldberg, E. Rogus, and J. Hagberg. Seven consecutive days of exercise lowers plasma insulin responses to an oral glucose challenge in sedentary elderly. *J. Am. Ger. Soc.* 42:394–398, 1994.

32. Cononie, C., J. Graves, M. Pollock, M. Phillips, C. Summers, and J. Hagberg. Effect of exercise training on blood pressure in 70–79 year old men and women. *Med. Sci. Sports Exerc.* 23:505–511, 1991.

33. Council on Exercise of the Am. Diabetes Association. Exercise and NIDDM. *Diabetes Care* 13:785–789, 1990.

34. Courtney, A., E. Wachtel, E. Myers, and W. Hayes. Effects of loading rate on strength of the proximal femur. *Calc. Tis. Internat.* 55:53–58, 1994.

35. Craig, B., J. Everhart, and R. Brown. The influence of high-resistance training on glucose tolerance in young and elderly subjects. *Mech. Aging Develop.* 49:147–157, 1989.

36. Cummings, S., J. Kelsey, and M. Nevitt. Epidemiology of osteoporosis and osteoporotic fractures. *Epidemiol. Review* 7:178–205, 1985.

37. Dalsky, G., K. Stocke, A. Ehsani, E. Slatopolsky, W. Lee, and S. Birge. Weight-bearing exercise training and lumbar bone mineral content in postmenopausal women. *Ann. Int. Med.* 108:824–828, 1988.

38. Davidson, M. The effect of aging on carbohydrate metabolism: a review of the English literature and a practical approach to the diagnosis of diabetes mellitus in the elderly. *Metabolism* 28:687–705, 1979.

39. Dela, F., K. Mikines, J. Larsen, and H. Galbo. Training-induced enhancement of insulin action in human skeletal muscle: the influence of aging. *J. Gerontol.* 51(Suppl 4): B247–B252, 1996.

40. Dengel, D., R. Pratley, J. Hagberg, E. Rogus, and A. Goldberg. Distinct effects of aerobic exercise training and weight loss on glucose homeostasis in obese sedentary men. *J. Appl. Physiol.* 81:318–325, 1996.

41. Despres, J. Abdominal obesity as important component of insulin-resistance syndrome. *Nutrition* 9:452–459, 1993.

42. Despres, J. Visceral obesity, insulin resistance, and dyslipidemia: contribution of endurance exercise training to the treatment of the plurimetabolic syndrome. *Exer. Sport Sci. Reviews.* 25:271–300, 1997.

43. Despres, J., B. Lamarche, P. Mauriege, et al. Hyperinsulinemia as an independent risk factor for ischemic heart disease. *New Eng. J. Med.* 334:952–957, 1996.

44. Donahue, R., R. Abbort, E. Bloom, D. Reed, and K. Yano. Central obesity and coronary heart disease in men. *Lancet* 1:822–824, 1987.

45. Douen, A., T. Ramlal, S. Rastogi, et al. Exercise induces recruitment of the "insulin-responsive glucose transporter." *J. Bio. Chem.* 265:13427–13430, 1990.

46. Durak, E., L. Jovanovis-Petersol, and C. Peterson. Randomized crossover study of effect of resistance training on glycemic control, muscular strength, and cholesterol in type I diabetic men. *Diabetes Care* 13:1039–1042, 1990.

47. Ehsani, A., T. Ogawa, T. Miller, R. Spina, and S. Jilka. Exercise training improves left ventricular systolic function in older men. *Circulation* 83:96–103, 1991.

48. Ezaki, O., M. Higuchi, H. Nakatsuka, K. Kawanaka, and H. Itakura. Exercise training increases glucose transporter content in skeletal muscles more efficiently from aged obese rats than young lean rats. *Diabetes* 41:920–926, 1992.

49. Fiatarone, M., E. O'Neill, N. Ryan, et al. Exercise training and nutritional supplementation for physical frailty in very elderly people. *New Eng. J. Med.* 330:1769–1775, 1994.

50. Friedewald, W. Introductory remarks. I. 18th Bethesda Conference Report: Cardiovascular disease in the elderly. *J. Am. Coll. Cardiol.* 10:7A, 1987.

51. Fripp, R., and J. Hodgson. Effect of resistive training on plasma lipid and lipoprotein levels in male adolescents. *J. Paediatrics* 11:926–931, 1987.

52. Frishman, W., J. Bauman, J. Soberman, J. Nadelmann, J. Wurzelmann, and M. Aronson. Treatment of ischemic heart disease in the elderly: Beta-adrenergic blockade and coronary artery bypass surpery. N.K. Wenger, C.D. Furberg, and E. Pitt (eds). *Coronary Heart Disease in the Elderly.* New York:Elsevier, 1986, pp. 153-197.

53. Frontera, W., C.N. Meredith, K. O'Reilly, H. Knuttgen, and W. Evans. Strength condition in older men: skeletal muscle hypertrophy and improved function. *J. Appl. Physiol.* 63:1038–1044, 1988.

54. Frontera, W., C.N. Meredith, K. O'Reilly, and W. Evans. Strength training and determinants of VO_{2max} in older men. *J. Appl. Physiol.* 68:329–333, 1990.

55. Frost, P., B. Davis, A. Burlando, et al. Serum lipids and incidence of coronary heart disease. *Circulation* 94:2381–2388, 1996.

56. Gardner, G. Effect of isometric and isotonic exercise on joint motion. *Arch. Phys. Med. Rehab.* 47:24–30, 1966.

57. Garraway, W., R. Stauffer, and J. Kurland. Limb fractures in a defined population: orthopedic treatment and utilization of health care. *Mayo Clinic Proceedings* 54:708–713, 1979.

58. Gehlsen, G., and M. Whaley. Falls in the elderly: part II, balance, strength, and flexibility. *Arch. Phys. Med. Rehab.* 71:739–741, 1990.

59. Germain, N., and S. Blair. Variability of shoulder flexion with age, activity and sex. *Am. Corrective Therapy J.* 37:156–160, 1983.

60. Girouard, C., and B. Hurley. Strength training inhibits gains in shoulder abduction from flexibility training. *Med. Sci. Sports Exerc.* 27:1444–1449, 1995.

61. Haapasalo, H., P. Kannus, H. Sievanen, A. Heinonen, P. Oja, and I. Vuori. Long-term unilateral loading and bone mineral density and content in female squash players. *Cal. Tiss. Internat.* 54:249–255, 1994.

62. Hagberg, J. Exercise, fitness, and hypertension. C. Bouchard, R.J. Shephard, T. Stephens, J.R. Sutton, and B.D. McPherson (eds). *Exercise, Fitness, and Health: A Consensus of Current Knowledge.* Champaign, IL:Human Kinetics Press, 1990, pp. 455-466.

63. Hagberg, J., S. Blair, A. Ehsani, et al. Position Stand: physical activity, physical fitness, and hypertension. *Med. Sci. Sports Exerc.* 25:I–x, 1993.

64. Hagberg, J., J. Graves, M. Limacher, et al. Cardiovascular responses of 70-79 year old men and women to exercise training. *J. Appl. Physiol.* 66:2589–2594, 1989.

65. Hagberg, J., S. Montain, W. Martin, and A. Ehsani. Effect of exercise training on 60 to 69 year old persons with essential hypertension. *Am. J. Cardiol.* 64:348–353, 1989.

66. Harris, M., W. Hadden, W. Knowler, and P. Bennett. Prevalence of diabetes and impaired glucose tolerance and plasma glucose levels in U.S. population aged 20–74 yr. *Diabetes* 36:523–534, 1987.

67. Heath, G., J. Hagberg, A. Ehsani, and J. Holloszy. A physiological comparison of young and older endurance athletes. *J. Appl. Physiol.* 51:634–640, 1981.

68. Helmrich, S., D. Ragland, R. Leung, and R. Paffenbarger Jr. Physical activity and reduced occurrence of non-insulin-dependent diabetes mellitus. *New England J. Med.* 325:147–152, 1991.

69. Hersey III, W., J. Graves, M. Pollock, et al. Endurance exercise training improves body composition and plasma insulin responses in 70- to 79–year–old men and women. *Metabolism* 43:847–854, 1994.

70. Hickson, R., M. Rosenkoetter, and M. Brown. Strength training effects on aerobic power and short-term endurance. *Med. Sci. Sports Exerc.* 12:336–339, 1980.

71. Hill, J., J. Thiel, P. Heller, C. Markon, G. Fletcher, and M. DiGirolamo. Differences in effects of aerobic exercise training on blood lipids in men and women. *Am. J. Cardiol.* 63:254–256, 1988.

72. Holbrook, T., K. Grazier, J. Kelsey, and R. Stauffer. Frequency of occurrence, impact, and cost of selected musculoskeletal conditions in the US. Chicago: Am. Academy of Orthopedic Surgery, 1984.

73. Hortobagyi, T., D. Zheng, M. Weidner, N. Lambert, Westbrook L, and J. Houmard. The influence of aging on muscle strength and muscle fiber characteristics with special reference to eccentric strength. *J. Gerontol.* 50A:B399–B406, 1995.

74. Houmard, J., M. Hickey, G. Tyndall, K. Gavigan, and G. Dohm. Seven days of exercise increase GLUT-4 protein content in human skeletal muscle. *J. Appl. Physiol.* 79:1936–1938, 1995.

75. Houmard, J., C. McCulley, L. Roy, R. Bruner, R. McCammon, and R. Israel. Effects of exercise training on absolute and relative measurements of regional adiposity. *Internat. J. Obesity* 18:243–248, 1994.

76. Hughes, V., M. Fiatarone, C. Ferrara, J. McNamara, J. Charnley, and W. Evans. Lipoprotein response to exercise training and a low-fat diet in older subjects with glucose intolerance. *Am. J. Clin. Nutrition* 59:820–826, 1994.

77. Hughes, V., M. Fiatarone, R. Fielding, et al. Exercise increases muscle GLUT-4 levels and insulin action in subjects with impaired glucose tolerance. *Am. J. Physiol.* 264:E855–E862, 1993.

78. Hughes, V., W. Frontera, G. Dallal, K. Lutz, E. Fisher, and W. Evans. Muscle strength and body composition: associations with bone density in older subjects. *Med. Sci. Sports Exerc.* 27:967–974, 1995.

79. Hurley, B. Effects of resistive training on lipoprotein-lipid profiles: a comparison to aerobic exercise training. *Med. Sci. Sports Exerc.* 21:689–693, 1989.

80. Hurley, B., J. Hagberg, A. Goldberg, et al. Resistive training can reduce coronary risk factors without altering VO$_2$max or percent body fat. *Med. Sci. Sports Exerc.* 20:150–154, 1988.

81. Hurley, B., J. Hagberg, D. Seals, A. Ehsani, A. Goldberg, and J. Holloszy. Glucose tolerance and lipid-lipoprotein levels in middle-aged powerlifters. *Clin. Physiol.* 7:11–19, 1987.

82. Hurley, B., R. Redmond, R. Pratley, M. Trueth, M. Rogers, and A. Goldberg. Effects of strength training on muscle hypertrophy and muscle cell disruption in older men. *Internat. J. Sports Med.* 16:380–386, 1995.

83. Johnson, C., M. Stone, Lopez-S A, J. Hebert, L. Kilgore, and R. Byrd. Diet and exercise in middle-aged men. *J. Am. Diet, Assoc.* 81:695–701, 1982.

84. Kahn, S., V. Larson, J. Beard, et al. Effect of exercise on insulin action, glucose tolerance and insulin secretion in aging. *Am. J. Physiol.* 21:E937–E943, 1990.

85. Kahn, S., V. Larson, R. Schwartz, et al. Exercise training delineates the importance of B-cell dysfunction to the glucose intolerance of human aging. *J. Clin. Endocrinol. Metabol.* 74:1336–1342, 1992.

86. Kannus, P., H. Haapasalo, H. Sievanen, P. Oja, and Vuori, I. Site-specific effects on long-term unilateral activity on bone mineral density and content. *Bone* 15:279–284, 1994.

87. Kaplan, N. *Clinical Hypertension* (5th Edition). Baltimore: Williams and Wilkins, 1990.

88. Karlsson, M., P. Vergnaud, P. Delmas, and K. Obrant. Indicators of bone formation in weight lifters. *Calc. Tiss. Internat.* 56:177–180, 1995.

89. Kelemen, M., M. Effron, S. Valenti, and K. Stewart. Exercise training combined with antihypertensive drug therapy. *JAMA.* 263:2766–2771, 1990.

90. King, D., G. Dalsky, W. Clutter, et al. Effects of exercise and lack of exercise on insulin sensitivity and responsiveness. *J. Appl. Physiol.* 64:1942–1946, 1988.

91. Kirwan, J., W. Kohrt, D. Wojta, R. Bourey, and J. Holloszy. Endurance exercise training reduces glucose-stimulated insulin levels in 60- to 70-year-old men and women. *J. Gerontol.* 48:M84–M90, 1993.

92. Kligman, E., and E. Pepin. Prescribing physical activity for older patients. *Geriatrics* 47: 33–47, 1992.

93. Kohl, H. I., N. Gordon, C. Scott, H. Vaandrager, and S. Blair. Musculoskeletal strength and serum lipid levels in men and women. *Med. Sci. Sports Exerc.* 24:1080–1087, 1992.

94. Kohrt, W., M. Malley, A. Coggan, et al. Effects of gender, age, and fitness level on response of VO_{2max} to training in 60–71 yr olds. *J. Appl. Physiol.* 71:2004–2011, 1991.

95. Kohrt, W., A. K. Obert, and J. Holloszy. Exercise training improves fat distribution patterns in 60- to 70-year-old men and women. *J. Gerontol.* 47:M99–M105, 1992.

96. Koivisto, V., H. Yki-Jarvinen, and R. DeFronzo. Physical training and insulin sensitivity. *Diabetes Metab. Review* 1:445–481, 1986.

97. Kokkinos, P., and B. Hurley. Strength training and lipoprotein-lipid profiles: a critical analysis and recommendations for further study. *Sports Med.* 9:266–272, 1990.

98. Kokkinos, P., B. Hurley, M. Smutok, et al. Strength training does not improve lipoprotein-lipid profiles in men at risk for CHD. *Med. Sci. Sports Exerc.* 123:1134–1139, 1991.

99. Kokkinos, P., P. Narayan, J. Colleran, et al. Effects of regular exercise on blood pressure and left ventricular hypertrophy in African-American men with severe hypertension. *New Eng. J. Med.* 333:1462–1467, 1995.

100. Krumholz, H., T. Seeman, S. Merrill, et al. Lack of association between cholesterol and coronary heart disease mortality and morbidity and all-cause mortality in persons older than 70 years. *JAMA.* 272:1335–1340, 1994.

101. Larsson, L., G. Grimby, and J. Karlsson. Muscle strength and speed of movement in relation to age and muscle morphology. *J. Appl. Physiol.* 46:451–456, 1979.

102. Lee, A., B. Craig, J. Lucas, R. Pohlman, and H. Stelling. The effect of endurance training, weight training and a combination of endurance and weight training upon the blood lipid profile of young male subjects. *J. Appl. Sports Sci. Research* 4:68–75, 1990.

103. Lehmann, R., A. Vokac, K. Niedermann, K. Agosti, and G. Spinas. Loss of abdominal fat and improvement of the cardiovascular risk profile by regular moderate exercise training in patients with NIDDM. *Diabetologia* 38:1313–1319, 1995.

104. Lindheim, S., M. Notelovitz, E. Feldman, S. Larsen, F. Khan, and R. Lobo. The independent effects of exercise and estrogen on lipids and lipoproteins in postmenopausal women. *Obstet. Gyn.* 83:167–172, 1994.

105. Lindle, R., E. Metter, N. Lynch, et al. Age and gender comparisons of muscle strength in 654 women and men aged 20-93. *J. Appl. Physiol.* 83:1581–1587, 1977.

106. Lindsay, R. *Osteoporosis.* Chicago: National Osteoporosis Foundation, 1992.

107. Lipsitz, L., I. Nakajima, M. Gagnon, T. Hirayama, C. Connelly, and H. Izumo. Muscle strength and fall rates among residents of Japanese and American. nursing homes: an international cross-cultural study. *J. Am. Ger. Soc.* 42:953–959, 1994.

108. Lombardi, V. *Beginning Weight Training.* Dubuque, Iowa: W. C. Brown Publishers, 1989.

109. MacRae, P., M. Feltner, and S. Reinsch. A 1-year exercise program for older women: effects on falls, injuries, and physical performance. *J. Aging Phys. Act.* 2:127–142, 1994.

110. Manning, J., C. Dooly-Manning, K. White, et al. Effects of a resistance training program on lipoprotein-lipid levels in obese women. *Med. Sci. Sports Exerc.* 23:1222–1226, 1991.

111. Marcinik, E., J. Hodgdon, K. Mittleman, and J. O'Brien. Aerobic/calisthenic and aerobic/circuit weight training programs for Navy men: a comparative study. *Med. Sci. Sports Exerc.* 17:482–487, 1985.

112. Marcinik, E., J. Potts, G. Schlabach, S. Will, P. Dawson, and B. Hurley. Effects of strength training on lactate threshold and endurance performance. *Med. Sci. Sports Exerc.* 23: 739–743, 1991.

113. Massey, B., and N. Chauder. Effects of systematic, heavy resistive exercise on range of joint movement in young male adults. *Research Quarterly* 27:41–51, 1956.

114. McCartney, N., R. McKelvie, J. Martin, D. Sale, and J. MacDougall. Weight-training-induced attenuation of the circulatory response of older males to weight lifting. *J. Appl. Physiol.* 74:1056–1060, 1993.

115. Means, K., D. Rodell, P. O'Sullivan, and L. Cranford. Rehabilitation of elderly fallers: Pilot study of a low to moderate intensity exercise program. *Arch. Phys. Med. Rehab.* 77: 1030–1036, 1996.

116. Menkes, A., S. Mazel, R. Redmond, et al. Strength trainings increase regional bone mineral density and bone remodeling in middle-aged and older men. *J. Appl. Physiol.* 74:2478–2484, 1993.

117. Meredith, C., W. Frontera, E. Fisher, et al. Peripheral effects of endurance training in young and old subjects. *J. Appl. Physiol.* 66:2844–2849, 1989.

118. Messier, S., C. Thompson, and W. Ettinger Jr. Effects of long-term aerobic or weight training regimens on gait in an older, osteoarthritic population. *J. Appl. Biomech.* 13: 205–225, 1997.

119. Miller, J., R. Pratley, A. Goldberg, et al. Strength training increases insulin action in healthy 50–65 year old men. *J. Appl. Physiol.* 77:1122–1127, 1994.

120. Miller, W., W. Sherman, and J. Ivy. Effect of strength training on glucose tolerance and post-glucose insulin response. *Med. Sci. Sports Exerc.* 16:539–543, 1984.

121. Morey, M., P. Cowper, J. Fuessner, et al. Evaluation of a supervised exercise program in a geriatric population. *J. Am. Ger. Soc.* 37:348–354, 1989.

122. Motoyama, M., Y. Sunami, F. Kinoshita, et al. The effects of long-term low intensity aerobic training and detraining on serum lipid and lipoprotein concentrations in elderly men and women. *Eur. J. Appl. Physiol.* 70:126–131, 1995.

123. Muller, D., D. Elahi, J. Tobin, and R. Andres. The effect of age on insulin resistance and secretion: a review. *Sem. Nephrol.* 16:289–298, 1996.

124. Myers, A., Y. Young, and J. Langlois. Prevention of falls in the elderly. *Bone* 18:87S–101S, 1996.

125. Narici, M., H. Hoppeler, B. Kayser, et al. Human quadriceps cross-sectional area, torque and neural activation during 6 months strength training. *Acta Physiol. Scand.* 157:175–186, 1996.

126. Narici, M., G. Roi, L. Landoni, A. Minetti, and P. Cerretelli. Changes in force, cross-sectional area and neural activation during strength training and detraining of human quadriceps. *Eur. J. Appl. Physiol.* 59:310–319, 1989.

127. National Center for Health Statistics. D. Dawson, P. Adams. Current estimates from the National Health Interview Survey, United States, 1986. Vital and Health Statistics, Series 10, No. 164, Hyattsville, MD: Public Health Service, 1987. (DHHS Pub #{PHS}87-1592).

128. National Center for Health Statistics. 1986 Summary: National Hospital Discharge Survey. Advance data from Vital and Health Statistics. No.145. Hyattsville, MD: Public Health Service, 1987; 6 (DHHS Pub # {PHS}87-1250).

129. Nelson, M., M. Fiatarone, C. Morganti, I. Trice, and W. Evans. Effects of high-intensity strength training on multiple risk factors for osteoporotic fractures. *JAMA* 272: 1909–1914, 1994.

130. Nieman, D., B. Warren, K. O'Donnell, and R. Dotson. Physical activity and serum lipids and lipoproteins in elderly women. *J. Am. Ger. Soc.* 41:1339–1344, 1993.

131. Ninimaa, V., and R. Shephard. Training and oxygen conductance in the elderly. I. The respiratory system. *J. Gerontol.* 33:354–361, 1978.

132. Notelovitz, M., D. Martin, and C. Probart. Estrogen therapy and variable-resistance weight training increase bone mineral in surgically menopausal women. *J. Bone Min. Res.* 6: 583–590, 1991.

133. Overend, T., D. Cunningham, D. Paterson, and M. Lefcoe. Thigh composition in young and elderly men determined by computed tomography. *Clin. Physiol.* 12:629–640, 1992.

134. Pacini, G., A. Valerio, F. Beccaro, R. Nosadini, C. Cobelli, and G. Crepaldi. Insulin sensitivity and beta-cell responsivity are not decreased in elderly subjects with normal OGTT. *J. Am. Ger. Soc.* 36:317–323, 1988.

135. Parker, N., G. Hunter, M. Treuth, et al. Effects of strength training on cardiovascular responses during a submaximal walk and a weight-loaded walking test in older females. *J. Cardio. Rehab.* 16:56–62, 1996.

136. Poehlman, E., E. Berke, J. Joseph, A. Gardner, S. Katzman-Rooks, and M. Goran. Influence of aerobic capacity, body composition, and thyroid hormones on the age-related decline in resting metabolic rate. *Metabolism* 41:915–921, 1992.

137. Poehlman, E., A. Gardner, P. Ades, et al. Resting energy metabolism and cardiovascular disease risk in resistance-trained and aerobically trained males. *Metabolism* 41:1351–1360, 1992.

138. Poehlman, E., A. Gardner, P. Arciero, M. Goran, and J. Calles-Escandon. Effects of endurance training on total fat oxidation in elderly persons. *J. Appl. Physiol.* 76:2281–2287, 1994.

139. Poehlman, E., A. Gardner, and M. Goran. Influence of endurance training on energy intake, norepinephrine kinetics, and metabolic rate in older individuals. *Metabolism* 41: 941–948, 1992.

140. Poehlman, E., M. Goran, A. Gardner, et al. Determinants of decline in resting metabolic rate in aging females. *Am. J. Physiol.* 264:E450–E455, 1993.

141. Poehlman, E., M. Toth, and G. Webb. Sodium-potassium pump activity contributes to the age-related decline in resting metabolic rate. *J. Clin. Endocrinol. Metabol.* 76: 1054–1057, 1993.

142. Pollare, T., H. Lithell, and C. Berne. Insulin resistance is a characteristic feature of primary hypertension independent of obesity. *Metabolism* 39:167–174, 1990.

143. Pollock, M., J. Carroll, J. Graves, et al. Injuries and adherence to walk/jog and resistance training programs in the elderly. *Med. Sci. Sports Exerc.* 23:1194–1200, 1991.

144. Pratley, R., B. Nicklas, M. Rubin, et al. Strength training increases resting metabolic rate and norepinephrine levels in healthy 50– to 65–yr–old men. *J. Appl. Physiol.* 76:133–137, 1994.

145. Province, M., E. Hadley, M. Hornbrook, et al. The effects of exercise on falls in elderly patients: a preplanned meta-analysis of the FICSIT Trials. *JAMA* 273:1341–1347, 1995.

146. Pruitt, L., R. Jackson, and R. Bartels. Weight-training effects on bone mineral density in postmenopausal women. *J. Bone Min. Res.* 7:179–185, 1992.

147. Raab, D., J. Agre, M. McAdam, and E. Smith. Light resistance and stretching exercise in elderly women: effect upon flexibility. *Arch. Phys. Med. Rehab.* 69:268–272, 1988.

148. Reed, R., L. Pearlmutter, K. Yochum, K. Meredith, and A. Mooradian. The relationship between muscle mass and muscle strength in the elderly. *J. Am. Ger. Soc.* 39:555–561, 1991.

149. Rhea, P., A. Ryan, L. Gordon, et al. Effects of strength training with and without weight loss on lipoprotein-lipid levels in postmenopausal women. Submitted for publication, *Internat. J. Sports Med.*, 1998.

150. Rockwell, J., A. Sorensen, S. Baker, et al. Weight training decreases vertebral bone density in premenopausal women: a prospective study. *J. Clin. Endocrinol. Metabol.* 71:988–993, 1990.

151. Roman, W., J. Fleckenstein, J. Stray-Gundersen, S. Alway, R. Peshock, and W. Gonyea. Adaptations in the elbow flexors of elderly males after heavy-resistance training. *J. Appl. Physiol.* 74:750–754, 1993.

152. Ross, R., and J. Rissanen. Mobilization of visceral and subcutaneous adipose tissue in response to energy restriction and exercise. *Am. J. Clin. Nut.* 60:695–703, 1994.

153. Ross, R., J. Rissanen, H. Pedwell, J. Clifford, and P. Shragge. Influence of diet and exercise on skeletal muscle and visceral adipose tissue in men. *J. Appl. Physiol.* 81:2445–2455, 1996.

154. Rowe, J., K. Minaker, J. Palotta, and J. Flier. Characterization of the insulin resistance of aging. *J. Clin. Invest.* 71:1581–1587, 1983.

155. Ryan, A., R. Pratley, D. Elahi, and A. Goldberg. Resistive training increases fat-free mass and maintains RMR despite weight loss in postmenopausal women. *J. Appl. Physiol.* 79: 818–823, 1995.

156. Ryan, A., R. Pratley, A. Goldberg, and D. Elahi. Resistive training increases insulin action in postmenopausal women. *J. Gerontol.* 51A:M199–M205, 1996.

157. Ryan, A., M. Treuth, M. Rubin, et al. Effects of strength training on bone mineral density. *J. Appl. Physiol.* 77:1678–1684, 1994.

158. Satler, L., C. Green, R. Wallace, and C. Rackley. Coronary artery disease in the elderly. *Am. J. Cardiol.* 63:245–248, 1989.

159. Schaefer, E., P. Moussa, W. Wilson, D. McGee, G. Dallal, and W. Castelli. Plasma lipoproteins in healthy octogenarians: lack of reduced high density lipoprotein cholesterol levels: results from the Framingham Heart Study. *Metabolism* 38:293–296, 1989.

160. Schwartz, R., K. Cain, W. Shuman, et al. Effect of intensive endurance training on lipoprotein profiles in young and older men. *Metabolism* 41:649–654, 1992.

161. Schwartz, R., W. Shuman, Larson, et al. The effect of intensive endurance exercise training on body fat distribution in young and older men. *Metabolism* 40:545–551, 1991.

162. Seals, D., J. Hagberg, W. Allen, et al. Glucose tolerance in young and older athletes and sedentary men. *J. Appl. Physiol.* 56:1521–1525, 1984.

163. Seals, D., J. Hagberg, B. Hurley, A. Ehsani, and J. Holloszy. Effects of endurance training on glucose tolerance and plasma lipid levels in older men and women. *JAMA* 252: 645–649, 1984.

164. Seals, D., J. Hagberg, B. Hurley, A. Ehsani, and J. Holloszy. Endurance training in older men and women. I. Cardiovascular responses to exercise. *J. Appl. Physiol.* 57:1024–1029, 1984.

165. Seals, D., J. Hagberg, R. Spina, M. Rogers, K. Schechtman, and A. Ehsani. Enhanced left ventricular performance in endurance trained older men. *Circulation* 89:198–205, 1994.

166. Seals, D., and M. Reiling. Effect of regular exercise on 24-hr arterial pressure in older hypertensive humans. *Hypertension* 18:583–592, 1991.

167. Shimokata, H., D. Muller, J. Fleg, J. Sorkin, A. Ziemba, and R. Andres. Age as an independent determinant of glucose tolerance. *Diabetes* 40:44–51, 1991.

168. Sipilä, S., J. Multanen, M. Kallinen, P. Era, and H. Suominen. Effects of strength and endurance training on isometric muscle strength and walking speed in elderly women. *Acta Physiol. Scand.* 156:457–464, 1996.

169. Sipilä, S., and H. Suominen. Effects of strength and endurance training on thigh and leg muscle mass and composition in elderly women. *J. Appl. Physiol.* 78:334–340, 1995.

170. Smith, A., L. Stroud, and C. McQueen. Flexibility and anterior knee pain in adolescent elite figure skaters. *J. Ped. Orthoped.* 11:77–82, 1991.

171. Smith, E., C. Gilligan, M. McAdam, C. Ensign, and P. Smith. Deterring bone loss by exercise. *Calc. Tiss. Internat.* 44:312–321, 1989.

172. Smith, E., W. Reddan, and P. Smith. Physical activity and calcium modalities for bone mineral increase in aged women. *Med. Sci. Sports Exerc.* 13:60–64, 1981.
173. Smutok, M., C. Reece, P. Kokkinos, et al. Aerobic vs. strength training for risk factor intervention in middle-aged men at high risk for coronary heart disease. *Metabolism* 42: 177–184, 1993.
174. Smutok, M., C. Reece, P. Kokkinos, et al. Effects of training modality on glucose regulation. *Internat. J. Sports Med.* 15:283–289, 1994.
175. Smutok, M., C. Reece, P. Kokkinos, et al. Effects of exercise training modality on glucose tolerance in men with abnormal glucose regulation. *Internat. J. Sports Med.* 15:283–289, 1994.
176. Soman, V., V. Koivisto, D. Deibert, P. Felig, and R. DeFronzo. Increased insulin sensitivity and insulin binding to monocytes after physical training. *New Eng. J. Med.* 301:1200–1204, 1979.
177. Spina, R., T. Ogawa, W. Kohrt, W. Martin III, J. Holloszy, and A. Ehsani. Differences in cardiovascular adaptations to endurance exercise training between older men and women. *J. Appl. Physiol.* 75:849–855, 1993.
178. Spina, R., T. Ogawa, T. Miller, W. Kohrt, and A. Ehsani. Effect of exercise training on left ventricular performance in older women free of cardiopulmonary disease. *Am. J. Cardiol.* 71:99–104, 1993.
179. Stone, M., S. Fleck, N. Triplett, and W. Kramer. Health and performance related potential of resistance training. *Sports Med.* 11:210–231, 1991.
180. Stout, R. Overview of the association between insulin and atherosclerosis. *Metabolism* 34: 7–12, 1984.
181. Taaffe, D., L. Pruitt, J. Reim, G. Butterfield, and R. Marcus. Effect of sustained resistance training on basal metabolic rate in older women. *J. Am. Ger. Soc.* 43:465–471, 1995.
182. Tataranni, P., and E. Ravussin. Variability in metabolic rate: biological sites of regulation. *Internat. J. Obesity.* 19:S102–S106, 1995.
183. Taunton, J., E. Rhodes, L. Wolski, et al. Effect of land-based and water-based fitness programs on the cardiovascular fitness, strength and flexibility of women aged 65–75 years. *J. Gerontol.* 42:204–210, 1996.
184. Tonino, R. Effect of physical training on the insulin resistance of aging. *Am. J. Physiol.* 256:E352–E356, 1989.
185. Treuth, M., G. Hunter, T. Kekes-Szabo, R. Weinsier, M. Goran, and L. Berland. Reduction in intra-abdominal adipose tissue after strength training in older women. *J. Appl. Physiol.* 78:1425–1431, 1995.
186. Treuth, M., G. Hunter, R. Weinsier, and S. Kell. Energy expenditure and substrate utilization in older women after strength training: 24-h calorimeter results. *J. Appl. Physiol.* 78: 2140–2146, 1995.
187. Treuth, M., A. Ryan, R. Pratley, et al. Effects of strength training on total and regional body composition in older men. *J. Appl. Physiol.* 77:614–620, 1994.
188. Tucker, L., and L. Silvester. Strength training and hypercholesterolemia: an epidemiologic study of 8499 employed men. *Phys. Health: Fitness* 11:35–41, 1996.
189. Van Etten, L., K. Westerterp, and F. Verstappen. Effect of weight-training on energy expenditure and substrate utilization during sleep. *Med. Sci. Sports Exerc.* 27:188–193, 1994.
190. Voorhips, L., K. Lemmunk, M. Van Heuvellon, P. Bult, and W. Van Stoveron. The physical condition of elderly women differing in habitual physical activity. *Med. Sci. Sports Exerc.* 25:1152–1157, 1993.
191. Vuori, I, A. Heinonen, H. Sievanen, P. Kannus, and P. Oja. Effects of unilateral strength training and detraining on bone mineral density in young women. *Calc. Tiss. Internat.* 55:59–67, 1994.
192. Welle, S., S. Totterman, and C. Thornton. Effect of age on muscle hypertrophy induced by resistance training. *J. Gerontol.* 51A:M270–M275, 1997.

193. Weltman, A., C. Janney, C. Rians, et al. Effects of hydraulic resistance strength training in pre-pubertal males. *Med. Sci. Sports Exerc.* 18:629–638, 1986.

194. Westerterp, K., G. Meijer, P. Schoffelen, and E. Janssen. Body mass, body composition and sleeping metabolic rate before, during and after endurance training. *Eur. J. Appl. Physiol.* 69:203–208, 1994.

195. Wilson, P., K. Anderson, T. Harris, W. Kannel, and W. Castelli. Determinants of change in total cholesterol and HDL-C with age: the Framingham study. *J. Gerontol.* 49:M252–M257, 1994.

196. Wosornu, D., D. Bedford, and D. Ballantyne. A comparison of the effects of strength and aerobic exercise training on exercise capacity and lipids after coronary artery bypass surgery. *Eur. Heart J.* 17:854–863, 1996.

197. Young, A., M. Strokes, and M. Crowe. Size and strength of the quadriceps muscles of old and young women. *Eur. J. Clin. Invest.* 14:282–287, 1984.

198. Young, A., M. Strokes, and M. Crowe. The size and strength of the quadriceps muscles of old and young men. *Clin. Physiol.* 5:145–154, 1985.

199. Zachwieja, J., G. Toffolo, C. Cobelli, D. Bier, and K. Yarasheski. Resistance exercise and growth hormone administration in older men: effects on insulin sensitivity and secretion during a stable-label intravenous glucose tolerance test. *Metabolism* 45:254–260, 1996.

200. Zavaroni, I, E. Bonoro, M. Pagliara, et al. Risk factors for coronary artery disease in healthy persons with hyperinsulinemia and normal glucose tolerance. *New Eng. J. Med.* 320:702–706, 1989.

4
A New Approach to Studying Muscle Fatigue and Factors Affecting Performance During Dynamic Exercise in Humans

STEVEN F. LEWIS, PH.D.
CHARLES S. FULCO, SC.D.

The physiological factors that determine human exercise performance have been studied extensively over the past century. Intense scrutiny of various types, intensities, and durations of physical effort established criteria for defining and measuring performance constructs such as strength, endurance, and work capacity. Voluntary muscle fatigue has, however, been more difficult to probe. A large portion of muscle fatigue research has focused primarily on static contractions of small, well-defined muscle groups in which muscle recruitment patterns are relatively simple and neither motion artifact nor changing muscle length impact electromyographic measurements. In contrast, much less attention has been allotted to fatigue of large muscle dynamic exercise, the primary interest for many exercise physiologists. Focus on dynamic exercise is dominated by studies of conventional treadmill and cycle ergometry, modes that do not readily permit quantitation of progressive muscle fatigue and its myoelectric manifestations. As a result, gradually increasing fatigue during constant work rate exercise has not been observable or systematically studied.

This review will present a newly developing approach to study muscle fatigue during dynamic exercise. Recent advances in isolating dynamic exercise to well-defined larger muscle groups [2, 78] and quantifying both the work performed and the rate of fatigue of the active muscles [36] provide a necessary framework. Our review will discuss the significance of this new approach to understanding dynamic exercise performance and muscle fatigue and the related impact of interventions likely to modify muscle function.

CONVENTIONAL APPROACHES TO STUDYING EXERCISE PERFORMANCE AND MUSCLE FATIGUE

Treadmills and cycle ergometers are used widely in the clinical and experimental study of human performance. These modes closely simulate spontaneous walking, running, and bicycling, common forms of human locomotion during which muscle energy demand is met primarily by oxidative metabolism. The oxygen cost of treadmill and cycle exercise is well characterized and normally predictable with minimal variation. Peak work rate and peak oxygen uptakes during these modes of large muscle effort are important performance criteria or predictors under a wide variety of conditions. Treadmill and cycle ergometry are also used extensively to characterize the limits of endurance (i.e. time of exercise performance to exhaustion at constant submaximal work intensities). These measurements contribute richly to identifying the factors that set upper limits to physical performance in sport and everyday life.

Peak oxygen uptake ($\dot{V}O_2$peak), peak work rate, and endurance time to exhaustion are, however, merely single indices of overall physical performance. Monitoring ongoing performance is more problematic. A progressive increase in difficulty of maintaining strenuous constant work rate exercise is reflected in gradual increases in electromyographic activity [7, 12, 17] and ratings of perceived exertion [69, 71]. However, an inability to make specific measurements of muscle performance serially during conventional dynamic exercise makes it virtually impossible to quantitate progressive fatigue. Thus, fatigue of dynamic exercise usually is defined as " . . . a failure to maintain the required or expected power output . . . " [26, 27]. This definition implies that fatigue does not occur until an individual is unable to continue exercising and, in effect, makes fatigue indistinguishable from exhaustion.

Several theoretical and methodological difficulties limit the feasibility of measuring progressively impaired muscle function during the complex, multi-joint movements involved in conventional ergometry. Many different muscles are involved and are likely working at very different percentages of their maximal capacities. Variations in intra- and intermuscular recruitment patterns (due partly to variations in leg position and range of movement) are a related concern. Thus, at any given time point, the degree of fatigue is likely to differ widely among specific muscles. As a result, human muscle fatigue often has been studied during sustained voluntary static contractions (constant contraction, no rest) or intermittent (precise intervals of contraction and rest) voluntary static contractions of small, isolated muscles or groups of muscles [12, 14, 17, 26, 66]. Periodic maximal voluntary static contractions (MVCs) integrated within the exercise period permit muscle fatigue to be measured as the slope of decline in MVC force relative to time (Figure 4.1). The small muscle static contraction approach features virtually complete overlap between the muscles used to produce fatigue and those used to measure falling MVC force. Highly motivated subjects typically will exercise until MVC force declines to equal the target force [14, 35, 105]. With this approach, fatigue has been defined as " . . . a gradual decline of muscle force generating capacity resulting from physical activ-

FIGURE 4.1.

Schematic of model for measuring progressive fatigue of intermittent static contractions. "Strength" is the highest maximal voluntary static contraction (MVC) force of rested muscle obtained at the start of exercise. The "target force" of submaximal contractions is set to a given percentage of strength. The durations of the target force contraction and the rest period following each contraction can each be adjusted to obtain any duty cycle. A MVC also is performed at the end of a specified time period or number of target-force contractions. "Rate of Fatigue" is defined as the rate of decline of MVC force resulting from the target force contractions. "Exhaustion" occurs when MVC force falls to the target force value or the target force cannot be maintained for a specified duration. "Endurance Time" is the time interval from the start of exercise to the exhaustion point. In the figure, the target force equals 50% of strength, both the MVC and target force contractions and rest periods last 5 sec (i.e., duty cycle = 0.5), and a MVC is performed at the end of each min (or every sixth contraction). Modified from Bigland-Ritchie and Woods [17].

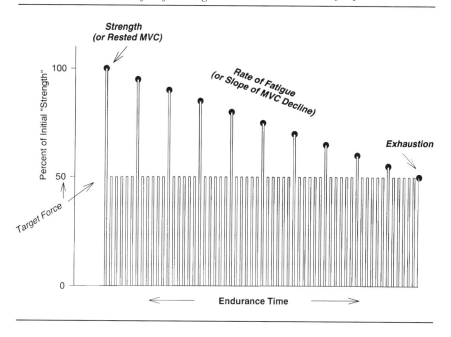

ity" [4, 17, 92]. Exhaustion, defined as the point at which force generating capacity (i.e., MVC force) has declined to the target force, can be clearly distinguished from fatigue. In contrast, studies of fatigue of dynamic effort have focused primarily on the moment a constant work rate can no longer be sustained, (i.e. the point of exhaustion).

Previous models of fatigue of dynamic exercise included the effects of cycling, running, or stepping exercise on MVC force during static knee extension [23, 45, 61, 73, 84, 91]. This approach is problematic because differences in muscle recruitment limit overlap between muscles used to produce and measure fatigue. Some workers studied the effects of dynamic exercise on force and/or endurance time during *sustained* static contractions [45, 61, 73], a fatigue assessment paradigm that itself induces marked fatigue. Furthermore, with few exceptions [18, 74, 84], fatigue was assessed after but not during dynamic exercise, and substantial delay in post-exercise measurement of MVC force in most [23, 24, 45, 91] if not all [84] studies has allowed at least partial force recovery. For some of these studies [45, 61, 73], emphasis was on how dynamic exercise affects static exercise performance rather than on the use of maximal effort static contractions to measure muscle fatigue of dynamic exercise.

A MODEL AND DEVICE FOR STUDYING FATIGUE OF DYNAMIC EXERCISE

In contrast to treadmill and cycle ergometry, dynamic knee extension exercise limited to the quadriceps femoris muscles involves little or no unnecessary muscle motion. This facilitates the ability to use a variety of noninvasive and invasive techniques to study muscle performance, myoelectric activity, metabolism, and blood flow during dynamic exercise [2, 3, 6, 36, 78, 81, 107]. During 1-leg dynamic knee extension, the active muscle mass is large enough to clearly distinguish the physiological responses to different work intensities. The active muscle mass, however, is sufficiently small to restrict systemic oxygen demand and cardiac output to submaximal levels at which local muscle perfusion and contractile performance are unlikely to be limited by cardiac pumping capacity [87]. Quadriceps muscle mass can be estimated from anthropometric measurements of the thigh [3], and quantification of oxygen uptake, quadriceps muscle force production, and power output, while local blood flow may be normalized to the active muscle mass.

Conventional cycle ergometers modified for performance of dynamic exercise localized to knee extensors are used to study cardiovascular, metabolic, and neuroendocrine regulation [2, 3, 5, 78, 79]. In contrast, a recently developed model and device were designed specifically to study progressive muscle fatigue during dynamic knee extension exercise [36]. The model features integration of dynamic knee extension contractions with serial measurement of maximal voluntary static contraction of the knee extensor muscles. This approach permits measurement of the rate of fall in maximal force generating capacity of the knee extensor muscles resulting from dynamic knee extension exercise [36, 37]. Together with other serially acquired physiological, biochemical and psychological measurements, the "frame-by-frame" examination of muscle fatigue permitted by this model allows detailed study of the factors responsible for gradually declining muscle performance during dynamic leg effort in humans. In contrast, previous work employing ordinary treadmill or cycle exercise largely center on a "snapshot" of physiological or biochemical events correlating with muscular exhaustion.

The knee extension exercise device was described in detail elsewhere [36]. Briefly, it consists of a platform on which the subject sits, an attached minimal-friction weight-pulley system with an ankle harness, transducers for measurement of force and ankle displacement during dynamic knee extension and, and separate transducers for measurement of static knee extension MVC force (Figure 4.2). In order to precisely control velocity of leg movement and work rate, two parallel columns of 14 light crystal diodes (LCDs) are placed in front of the subject at eye level. One LCD column is wired in series to the displacement transducer, such that the number of LCDs lighted is propor-

FIGURE 4.2.

Front and rear views of the knee extension device. For each leg, a transducer for measurement of maximal voluntary contraction (MVC) force is anchored to a cross member on the device, and a transducer for measurement of dynamic force is attached between the back of the ankle harness and a cord connected to the weight platform. This arrangement permits dynamic knee extension and MVC force recordings during one- or two-leg exercise. In experiments to date, MVC has been measured at a knee angle of 90°. Distance of ankle displacement and rate of knee extension are precisely monitored using a position transducer attached by fine wire to the bottom of the weight platform. As the leg is extended from a 90° to 150° knee angle, the position transducer provides a voltage output proportional to the wire displacement. The resulting voltages are used to light from one to 14 light crystal diodes (LCDs) that provide visual feedback to control work rate and contraction velocity. See text for details. Modified from Fulco et al. [36].

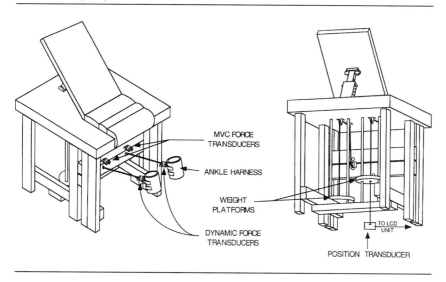

tional to ankle displacement during knee extension. The other LCD column is connected to a synthesizer/function generator, which automatically and sequentially lights from one LCD (at the 90^0 knee angle starting position) to 14 LCDs (corresponding to ankle displacement on reaching 150^0 of knee extension) to one LCD (return to 90^0 starting position) at a pre-determined knee extension rate of 1 Hz. To maintain correct distance and rate of dynamic knee extension, the subject continuously matches the column of LCDs controlled by leg movement with the LCD column controlled by the synthesizer/function generator. The LCD units simplify subject and investigator monitoring of adherence to the required work rate and permit control of contraction velocity within relatively narrow limits. Since one knee extension is performed each second, movement from a knee angle of 90° to 150° consumes 0.5 sec and from 150° to 90° another 0.5 sec. Thus, knee extension velocity is controlled at $120° \times sec^{-1}$. Because the knee extension movement encompasses 60° and there are 13 intervals between LCDs, the maximum allowable difference between the desired and actual knee extension angle is 4.62°. Muscle exhaustion is defined as a mismatch of only one LCD between the right and left LCD columns — usually the 14th LCD— for three consecutive knee extensions. This effectively means that exhaustion is associated with an inability to complete the last 5^0 of knee extension— from 145° to 150°— at the required contraction rate. Force and ankle displacements are continuously recorded. Work rate (watts) is determined by multiplying mean force developed per contraction, distance of ankle movement during knee extension from 90° to 150° and rate of knee extension (1 Hz). The quadriceps muscles also act eccentrically in moving from a knee angle of 150° to 90° to lower the weight. Because little or no increase in energy expenditure, muscle fatigue, or intramuscular pressure is associated with this eccentric component [16, 22, 43, 55, 99], eccentric action is omitted from the calculation of work rate.

To assess muscle fatigue rate as a decline in force generating capacity relative to duration of dynamic exercise, the dynamic knee extension device facilitates performance of maximal voluntary static contractions of the knee extensor muscles during brief (≤ 5 sec) pauses in dynamic exercise (Figure 4.3). This procedure involves the following: Interruption of dynamic knee extension and rapid disconnection of the ankle harness from the weight-pulley system (< 1 sec); connection to a force transducer dedicated to measurement of knee extensor MVC force (< 1 sec); actual measurement of MVC force (2.5 sec—as cued by an auditory device triggered by a voltage from the transducer used to measure MVC force); and reconnection to the weight-pulley system and resumption of dynamic knee extension (< 1 sec). The momentary pause between interruption of dynamic knee extension and measurement of MVC force virtually eliminates impact of inadvertent recovery from assessment of fatigue rate. However, the equally brief pause between completion of MVC and resumption of dynamic knee extension allows potential carry-over of fatigue from the MVC. In experiments per-

FIGURE 4.3.

Schematic of dynamic knee extension fatigue model. "Strength" *or maximal voluntary static contraction (MVC) force of rested muscle is the highest MVC force obtained prior to the start of dynamic exercise. Peak force during each dynamic knee extension is the product of the amount of weight lifted and the speed with which the weight is displaced. Also, MVCs are repeated at specific points in time (typically every 2 to 4 min) during dynamic exercise.* "Rate of Fatigue" *is defined as the rate of decline of MVC force resulting from dynamic knee extension exercise.* "Exhaustion" *occurs when an individual is unable for three consecutive contractions to maintain the rate of knee extension and/or the distance of ankle movement. In the figure, peak force during each submaximal contraction equals 20% of MVC force of rested muscle, a MVC is performed every third min of dynamic knee extension, and at exhaustion, the percent MVC force equals 50% that of rested muscle. In contrast to the static contraction fatigue model depicted in Figure 1, the point of exhaustion for dynamic knee extension occurs with MVC force remaining substantially above the level of peak force during submaximal contractions. See the* "Point of Exhaustion" *section in the text for details.*

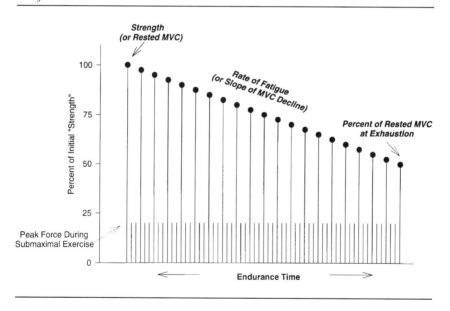

formed to date, MVC force was measured at 2 or 4-min intervals during dynamic knee extension. Repetition of MVC for 2 to 3 sec as often as once per min for 30 min in the absence of dynamic exercise results in no diminution of force generating capacity [37]. However, the specific impact on endurance performance or fatigue rate of knee extensor MVCs performed periodically during dynamic knee extension has not been studied.

FIGURE 4.4.

Force during one-leg dynamic knee extension exercise as a percentage of maximal voluntary contraction (MVC) force of rested (•) *and* exercising (○) *knee extensor muscles. Values are means ± SE. (A) Constant work rate exercise: Dynamic force as a percentage MVC force of rested muscle remained constant at 18 ± 1% throughout dynamic exercise performed to exhaustion at 79% of peak one-leg oxygen uptake. In contrast, dynamic force as a percentage of the progressively declining MVC force (i.e., MVC force of exercising muscle), increased from 18 ± 1% at the start of dynamic exercise to 42 ± 5% at the point of exhaustion. *P < 0.05, rested vs. exercising MVC force). EXH = exhaustion. (B) Graded exercise: MVC forces of exercising muscle were measured immediately following 4 min of knee extension at work rates approximating 66%, 78%, 100% of peak one-leg oxygen uptake. *P < 0.01 compared to percent MVC force at lower percentages of peak oxygen uptake for rested and exercising muscle, respectively. At the end of the work rate eliciting 100% of peak one-leg oxygen uptake, peak force of dynamic knee extension reached 47 ± 6% of MVC force of exercising muscle. Modified from Fulco et al. [36, 37].*

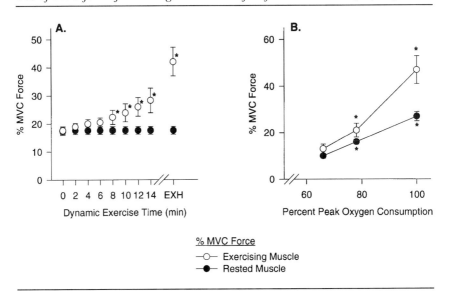

In addition to providing the novel ability to track—during dynamic leg exercise—the decline in force generating capacity expressed in absolute terms or as a percentage of MVC force of *rested* muscle, the dynamic knee extension model permits study of the force exerted during dynamic knee extension as a fraction of the "current" MVC force available to *exercising* muscle (Figure 4.4). Commensurate with progressively falling MVC force during dynamic exercise, there is a gradual rise in the percentage MVC force of *exercising* muscle represented by the force of dynamic contractions. We are unaware of previous study of dynamic contraction force during submaximal exercise as a function of MVC of *exercising* muscle. This approach is likely to provide important insights regarding physiological and perceptual factors associated with exhaustion [36, 37]. (See *"The Point of Exhaustion"* below).

In general, the ergometric characteristics of the weight-pulley system for dynamic knee extension are similar to those for friction-braked cycle ergometers modified for knee extension exercise. The same tight linear relationship between oxygen uptake and work rate during dynamic knee extension is achieved using both the weight-pulley and friction-braked ergometers (Figure 4.5). In addition, there was minimal day-to day variation in oxygen

FIGURE 4.5.

Relationship between oxygen uptake and work rate during one-leg dynamic knee extension exercise. Open circles represent individual data using our knee extension exercise device [36] during graded dynamic knee extension to peak oxygen uptake. Regression line for these data is the solid line. Dashed and dotted lines are regression lines calculated from figures published by Andersen et al. [2] and Richardson et al. [78], respectively. Regression line of Richardson et al. only includes a range of work rates similar to that used by our subjects [36]. From Fulco et al. [36].

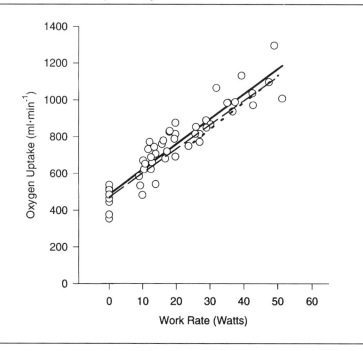

uptake for a given work rate during knee extension using the weight-pulley device [36]. The weight-pulley device does, however, include a slightly greater static component to dynamic knee extension than modified friction-braked ergometers [36]. This relates to the force required to overcome inertia of the weight stack at the instant of return of the knee angle to $90°$ and initiation of the next knee extension, and may result in a transiently higher intramuscular pressure and commensurately greater local muscle ischemia for dynamic knee extension using the weight-pulley device.

In contrast to dynamic exercise, muscle ischemia during high-intensity static exercise is well established. In static exercise, sustained elevations in intramuscular pressure approach or exceed perfusion pressure [28, 89], thereby reducing muscle blood flow. For a given individual, intramuscular pressure increases linearly with increasing percentage of MVC exerted during static knee extension [28, 89]. Intramuscular pressure measurements imply partial occlusion of arterial inflow to the human quadriceps during static knee extension at tensions equivalent to 20% of MVC. Occlusion may be nearly or totally complete at 50% of MVC [28, 82, 89]. However, muscle microcirculation and, hence, oxygen delivery may be compromised at tensions <15% of MVC [90]. Similarly, during dynamic exercise, markedly reduced muscle blood flow was observed during the phase of contraction that elicits peak force development [3, 107]. In our fatigue model, expression of the force of dynamic contractions as a percentage of MVC force of rested knee extensor muscles permits noninvasive estimation of the extent and duration of transient quadriceps muscle ischemia during dynamic knee extension. In turn, the estimated degree of ischemia is likely to provide important clues to the nature of the observed fatigue. There are limited published data relating intensity of dynamic exercise to force generation expressed as a percentage of MVC force. In ordinary cycle ergometry, approximately 9%, 12%, and 15% of MVC force were exerted per pedal thrust at work intensities of 60, 80, and 100% of peak oxygen uptake [86, 93]. In contrast, for 1-leg dynamic knee extension, mean values of 10%, 16%, and 27% of MVC force of *rested* muscle were exerted at 66%, 78%, and 100% of peak 1-leg oxygen uptake [36]. The relationship between percentage of MVC force of rested muscle and percentage of peak oxygen uptake (Figure 4.4, Panel B) provides a framework for studying the impact of transient muscle ischemia on fatigue of dynamic exercise.

MYOELECTRIC MANIFESTATIONS OF FATIGUE

The magnitude of electromyographic (EMG) activity in active muscle is determined by the number of muscle fibers recruited and their frequency of excitation— the same factors that determine muscle force. In unfatigued muscle, the amplitude of the rectified integrated EMG activity is directly proportional to muscle force development [12, 15, 16, 72]. During submaximal exercise performed to exhaustion, the effects of fatigue [12, 39, 56, 72, 99, 104] alter this relationship between EMG and muscle force development. Gradually increasing EMG activity during constant force static muscle contraction is a classical correlate of progressive fatigue usually attributed to recruitment of additional motor units and/or increased motoneuron discharge to compensate for gradual contractile failure of active muscle fibers [12].

In contrast to voluminous literature on EMG activity during static contraction, much less attention has been paid to EMG changes during dynamic exercise [15, 16, 39, 56, 88, 99]. This relates partly to effects on the EMG signal of changes in muscle length, variations in movement velocity, and movement of muscle under surface electrodes during dynamic exercise [10]. In addition, interpretation of EMG changes during conventional dynamic exercise is limited by an inability to quantify muscle fatigue. An exception involves measurement of muscle force and EMG activity for repeated isokinetic maximal voluntary concentric contractions during very short duration exercise bouts in which muscular fatigue and exhaustion are rapidly induced [39, 56, 99].

Our knee extension model minimizes several of these concerns, thereby enhancing study of the myoelectric manifestations of gradually increasing fatigue during dynamic contractions. Feedback from the LCD column facilitates precise control of velocity of movement and contraction/relaxation length of the quadriceps muscles throughout the range of motion during each knee extension. Moreover, signals from the inline position transducer allow quantitation of EMG activity at specified knee angles throughout the range of motion. This virtually eliminates potential EMG variation due to muscle length changes and permits tracking—with increasing duration of exercise—of progressive changes in angle-specific EMG activity during dynamic knee extension in addition to progressive changes in force generating capacity and EMG activity during MVC.

The progressive fall in integrated (I) EMG activity during MVCs performed periodically during dynamic knee extension [37] is analogous to falling IEMG activity observed during continuous maximal effort static contractions held to exhaustion [11] and during brief MVCs performed periodically during fatiguing sustained submaximal contractions [60]. Measurement of IEMG during periodic MVCs permits study of gradual changes in both maximal muscle excitation and force generating capacity resulting from fatiguing constant work rate submaximal dynamic exercise. The relationship between maximal muscle excitation and force generating capacity has important implications for the specific mechanisms of muscle fatigue. In our knee extension studies, [37] the gradual fall in maximal IEMG activity during MVC with duration of submaximal dynamic exercise closely overlapped the fall in MVC force (Figure 4.6). This observation supports the view that fatigue of dynamic knee extension was tightly coupled to dimin-

FIGURE 4.6.

Decline in percentage of maximal voluntary contraction (MVC) force (○) and integrated (I) electromyographic (EMG) activity (□) during knee extensor MVC relative to duration of constant work rate knee extension expressed as a percentage of endurance time. Force and IEMG activity are expressed as percentages of maximal values observed during MVC of rested muscle. Lines show average (n = 8 males) declines in MVC force and IEMG derived from average slope of individual regression equations relating percentage changes in MVC force and maximal IEMG activity to percentage of endurance time. Modified from Fulco et al. [37].

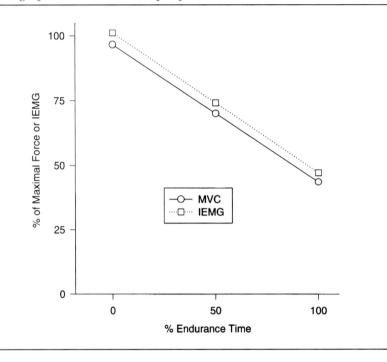

ished muscle excitation. Diminished muscle excitation may relate to a reduced central motor drive [4], an impaired neuromuscular propagation [96], a decline in sarcolemmal conduction velocity [66], and/or a reflex-induced fall in motoneuron firing rate [13, 62]. Additional experiments are needed to define in detail the precise mechanisms involved.

THE POINT OF EXHAUSTION

Emphasis on progressively declining muscle function in the present review contrasts with published physiological and biochemical correlates of impaired dynamic exercise performance relating almost exclusively to the point of exhaustion. For static exercise, in which exhaustion is defined as the inability to maintain a given target force, it is relatively straightforward to relate changes in muscle chemistry, for example, to a specific degree of muscle force failure. This is because the degree of force failure in exhaustive sustained submaximal static exercise is equal to the MVC force expressed as 100% minus the target force expressed as a percent of MVC [80]. In contrast, there is little or no systematic study of the extent to which muscle function is impaired at exhaustion during different intensities and durations of constant work rate dynamic exercise.

Measurement of MVC force at the point of exhaustion using the dynamic knee extension fatigue model provided an initial means of addressing this problem. In healthy young men, MVC force was measured at the point of exhaustion from both constant and graded work rate knee extension [37]. For constant work rate and graded work rate dynamic knee extension, the point of exhaustion corresponded to a similar, approximately 50%, mean fall in MVC force from that of rested muscle. Constant work rate exercise ended at a lower absolute work rate but longer duration than graded work rate exercise. Thus, the point of exhaustion from dynamic knee extension was more closely related to the extent of decline in force generating capacity than to absolute work rate or exercise duration. In healthy young women, MVC force measured at the point of exhaustion from constant work rate dynamic knee extension was somewhat higher than that of men, averaging approximately 60–65% of MVC force of rested muscle (C.S. Fulco, P.B. Rock, and S.F. Lewis, unpublished observations).

At the point of exhaustion from constant work rate exercise, corresponding to an inability to extend the knee from 145° to 150° at the required contraction rate of 1 Hz, knee extensor MVC force was nearly threefold greater than peak dynamic force of submaximal knee extension in men. In our exercise model, peak force of dynamic contraction is achieved at approximately the same knee angle at which static MVC is measured (i.e., 90°), and falls gradually to near zero as the knee angle approaches 150° [36]. Maximal force of dynamic or static MVC was not measured at knee angles approaching 150°. However, at the contraction velocity of $120° \times sec^{-1}$, maximum possible dynamic knee extension force at a knee angle of approximately 150° is likely to be only 35–40% lower than that of static MVC at a similar knee angle [53, 99, 100]. Thus, at the extended knee position, force of submaximal dynamic contraction at the time of exhaustion probably represented a low percentage of remaining force generating capacity, making force failure an unlikely explanation for exhaustion. An inability to extend the knee at angles at which diminished force is unlikely to cause exhaustion implies a failure of knee extensor muscle shortening. Thus, it is reasonable to postulate that muscle exhaustion in men is more closely linked with impaired shortening velocity than with decreased force generating capacity. In agreement, after reaching exhaustion, each male subject (when requested) was able to extend his knee from 90° to 150° at a contraction rate slower than 1 Hz.

SIGNIFICANCE OF THE DYNAMIC KNEE EXTENSION FATIGUE MODEL FOR STUDYING THE EFFECTS OF EXPERIMENTAL INTERVENTIONS ON EXERCISE PERFORMANCE

Unique features of the knee extension model enhance the ability to define in detail the effects of a given intervention on several specific measures of voluntary muscle function during *a single bout of constant work rate exercise.* Experiments using the knee extension model routinely include each of the four following primary performance measures: MVC force of rested muscle (i.e., strength); rate of decline in MVC force during dynamic exercise (i.e., fatigue); time to exhaustion (i.e., endurance); and, percentage of rested MVC force reached at the limit of endurance (i.e., the point of exhaustion). For each of these four measures, any given experimental intervention will elicit three possible effects: An increase, decrease, or no change. This theoretically permits 4^3 or 64 different specific combinations of effects of an acute or chronic intervention on knee extensor muscle performance. In contrast, for conventional constant work rate cycle or treadmill exercise, endurance time to exhaustion frequently serves as the sole measure of performance, and only three overall effects—an increase, decrease, or no change—are observable.

The ability to demonstrate multiple effects of different experimental interventions is likely to provide the knee extensor fatigue approach with potential for novel insights into primary determinants of muscle performance and their potential interactions. This concept is illustrated in Figure 4.7, panels A-D. Panel A shows a comparison of knee extension exercise under conditions of normoxia versus acute exposure to hypobaric hypoxia. In response to the same absolute constant work rate, hypoxia resulted in no change in MVC force of rested muscle, an increase in fatigue rate, a decrease in endurance time, and no change in percentage of rested MVC force reached at the point of exhaustion [37]. Panel B shows the postulated outcome of a comparison of subjects studied before and after significant loss of lean body weight through prolonged semi-starvation. In response to the same absolute constant work rate, underfeeding may be postulated to result in a drop in MVC force of rested muscle, no change in fatigue rate, a decrease in endurance time, and no change in percentage of rested MVC force reached at the point of exhaustion. Panel C depicts the postulated outcome of a comparison of subjects studied before and after strength training of the knee extensor muscles. In response to the same absolute constant work rate, strength training is postulated to result in a marked increase in MVC force of rested muscle, a little or no decline in fatigue rate, a longer endurance time, and a similar or lower percentage of rested

FIGURE 4.7.

Interaction of muscle strength, fatigue rate, endurance time to exhaustion, and percentage MVC force recorded at the point of exhaustion during hypobaric hypoxia (A); lean body weight loss (B); strength training (C); and endurance training (D). Relative to baseline values, muscle performance changes during hypobaric hypoxia exposure were demonstrated experimentally [37] while the effects of the other interventions are postulated. A and B depict reduced endurance time to exhaustion during acute hypoxia and after substantial lean body weight loss due to prolonged semi-starvation. Use of the leg extension exercise model is likely to reveal whether shortened endurance times are due to decreased strength, increased fatigue rate, a difference in maximal voluntary contraction (MVC) force at the point of exhaustion, or a combination of these factors. For hypobaric hypoxia, strength was not altered but rate of fatigue was accelerated [37]. In contrast, a reduction in muscle mass due to prolonged semi-starvation is likely to cause a loss in strength and endurance [97] without a marked change in rate of fatigue. Neither hypoxia exposure nor loss of lean body weight is likely to alter the percentage of MVC force of rested muscle measured at the point of exhaustion. C and D illustrate postulated increases in endurance times to exhaustion resulting from strength and endurance training, respectively. For strength training, an increase in time to exhaustion is likely to be associated with an increase in strength and little change in rate of fatigue. In contrast, the increase in time to exhaustion following endurance training is likely to be associated with no change in strength and an attenuated fatigue rate. For these interventions involving physical conditioning, exhaustion is postulated to occur at a slightly lower percentage of rested MVC force.

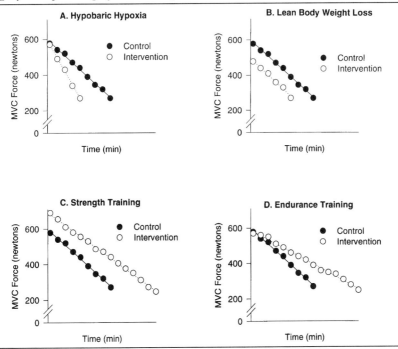

MVC force reached at the point of exhaustion. Panel D shows the potential outcome of a comparison of subjects studied before and after endurance training of the knee extensor muscles. In response to the same absolute constant work rate, endurance training is postulated to result in no change in MVC force of rested muscle, a marked decline in fatigue rate, a marked increase in endurance time, and about the same percentage of rested MVC force reached at the point of exhaustion. A basic tenet of these examples is that the physiological links between such familiar performance constructs as strength, endurance, fatigue and, exhaustion are poorly defined [64, 67, 68, 103], and that the knee extension model is likely to provide a valuable experimental probe. Dissection of the synergistic versus antagonistic effects on performance of combined strength and endurance training [25, 44, 85] is one potential application.

The value of the dynamic knee extension model in studying intervention-related changes in performance is underscored by observations of relatively minor intra-individual test-retest variation in each of the knee extensor performance measures (i.e., MVC force of rested muscle, fatigue rate, endurance time, and percentage of rested MVC force achieved at the point of exhaustion in untrained subjects) (Figure 4.8). Reproducibility of knee extensor MVC force as measured by correlation coefficient (R) or test-retest percentage variation is similar to that reported previously [58, 63, 102]. In contrast, test-retest percentage variation in endurance time to exhaustion for dynamic knee extension tends to be less than that for constant work rate cycle ergometry [41, 50, 57] (Figure 4.9). Marked within-subject variation in cycle endurance time has been reported even in subjects familiar with exhaustive leg exercise, such as well-trained long distance cyclists [50]. For trained cyclists, intra-individual performance variation tends to be smaller for time-trial cycling in which subjects are asked to perform a given quantity of work in the shortest possible time than for endurance time to exhaustion at a constant work rate [50]. Nevertheless, time-trial testing, like endurance time testing, typically provides only a single measurement of muscle performance. In addition, individual variation in pacing during time-trial testing renders serial measurement of performance impractical.

Minimization of test-retest variability of knee extension exercise performance measurements improves the resolution for detecting potential changes caused by a given intervention. For example, a power analysis (n = 15; α = 0.05; β = 0.25) [112] indicated that in order to demonstrate statistical significance, an intervention would have to improve endurance time to exhaustion by more than 17% during conventional cycling [50] but by less than 11% during dynamic knee extension. Another advantage to the dynamic knee extension model is that the muscle fatigue rate, calculated from multiple periodic measurements of MVC force from rest to exhaustion, is unlikely to be markedly affected by an occasional poorly per-

FIGURE 4.8.

Test-retest data for (A) maximal voluntary contraction (MVC) force, (B) fatigue rate, (C) endurance time to exhaustion, and (D) percentage of MVC force of rested muscle reached at exhaustion in 11 young, healthy women during two identical constant work rate, one-leg dynamic knee extension tests performed with a 4 to 8 day interval. To minimize the effects on performance of physical conditioning and habituation to the laboratory environment, each subject completed at least two preliminary exercise sessions prior to the two definitive tests. Data are from C.S. Fulco, P.B. Rock, and S.F. Lewis (unpublished observations).

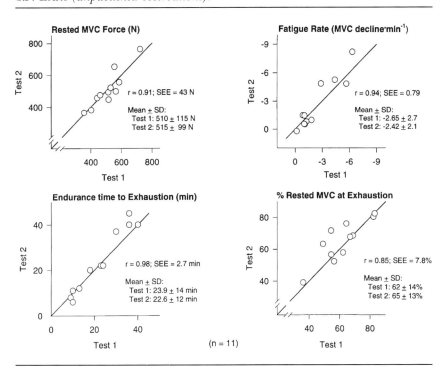

formed MVC due to a momentary lapse in motivation or concentration, or by a nonrecorded MVC due to technical problems.

APPLICATION OF THE KNEE EXTENSION MODEL TO STUDY IMPAIRED EXERCISE PERFORMANCE IN HYPOBARIC HYPOXIA

Recently, we used the 1-leg knee extension fatigue model to compare exercise performance under conditions of normoxia versus acute hypobaric hypoxia (464 torr) in healthy young men [37]. The knee extension model was employed in an attempt to resolve discrepancies relating to previous

FIGURE 4.9.

Test-retest variability in endurance time to exhaustion for dynamic knee extension and conventional cycle ergometry. Cycle data are from: Table 2, test 3 vs test 4, test 4 vs test 5, and test 3 vs test 5, respectively, of Jeukendrup et al. [50]; Krebs and Powers [57]; and Table 3, "no rest" tests conducted during weeks 1 and 6 of Gleser and Vogel [41]. Values are means ± standard deviation (SD) of the absolute test-retest differences in endurance time to exhaustion.

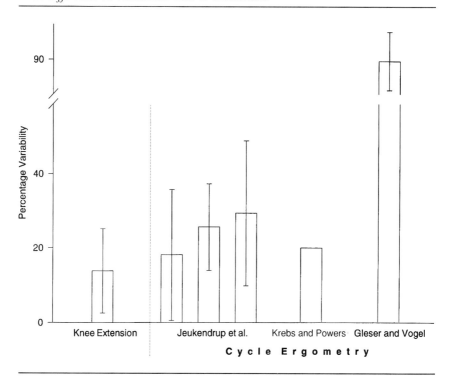

findings in hypoxia of a marked diminution of submaximal treadmill or cycle exercise performance [38, 42, 48, 95], an increase in MVC force of rested muscle [21, 110], and a lack of consistently impaired performance [19, 29, 52, 110]. As found by some workers [21, 110], without serial measurements of MVC force during exercise, a similar endurance time to exhaustion in normoxia and hypobaria may relate to a higher MVC force of rested muscle in hypobaria that obscures a faster rate of decline in force generating capacity. Our subjects performed the same constant work rate (21 ± 3 W, 79 ± 2% and 87 ± 2% of 1-leg knee extension $\dot{V}O_2$peak for normoxia and hypobaria, respectively), eliciting 18 ± 1% of MVC force of rested muscle under normoxic and hypobaric conditions. Endurance time to exhaustion was more than 50% shorter in hypobaria than in normoxia, but strength of rested muscle was similar for both conditions. Quadriceps muscle force generating capacity declined at a nearly twofold faster rate for hypobaria than for normoxia (depicted schematically in Figure 4.7, panel A). At the point of exhaustion, subjects reached approximately the same strength decrement and level of perceived difficulty under each condition. For both normoxia and hypoxia, MVC force fell to approximately 50% of that of rested muscle, the percentage of MVC force represented by the peak force of each dynamic contraction was approximately 38% of MVC force of exercising muscle, and ratings of perceived exertion localized to active muscle were similar. Consistent with the faster rate of fatigue in hypobaria, these findings imply that the shorter endurance time for hypobaria was closely linked to diminished muscle performance, per se, and not due simply to a decline in motivation, a poorer tolerance of physical discomfort, or a reduced ability to ignore perceptual cues associated with impending exhaustion.

We also observed that the difference in knee extensor force generating capacity between normoxia and hypobaria did not reach statistical significance until the fourth min of dynamic knee extension. In agreement are previous experimental findings of no difference between normoxia and hypoxia in muscle performance during very high intensity, short duration contractions [29, 46, 47, 52], and a lack of effect of hypoxia on competitive running times in races lasting less than three minutes [34]. In contrast to a 25–30% lower $\dot{V}O_2$ peak reported for treadmill or cycle ergometer exercise in hypoxia [31, 111], we observed that peak 1-leg knee extension oxygen uptake was only 9% lower in hypobaric hypoxia than in normoxia [37]. Accordingly, we found a much smaller fall in arterial oxygen saturation for 1-leg knee extension than seen previously for cycle ergometer exercise at a similar degree of hypobaria. The markedly greater muscle fatigue during constant work rate 1-leg knee extension in hypobaria was thus postulated to relate more closely to a reduced local muscle capillary-to-mitochondrial oxygen gradient that in turn, modified regulation of muscle oxidative phosphorylation, than simply to reduced arterial oxygen content. In view of the above discussion, the ability of our model to provide performance data on strength, fatigue, endurance, exhaustion, and peak oxygen uptake with the same muscle group seems advantageous in interpreting the specific impact of hypobaria on muscle fatigue and exercise performance.

UNSOLVED PROBLEMS AND DIRECTIONS FOR NEW RESEARCH

To date, the dynamic knee extension fatigue model has focused exclusively on declining force of maximal voluntary static contractions as an index of gradual impairment in muscle performance during constant work rate exercise. Emphasis on impaired force production as an index of fatigue in dynamic exercise derives in part from use of isokinetic contractions to track progressive changes in peak torque and power [8, 40, 54]. During isokinetic contractions, the angular velocity of the lever arm is maintained constant throughout the range of motion, thereby obscuring the potential contribution of diminished peak muscle shortening velocity to declining power output. Isokinetic exercise has, nevertheless, provided important information regarding the torque component of the rapid *power failure* characteristic of very high intensity dynamic exercise [8, 29, 53, 59, 65, 70, 101, 108]. Thusly used, conventional isokinetic exercise, per se, does not permit study of the declining force generating capacity during dynamic exercise at constant work rate. Apparatus specialized for performance of peak effort isokinetic contractions periodically during conventional cycle ergometry [49] does, however, allow quantitation of progressive loss in peak force and power during constant work rate exercise. Nevertheless, peak power output is a function of both strength, i.e., MVC force and speed of movement, and it is likely that power loss associated with fatiguing dynamic exercise is due to impairments in generation of both peak muscle force and velocity [32, 77]. However, a remarkable paucity of published data exists on peak voluntary movement velocity as an expression of peak velocity of shortening of intact human muscle [20, 51, 76, 109]. The significance of this omission is punctuated by the Fenn effect (i.e., the marked increase in adenosine triphosphate—ATP—cost of contractions involving both shortening and force development above those involving only isometric force development) [30, 75], and the large body of data linking fatigue of dynamic exercise to cellular events associated with very high rates of contractile ATP utilization compared to slower ATP production via muscle oxidative metabolism [1, 6, 33, 83, 94, 98, 106]. Additional research is therefore needed to define in detail the time courses of change in both peak force generating capacity and peak velocity of shortening as functions of intensity and duration of dynamic exercise, as well as to identify the contributions of both force and velocity to the inability to maintain a constant work rate (i.e., the point of exhaustion).

ACKNOWLEDGEMENTS

Work related to this review was performed in part while S.F. Lewis was a Senior Research Associate of the National Research Council, in the Military Nutrition and Biochemistry Division, United States Army Research Institute of Environmental Medicine (USARIEM), Natick, MA. Some studies conducted by C.S. Fulco were supported in part by the USARIEM Defense Women's Health Research Program (DWHRP), #DI950050, and/or were done in collaboration with the following colleagues to whom the authors are most grateful: B. Braun, G. Butterfield, A. Cymerman, P. Frykman, E.A.

Harmon, K.W. Kambis, E. Lammi, L.G. Moore, S.R. Muza, K.B. Pandolf, J.T. Reeves, P.B. Rock, and S. Zamudio.

REFERENCES

1. Allen, D.G., H. Westerblad, and J. Lannergren. The role of intracellular acidosis in muscle fatigue. S.C. Gandevia, R.M. Enoka, A.J. McComas, D.G. Stuart, and C.K. Thomas (eds). *Fatigue: Neural and Muscular Mechanisms*. New York: Plenum Press, 1995, pp. 57–68.

2. Andersen, P., R. P. Adams, G. Sjogaard, A. Thorboe, and B. Saltin. Dynamic knee extension as model for study of isolated exercising muscle in humans. *J. Appl. Physiol.* 59: 1647–1653, 1985.

3. Andersen, P., and B. Saltin. Maximal perfusion to skeletal muscle in man. *J. Physiol. (London)* 366:233–249, 1985.

4. Asmussen, E. Muscle fatigue. *Med. Sci. Sports* 11:313–321, 1979.

5. Bangsbo, J., L. Johansen, T. Graham, and B. Saltin. Lactate and H$^+$ effluxes from human skeletal muscles during intense, dynamic exercise. *J. Physiol. (London)* 462:115–133, 1993.

6. Bangsbo, J., K. Madsen, B. Kiens, and E.A. Richter. Effect of muscle acidity on muscle metabolism and fatigue during intense exercise in man. *J. Physiol. (London)* 495:587–596, 1996.

7. Basmajian, J.V., and C.J. DeLuca. Muscle fatigue and time-dependent parameters of the surface EMG signal. J. V. Basmajian and C.J. DeLuca (eds). *Muscle Alive: Their Functions Revealed by Electromyography*. Baltimore, MD:Waverly Press, Inc, 1985, pp. 201–222.

8. Beelen, A., A.J. Sargeant, and F. Wijkhuizen. Measurement of directional force and power during human submaximal and maximal isokinetic exercise. *Eur. J. Appl. Physiol.* 68: 177–181, 1994.

9. Bigland, B., and O.C.J. Lippold. The relation between force, velocity and integrated electrical activity in human muscles. *J. Physiol. (London)* 123:214–224, 1954.

10. Bigland-Ritchie, B. EMG and fatigue of human voluntary and stimulated contractions. Ciba Foundation (ed). *Human Muscle Fatigue: Physiological Mechanisms*. London:Pitman Medical, 1981, pp. 130–156.

11. Bigland-Ritchie, B. EMG/force relations and fatigue of human voluntary contractions. D. I. Miller (ed). *Exercise and Sport Sciences Reviews*. The Franklin Institute, 1981, pp. 75–117.

12. Bigland-Ritchie, B., N.J. Dawson, R.S. Johansson, and O.C.J. Lippold. Reflex origin for the slowing of motoneurone firing rates in fatigue of human voluntary contractions. *J. Physiol. (London)* 379:451–459, 1986.

13. Bigland-Ritchie, B., F. Furbush, and J.J. Woods. Fatigue of intermittent submaximal voluntary contractions: central and peripheral factors. *J. Appl. Physiol.* 61:421–429, 1986.

14. Bigland-Ritchie, B., R. Johansson, O.C. J. Lippold, and J.J. Woods. Contractile speed and EMG changes during fatigue of sustained maximal voluntary contractions. *J. Neurophysiol.* 50:313–324, 1983.

15. Bigland-Ritchie, B., and J.J. Woods. Integrated EMG and oxygen uptake during dynamic contractions of human muscles. *J. Appl. Physiol.* 36:475–479, 1974.

16. Bigland-Ritchie, B., and J.J. Woods. Integrated electromyogram and oxygen uptake during positive and negative work. *J. Physiol. (London)* 260:267–277, 1976.

17. Bigland-Ritchie, B., and J J. Woods. Changes in muscle contractile properties and neural control during human muscular fatigue. *Muscle Nerve* 7:691–699, 1984.

18. Bourguignon, A., R. Marty, and J. Scherrer. Etude du travail musculaire et de la fatigue. Il donnees dynamographiques obtenues chez l'homme. *J. Physiol. (Paris)* 51:93–110, 1959.

19. Bowie, W., and G.R. Cumming. Sustained handgrip-reproducibility: effects of hypoxia. *Med. Sci. Sports* 3: 24–31, 1971.

20. Brozek, J., E. Simonson, and A. Keys. A test of speed of leg and arm movements. *J. Appl. Physiol.* 4:753–760, 1952.

21. Burse, R.L., A. Cymerman, and A.J. Young. Respiratory response and muscle function during isometric handgrip exercise at high altitude. *Av. Space Environ. Med.* 58:39–46, 1987.

22. Crenshaw, A.G., S. Karlsson, J. Styf, T. Backlund, and J. Friden. Knee extension torque and intramuscular pressure of the vastus lateralis muscle during eccentric and concentric activities. *Eur. J. Appl. Physiol.* 70:13–19, 1995.

23. Davies, C.T.M., and M.W. Thompson. Physiological responses to prolonged exercise in ultramarathon athletes. *J. Appl. Physiol.* 61:611–617, 1986.

24. Davies, C.T.M., and M.J. White. Muscle weakness following dynamic exercise in humans. *J. Appl. Physiol.* 53:236–241, 1982.

25. Dudley, G.A., and R. Djamil. Incompatibility of endurance- and strength-training modes of exercise. *J. Appl. Physiol.* 59:1446–1451, 1985.

26. Edwards, R.H.T. Human muscle function and fatigue. R. Porter and J. Whelan (eds). *Human Muscle Fatigue: Physiological Mechanisms.* London: Pitman Medical, 1981, pp. 1–18.

27. Edwards, R.H.T., and H. Gibson. Perspectives in the study of normal and pathological skeletal muscle. G. Altan, L. Beliveau, and P. Bouissou (eds). *Muscle Fatigue: Biochemical and Physiological Aspects.* Paris: Masson, 1991, pp. 3–15.

28. Edwards, R.H.T., D.K. Hill, and M. McDonnell. Myothermal and intramuscular pressure measurements during isometric contractions of the human quadriceps muscle. *J. Physiol. (London)* 224:58P–59P, 1972. (Abstract)

29. Eiken, O., and P.A. Tesch. Effects of hyperoxia and hypoxia on dynamic and sustained static performance of the human quadriceps muscle. *Acta Physiol. Scand.* 122:629–633, 1984.

30. Fenn, W.O. A quantitative comparison between the energy liberated and the work performed by isolated sartorius muscle of the frog. *J. Physiol. (London)* 58:175–203, 1923.

31. Ferretti, G., C. Moia, J.M. Thomet, and B. Kayser. The decrease of maximal oxygen consumption during hypoxia in man: a mirror image of the oxygen equilibrium curve. *J. Physiol. (London)* 498.1:231–237, 1997.

32. Fitts, R.H. Cellular mechanisms of muscle fatigue. *Physiol. Rev.* 74:49–94, 1994.

33. Fitts, R.H., and E.M. Balog. Effect of intracellular and extracellular ion changes on E-C coupling and skeletal muscle fatigue. *Acta Physiol. Scand.* 156:169–181, 1995.

34. Fulco, C.S., and A. Cymerman. Physical performance at varying altitudes. P.B. Rock and R. Pozos (eds). *Textbook of Military Medicine: Medical Aspects of Deployment to Harsh Environments.* Washington, D.C.:Borden Institute, 1998.

35. Fulco, C.S., A. Cymerman, S.R. Muza, P.B. Rock, K.B. Pandolf, and S.F. Lewis. Adductor pollicis muscle fatigue during acute and chronic altitude exposure and return to sea level. *J. Appl. Physiol.* 77:179–183, 1994.

36. Fulco, C.S., S.F. Lewis, P. Frykman, et al.. Quantitation of progressive muscle fatigue during dynamic leg exercise in humans. *J. Appl. Physiol.* 79:2154–2162, 1995.

37. Fulco, C.S., S.F. Lewis, P. Frykman, et al. Muscle fatigue and exhaustion during dynamic leg exercise in normoxia and hypobaric hypoxia. *J. Appl. Physiol.* 81:1891–1900, 1996.

38. Fulco, C.S., P.B. Rock, L. Trad, V. Forte, Jr., and A. Cymerman. Maximal cardiorespiratory responses to one- and two-legged cycling during acute and long-term exposure to 4300 meters altitude. *Eur. J. Appl. Physiol.* 57:761–766, 1988.

39. Gerdle, B., and J. Elert. The temporal occurrence of the mean power frequency shift of the electromyogram during maximal prolonged dynamic and static working cycles. *Int. J. Sports Med.* 15 Suppl. 1:S32–S37, 1994.

40. Gleeson, N.P., and T.H. Mercer. The utility of isokinetic dynamometry in the assessment of human muscle function. *Sports Med.* 21:18–34, 1996.

41. Gleser, M.A., and J.A. Vogel. Endurance exercise: effect of work-rest schedules and repeated testing. *J. Appl. Physiol.* 31:735–739, 1971.

42. Gleser, M.A., and J.A. Vogel. Effects of acute alterations of V̇O2max on endurance capacity of men. *J. Appl. Physiol.* 34:443–447, 1973.

43. Gray, J.C., and J.M. Chandler. Percent decline in peak torque production during repeated concentric and eccentric contractions of the quadriceps femoris muscle. *J. Orthop. Sports Phys. Ther.* 10:309–314, 1989.

44. Hickson, R.C. Interference of strength development by simultaneously training for strength and endurance. *Eur. J. Appl. Physiol.* 45:255–263, 1980.

45. Hoffman, M.D., C.A. Williams, and A.R. Lind. Changes in isometric function following rhythmic exercise. *Eur. J. Appl. Physiol.* 54:177–183, 1985.

46. Hogan, M.C., J. Roca, P.D. Wagner, and J.B. West. Limitation of maximal O2 uptake and performance by acute hypoxia in dog muscle in situ. *J. Appl. Physiol.* 65:815–821, 1988.

47. Hogan, M.C., and H.G. Welch. Effect of altered arterial O2 tensions on muscle metabolism in dog skeletal muscle during fatiguing work. *Am. J. Physiol.* 251:C216–C222, 1986.

48. Horstman, D., R. Weiskoff, and R.E. Jackson. Work capacity during 3-wk sojourn at 4,300 m: effects of relative polycythemia. *J. Appl. Physiol.* 49:311–318, 1980.

49. James, C., P. Sacco, and D.A. Jones. Loss of power during fatigue of human leg muscles. *J. Physiol. (London)* 484.1:237–246, 1995.

50. Jeukendrup, A., W.H.M. Saris, F. Brouns, and A.D.M. Kester. A new validated endurance performance test. *Med. Sci. Sports Exerc.* 28:266–270, 1996.

51. Jones, D.A., H.M. Seymour, S. Ward, and J. Rowbury. Changes in the force/velocity relationship of the fatigued human adductor pollicis muscle. *J. Physiol. (London)* 473: 89P, 1993. (Abstract)

52. Kaijser, L. Limiting factors for aerobic muscle performance: the influence of varying oxygen pressure and temperature. *Acta Physiol. Scand.* 346:S1–S96, 1970.

53. Knapik, J.J., J.E. Wright, R.H. Mawdsley, and J. Braun. Isometric, isotonic and isokinetic torque variations in four muscle groups through a range of motion. *J. Am. Phys. Ther. Assoc.* 63:838–847, 1983.

54. Knapik, J.J., J.E. Wright, R.H. Mawdsley, and J.M. Braun. Isokinetic, isometric and isotonic strength relationships. *Arch. Phys. Med. Rehab.* 64:77–80, 1983.

55. Knuttgen, H.G., F.B. Petersen, and K. Klausen. Exercise with concentric and eccentric muscle contractions. *Acta Paediat. Scand. Suppl.* 217:42–46, 1971.

56. Komi, P.V., and P. Tesch. EMG frequency spectrum, muscle structure, and fatigue during dynamic contractions in man. *Eur. J. Appl. Physiol.* 42:41–50, 1979.

57. Krebs, P.S., and S.K. Powers. Reliability of laboratory endurance tests. *Med. Sci. Sports Exerc.* 31:S10, 1989. (Abstract)

58. Kroll, W. Reliability variations of strength in test-retest situations. *Res. Quart.* 34:50–55, 1963.

59. Lands, L.C., L. Hornby, G. Desrocher, T. Iler, and J. F. Heigenhauser. A simple isokinetic cycle for measurement of leg muscle function. *J. Appl. Physiol.* 77:2506–2510, 1994.

60. Lind, A.R., and J.S. Petrofsky. Amplitude of the surface electromyogram during fatiguing isometric contractions. *Muscle Nerve* 2:257–264, 1979.

61. Lind, A.R., R.R. Rochelle, J.S. Rinehart, J S. Petrofsky, and R.L. Burse. Isometric fatigue induced by different levels of rhythmic exercise. *Eur. J. Appl. Physiol.* 49:243–254, 1982.

62. Macefield, G., K.E. Hagbarth, R. Gorman, S.C. Gandevia, and D. Burke. Decline in spindle support to α-motoneurones during sustained voluntary contractions. *J. Physiol. (London)* 440:497–512, 1991.

63. Mannion, A.F., P.M. Jakeman, and P.L.T. Willan. Effects of isokinetic training of the knee extensors on isometric strength and peak power output during cycling. *Eur. J. Appl. Physiol.* 65:370–375, 1992.

64. Maughan, R.J., M.A. Nimmo, and M. Harmon. The relationship between muscle myosin ATP-ase activity and isometric endurance in untrained male subjects. *Eur. J. Appl. Physiol.* 54:291–296, 1985.

65. McCartney, N., J.F. Heigenhauser, A.J. Sargeant, and N.L. Jones. A constant-velocity cycle ergometer for the study of dynamic muscle function. *J. Appl. Physiol.* 55:212–217, 1983.

66. Milner-Brown, H.S., and R.G. Miller. Muscle membrane excitation and impulse propagation velocity are reduced during muscle fatigue. *Muscle Nerve* 9:367–374, 1986.

67. Monod, H. How muscles are used in the body. G. H. Bourne (ed). *The Structure and Function of Muscle.* New York: Academic Press, 1972, pp. 23–74.

68. Mundale, M.O. The relationship of intermittent isometric exercise to fatigue of hand grip. *Arch. Phys. Med. Rehab.* 51: 32–539, 1950.

69. Noble, B.J. Clinical applications of perceived exertion. *Med. Sci. Sports Exerc.* 14:406–411, 1992.

70. Osternig, L.R. Isokinetic Dynamometry: Implications for muscle testing and rehabilitation. K. B. Pandolf (ed.). *Exercise and Sport Sciences Reviews.* New York: Macmillan Publishing Company, 1986, pp. 45–80.

71. Pandolf, K.B. Differential ratings of perceived exertion during physical exercise. *Med. Sci. Sports Exerc.* 14:397–405, 1982.

72. Petrofsky, J.S., and C.A. Phillips. The physiology of static exercise. K. B. Pandolf (ed.). *Exercise and Sport Sciences Reviews.* New York: Macmillan Publishing Company, 1986, pp. 1–44.

73. Petrofsky, J.S., R.R. Rochelle, J.S. Rinehart, R.L. Burse, and A.R. Lind. The assessment of the static component in rhythmic exercise. *Eur. J. Appl. Physiol.* 34:55–63, 1975.

74. Potvin, J.R., and R.W. Norman. Quantification of erector spinae muscle fatigue during prolonged, dynamic lifting tasks. *Eur. J. Appl. Physiol.* 67: 554–562, 1993.

75. Rall, J.A. Sense and nonsense about the Fenn effect. *Am. J. Physiol.* 242: H1–H6, 1982.

76. Ralston, H.J., M.J. Polissar, V.T. Inman, J.R. Close, and B. Feinstein. Dynamic features of human isolated voluntary muscle in isometric and free contractions. *J. Appl. Physiol.* 1:526–533, 1949.

77. Report of the Respiratory Muscle Fatigue Workshop Group. Respiratory Muscle Fatigue. *Ann. Rev. Respir. Dis.* 142:474–480, 1990.

78. Richardson, R.S., D.C. Poole, D.R. Knight, S.S., et al. High blood flow in man: is maximal O_2 extraction compromised? *J. Appl. Physiol.* 75:1911–1916, 1993.

79. Richter, E.A., B. Kiens, and B. Saltin. Skeletal muscle glucose uptake during dynamic exercise in humans: Role of muscle mass. *Am. J. Physiol.* 254:E555–E561, 1988.

80. Rohmert, W. Physiologische grundlagen der erholungszeitbestimmung. *Zbl. Arbeit. Wiss.* 26:363–369, 1965.

81. Rowell, L B., B. Saltin, B. Kiens, and N. Juel Christensen. Is peak quadriceps blood flow in humans even higher during exercise with hypoxemia? *Am. J. Physiol.* 251: H1038–H1044, 1986.

82. Sadamoto, T., F. Bonde-Petersen, and Y. Suzuki. Skeletal muscle tension, flow, pressure, and EMG during sustained isometric contractions in humans. *Eur. J. Appl. Physiol.* 51: 395–408, 1983.

83. Sahlin, K. Metabolic changes limiting muscle performance. B. Saltin (ed.). *Biochemistry of Exercise VI*, Champaign, IL: Human Kinetics, 1986, pp. 323–343.

84. Sahlin, K., and J.Y. Seger. Effects of prolonged exercise on the contractile properties of human quadriceps muscle. *Eur. J. Appl. Physiol.* 71:180–186, 1995.

85. Sale, D.G., J.D. MacDougall, I. Jacobs, and S. Garner. Interaction between concurrent strength and endurance training. *J. Appl. Physiol.* 68:260–270, 1990.

86. Saltin, B. Muscle fiber recruitment and metabolism in exhaustive dynamic exercise. R. Porter and J. Whelan (eds.). *Human Muscle Fatigue: Physiological Mechanisms.* London: Pitman, 1981, pp. 41–58.

87. Saltin, B. Hemodynamic adaptations to exercise. *Am. J. Cardiology* 55:42–47, 1985.

88. Scherrer, J., and A. Bourguignon. Changes in the electromyogram produced by fatigue in man. *Am. J. Phys. Med.* 38:148–158, 1959.

89. Sejersted, O.M., A.R. Haggens, K.R. Kardel, P. Blom, O. Jensen, and L. Hermansen. Intramuscular fluid pressure during isometric contraction of human skeletal muscle. *J. Appl. Physiol.* 56:287–295, 1984.

90. Sejersted, O.M., and A.R. Hargens. Intramuscular pressures for monitoring different tasks and muscle conditions. S.C. Gandevia, R.M. Enoka, A.J. McComas, D.G. Stuart, and C.K. Thomas (eds). *Fatigue: Neural and Muscular Mechanisms.* New York:Plenum Press, 1995, pp. 361–380.

91. Sherman, W.M., L.E. Armstrong, T.M. Murray, et al. Effect of a 42.2-km footrace and subsequent rest or exercise on muscular strength and work capacity. *J. Appl. Physiol.* 57: 1668–1673, 1984.

92. Simonson, E. Introduction. E. Simonson (ed). *Physiology of Work Capacity and Fatigue.* Springfield, IL:Charles C. Thomas, 1971, pp. xi–xviii.

93. Sjøgaard, G. Force-velocity curve for bicycle work. E. Asmussen and K. Jorgensen (eds). *Biomechanics VI.* Baltimore, MD:University Park Press, 1978, pp. 93–99.

94. Sjøgaard, G., and A.J. McComas. Role of interstitial potassium. S.C. Gandevia, R.M. Enoka, A.J. McComas, D.G. Stuart, and C.K. Thomas (eds). *Fatigue: Neural and Muscular Mechanisms.* New York:Plenum Press, 1995, pp. 69–80.

95. Stenberg, J., B. Ekblom, and R. Messin. Hemodynamic response to work at simulated altitude, 4,000 m. *J. Appl. Physiol.* 21:1589–1594, 1966.

96. Stephens, J.A., and A. Taylor. Fatigue of maintained voluntary muscle contraction in man. *J. Physiol. (London)* 220:1–18, 1972.

97. Taylor, H.L., E.R. Buskirk, J. Brozek, J.T. Anderson, and F. Grande. Performance capacity and effects of caloric restriction with hard physical work on young men. *J. Appl. Physiol.* 10: 421–429, 1957.

98. Tesch, P. Muscle fatigue in man. With special reference to lactate accumulation during short term intense exercise. *Acta Physiol. Scand. Suppl.* 480:1–40, 1980.

99. Tesch, P. A., G. A. Dudley, M. R. Duvoisin, B. M. Hather, and R. T. Harris. Force and EMG signal patterns during repeated bouts of concentric or eccentric muscle actions. *Acta Physiol. Scand.* 138:263–271, 1990.

100. Thorstensson, A., G. Grimby, and J. Karlsson. Force-velocity and fiber composition in human knee extensor muscles. *J. Appl. Physiol.* 40:12–16, 1976.

101. Tihanyi, J., P. Apor, and G.Y. Fekete. Force-velocity-power characteristics and fiber composition in human knee extensor muscles. *Eur. J. Appl. Physiol.* 48:331–343, 1982.

102. Tornvall, G. Assessment of physical capabilities (with special reference to the evaluation of maximal voluntary isometric muscle strength and maximal working capacity). *Acta Physiol. Scand.* 58:1–101, 1963.

103. Tuttle, W.W., C.D. Janney, and C.W. Thompson. Relation of maximum grip strength to grip strength endurance. *J. Appl. Physiol.* 2:663–670, 1950.

104. Viitasalo, J.H.T., and P.V. Komi. Signal characteristics of the EMG during fatigue. *Eur. J. Appl. Physiol.* 37:111–121, 1977.

105. Vollestad, K.K., O.M. Sejersted, R. Bahr, J.J. Woods, and B. Bigland-Ritchie. Motor drive and metabolic responses during repeated submaximal contractions in humans. *J. Appl. Physiol.* 64:1421–1427, 1988.

106. Vollestad, N.K. Metabolic Correlates of Fatigue from Different Types of Exercise in Man. S.C. Gandevia, R.M. Enoka, A.J. McComas, D.G. Stuart, and C.K. Thomas (eds). *Fatigue: Neural and Muscular Mechanism.* New York:Plenum Press, 1995, pp. 185–194.

107. Walloe, L., and J. Wesche. Time course and magnitude of blood flow changes in the human quadriceps muscles during and following rhythmic exercise. *J. Physiol. (London)* 405:257–273, 1988.

108. Westing, S.H., A.G. Cresswell, and A. Thorstensson. Muscle activation during maximal voluntary eccentric and concentric knee extension. *Eur. J. Appl. Physiol.* 62:104–108, 1991.

109. Wilkie, D.R. The relation between force and velocity in human muscle. *J. Physiol. (London)* 110:249–280, 1950.

110. Young, A., J. Wright, J. Knapik, and A. Cymerman. Skeletal muscle strength during exposure to hypobaric hypoxia. *Med. Sci. Sports Exerc.* 12:330–335, 1980.
111. Young, A.J., A. Cymerman, and R.L. Burse. The influence of cardiorespiratory fitness on the decrement in maximal aerobic power at high altitude. *Eur. J. Appl. Physiol.* 54: 12–15, 1985.
112. Zar, J.H. *Biostatistical Analysis.* Englewood Cliffs, N.J.:PrenticeHall, 1984.

5
Malonyl-CoA—Regulator of Fatty Acid Oxidation in Muscle During Exercise

WILLIAM W. WINDER, PH.D.

FATTY ACID OXIDATION INCREASES DURING EXERCISE

The increased energy requirements during exercise are met by an increase in both carbohydrate and fat oxidation [13, 16, 24, 30, 40, 46, 49]. At rest, the rate of fatty acid oxidation in both endurance-trained and non-trained human subjects is approximately 3–5 μmol/kg/min [21,33]. When exercising, the rate of fatty acid oxidation differs between non-trained and trained subjects. During exercise that required an oxygen uptake of 20 ml/kg/min, fatty acid oxidation in non-trained subjects increased to 12 μmol/kg/min after 15 min of exercise, and to 20 μmol/kg/min after 3–4 hr of exercise at this low work-rate [21]. The rate of fat oxidation was higher in trained subjects working at the same absolute work-rate [21]. In a study with trained cyclists, the rate of fat oxidation increased over resting values (reported in other studies in the same laboratory) at all work rates studied. When subjects worked for 30 min, the rate of fat oxidation was 26.8 μmol/kg/min at 25% of Vo_{2max}, 42.8 μmol/kg/min at 65% of $Vo_{2max,}$ and 29.6 μmol/kg/min at 85% of Vo_{2max} [32]. In fact, fat oxidation increased 5–8 fold relative to resting values at all work-rates studied. At the highest work-rate (85%), carbohydrate oxidation was responsible for a greater proportion of the total energy requirements, but the absolute rate of fat oxidation was still markedly elevated compared to the resting value. Fatty acids may be derived from enzymatic hydrolysis of triglycerides in adipose tissue, from triglycerides in the blood, or from intramuscular triglycerides [13, 16, 24, 30, 40, 46, 49]. Plasma fatty acids derived from hydrolysis of triglycerides in adipose tissue are the principal fat substrates for muscle during low intensity exercise, whereas hydrolysis of intramuscular triglycerides become more important at higher work-rates (i.e., 65% and 85%) [33].

The increase in fat utilization during exercise seen in numerous human studies has been verified in rat hindlimb perfusion models, as well. Turcotte et al. [44, 45] demonstrated a 6–10 fold increase in palmitate oxidation (compared to non-contracting muscle) in the perfused rat hindlimb in response to muscle contraction induced by electrical stimulation.

POSSIBLE RATE-LIMITING SITES OF FATTY ACID OXIDATION

During exercise, a number of sites could possibly be rate-limiting for fatty acid utilization (Figure 5.1). These include: (1) Availability of fatty acids as determined by rate of lipolysis in adipose tissue and muscle or by activation of the lipoprotein lipase in capillaries of the muscle; (2) Rate of transport of fatty acids across the sarcolemma into skeletal muscle fibers; (3) Rate of formation of the coenzyme-A (Co-A) derivatives of fatty acids catalyzed by fatty acyl-CoA synthetase. (4) Rate of transport of fatty acyl-CoA into the mitochondria by the carnitine palmitoyl-transferase (CPT) system. This reaction can be limited by the amount of CPT, the concentration of substrates, and the concentration of the inhibitor, malonyl-CoA; (5) Rate of oxidation of intramitochondrial fatty acyl-CoA to acetyl-CoA as determined by the activity of the enzymes of β-oxidation. This process can be limited by the quantity of enzymes, by concentration of substrates for any one of the reactions, and by feedback inhibition by acetyl-CoA; (6) Rate of oxidation of acetyl-CoA generated by the β-oxidation enzymes. This process is coupled to the prevailing energy requirements of the muscle fiber.

FIGURE 5.1.

Mobilization and oxidation of fatty acids.

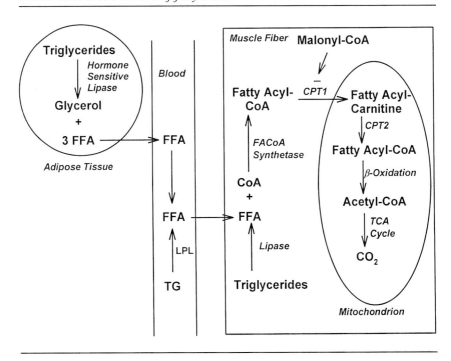

Several levels of control may exist for determining the final rate of fatty acid oxidation. It is conceivable that the rate-limiting step is not always the same under different physiological conditions. That is, the rate-limiting step may be different at rest or at low work-rates vs. work-rates above 65% of maximal oxygen consumption. This review will focus on the control of uptake of the CoA derivative of long-chain fatty acids into muscle mitochondria, or, in other words, the control of fatty acyl-CoA transport into the mitochondria by malonyl-CoA. It should be emphasized that this is not the only control point in the metabolic scheme, and that additional control mechanisms are likely, as suggested previously [17].

CARNITINE PALMITOYL TRANSFERASE

The carnitine palmitoyl transferase (CPT) system for transport of fatty acyl-CoA into mitochondria consists of CPT 1 and CPT 2 [25, 26, 35] (Figure 5.1). CPT 1 catalyzes formation of fatty acyl carnitine, which moves across the inner mitochondrial membrane. There, fatty acyl-CoA is regenerated and carnitine is released and catalyzed by CPT 2. Once inside the lumen of the mitochondrion, the fatty acyl-CoA can undergo β-oxidation, thus generating NADH, FADH2, and acetyl-CoA for oxidation in the citric acid cycle. Over 25 years ago, Mole et al. [28] demonstrated some of the important factors that determine the rate of fatty acid oxidation using mitochondria isolated from hindlimb muscle of trained and non-trained rats. They showed that the oxidation of palmitate increased as a function of fatty acid concentration. Both coenzyme A and carnitine were required to produce optimal rates of palmitate oxidation, thus demonstrating the importance of the CPT fatty acyl-CoA transport system. In the absence of carnitine (and with other substrates and cofactors non-limiting), the mitochondrial oxygen uptake was 69 μl oxygen/hr/g. With the addition of 1 mM carnitine, the rate increased to 543 μl oxygen/hr/g. Mitochondria isolated from the same amount of skeletal muscle of endurance-trained rats (2 hr/d for 3 mon) oxidized fatty acids at about twice the rate as mitochondria from sedentary rats. The requirement for carnitine clearly demonstrates the rate-limiting nature of the CPT system for governing the rate of fatty acid oxidation at the mitochondrial level. It also shows that at the same carnitine concentration and under optimal conditions, an increase in the amount of CPT 1 enzyme can also increase fatty acid oxidation. More recently, the importance of a decrease in malonyl-CoA in providing a rapid mechanism for increasing the fatty acid oxidation rate in response to increased energy needs was proposed.

SIGNIFICANCE OF MALONYL-CoA IN LIVER

In the liver, malonyl-CoA is the first committed intermediate in the pathway for fatty acid synthesis from glucose and other carbohydrate precursors

[25]. This compound is not only a source of two carbon units for synthesis of fatty acids, but also is important as a regulator of fatty acid oxidation. Malonyl-CoA is a potent inhibitor of carnitine palmitoyl transferase 1 (CPT 1), the rate-limiting enzyme of fatty acid oxidation and ketogenesis. When glucose is present in abundance, hepatic glycolysis is stimulated and mitochondrial citrate synthesis is enhanced. Citrate diffuses out of the mitochondria and is cleaved by citrate lyase to acetyl-CoA and oxaloacetate. The acetyl-CoA then becomes a substrate for malonyl-CoA synthesis by acetyl-CoA carboxylase (ACC). The consequent elevation in malonyl-CoA inhibits the CPT 1 enzyme, thereby preventing fatty acid oxidation and ketogenesis at a time when fatty acid synthesis is occurring at a high rate. During periods of fasting or prolonged exercise, hepatic glycolysis is inhibited along with mitochondrial citrate production. The consequent reduction in rate of production of extramitochondrial acetyl-CoA, coupled with phosphorylation-induced decrease in ACC activity, causes a reduction in malonyl-CoA [2, 3, 25, 27]. This relieves inhibition of the CPT 1 enzyme, thereby allowing increased rates of fatty acid oxidation and ketogenesis. In the liver, therefore, malonyl-CoA not only is a major substrate for fatty acid synthesis, but also serves as a signal molecule to decrease the rate of fatty acid oxidation by liver mitochondria when fat is being synthesized.

MALONYL-CoA IN SKELETAL MUSCLE

Skeletal muscle is not considered to be a lipogenic tissue, yet malonyl-CoA can be detected in muscle at a level approximately 20% of that found in livers of fed rats [26, 54, 56]. The highest concentration of malonyl-CoA is found in the red Type I and Type IIA hindlimb muscle fibers [56]. Type IIB has a lower malonyl-CoA concentration.

Like liver CPT 1, muscle CPT 1 is also sensitive to inhibition by malonyl-CoA. In fact, lower concentrations are required to inhibit CPT 1 activity in isolated mitochondria from muscle, as compared to those required to inhibit CPT 1 activity in isolated liver mitochondria [26, 35]. This difference is due to the existence of a different isoform in muscle vs. liver. The concentration of malonyl-CoA which produces 50% inhibition (I_{50}) of CPT 1 in isolated mitochondria was reported to be 2.7 ± 0.4 μM for liver and 0.034 ± 0.006 μM for skeletal muscle [26]. Heart mitochondria appear to have an I_{50} for malonyl-CoA inhibition of CPT 1 intermediate between liver and skeletal muscle. This is due to the presence of a mixture of both isoforms [51, 52]. Since the concentration of malonyl-CoA in muscle does not decrease below approximately 0.2 nmol/g, even after prolonged fasting or after prolonged exercise, it would appear that CPT 1 is always inhibited. Fatty acid oxidation does occur in muscle during fasting and exercise, however. It has been suggested that not all the malonyl-CoA of muscle is in the sarcoplasmic compartment, or that much of the malonyl-CoA is not free in solution, but is bound to proteins in the sarcoplasm. Only the free malo-nyl-CoA in the sarcoplasm would be available for inhibition of CPT 1. This compartmentalization idea is certainly possible, but another explanation has become apparent as a result of recent experiments in our laboratory. These preliminary studies demonstrate that the I_{50} for malonyl-CoA inhibition of CPT 1 in isolated skeletal muscle mitochondria can be shifted into the physiological range of malonyl-CoA concentrations by changing the incubation conditions. The incubation conditions chosen by McGarry et al. [26] for measurement of inhibition of CPT 1 by malonyl-CoA were never meant to duplicate conditions inside the muscle fiber, but were utilized for comparison of the liver, muscle, and other tissue isoforms. Using the incubation conditions employed, a distinct difference was noted between the liver and muscle isoforms, but again, conditions inside the cell may shift the I_{50} markedly, as compared to the somewhat arbitrarily selected conditions of the *in vitro* assay.

MALONYL-CoA DECREASES IN MUSCLE DURING EXERCISE OR FASTING

The concentration of malonyl-CoA decreases in muscle in response to fasting and in response to treadmill exercise [26, 55, 56]. A significant decrease can be observed after 5 min of submaximal exercise in the Type IIA fibers of the quadriceps of the rat [56]. Malonyl-CoA continues to decrease as exercise continues. Changes in Type IIB fibers appear to occur after more prolonged bouts of exercise at submaximal rates. Electrical stimulation of the sciatic nerve of anesthetized rats causes a significant decline in muscle malonyl-CoA [10, 18, 29, 47]. Infusion of glucose into rats during exercise causes a partial attenuation of the decline in gastrocnemius malonyl-CoA [12]. The decrease in muscle malonyl-CoA during exercise is not dependent on the increase in epinephrine [57].

One study on the effect of exercise on malonyl-CoA in human skeletal muscle is available. Odland et al. [29] reported malonyl-CoA to be much lower in concentration in human skeletal muscle vs. rat skeletal muscle. In that study, no definite negative correlation was observed between malonyl-CoA and the rate of fat oxidation. The reason for this apparent discrepancy between studies performed using rats and humans is not clear at this time. Recent studies in our laboratory, however, indicate that malonyl-CoA in rat skeletal muscle does not recover for at least 30–90 min after cessation of an exercise bout. It may be important in future human studies to have subjects resting for a prolonged period prior to obtaining the resting muscle biopsy. Whether this is the reason for the discrepancy between the rat and human work is yet to be determined.

As indicated previously, exercise at rates up to at least 85% of Vo_{2max} cause up to an 8–fold increase in the rate of fat oxidation compared to rest. If the fatty acid oxidation rate increases 8–fold, the rate of entry of fatty acyl-CoA into the mitochondria must also increase correspondingly. Skeletal muscle is not considered to be a lipogenic tissue (i.e., capable of synthesizing fatty acids from glucose), yet malonyl-CoA is present in this tissue. Malonyl-CoA is an inhibitor of CPT 1 in mitochondria isolated from skeletal muscle. Together, these facts raise the question of the physiological role of malonyl-CoA in skeletal muscle. Is it there primarily as a regulatory molecule with the role of governing the rate of fatty acid oxidation by muscle mitochondria?

SYNTHESIS OF MALONYL-CoA IN SKELETAL MUSCLE BY ACC

Experiments in our laboratory indicated the presence of an avidin-sensitive ACC in the 50,000 X g supernatant of hindlimb skeletal muscle of the rat [42]. Avidin is a protein found in eggs that binds to biotin, a component of all carboxylases. The avidin sensitivity was reversible with high concentrations of biotin. Citrate, bicarbonate, acetyl CoA, and adenosine triphosphate (ATP) are all required for full activity. Two immunologically distinct isoforms of the ACC had been identified, one with a molecular weight of 265 kDa (ACC265), and one with a molecular weight of 280 kDa (ACC280) [4, 19]. Both are present in liver, but the 265 kDa is by far the predominant isoform. Only the ACC265 is present in white adipose tissue [19]. Thampy reported that the principal heart isoform has a molecular weight of approximately 280 kDa [41]. In our laboratory, we found rat hindlimb skeletal muscle to contain a unique isoform. In SDS-PAGE, the muscle ACC migrates midway between the ACC265 and ACC280 at approximately 272 kDa [43]. Witter's group reported human skeletal muscle ACC to have a molecular weight of 275 kDa, similar to values we later reported for the rat [62]. This isoform was more recently given the designation of ACC-β. At least two genes are responsible for coding for synthesis of the two major isoforms [53]. At this time, it is not clear whether the heart and skeletal muscle isoforms are identical. Although many similarities exist between heart and muscle ACC (i.e., both are regulated by 5'AMP-activated protein kinase—AMPK), significant differences do exist in regulation (i.e., heart ACC appears to be less citrate dependent) [1, 22, 23, 34].

In the isolated resting perfused rat hindlimb, both insulin and glucose are required to maintain high levels of malonyl-CoA [11]. If either glucose or insulin is left out of the medium, malonyl-CoA decreases. Saha et al. [36] reported a marked increase in malonyl-CoA content of soleus muscles incubated *in vitro* in the presence of high concentrations of glucose and insulin, thus clearly demonstrating the importance of the availability of carbohydrate in governing the malonyl-CoA concentration.

Saha et al. [37] also recently provided evidence that the precursor of sarcoplasmic acetyl-CoA for malonyl-CoA synthesis is citrate. Acetyl-CoA does not cross the mitochondrial membrane. Acetyl-CoA generated by the pyruvate dehydrogenase reaction must therefore condense with oxaloacetate to form citrate in the citrate synthase reaction. Citrate may then be transferred out of the mitochondria into the sarcoplasm, where citrate lyase catalyzes cleavage of citrate to form acetyl-CoA and oxaloacetate. Oxaloacetate is reduced to malate, an antiporter for citrate efflux from the mitochondria. The sarcoplasmic acetyl-CoA may then be utilized for malonyl-CoA synthesis. The increase in malonyl-CoA in incubated soleus muscles that is induced by glucose and insulin can be prevented with hydroxycitrate, an inhibitor of citrate lyase [37]. An alternative source of sarcoplasmic acetyl-CoA may be derived from acetyl-carnitine, which is formed in the mitochondria and which may enter the sarcoplasm and be cleaved to acetyl-CoA and carnitine [17].

REGULATION OF LIVER ACC

The liver ACC activity is regulated by short-term allosteric and covalent modification mechanisms, as well as by long-term mechanisms involving modulation of the amount of enzyme present [15, 20, 61]. Citrate is an allosteric activator. Long-chain fatty acyl-CoAs and malonyl-CoA inhibit the activity of the enzyme. Phosphorylation by AMPK and cAMP-dependent protein kinase (PKA) causes a reduction in enzyme activity [5, 9, 14, 15, 20]. An upstream kinase (AMPK kinase) is also activated by AMP [50]. Activity of liver ACC is decreased in response to glucagon and increased in response to insulin [15, 20, 38, 61]. Therefore, during fasting, prolonged exercise, and diabetes the ACC activity is reduced, malonyl-CoA concentration declines, the inhibition of CPT 1 is relieved, and fatty acid oxidation and ketogenesis proceed at a high rate. The opposite occurs when glucose and insulin are present in high concentrations. Malonyl-CoA concentration increases, CPT 1 is inhibited, and fatty acid synthesis from glucose carbons occurs at a high rate. The total amount of ACC activity increases in response to high carbohydrate diets and decreases in response to fasting and experimental diabetes mellitus.

REGULATION OF SKELETAL MUSCLE ACC

Regulation of skeletal muscle ACC has been studied recently. These studies indicate that the muscle ACC does not fluctuate as a function of dietary or hormonal manipulations, including fasting and refeeding [59]. This marks a distinct difference in long-term regulation of muscle and liver enzymes. We demonstrated that the skeletal muscle isoform of ACC has distinct kinetic properties compared to the 265 kDa isoform found in adipose tissue [42]. The Km for acetyl-CoA was found to be 32 μM for skeletal muscle ACC, as compared to 22 μM for the adipose

FIGURE 5.2.

Effect of phosphorylation by AMPK on citrate activation of purified skeletal muscle ACC. (See Am. J. Physiol. *270:E299-E304, 1996.)*

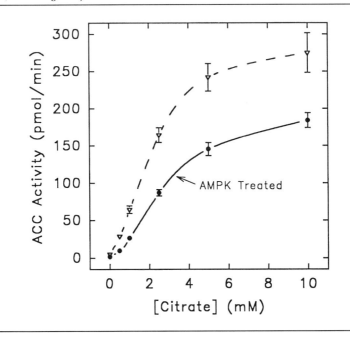

ACC. The Km for ATP was 58 μM vs. 107 μM. The Km for bicarbonate was not significantly different. The $K_{0.5}$ for citrate activation of ACC was 2.1 mM for the muscle and 3.0 mM for the adipose tissue isoforms. As with the liver and adipose isoforms of the enzyme, palmitoyl-CoA and malonyl-CoA were found to be competitive inhibitors [42].

Recent studies in our laboratory [58, 60] demonstrated that the purified muscle ACC can be phosphorylated by AMPK. Phosphorylation by AMPK causes a marked decrease in activity of the ACC at physiological concentrations of citrate (Figure 5.2). The Ka for citrate increases from 3.6 to 6.8 mM as a consequence of phosphorylation. The Kms for acetyl-CoA and for ATP also increase in consequence of phosphorylation. The net effect of these kinetic changes in the enzyme due to phosphorylation would be a decrease in the rate of malonyl-CoA formation. The ACC would become much less sensitive to activation by citrate, particularly in the physiological range of citrate concentrations. AMPK appears to be abundant in skeletal muscle, although measured activity is much less than in liver [7, 39, 48]. *In vitro* phosphorylation by PKA does not result in any detectable change in activity of ACC [60]. This appears to be another distinct difference between the principal liver and muscle iso-forms.

REGULATION OF ACC DURING EXERCISE OR IN RESPONSE TO MUSCLE CONTRACTION.

Previous studies demonstrated that malonyl-CoA decreases in muscle in response to exercise [56]. The mechanism of this decrease was recently investigated [58]. Rats were killed at rest or after running on the treadmill for 5 min or 30 min. Muscles were quickly removed and frozen. Muscle homogenates were prepared and subjected to ammonium sulfate precipitation to partially purify ACC and AMPK. The resuspended precipitates were analyzed for ACC in the presence of variable citrate concentrations and for AMPK activity. Figure 5.3 shows that AMPK is activated as soon as 5 min after the beginning of exercise, and that it remains active throughout the course of the exercise. Concurrent with the increase in AMPK activity is a decrease in ACC activity at 0.2 mM citrate, which is close to the concentration of citrate in muscle. The citrate activation curve for ACC shows a change similar to that observed when purified skeletal muscle ACC is phosphorylated by AMPK *in vitro* (Figure 5.4). That is, the ACC shows a decrease in the maximal velocity of the reaction (as a function of citrate concentration), and an increase in the activation constant (Ka) for citrate. Thus, the changes in the kinetic values measured for ACC provide an indirect measure of phosphorylation. In other words, since the Ka and Vmax values for skeletal muscle ACC change similarly to those observed during phosphorylation *in vitro*, this provides evidence that the mechanism of the decrease in malonyl-CoA during exercise is phosphorylation and inactivation of ACC by AMPK.

Additional information concerning this control system comes from *in situ* muscle stimulation studies. Induction of muscle contraction by stimulating the sciatic nerve of anesthetized rats also results in a decrease in malonyl-CoA [10], accompanied by activation of AMPK and inactivation of ACC [18]. There also is an increase in the estimated free 5'-AMP concentration in the muscle. At low frequency stimulation, the time course of activation of AMPK does not precisely precede the inactivation of ACC. It must be remembered that 5'-AMP can activate AMPK allosterically, as well as activating the kinase (AMPK kinase), which phosphorylates and activates AMPK. Only the phosphorylation-induced activation would be detected in the re-suspended ammonium sulfate precipitate. Most of the AMP present in the muscle homogenates would have been discarded in the supernatant after centrifugation. Yet, in the contracting muscle, the increase in AMP would have immediately activated the AMPK.

More recently, Vavvas et al. [47] confirmed and extended these observations. Rat hindlimb muscles stimulated to contract *in situ* via the sciatic

FIGURE 5.3.

Effect of treadmill exercise (21 m/min, 15% grade) on the time course of AMPK activity, ACC activity at 0.2 mM citrate, and malonyl-CoA in red quadriceps muscle. (See Am. J. Physiol. 270:E299-E304, 1996).

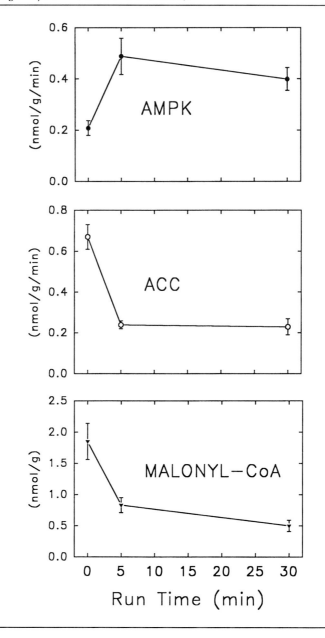

FIGURE 5.4.

Effect of 5 min or 30 min of treadmill exercise (21 m/min, 15% grade) on citrate activation of ACC partially purified from red quadriceps muscle. (See Am. J. Physiol. *270:E299-E304, 1996).*

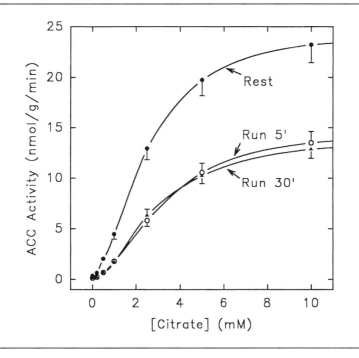

nerve for 5 min also showed a decrease in malonyl-CoA, an increase in AMPK, and a decrease in ACC activity. A 5–6 fold increase in the activity of the $\alpha2$ isoform of AMPK was observed to occur within 30 sec after beginning electrical stimulation (5 pps, 100 ms trains of 2.5 V, 50 Hz, and 10 ms duration). The activity remained elevated for at least 30 min after cessation of stimulation. ACC from the electrically stimulated muscle showed an electrophoretic mobility shift, which provides additional evidence of phosphorylation. Treatment of the immunologically purified ACC with phosphatases reversed the activity change caused by the electrical stimulation.

EFFECT OF EXERCISE INTENSITY ON ACTIVATION OF AMPK, INACTIVATION OF ACC, AND DECREASE IN MALONYL-CoA

The activation of AMPK, inactivation of ACC, and decrease in malonyl-CoA were recently determined to be dependent on exercise intensity [31]. Rats were run on the treadmill for 5 min at 10, 20, 30, and 40 m/min up a 5%

grade. The faster the speed of running, the greater the decrease in malonyl-CoA, and the greater the activation of AMPK and inactivation of ACC. If the trigger for activation of AMPK and consequent inactivation of ACC is contraction, only those fibers contracting would exhibit activation of the AMPK and inactivation of ACC. This appeared to be the case, since ACC isolated from superficial white quadriceps was unchanged except at the highest work rate (40 m/min). This system appears to be designed to decrease malonyl-CoA any time the muscle contracts, thus allowing increased fatty acid oxidation as fatty acids become available. Because the muscle appears to use carbohydrate for a greater percentage of energy needs at high work rates, this implies that factors other than a low malonyl-CoA concentration become rate-limiting for fatty acid oxidation. It should be remembered, however, that human subjects working at work rates as high as 85% of maximal oxygen consumption are still oxidizing fatty acids at a rate 5–6 fold above that seen in the resting condition [32, 33]. A reduction in malonyl-CoA in the environment of CPT 1 is likely essential for sustaining these higher fat utilization rates.

SUMMARY

As muscle goes from a resting state to exercise, the following sequence of events occurs (Figure 5.5): (1) The rise in AMP accompanying contraction

FIGURE 5.5.

Postulated sequence of events that leads to a decrease in malonyl-CoA and an increased rate of fatty acid oxidation by muscle during exercise.

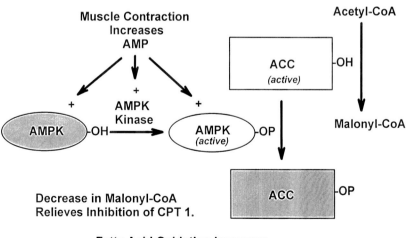

allosterically activates AMPK and an AMPK kinase; (2) The activated AMPK kinase phosphorylates and further activates AMPK; (3) The activated AMPK phosphorylates and inactivates ACC; and (4) The consequent decline in malonyl-CoA (product of ACC reaction) relieves inhibition of CPT-1 and allows an increased rate of fatty acid oxidation when fatty acids become available.

ACKNOWLEDGEMENTS

This work was supported by National Institute of Arthritis and Musculoskeletal and Skin Diseases Grant AR-41438.

REFERENCES

1. Awan, M.M., and E.D. Saggerson. Malonyl-CoA metabolism in cardiac myocytes and its relevance to the control of fatty acid oxidation. *Biochem. J.* 295:61–66, 1993.
2. Beattie, M.A., and W.W. Winder. Mechanism of training-induced attenuation of post-exercise ketosis. *Am. J. Physiol.* 247:R780–R785, 1984.
3. Beattie, M.A., and W.W. Winder. Attenuation of post-exercise ketosis in fasted endurance-trained rats. *Am. J. Physiol.* 248:R63–R67, 1985.
4. Bianchi, A., J.L. Evans, A.J. Iverson, A. Nordlund, T.D.Watts, and L.A.Witters. Identification of an isozymic form of acetyl-CoA carboxylase. *J. Biol. Chem.* 265:1502–1509, 1990.
5. Carling, D., P.R. Clarke, V.A. Zammit, and D.G. Hardie. Purification and characterization of the AMP-activated protein kinase. *Eur. J. Biochem.* 186:129–136, 1989.
6. Corton, J.M., J.G. Gillespie, and D.G. Hardie. Role of the AMP-activated protein kinase in the cellular stress-response. *Cur. Bio.* 4:315–324, 1994.
7. Davies, S.P., D. Carling, and D.G. Hardie. Tissue distribution of the AMP-activated protein kinase and lack of activation by cyclic-AMP-dependent protein kinase, studied using a specific and sensitive peptide assay. *Eur. J. Biochem.* 186:123–128, 1989.
8. Davies, S.P., N.R. Helps, P.T.W. Cohen, and D.G. Hardie. 5'–AMP inhibits dephosphorylation, as well as promoting phosphorylation, of the AMP-activated protein kinase. Studies using bacterially expressed human protein phosphatase-2Cα and native bovine protein phosphatase-2A$_C$. *FEBS Letters.* 377:421–425, 1995.
9. Davies, S.P., A.T.R. Sim, and D.G. Hardie. Location and function of three sites phosphorylated on rat acetyl-CoA carboxylase by the AMP-activated protein kinase. *Eur. J. Biochem.* 187:183–190, 1990.
10. Duan, C., and W.W. Winder. Nerve stimulation decreases malonyl-CoA in skeletal muscle. *J. Appl. Physiol.* 72:901–904, 1992.
11. Duan, C., and W.W. Winder. Control of malonyl-CoA by glucose and insulin in perfused skeletal muscle. *J. Appl. Physiol.* 74:2543–2547, 1993.
12. Elayan, I.M., and W.W. Winder. Effect of glucose infusion on muscle malonyl-CoA during exercise. *J. Appl. Physiol.* 70:1495–1499, 1991.
13. Galbo, H., and B. Stallknecht. Regulation of fat metabolism in exercise. R.J. Maughan and S.M. Shirreffs (eds.). *Biochemistry of Exercise IX.* Human Kinetics:Champaign, 1996, pp. 63–72.
14. Ha, J., S. Daniel, S.S. Broyles, and K.H. Kim. Critical phosphorylation sites for acetyl-CoA carboxylase activity. *J. Biol. Chem.* 269:22162–22168, 1994.
15. Hardie, D.G. Regulation of fatty acid synthesis via phosphorylation of acetyl-CoA carboxylase. *Prog. Lipid Res.* 28:117–146, 1989.

16. Holloszy, J.O., and W.M. Kohrt. Regulation of carbohydrate and fat metabolism during and after exercise. *Ann. Rev. Nut.* 16:121–138, 1996.

17. Hultman, E. Pyruvate dehydrogenase as a regulator of substrate utilization in skeletal muscle. R.J. Maughan and S.M. Shirreffs (eds.). *Biochemistry of Exercise IX.* Human Kinetics: Champaign, 1996, pp. 157–171.

18. Hutber, C., Adrian, D.G. Hardie, and W.W. Winder. Electrical stimulation inactivates muscle acetyl-CoA carboxylase and increases AMP-activated protein kinase. *Am. J. Physiol.* 272:E262–E266, 1997.

19. Iverson, A.J., A. Bianchi, A.C. Nordlund, and L.A. Witters. Immunological analysis of acetyl-CoA carboxylase mass, tissue distribution, and subunit composition. *Biochem. J.* 269: 365–371, 1990.

20. Kim, K.H., F. Lopez-Casillas, D.H. Bai, X. Luo, and M.E. Pape. Role of reversible phosphorylation of acetyl-CoA carboxylase in long-chain fatty acid synthesis. *FASEB J.* 3:2250–2256, 1989.

21. Klein, S., E.F. Coyle, and R.R. Wolfe. Fat metabolism during low-intensity exercise in endurance-trained and untrained men. *Am. J. Physiol.* 267:E934–E940, 1994.

22. Kudo, N., A.J. Barr, R.L. Barr, S. Desai, and G.D. Lopaschuk. High rates of fatty acid oxidation during reperfusion of ischemic hearts are associated with a decrease in malonyl-CoA levels due to an increase in 5'-AMP-activated protein kinase inhibition of acetyl-CoA carboxylase. *J. Biol. Chem.* 270:7513–17520, 1995.

23. Lopaschuk, G.D., and J. Gamble. Acetyl-CoA carboxylase: an important regulator of fatty acid oxidation in the heart. *Can. J. Physiol. Pharmacol.* 72:1101–1109, 1994.

24. Martin, W.H. Effects of acute and chronic exercise on fat metabolism. *Exerc. Sports Sci. Rev.* 24:203–231, 1996.

25. McGarry, J.D., and D. W. Foster. Regulation of hepatic fatty acid oxidation and ketone body production. *Ann. Rev. Biochem.* 49:395–420, 1980.

26. McGarry, J.D., S.E. Mills, C.S. Long, and D.W. Foster. Observations on the affinity for carnitine, and malonyl-CoA sensitivity, of carnitine palmitoyltransferase I in animal and human tissues. *Biochem. J.* 214:21–28, 1983.

27. McGarry, J.D., M.J. Stark, and D.W. Foster. Hepatic malonyl-CoA levels of fed, fasted and diabetic rats as measured using a simple radioisotopic assay. *J. Biol. Chem.* 253:8291–8293, 1978.

28. Mole, P.A., L.B. Oscai, and J.O. Holloszy. Adaptation of muscle to exercise. Increase in levels of palmityl CoA synthetase, carnitine palmityltransferase, and palmityl CoA dehydrogenase, and in the capacity to oxidize fatty acids. *J. Clin. Invest.* 50:2323–2330, 1971.

29. Odland, L.M., G.J.F. Heigenhauser, G.D. Lopaschuk, and L.L. Spriet. Human skeletal muscle malonyl-CoA at rest and during prolonged submaximal exercise. *Am. J. Physiol.* 270:E541–E544, 1996.

30. Oscai, L.B., and K. Esser. Regulation of muscle triglyceride metabolism in exercise. R.J. Maughan and S. M. Shirreffs (eds.). *Biochemistry of Exercise IX.* Human Kinetics: Champaign, 1996, pp. 105–115.

31. Rasmussen, B.B., and W.W. Winder. Effect of exercise intensity on skeletal muscle malonyl-CoA and acetyl-CoA carboxylase. *J. Appl. Physiol.* 83:1104—1109, 1997.

32. Romijn, J.A., E.F. Coyle, L.S. Sidossis, et al. Regulation of endogenous fat and carbohydrate metabolism in relation to exercise intensity and duration. *Am. J. Physiol.* 265:E380–E391, 1993.

33. Romijn, J.A., E.F. Coyle, L.S. Sidossis, X.J. Zhang, and R.R. Wolfe. Relationship between fatty acid delivery and fatty acid oxidation during strenuous exercise. *J. Appl. Physiol.* 79: 1939–1945, 1995.

34. Saddik, M., J. Gamble, L.A. Witters, and G.D. Lopaschuk. Acetyl-CoA carboxylase regulation of fatty acid oxidation in the heart. *J. Biol. Chem.* 268:25836–25845, 1993.

35. Saggerson, D., I. Ghadiminejad, and M. Awan. Regulation of mitochondrial carnitine palmitoyl transferases from liver and extrahepatic tissues. *Adv. Enzyme Regul.* 32: 285–306, 1992.

36. Saha, A.K., T.G. Kurowski, and N.B. Ruderman. A malonyl-CoA fuel-sensing mechanism in muscle: effects of insulin, glucose, and denervation. *Am. J. Physiol.* 269:E283–E289, 1995.

37. Saha, A.D., D. Vavvas, T.G. Kurowski, et. al. Malonyl-CoA regulation in skeletal muscle: its link to cell citrate and the glucose-fatty acid cycle. *Am. J. Physiol.* 272:E641–E648, 1997.

38. Sim, A.T.R., and D.G. Hardie. The low activity of acetyl-CoA carboxylase in basal and glucagon-stimulated hepatocytes is due to phosphorylation by the AMP-activated protein kinase and not cyclic AMP-dependent protein kinase. *FEBS Lett.* 233: 294–298, 1988.

39. Stapleton, D., K.I. Mitchelhill, G. Gao, et al. Mammalian AMP-activated protein kinase subfamily. *J. Biol. Chem.* 271:611—614, 1966.

40. Terjung, R.L., and H. Kaciuba-Uscilko. Lipid metabolism during exercise: influence of training. *Diab. Metab. Rev.* 2:35–51, 1986.

41. Thampy, K.G. Formation of malonyl coenzyme A in rat heart. *J. Biol. Chem.* 264: 17631–17634, 1989.

42. Trumble, G.E., M.A. Smith, and W.W. Winder. Evidence of a biotin dependent acetyl-coenzyme A carboxylase in rat muscle. *Life Sci.* 49:39–43, 1991.

43. Trumble, G.E., M.A. Smith, and W.W. Winder. Purification and characterization of rat skeletal muscle acetyl-CoA carboxylase. *Eur. J. Biochem.* 231:192–198, 1995.

44. Turcotte, L.P., P.J.L. Hespel, T.E. Graham, and E.A. Richter. Impaired plasma FFA oxidation imposed by extreme CHO deficiency in contracting rat skeletal muscle. *J. Appl. Physiol.* 77:517–525, 1994.

45. Turcotte, L.P., P. Hespel, and E.A. Richter. Circulating palmitate uptake and oxidation are not altered by glycogen depletion in contracting skeletal muscle. *J. Appl. Physiol.* 78: 1266–1272, 1995.

46. Van der Vusse, G.J., and R.S. Reneman. Lipid metabolism in muscle. L.B. Rowell and J.T. Shepherd (eds.). *Handbook of Physiology, Section 12: Exercise: Regulation and Integration of Multiple Systems.* New York: Oxford University Press, 1996, pp. 952–994.

47. Vavvas, D., A. Apazidis, A.K. Saha, et al. Contraction-induced changes in acetyl-CoA carboxylase and 5'-AMP-activated kinase in skeletal muscle. *J. Biol. Chem.* 272:13256–13261, 1997.

48. Verhoeven, A.J.M., A. Woods, C.H. Brennan, et al. The AMP-activated protein kinase gene is highly expressed in rat skeletal muscle. *Eur. J. Biochem.* 228: 236–243, 1995.

49. Wasserman, D.H., and A.D. Cherrington. Regulation of extramuscular fuel sources during exercise. L.B. Rowell and J.T. Shepherd (eds.). *Handbook of Physiology, Section 12: Exercise: Regulation and Integration of Multiple Systems,* New York: Oxford University Press, 1996, pp. 1036–1074.

50. Weekes, J., S.A. Hawley, J. Corton, D. Shugar, and D.G. Hardie. Activation of rat liver AMP-activated protein kinase by kinase in a purified, reconstituted system: effects of AMP and AMP analogues. *Eur. J. Biochem.* 219:751–757, 1994.

51. Weis, B.C., A.T. Cowan, N. Brown, D.W. Foster, and J.D. McGarry. Use of a selective inhibitor of liver carnitine palmitoyltransferase I (CPT 1) allows quantification of its contribution to total CPT 1 activity in rat heart. *J. Biol. Chem.* 269:26443–26448, 1994.

52. Weis, B.C., V. Esser, D.W. Foster, and J.D. McGarry. Rat heart expresses two forms of mitochondrial carnitine palmitoyltransferase I. *J. Biol. Chem.* 269:8712–18715, 1994.

53. Widmer, J., K.S. Fassihi, S.C. Schlichter, et al. Identification of a second human acetyl-CoA carboxylase gene. *Biochem. J.* 316:915–922, 1996.

54. Winder, W.W. Malonyl-CoA as a metabolic regulator. R.J. Maughn (ed.). *Biochemistry of Exercise IX Conference Proceedings.* Champaign, IL: Human Kinetics, 1996, pp. 163–174.

55. Winder, W.W., J. Arogyasami, R.J. Barton, I.M. Elayan, and P.R. Vehrs. Muscle malonyl-CoA decreases during exercise. *J. Appl. Physiol.* 67:2230–2233, 1989.

56. Winder, W.W., J. Arogyasami, I.M. Elayan, and D. Cartmill. Time course of the exercise-induced decline in malonyl-CoA in different muscle types. *Am. J. Physiol.* 259:E266–E271, 1990.

57. Winder, W.W., R.W. Braiden, D.C. Cartmill, C.A. Hutber, and J.P. Jones. Effect of adreno-demedullation on decline in muscle malonyl-CoA during exercise. *J. Appl. Physiol.* 74: 2548–2551, 1993.

58. Winder, W.W., and D.G. Hardie. Inactivation of acetyl-CoA carboxylase and activation of AMP-activated protein kinase in muscle during exercise. *Am. J. Physiol.* 270:E299–E304, 1996.

59. Winder, W.W., P.S. MacLean, J.C. Lucas, J.E. Fernley, and G.E. Trumble. Effect of fasting and refeedng on acetyl-CoA carboxylase in rat hindlimb muscle. *J. Appl. Physiol.* 78: 578–582, 1995.

60. Winder, W.W., H.A. Wilson, D.G. Hardie, et al. Phosphorylation of rat muscle acetyl-CoA carboxylase by AMP-activated protein kinase and protein kinase A. *J. Appl. Physiol.* 82: 219–225, 1997.

61. Witters, L.A., D. Moriarity, and D.B. Martin. Regulation of hepatic acetyl-coenzyme A carboxylase by insulin and glucagon. *J. Biol. Chem.* 254:6644–6649, 1979.

62. Witters, L.A., J. Widmer, A.N. King, K. Fassihi, and F. Kuhajda. Identification of human acetyl-CoA carboxylase isozymes in tissue and in breast cancer cells. *Int. J. Biochem.* 26: 589–594, 1994.

6
Physical Self-Concept: Assessment and External Validity

ROBERT J. SONSTROEM, PH.D., FASCM

Currently, the theory of the self-concept is studied as a collection of specific facets of the self, such as academic self-concept, social self-concept, or physical self-concept [46, 118]. These facets are commonly regarded as components of global self-esteem, the overall evaluation of the self. Exercise and sport psychologists have followed this general trend in psychology and have developed a variety of physical self-concept measures that they have related to sport and exercise participation. In terms of the success experienced by these measures and the new approaches they provide in studying people engaged in physical activity, a review of the physical self-concept construct would seem to be important. Other reviews have examined "self-confidence" and its relationship with physical activity participation and performance, as evaluated from theoretical [22] and gender [64] perspectives. Gruber [42] conducted a meta-analysis of global self-concept/exercise interventions conducted with elementary school children, and Sonstroem [123] summarized studies attempting to document self-esteem change via exercise.

This chapter will summarize knowledge about the physical self-concept in relevant topical areas, as well as recommend principles of measurement that seem advantageous to the acquisition of further knowledge. As such, the following will be discussed: (1) self-conception (structure and measurement); (2) advantages of employing component scales; (3) a brief review of the most frequently used physical self-concept scales; (4) measurement considerations; (5) development of the physical self-concept; (6) age and gender effects; (7) skill development research; (8) self-enhancement research; (9) relationships with mental health; and (10) suggested directions. Parameters of the chapter preclude the consideration of projective assessments [27] and identity measures [58].

SELF-CONCEPTION: STRUCTURE AND MEASUREMENT

Definitions

Self-concept (SC) refers to "an organized configuration of perceptions of the self which are admissible to awareness" [107]. It may be thought of

FIGURE 6.1.
Self-esteem interactions with the environment.

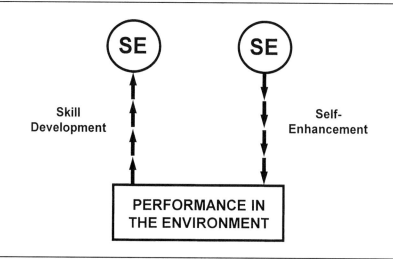

as a personal picture or self-description. Self-esteem (SE) refers to the evaluation and affect one holds for this personal picture. However, since it is difficult to describe one's self without experiencing evaluation and affect, the two terms are often used interchangeably [146]. Moreover, empirical attempts to distinguish the two have met with frequent failure [10]. Within this chapter the terms are used interchangeably. SE appears to consist of at least two senses or dimensions—competence and self-acceptance [134, 146]. Feelings of competence tend to be reinforced in Western society with its emphasis on success. Additionally, positive SE implies that one should like or, at the very least, be satisfied with one's self.

The interaction of SE with the environment may be understood by dichotomizing directional influence into the separate pathways of self-enhancement and skill development [66] (Figure 6.1). The first refers to the influence of SE on the environment (our SE directs our behavior within the environment). We tend to act as we perceive ourselves to be. As society rewards achievement, we engage in activities that we believe will lead to success, thus enhancing our SE. The skill development path refers to the influence of environmental activities and forces on our SE. Our behavior in the environment increases our SE by means of success experiences. This latter hypothesis has been tested frequently in the exercise/SE literature, with many physical activity programs seeking to validate psychological worth by demonstrating SE change.

With the newer emphases on a multidimensional SC, a variety of self-system structures have been advanced [10, 74]. A majority of these models are hierarchical, with more general constructs at the apex of the hierarchy, and with specificity increasing down to the lowest, most situation-specific level as proposed by Shavelson [118]. This organized self-system operates on the premise that constructs depend on " . . . secondary ones, which are in turn determined by lower order components representing more specific competencies" [29]. It can then be hypothesized that changes in lower level constructs influence change in more general constructs.

An example is shown in Figure 6.2. This hierarchical Exercise and Self-Esteem Model (EXSEM) [126] expands the competence dimension of the original Exercise and Self-Esteem Model [129]. It proposes that one of global SE's domains is that of physical self-worth. In turn, this latter construct may be divided into subdomains of sport competence, physical condi-

FIGURE 6.2.
Expanded Exercise and Self-Esteem Model (EXSEM).

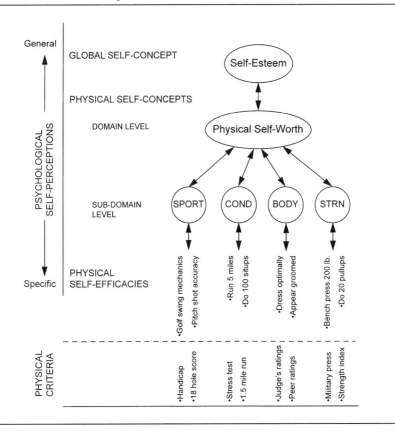

tion, attractive body, and strength, as advanced by Fox [31]. EXSEM goes further in that it assesses more specific performance self-efficacies directly related to the skills practiced in athletic or physical training programs. Physical self-efficacy is the expectation that right now one can perform a specific physical skill. The lowest level of the model, actual measured physical skill, assists in studying the manner in which program physical performance generalizes to psychological self-efficacies specific to that performance and then to more abstract feelings of well-being.

It would seem that the reception of psychological benefit from human behavior often represents generalizations from more narrow specific behaviors to broader mental conceptualizations. The nature of this process is seen to parallel that of generalization within a SE hierarchy. Therefore, this chapter proposes that proper operationalizations of hierarchical self-perception models provide excellent opportunities to study the manner in which real-life generalizations function. The manner in which previous values and changes in components at one level of the SC hierarchy affect components and their changes at other levels of SC seems able to provide knowledge regarding internal processes of change. Higher levels of SC are consistent, of course, with the reception of psychological benefit. Additionally, the employment of hierarchical models can increase understanding of the effects of extrinsic variables, such as socialization or goal attainment, when they are included in the design. The use of hierarchical self-systems is recommended for self-enhancement research and for studying associations with variables such as autonomy, anxiety, and intrinsic motivation. Physical SCs are provided with additional use by hierarchical models such as EXSEM. They are situated within multi-level self-systems as mediators between the environment and global SE. They should be relevant and related to environmental variables, and capable of transferring this association to global SE by virtue of their own robust associations with SE. This is especially true when more specific assessments (e.g., physical self-efficacies) are not present in the design.

Measurement

Marsh [72] emphasized the importance of relying on item characteristics to define a scale and the perils involved in relying on a scale name. While SC assessment items can differ in many ways, two factors are of special concern in this review. The first factor is *relevance*. At more specific levels of the SC hierarchy, referents in an assessment statement should correspond as closely as possible to appropriate stimuli (e.g., skills, activities) within the setting. For example, it would be foolish to attempt to predict baseball batting averages with the item "I am not agile and graceful." An item such as "I have an excellent eye for hitting a baseball" corresponds better to the environmental stimulus, baseball batting.

TABLE 6.1.
Levels of Generality/Specificity in Self-Concept Items

SE1	On the whole, I am satisfied with myself.
SE2	I feel I do not have much to be proud of.
BI1	On the following pages are listed a number of things characteristic of yourself or related to you. Consider each item listed and circle the number of each item that best represents your feelings according to the following scale:

1. Have strong positive feelings.
2. Have moderate positive feelings.
3. Have no feeling one way or the other.
4. Have moderate negative feelings.
5. Have strong negative feelings.

1 2 3 4 5 teeth	1 2 3 4 5 hair	
1 2 3 4 5 body	1 2 3 4 5 muscles	

PSC1	Some people do not feel very **BUT** Other people realy feel good confident about themselves about themselves physically. physically.
PSC2	Physically, I am happy with myself.
PSC3	I play sports well.
PPC4	I could jog 5 kilometers without stopping.
Self-Eff.	Indicate which of the tasks below you feel you can perform now. Beside each task selected, assess your probabilities (10% to 100%) of completing the tasks.

Jogging	*Confidence*
Jog 200 yards	_____
Jog ¼ mile	_____
Jog ½ mile	_____
Jog 1 mile	_____

The second factor of concern refers to the *specificity/generality* level of the item. Very specific statements that correspond directly to the immediately relevant environment provide a valid and reliable origin for initiating study of the process of generalization from specific, narrowly defined constructs, to broad constructs encompassing larger amounts of individual personality and behavior. Utilizing our baseball paradigm, this might involve progress on the specificity/generality continuum from "I have an excellent eye for hitting a baseball" to "I am an excellent baseball player" to "I am an excellent athlete" to "I am an excellent person."

Table 6.1 provides the opportunity to relate item characteristics to physical SC constructs such as those contained in Figure 1. Global SC items describe the self without application to a context within the environment. Examples of global SC items from the Rosenberg scale [109] are represented by the top two items (SE1 and SE2) in Table 1. A body image 1 (BI1) item becomes more specific in that it refers to features such as face, hair, and waist, but with no consideration of referents, such as behavior or situational context. Items labeled PSC1 (Physical Self-Concept 1) and PSC2 (Physical Self-Concept 2) of Table 1 are general measures of the physical SC taken from Fox's Physical Self-Perception Profile (PSPP) [33] and Marsh's Physical Self-Description Questionnaire (PSDQ) [83], respectively. PSC1 represents an item assessing physical self-worth (Figure 6.2) and employs an alternative response format. Respondents first select which of the statements is more like them and then indicate the degree ("1" or "2") to which the statement categorizes them. Responses are scored 1 through 4, with a high score representing a high positive evaluation. PSC3 and PSC4 refer to performances at particular motor tasks and are increasingly more specific than PSC1 or PSC2. A person who agreed with PSC3 would probably agree with PSC4, but the reverse might not be true. Items such as these from the PSDQ could be employed in the assessment of the subdomains of sport competence and physical condition, respectively, in Figure 2. While PSC3 and PSC4 would be expected to relate better to athletic behaviors in the environment, PSC1 and PSC2 would be expected to relate better to variables such as global SE. A point emphasized by Harter [46] and again by Fox [31] is that broader constructs, such as indicated by PSC1 and PSC2, should be assessed by direct statements, rather than by summing responses to more specific statements (e.g., PSC3 and PSC4) believed to be contained within the first construct.

The bottom category of Table 1 represents our most specific assessment and provides an example of a self-efficacy statement. It is more specific than PSC3 and PSC4 because it includes actual performance levels at a particular task. While self-efficacy was developed from social cognitive theory [2], it does involve self-evaluations of specific competencies. Subjects are provided with 10–16 levels of a particular task, are asked to check which levels they can currently complete, and should then indicate their degree of certainty (10% to 100%) for completing each level they have checked. Summing the probabilities and dividing by the number of levels provided develops strength of self-efficacy scores.

In summary, Table 1 is organized on an approximate continuum ranging from very broad items and corresponding constructs at the top of the table, to items and constructs specific to behaviors in the immediate environment at the bottom of the table. Following the principles proposed by Shavelson et al. in their hierarchical model [118], it is suggested here that associations between measures of self-concept and external criteria will be larger for relevant component scales, and smaller for scales assessing broad, general constructs. Furthermore, experiments should attempt to utilize as many hierarchical levels as possible. If contingencies do not permit this, constructs and items that relate well to both environmental stimuli and higher levels of self-perception should be employed. Appropriate use and operationalization of hierarchical constructs is seen as a means of studying the process of generalization.

ADVANTAGES OF EMPLOYING COMPONENT SCALES

There are many advantages to using component scales for research purposes, as opposed to global self-concept scales alone. The research attempting to link SE improvement to exercise participation illustrates very well the limitations of employing a single outcome variable, such as global SE. When a positive effect occurs, we are hard pressed to deduce why or how it occurred. Contrast this with research where component scales as well as global SE are employed, such as in the Tennessee Self-Concept Scale (TSCS) [28]. TSCS scores of adolescent idiopathic scoliosis (AIS) subjects (n = 140) were compared to an approximately equal number of healthy adolescents [15]. Based on self-reports, groups were divided into sedentary, moderate, and extensive physical activity groups. In both study groups, subjects who exercised moderately or extensively had significantly larger ($p <$ .007) physical SC and global SC scores than subjects who failed to exercise. While longitudinal data would provide more definitive support, this simple analysis, because of the presence of the physical SC variable, is able to support tentative inferences regarding the mechanisms of change. That is, physical SC represents a mediating or bridging mechanism between activity experiences and the SC.

It seems obvious that four or five scales will provide more information regarding possible causes, outcomes, and associations, as compared to a single scale. In longitudinal research, studying changes and covariation in specific self-perception and global SC provides opportunities for studying a variety of change mechanism. Blascovich and Tomaka suggest that investigators should "focus on more specific self-evaluations which are closely related to the achievement task at hand and show associations between these self-evaluations and global self-esteem" [6].

Second, employing multiple components in a research design provides opportunities to display discriminant as well as convergent validity. For example, if exercise groups in the study above had differed significantly on the moral, family, and physical scales of the TSCS, support for exercise as the cause for group differences would have been weakened considerably. Also, it would be possible to suspect the presence of confounding variables, such as the Hawthorne effect. Marsh et al. [81] administered the Self-Description Questionnaire III (SDQIII) to 361 participants before and after a series of Outward Bound programs. Apprehensive about possible future post-group "euphoria effects," the investigators a priori asked the program director to identify several self-concept components that would not be expected to change as a result of program activities. At program end, it was found that scores had increased significantly on all 13 SDQIII scales. However, the magnitude of increases for the 4 identified scales (Religion, Mathematics, Academic, and Relationships with Opposite Sex) was significantly less than that for the other 9 scales ($p <$ .001), with an average increase of less than 50% that of the others. While post-group euphoria undoubtedly exerted some influence on scores at the second testing, the presence of convergent and discriminant validity also was indicated. This conclusion is supported by the above analysis, by the fact that results tended to be similar across the study's 26 different sites and time periods, and by the relative stability of results assessed after 18 months [82]. The scales that best reflected the intervention were Physical Appearance, Honesty, Parents, Physical Abilities, and General SC.

Buss [9] stated that narrow traits are more homogenous than broad traits. Therefore, narrow traits tend to be better predictors of particular and relevant behaviors. Besides being a tenet of the generic hierarchical model of SC structure [118], this principle has received repeated empirical support [44]. A recent investigation tested the ability of component scales, as opposed to global SC, to differentiate between groups known to differ in actual academic ability [138]. Study 1 compared talented (n = 65) and regular (n = 69) students in grades 4 to 6 on responses to Harter's Perceived Competence scales. Scores on Cognitive Competence significantly discriminated the groups, while scores on General SE as well as Social and Athletic competence did not. A second comparison separated teenage swimmers (age M = 13.6) into nationally ranked and regular swimming club members. A 7-item perceived competence at swimming scale was administered along with Harter's Perceived Competence Scales. Significant differences were obtained for the swimming ($p < .001$) and for Harter's athletic ($p < .04$) scales, but not for other scales, including the general SC scale. Recent research [85] documented that components of SC, such as perceived physical condition, developed significant associations with self-reports of exercise participation, while global SC did not. Earlier, it was emphasized that theory and empirical data failed to support a reliable relationship between physical fitness and global SC across people. Perceived physical ability, regarded as a component of global SC, developed significant and moderate relationships with both fitness and SC [122].

Stability represents a fourth factor arguing against the use of global SC alone in research designs. Since global SE is a relatively stable characteristic, especially in adults, meaningful changes are difficult to detect when global SE is employed in an experiment. For example, experimentally manipulated success or failure experiences are unlikely to have any measurable impact when assessed against a lifetime of self-evaluative experiences [6].

As discussed by Blascovich and Tomaka [6], an expedient approach is to focus on more specific self-evaluations closely related to the achievement task at hand. Because of their greater correspondence with the criterion task, these specific perceptions would be expected to reflect changes in the criterion task more readily than global SC [85, 118].

Finally, it is suggested [146] that broad traits, because of their greater inclusiveness, are more apt to be influenced by mood and non-objective influences, such as social desirability. This principle has been repeatedly verified with the physical SC. This construct has developed considerably smaller associations than global SC with a variety of social desirability measures [35, 121, 127, 130]. Moreover, the significance of associations with validity criteria has not been extinguished when statistically controlled for social desirability [121, 130]. McKinmon and Berger [91] found that mood scores correlated most highly with global SE then with components of emotional stability and physical appearance. Other components, including physical ability SC, did not relate significantly to mood.

A BRIEF REVIEW OF PHYSICAL SC SCALES

Physical self-concept scales that have received predominant use to this point are discussed in this section. The review is roughly historical in nature with continued improvements in assessment noticeable over time. Reviews of individual inventories include only a brief discussion of scale development and item characteristics. Table 6.2 contains descriptive data on those scales that are recommended under the guidelines of this review.

Body Image

''It seems intuitively obvious that attitudes toward the body are important aspects of self-regard,'' asserted Ruth Wylie [150] in her classic review of the SC. This appeal was buttressed by medical and psychiatric theories of the early 20th Century. Hall [43] pointed to young children's preoccupation with body parts. Freud stated, ''The ego is first and foremost a body ego'' [38]. The medical community became increasingly impressed with the alteration of body part perceptions often accompanying psychopathology. Neurologists came to study these deviations, as well as phenomena such as the ''phantom limb'' that can occur after amputation. Working with projective measures, Fisher and Cleveland [27] showed that the perception of individual body boundaries was related to behavior beyond the body's boundaries.

The development of the Body Cathexis Scale [117] provided an objective assessment of body image that emphasized responses based on affect rather than perception. Cathexis has been defined as, ''the degree of satisfaction or dissatisfaction with the various parts or processes of the body'' [117]. Body cathexis items would not seem to relate to the criterion behaviors of this chapter, as well as items from many of the physical self-concept scales to follow. It appears logical to believe that physical activity participation would be more directly related to scores on a perceived physical condition scale than to evaluations of one's lips, fingers, or digestion. While physical activity is often associated with positive body image [7, 51], subpopulations of active people have been identified as possessing body dissatisfaction and eating disorders [14, 96, 106, 136]. While space precludes a review of the vast amounts of body image literature, the Body Esteem Scale, which has received increasing use in exercise and fitness research, will be addressed later in this chapter.

TABLE 6.2.
Frequently Employed Physical Self-Concept Scales

Inventory [Citation]	Scales (No. of Items)	Ages[a]	Type of Item	Referents
a. Physical Self-Efficacy Scale [114]	Physical Self-Presentation Confidence [12]	17–adult		
	*Perceived Physical Ability (PPA) [10]		PSC3, PSC4	Reflexes, agility, physique, muscle tone, running speed
b. Self-Perception Profile for Children [47]	Global Self-Worth [6]	8–14		
	Scholastic Competence [6]			
	Social Acceptance [6]			
	Behavioral Conduct [6]			
	Physical Appearance [6]		PSC2	Satisfaction with looks, face, body, ht, and wt
	*Athletic Competence [6]		PSC2	Competence in and satisfaction with athletic competence, learning, and new games
c. Self-Desription Questionnaire (SDQ) [84]	General Self	6–12	[b]	
	General School			
	Reading			
	Mathematics			
	Peer Relations			
	Parent Relations			
	Appearance			
	*Physical Ability			
d. Self-Description Questionnaire III (SDQIII) [76]	General Self	Late adol.	[b]	
	Academic			
	Mathematics			
	Verbal			
	Problem Solving			
	Same Sex Relations			
	Opposite Sex Relations			
	Relations with Parents			
	Religion/Spirituality			
	Honesty/Reliability			
	Emotional Stability			
	*Physical Appearance		PSC3	Evaluation and satisfaction with attractiveness, body, wt., and face
	*Physical Abilities		PSC3	Competence in coordination, sports ability, body build, physical energy, plus liking for physical activity
e. Body Esteem Scale [37]	Males: *Physical Attractiveness [11]	College to adult	B1	Satisfaction with body parts
	*Upper Body Strength [9]		"	"
	*Physical Condition [13]		"	"
	Females: *Sexual Attractiveness [13]		"	"
	*Weight Concern [10]		"	"
	*Physical Condition [9]		"	"

(continued)

TABLE 6.2.
(continued)

Inventory [Citation]	Scales (No. of Items)	Ages[a]	Type of Item	References
f. Physical Self-Perception Profile (PSPP) [32]	*Physical Self-Worth [6]	College to adult	PSC1	Satisfaction with one's general physical self
	*Sport Competence [6]		PSC3[c]	Competence in and confidence at possessing these traits
	*Physical Condition [6]	"	"	"
	*Attractive Body [6]	"	"	"
	*Strength	"	"	"
g. Physical Self-Description Questionnaire (PSDQ) [83]	Esteem [8]	12–18		Global self-acceptance and self-competence
	*Global Physical [6]		PSC3	Satisfaction with one's general physical self
	*Health [8]		PSC3, PSC4	Competence in 9 physical subdomains
	*Coordination [6]	"	"	"	"
	*Physical Activity [6]	"	"	"	"
	*Sports Competence [6]	"	"	"	"
	*Body Fat [6]	"	"	"	"
	*Appearance [6]	"	"	"	"
	*Strength [6]	"	"	"	"
	*Flexibility [6]	"	"	"	"
	*Endurance [6]	"	"	"	"

* Primary interest scale.
[a] Ages are approximate. At times, scales have been utilized with older Ss (e.g., the SDQ).
[b] Complete information on all SDQ inventories may be obtained from Herbert W. Marsh.
[c] In alternative response format.

Physical SC Scales

The Estimation scale [120, 122] provided the first assessment of perceived capabilities at exercise and sport, as opposed to the prior use of body parts as referents. This scale was developed as a mediating variable in an early model explaining the psychological benefits of exercise and predicting participation in physical activity. Sonstroem [122] emphasized that while global SE was not related to physical fitness across people (or could not be expected to be sizably related by theory), estimation was significantly related to both fitness and global SE. Across 13 samples grouped by gender and grade (grades 6 to college), correlation coefficients between estimation and fitness ranged from .21 to .53 (median = .37) [17, 34, 104, 122]. In these studies, coefficients between estimation and global SE ranged from .30 to .61 (median = .51). The 33-item Estimation measure utilizes items similar to PSC3 and PSC4, and is contained in the Physical Estimation and Attraction Scales (PEAS) [120, 122]. A major limitation precluding continued use of the Estimation scale concerns its wide assortment of statement referents. These include strength, coordination, aerobic fitness, abilities, and aptitudes at gymnastics, tennis, golf, and sport leadership. As suggested by the thesis of this chapter, when disparate elements like those above are summed to provide a single score, this score's subsequent association with a specific criterion, such as exercise participation, will tend to be vitiated. Also, the investigator is unable to determine the contribution of each of these elements to the association.

The Physical Self-Efficacy Scale [114] (Table 2) contains items similar to those at the PSC3 and PSC4 level in Table 1. In terms of chapter specifications, this inventory is recognized as a physical SC scale. It was developed in the context of 6 studies that included principal component analyses, tests of internal consistency and stability, and correlations with global SE, other personality scales, and indices of physical activity participation. Factor analyses produced a 10-item Perceived Physical Ability scale (PPA), and a 12-item Physical Self-Presentation Confidence scale. The developmental study showed that PPA scores were positively related to mesomorphy ($r = .19$, $p < .03$), reaction time ($r = -.40$, $p < .03$), performance on a motor coordination task ($r = .40$, $p < .04$), and negatively related to social anxiety ($r = .32$, $p < .001$) [114].

The following three multidimensional inventories (Tennesse Self-Concept Scale, Self-Perception Profile for Children, and Self-Description Questionnaire) possess 1 or 2 scales that can be regarded as physical SC measures. Their other scales assess a variety of specific SCs, such as academic, social, family, and health concepts. These inventories are useful in characterizing subjects from a more complete perspective in school, family, or social settings.

The TSCS represents a pioneer multidimensional inventory developed in 1965 [28], with recent minor modifications and new norms [108]. It remains the most frequently employed multidimensional SE inventory [6]. The 100-item inventory possesses five external and three internal frames of reference, as well as clinical and response distortion scales. Items contain a 5-point Likert response format and are written at a mid-range level of specificity (PSC2-PSC3 in Table 2). The five external frames of reference include Physical, Moral, Personal, Family, and Social SCs.

Following theory proposed by James [56] and White [147], Susan Harter's seminal research has emphasized competence as a personal trait, as well as the multidimensionality of self-conception. Avoiding the label "self-esteem," her first scale was titled The Perceived Competence Scale for Children [45] (Table 2). It contained a global SE scale labeled Global Self-Worth and three specific domain scales assessing cognitive, physical, and social competencies. This was replaced by the Self-Perception Profile for Children [47], which added scales for Physical Appearance and Behavioral Conduct and replaced competence with self-adequacy as the underlying dimension for 4 of the 6 scales. The Physical Competence scale is now referred to as Athletic Competence to better reflect item content. These scales, primarily for grades 3–8, possess a structured alternative response format (see PSC1 in Table 1). The manual [47] provides means and standard deviations by gender for grades 3–8.

Based on the original Shavelson model [118], the Self-Description Questionnaire (SDQ) (Table 2) assesses three academic content areas (Reading, Mathematics, and General-School) and four non-academic content areas (Physical Ability, Physical Appearance, Peer Relations, and Parent Relationships) [84]. The SDQII [70] and the SDQIII [76] contain similar and additional scales and were developed for early and late adolescence, respectively.

The following three multidimensional physical SC inventories offer increased opportunities to study both discriminant validity and the manner in which experimental effects generalize to related components.

A major limitation of the Body Cathexis Scale is its assessment of body image as a unidimensional concept, an idea which has been consistently disconfirmed [27, 65]. The Body Esteem Scale (BES) [37] was developed over three separate administrations to large samples of college male and female students. Over these three data analyses involving principal component analysis with mainly oblique rotation, the 40 items from the Body Cathexis Scale (plus 16 new items) were reduced to 35 items involving three components for each sex [37].

Franzoi's research is important because it allowed for gender differences in components and test items [37]. The three female scales are labeled Sexual Attractiveness, Weight Concern, and Physical Condition. Larger scores on the second scale indicate a lack of weight concern. Male scales are labeled Physical Attractiveness, Upper Body Strength, and Physical Condition. This and a subsequent study [36] supported the independence of components, with none of the between-component coefficients exceeding .65 (most were considerably lower). Subtracting an effect size ($r^2 \times 100$) from 1.00 indicates that a majority of the component variance represented independent, rather than shared, variance for all components.

Study of the physical self was greatly advanced by the development of the PSPP [33]. This is a physical SC inventory that satisfies content validity criteria very well. An open-ended questionnaire that asked respondents to list reasons why people feel good about their physical selves was administered to 63 male and 84 female college students. Based upon their responses, 6-item scales were developed for components of sport competence, physical condition, attractive body, and strength. These factors persisted over a multi-sample series of principle component analyses with college students. A superordinate, more general Physical Self-Worth Scale was added to form the 5-scale PSPP (the two PSPP levels may be seen as the middle levels in Figure 1). A confirmatory factor analysis with 216 adult females established that all items loaded significantly on hypothesized factors with no crossovers [126]. Subsequent covariance analyses testing a variety of models established the importance of retaining Physical Self-Worth (PSW) as a mediator with global SE, and validated the EXSEM model structure, as seen in Figure 1. The PSPP has been validated for use with high school athletes [145], and a Children's PSPP was developed for use with seventh and eighth graders [148].

The most comprehensive multidimensional physical SC instrument was developed in 1994 with two large samples of Australian students, ages 12–18 [83]. This instrument contains 11 scales with 70 items representing scales from Marsh's SDQ inventories or measures that were developed to assess multiple physical fitness components. It contains global scales rating Esteem and Physical Ability and 9 physical subdomain scales encompassing health, coordination, physical activity, body fat, sport competence, appearance, strength, flexibility, and endurance. Confirmatory factor analyses replicated component structure across samples and structure. Additionally, extensive subsequent research has provided excellent intra-structure information regarding associations among components, as well as extra-structure relationships with criteria such as physical fitness tests and athletic participation [73]. All scales included in this review contain adequate to excellent values for both internal consistency and stability.

Measurement Considerations

The relatively large amount of criterion validity developed by the PPA makes it a likely candidate for use when a single general physical SC scale is wanted for research in an athletic setting. While it is possible to utilize global SC and other scales with the PPA, heuristic motives suggest that exercise and sport scientists may wish to employ multidimensional physical SC inventories when studying discriminant and convergent validity, and the manner in which personal evaluations generalize to neighboring and to higher levels of regard. The Self-Perception Profile for Children of Harter [47] or the SDQs of Marsh [70, 76, 84] are recommended, especially in educational settings where more complete profiles of students may be desired. Harter's Athletic scale is more relevant for athletic settings, whereas the SDQ Physical Abilities scale possesses stimuli relevant to both sport and exercise.

The TSCS is criticized because many of its items are scored on multiple scales, which creates collinearity among constructs [4]. Reports examining the skill development hypothesis often identify significant changes in 5 or more scales, which limits discriminant validity and impedes an understanding of the mechanisms of change [25, 26, 50, 101]. In a definitive study employing both exploratory and confirmatory factor analysis, Marsh and Richards [80] found consistent support for the external scales of Family, Physical, and Social, as well as Total Positive Score. However, the authors concluded that none of the external scales were clearly unidimensional. In reference to the Physical scale, this is not at all surprising. The items in this scale refer to appearance, body build, state of health, sexuality, and skills, with a special concentration on appearance. Not surprisingly, the Marsh and Richards study found that the Physical scale related more closely with the Physical Appearance scale than with the Physical Abilities scale of the SDQIII.

At this stage in our understanding of physical SC structure, continued use of multidimensional physical SC scales is strongly encouraged. Both the PSPP [33] and the PSDQ [83] can define the self-processes involved in exercise and athletic experiences. However, limitations of the PSPP include occasional difficulties at understanding the response format (especially in children and the elderly) [125]. Additionally, its physical condition scale is criticized for a lack of unidimensionality in that items refer to both physical condition and maintenance of exercise [83]. The PSDQ was developed by an experienced psychometrician and presents itself as a very promising inventory, with the limitation that it has not been employed in the US. In his recently published text, Fox and chapter authors [32] provide more information on the PSPP and the PSDQ.

PHYSICAL SC DEVELOPMENT

Hattie [49] endorses the idea that the self is born in the communication processes of the mother-child dyad. Self-identity develops from the additional processes of separating one's self from the environment and others, discovering personal causation, learning more about the self from environmental testing, and learning from the responses of others. Studies show that younger children describe themselves in concrete, behavioristic terms rather than in abstract trait-like reports [46]. Self-appraisals of younger children tend to be unrealistic, and are labeled egocentric by Marsh [68]. They do, however, improve in accuracy over time, as the child tests reality and compares abilities with peers.

While many forces potentially can influence the SC, sources of information about the self tend to be contained within two external sources (reflected appraisals and social comparisons), and an internal source (self-perceptions of competence). Reflected appraisals is a postulate of symbolic interactionism theory and is exemplified in Cooley's "looking glass theory" [12]. Briefly, it posits that SC is formed by how we think important others see us. If we believe that they think highly of us and expect big things from us, the self-fulfillment prophecy is apt to be supported. This concept is of salient importance in social communication and is a cornerstone of Rogerian counseling psychology. Horn and Lox [54] described the disparate effects produced by a coach's high and low expectations for different athletes. Conversely, it has been established that important others, and especially coaches, have the power to increase SC in young athletes by virtue of feedback and praise contingent on performance [5, 53, 119, 143]. "Pygmalion in the classroom" documents the positive academic achievements of elementary school students whose teachers held high expectations of them [112]. While research sometimes has failed to support the power of reflected appraisals, it continues to be regarded as a vital force in SC development. Mboya [87] asked 276 South African adolescents to rate their teachers on a scale encompassing support, interest, and encouragement. These teacher ratings correlated positively with multiples SCs, and values ranged to .61 for general school SC and .47 for global SC.

We also learn about ourselves by observing others, and by comparing ourselves to our perceptions of their strengths and weaknesses. Because of the importance of sports ability in establishing peer status in youth, particularly in younger boys, it would seem that children get early and extensive information about physical abilities through reflected appraisals and social comparisons [13, 21, 141]. Preferred sources of information concerning one's athletic abilities appear to gravitate from reliance on parents at younger ages, to appreciation of peer comparisons at about ages 12–15 [53, 143]. Unfavorable social comparisons will impinge on the development of a positive SC. Marsh's research addressed the phenomenon of the "Big Fish, Little Pond" and its powerful effects in society [69, 77]. He determined that positive SCs are fostered by environments where positive self-other comparisons can be established, rather than by more select settings where negative comparisons are more probable [69]. A series of studies compared Australian students assigned to programs for the gifted and talented with equally talented students assigned to regular classes. Those in the gifted and talented programs decreased SCs in Reading, Math, and School over time, whereas SC scores on Physical Abilities, Physical Appearance, Peer Relations, and Parent Relations were unaffected [75]. It has been suggested that similar frames of reference may impede the progress of elite athletes [79]. Conceivably, this may indicate that the prevalence of task-orientation as opposed to ego-orientation in better young athletes represents a motivation to avoid negative self-other comparisons.

By self-perceptions, we refer to personal evaluations of self and behavior in the environment. With age and experience, children develop internalized standards regarding competencies, control of performance, effort exerted, and enjoyment when participating at specific activities [44, 144]. Within the athletic milieu, establishment of these internal perceptions is influenced by referred appraisals and social comparisons, as well as by task mastery, degree of improvement over time, goal achievement, and actual performance statistics, such as batting average, won-lost percentage, etc. [44, 53]. Additionally, internal standards are associated with positive physical SCs [143].

Physical SC tends to be formed in youth in relation to one's peers (in similar grades in the same school and the same gender) [71]. Perceived physical competence is usually more highly related to certain components of fitness (e.g., cardiovascular endurance, body composition, dynamic strength, and power) [71]. Of the physical SC components, appearance tends to be the most closely associated with higher hierarchical levels, such as global physical SC [33, 126, 131] and global SE [33, 48, 126, 131]. This effect is found across all ages and both genders [33, 47, 131]. While body weight invariably has been negatively associated with SE in children, a recent longitudinal design paired increases in body mass index with declines in perceived physical competence and with unfavorable changes in attitudes toward physical activity and activity preferences [62].

AGE AND GENDER EFFECTS

Gender differences in global SE do not appear to be consistent at any age level [10, 151]. However, gender differences in component scores have been reliably identified. This fact suggests a multidimensional perspective when studying age and gender effects across the life span.

Preadolescence

Most investigations have found a steady linear decrease in both component and general SE scores from about grade 2 to about grade 7, with an amount of individual variation [68, 95, 110]. Marsh [68] employed 12,266 responses to SDQ, SDQII, and SDQIII inventories to study age and sex effects in Australian children. SDQ data revealed a significant linear decrease in all scores from grade 2 to grade 9. A partial explanation for these decreases may be blamed on the inaccurate evaluations of younger children. As indicated previously, this may be a factor of unrealistically high SCs that lacks sufficient comparisons to external criteria. This age effect included decreased scores on Physical SC and Physical Appearance SC. Boys had significantly larger Physical SC scores than girls, with a significant interaction effect ($p < .01$), indicating an increased male effect with age. A significant quadratic function by age interaction found this differential to be most pronounced at the polarities of the age range. Physical Appearance scores were significantly larger for boys ($p < .001$), and a significant sex X linear age interaction ($p < .01$) indicated that this differential increased with age. At the preadolescent age level, boys had significantly larger scores on all scales, with the exception of the Parent Relationships and School scales. Similar trends were observed in an American sample [149].

Adolescence

Theorists and investigators tend to agree that somewhere in the early to middle teen years, decreases in SC tend to be corrected, and SC scores increase or remain level for a period of time before rising into adulthood. This reversal in trend varies considerably in terms of time of onset, sex, and component effects. Additionally, the direction of subsequent age effects is not clear. Parent Relationships show decreases at this age level, whereas Opposite Sex Relationships tend to increase.

Marsh's [68] examination of SDQII responses in grades 7–11 identified significant decreases in Physical SC ($p < .001$) and significant increases in Physical Appearance ($p < .001$). Again, males scored significantly higher than females ($p < .001$) on both of these scales. Girls scored significantly more favorably than boys ($p < .001$) on the Verbal, Honesty, and Same Sex Relationships scales.

Late Adolescence-Early Adulthood

Two large studies utilized longitudinal data in reaching similar conclusions. Bachman and O'Malley [1] found that global SE increased in boys by about one standard deviation from 10th grade to 5 years post high school. Another study utilized girls as well as boys in finding that SE increased about .1 standard deviation per year in the 2 years following high school [97]. In Australian students ages 15–19, significant linear score increases were obtained across the age range for a majority of components, including physical and physical appearance SCs. Again, males scored significantly more favorably ($p < .001$) than females on both of these scales. However, significant interaction effects ($p < .001$) found that with age, females were decreasing this difference in scores [68]. Very similar results were obtained in a large US sample [55]. Transition from single sex to coeducational high schools failed to adversely affect multidimensional scores or gender differences in scores [67].

Adulthood

In adults, relatively little research has examined the effect of age and gender on SC, particularly physical SC. Godin and Shephard [41] failed to obtain significant differences in PPA scores among three age categories of adults whose ages ranged from 45–74. However, they found significant gender differences favoring the men ($p < .01$). It is theorized that with increasing age, people develop an increase in the number of SC components they use to define themselves. Mean levels of SE tend to remain stable, however, and changes tend to be influenced by social and environmental factors rather than by maturation [3]. Notwithstanding psychology's continued emphasis on factors influencing SC development, a recent large twin-pair study concluded that SC crystallizes in early adulthood and is heavily influenced by genetics [90].

Female Scores

A superiority in male Physical SC scores over those of females at all age levels was previously noted. A meta-analysis of 35 studies with 46 effect sizes in young athletes verified this conclusion and attempted to identify reasons for this difference [64]. Instruments utilized in these 35 studies included Vealey's Sport-Confidence Scale [140], Ryckman's Perceived Physical Ability subscale [114], the Sport Competence subscale of the PSPP [33], the Perceived Athletic Competence subscale [45], and the Estimation scale of the PEAS [120]. Results showed an average gender effect size of .40 favoring men. However, individual study results were extremely variable, thus limiting the reliability of this effect size. Results tended to show that the differential athlete effect was more prevalent in male-oriented sports. However, only a single feminine task was encountered within the study. As is so often the case with the female SC, as well as with female sport participation, the influences exerted by stereotypical perspectives within society must be considered.

SKILL DEVELOPMENT RESEARCH

Physical Activity

Many studies with adults have documented changes in physical SC following aerobic or strength conditioning programs. [8, 59, 98, 101, 132, 137]. McAuley et al. [88] documented self-efficacy increases at bicycling, walk/jog, and sit-ups in 45–64 year olds after 20 weeks of structured training. Female scores were inferior to those of males at preprogram testing but made significantly greater improvements over the 20 weeks. This study and others [59, 82, 98] have documented the stability of results, with follow-up testing ranging up to 18 months after program cessation. Marsh and Peart [78] found that fitness programs based on cooperation and improvement manifested positive changes in perceived physical ability, whereas programs based on competition did not.

A review of 16 studies concluded that SE scores were significantly associated with participation in exercise programs [123]. However, incomplete or relatively simple designs and a failure to provide controls for confounding variables, such as perceived task demands and response distortion, made it impossible to conclude why or how change occurred. It was evident that a majority of the research tacitly assumed that increases in physical fitness caused the change. Efforts generally were not made or were unsuccessful in supporting this inference. Recently, it was concluded that increases in physical fitness are not the causal factor, per se, in SE changes following exercise [124]. Significant SE increases very often followed programs lacking significant fitness change [98, 101], and failed to appear in other programs where fitness increased [94, 103].

As indicated earlier, the relative stability of global SE limits the probabilities of effecting true SE change via exercise. Identifying causal agents may be difficult because of a host of possible factors (some of them potentially confounding) that reside within exercise programs [93, 123]. One of these pervasive factors is expectancy (placebo effect) [16]. Once people are told that exercise will make them feel better about themselves, expectancy for SE change becomes irrevocably rooted in the experimental process. Realistically, it is recognized also that expectancies can energize the therapeutic process.

As discussed by Blaskovich and Tomaka [6], one approach to studying SE change is to employ specific evaluations closely related to the achievement task at hand, and to show associations between changes in these evaluations and those of global SE. The EXSEM model followed earlier proscriptions [6, 123], and was developed as a means of documenting psychological change via interactions between self-efficacies and changes in actual physical competencies. Additional mechanisms of change can be added to the model, and their interactions with self-efficacies and physical SC can be examined. Use of multiple variables in either this or other multidimensional models is encouraged as a means to better identify the psycho-social factors (including expectancies) that may be involved in SE change via physical activity.

Athletics

Perceived physical SC differences were found between participants and non-participants in youth sports [24], and between high school athletes and non-athletes [145]. Perceived athletic competence scores related significantly to a physical skills composite score in 8–13 year old soccer players; however, the largest association of self-perception scales was developed by a more specific soccer competence scale [23]. Athletic SC scores in 8–14 yr olds increased significantly after 1 week of soccer [52] and 5 weeks of swimming instruction [92]. The athletic SC in young competitive athletes (ages 12–18) was found to be related to coaches' praise and feedback following desirable performance [5, 119].

Conclusions

We remain unable to explain why chronic SE benefits often occur after programs of physical fitness. Youth programs in athletic settings have learned a great deal more comparatively about the motives and attributions of their subjects (see next section). Much of this athletic research can be characterized as possessing multiple measures linked by carefully constructed hypotheses.

SELF-ENHANCEMENT RESEARCH

Physical Activity

While the self-enhancement hypothesis functions as a favorite credo of SC enthusiasts, little research at the global level supports this hypothesis. [116]. The converse seems to be true at the more micro levels of assessment [e.g., 66, 85, 102, 114, 127, 128]. A lower level of statistical evidence relies on associations between SC variables and criterion measures where both assessments are obtained at the same point in time. PSPP subscales are proven effective in developing large correlations with self-reports of physical activity

[33, 126, 131]. Convergent validity was established in that physical condition developed the largest relationships of the 5 PSPP scales in the above studies. Discriminant validity was provided by showing that other less relevant scales failed to associate significantly [126], and especially by the canonical correlation analyses of Fox and Corbin [33]. Using hierarchical regression analysis, Ryckman et al. [114] showed that the PPA developed significant and large associations with weighted sport participation indices beyond those explained by the physical scale of the TSCS.

A structural modeling analysis of 219 adult females found that the EXSEM explained 26% of aerobic class attendance and 27.6% of exercise outside of class. The PSPP scales of Physical Condition and Attractive Body were significant predictors and were positively and negatively related, respectively, to the dependent variables [126].

Several studies have employed physical SCs to predict subsequent actual behaviors. Perceived physical ability scores obtained during the first week of school from 467 junior high school boys significantly predicted those who would enroll a week later in intramural sports [128]. While scores were not significantly related to subsequent 8-week program adherence, the authors pointed to many social and personal problems that served to confound an accurate prediction. Earlier research by Dishman [18] found that estimation was unable to predict the adherence of middle-aged men to a university exercise program. Additionally, the PPA scale of the Physical Self-Efficacy Scale was unable to predict either short or long-term exercise behavior in 240 adults [139]. However, it is emphasized that these scales are not truly relevant for this use. Both studies contained middle-aged subjects engaged in formal exercise programs. The Estimation scale was developed for adolescent boys and contains more items of an athletic nature, as opposed to a fitness or exercise nature. The author located only 2 items in the 10-item PPA scale that were relevant to exercise rather than athletics. It is hoped that today these same hypotheses could be tested with newer, more relevant scales, such as the Condition and Strength scales of the PSPP or the Physical Activity, Endurance, Strength, Body Fat, and Health scales of the PSDQ.

Athletics

In youth, physical SCs are positively associated with participation in sport programs [105] and negatively associated with dropping out of sports programs [24]. Motives for participation can be related to physical SCs. Children high in perceived physical ability make attributions for their own performance that are more stable, internal, and higher in control than children low in perceived physical ability [144]. The children high in perceived physical ability believe that they are successful at sport and they manifest higher expectations for future athletic success. They rank skill development, team affiliation, and having fun as major reasons for their participation [61, 113]. Results such as these are a basis for concluding that high intrinsic motivation is present in athletes with favorable physical SCs.

A study supporting the self-enhancement theory found that three TSCS scales, combined with locus of control and trait anxiety, predicted competition scores after 8 months of gymnastics training [102]. A path analysis across a high school varsity swimming season [127] found that November perceived physical competence scores, as assessed by estimation items, significantly predicted January swim times ($p < .05$). Subsequently, January estimation scores approached traditional significance levels in predicting March swim times ($p < .12$). Prerace scores of a 12-item version of the estimation scale [115] significantly predicted race times of 49 marathoners ($r = -.28$, $p < .05$) [40]. Gayton et al. [39] found that prerace PPA scores predicted marathon finish times ($r = -.55$, $p < .001$) in 33 runners. PPA scores also predicted pace times in three subsequent 1 mile to 10 kilometer races, with correlations ranging from $-.32$ ($p < .05$) to $-.40$ ($p < .01$) [63]. As could be expected, a task-specific perceived ability scale developed larger coefficients ranging from .49 ($p < .001$) to .50 in this latter study. A similar effect was obtained with 52 university female gymnasts, where PPA scores significantly predicted subsequent performance in only one of four events, while a task-specific self-efficacy scale predicted performance in all events [89].

Conclusions

Even though research has been slow in supporting the self-enhancement hypothesis where global SE is concerned, research on physical and athletic SCs has been quite successful in supporting this hypothesis. Much of this research supports the merit of employing hierarchical models. It can be concluded that physical SCs are valid predictors of physical activity and especially of athletic participation. Through their employment with youth in sport settings, we have been able to study the development of physical SCs and the manner in which they relate to participation motives and attributions. Their use in eclectic models predicting physical activity participation and adherence is encouraged [124, 125].

PHYSICAL SCS AND LIFE ADJUSTMENT

Since global SC is recognized as *the* psychological variable most indicative of emotional and life adjustment, it seems apparent that these desirable attributes may be vested in SC components as well. Social and peer acceptance is recognized as an important correlate of adjustment in children [21]. Competence in athletics represents the major criterion for status in adolescent boys [20]. Moreover, active engagement in physical and sport skills is believed to represent both a social asset [11] and a medium for utilizing social comparison processes [60, 141]. While working in a summer sports program with 126 children (ages 8–13), Weiss and Duncan [142] showed that perceived physical competence was highly related to perceived peer acceptance and to teachers' ratings of peer acceptance.

Depression has been negatively associated with an adolescent's perceived physical competence. [19]. On the other hand, other correlational research has associated perceived physical ability scores in college students with optimism [57] and with self-actualization [133]. These last three studies all employed the PPA scale [114]. Meanwhile, Tappe and Duda [135] found that a personal sense of physical competence was the best predictor of life satisfaction in the elderly.

A recent study of 119 female and 126 male undergraduates representing 23 academic disciplines employed positive and negative affect, depressive symptoms, and health complaints as adjustment measures [130]. Two measures of social desirability were entered first in the hierarchical regression analysis followed by global SE, and then by Fox's [33] 5 physical SC scales. Even with the effects of social desirability and global SE accounted for, three of the eight associations (across sex) between adjustment measures and physical SCs remained significant, with effect sizes ranging to 16% (median = 6% across the eight associations). This research replicates earlier work [121] where response distortion was also assessed and controlled for. It provides greater evidence that of themselves, positive perceptions of physical competence are associated with favorable life adjustment.

Conclusion

It can be concluded that satisfaction and pride in one's physical capabilities are related to a positive mental outlook and to life adjustment. These results occurred after tendencies to exaggerate and to create false impressions were already considered and controlled for. This implies that future skill development research may employ physical SCs not only as variables mediating global SC change, but also as primary outcome variables of themselves.

SUGGESTED DIRECTIONS

A limitation of this chapter is that it fails to present more of the newer knowledge involving component associations within a hierarchical SC structure. Also, the author is unable to address the importance individuals may place on the physical SC and its particular components. There are many sources the interested reader can refer to [31–33, 74, 83, 125, 126].

To the degree that item-criterion congruence may represent a tenuous principle across people, certain conclusions within the chapter become invalid. The validity of item-criterion specificity has not always been supported in the research. The fact that scales of the TSCS, other than the Physical, developed as large or larger relationships with activity criteria has been discussed. Also, other scales sometimes encounter a lack of consistent discriminant ability. While a lack of scale sensitivity may be blamed, other possible causes should be noted. One cause concerns the manner in which people may generalize success at an activity to a variety of SC components—both those on the same level of generality as the "target SC," and those that are positioned at a higher level of generality in the hierarchy. For example, someone who becomes successful at a golf skill (Figure 2) may generalize this competence to the sport competence level, while bypassing the self-efficacy level. Or, a woman who has spent 12 months in a diet exercise program may become very satisfied with aspects of her body image, while never thinking about physical self-efficacies or the physical condition SC. Although this may be used as an argument against relying on item-criterion specificity, it is also logical to state that principles of generalization may not become understood without operationalizing principles of item-criterion specificity.

Perhaps a major limitation present in contemporary SC items results from the lack of attempts to differentiate between the generally recognized SE dimensions of competence and self-acceptance. Self-acceptance refers to the self-liking or unconditional positive regard of an individual [46, 134, 146]. Self-accepting people recognize personal imperfections and faults, but they continue to like and to respect themselves while they work to erase or to minimize these flaws. While a great deal of attention in the 1980s and 1990s has been directed toward the competence dimension, self-acceptance has been largely ignored. Using confirmatory factor analysis, Tafaradi and Swann [134] recently validated a two-dimensional model and developed the Self-Liking/Self Competence Scale. External validity for this global measure was obtained by showing that depression scores correlated negatively and significantly with self-liking, but failed to associate significantly with self-competence. An example of their competence and self-acceptance items is found in the first two rows of Table 6.3.

The original Exercise and Self-Esteem Model included physical self-acceptance at the domain level. Recent research, emanating from a disserta-

TABLE 6.3.
Examples of Competence and Self-Acceptance Items

Component	Dimension	Item
SC	Comp.	I am a capable person.
	S. Acc.	I like the kind of person I am.
END/F	Comp.	I can run a long way without stopping.
	S. Acc.	I feel good about my level of fitness/endurance.
STRE	Comp.	I am stronger than most people my age.
	S. Acc.	I am embarrassed about my physical strength.

SC, Global Self-Concept; COMP, competence item; S. Acc., self-acceptance item; END/F, endurance/fitness sub-domain; STRE, strength sub-domain.

tion in psychology, has attempted to develop scales for assessing competence and self-acceptance at the physical domain level and five subdomains (sports ability, strength, fitness/endurance, appearance, and body fat) [100]. Competence items assessed the quality of personal abilities or performances as compared to an implied or stated standard. Some of these items were taken or adapted from the PSDQ inventory [83]. Self-acceptance items assessed feelings of satisfaction in or acceptance of personal abilities or performances. Examples of items from the different scales are listed in rows 3–6 of Table 3. While confirmatory factor analysis revealed a very good fit of the model to data, three of the paths from subdomains to general physical acceptance failed to achieve significance. These results confirm that assessment of both competence and self-acceptance in physical SC components is possible, and encourage further research in this area.

It is challenging that a majority of SE items measuring higher structural levels, such as Physical Self-Worth, General Physical SC, or global SE, consist of self-acceptance statements. Rosenberg et al., always a proponent of global SE, concluded that global SE is especially relevant to psychological well-being, while specific SE is relevant to behavior [111]. Perhaps this interpretation is caused by the fact that many current assessments involve competence evaluations at the specific end of the continuum and self-acceptance evaluations at more global levels. However, this condition is seldom recognized in the literature and the two dimensions are often mixed in random fashion across levels of specificity/generality. It is obvious that the dimensions of competence and self-acceptance are related, perhaps in both causative and reciprocal fashions. The SC knowledge area has made outstanding progress in assessment over the past 10 years. As scientists, we remain interested in sharpening the tools of our exploration. Studying dimensions of competence and self-acceptance, along the specificity-generality continuum, may provide us with the knowledge of how physical and athletic skills generalize to positive feelings about one's self.

SUMMARY

This chapter summarized knowledge about the physical SC, a variable that has assumed great importance in studying how self-esteem is related to physical activity participation. It discussed the advantages of employing component scales such as physical SCs, and reviewed research and theory on the development of the physical SC, age and sex differences, and relationships with life adjustment. Skill development and self-enhancement research were summarized. Leading physical SC scales were briefly reviewed. A thesis of the chapter is that SE and its associations with physical activity participation can be studied best by the employment of models that are hierarchical in their structure, and which contain SC components ranging from very specific to very broad constructs. This has implications for item and inventory selection and for an ultimate understanding of how physical activity leads to mental and emotional benefits.

REFERENCES

1. Bachman, J.G., and P.M. O'Malley. Self-esteem in young men: a longitudinal analysis of the impact of educational and occupational attainment. *J. Pers. Soc. Psychol.* 35:365–380, 1977.

2. Bandura, A. *Social Foundations of Thought and Action.* Englewood Cliffs, NJ: Prentice-Hall, 1986.

3. Bengston, V.I., M.N. Reedy, and C. Gordon. Aging and Self-Conceptions: personality processes and social content. J.E. Birren and K.W. Schaie (eds.). *Handbook of the Psychology of Aging (2nd edition).* New York: Van Nostrand Reinhold, 1985, pp. 544–593.

4. Bentler, P.M. Review of the Tennessee Self-Concept Scale. O.K. Buros (ed.). *The Seventh Mental Measurements Yearbook.* Highland Park, NJ: Gryphon Press, 1972, pp. 366–367.

5. Black, S.J., and M.R. Weiss. The relationships among perceived coaching behaviors, perceptions of ability, and motivation in competitive age-group swimmers. *J. Sport Exerc. Psychol.* 14:309–325, 1992.

6. Blascovich, J., and J. Tomaka. Measures of self-esteem. J.P. Robinson, P.R. Shaver, and L.S. Wrightsman (eds). *Measures of Personality and Social Psychology.* San Diego: Academic Press, 1994, pp. 115–160.

7. Bosscher, R.J. Running and mixed physical exercises with psychiatric patients. *Int. J. Sport. Psychol.* 24:170–184, 1993.

8. Brown, R. D., and Harrison, J. M. The effects of a strength training program on the strength and self-concept of two female age groups. *Res. Q. Exerc. Sport.* 57:315–320, 1986.

9. Buss, A. H. Personality as traits. *Am. Psychol.* 44:1378–1388, 1989.

10. Byrne, B. M. *Measuring Self-Concept Across the Life Span.* Washington, D.C.: American Psychological Association, 1996.

11. Coie, D.J., K.A. Dodge, and J. Kupersmidt. Peer group behavior and social status. S.R. Asher, and J.D. Coie (eds.). *Peer Rejection in Childhood.* New York: Cambridge University Press, 1991, pp. 17–59.

12. Cooley, C.H. *Human Nature and the Social Order.* New York: Scribners, 1902.

13. Cowell, C.C., and A.H. Ismail. Relationships between selected social and physical factors. *Res. Q. Exerc. Sport.* 33:40–43, 1962.

14. Davis, C., S.H. Kennedy, E. Ralevski, and M. Dionne. The role of physical activity in the development and maintenance of eating disorders. *Psychol. Med.* 24:957–967, 1994.

15. Dekeel, Y.G., G. Tenenbaum, and K. Kudar. An exploratory study on the relationship between postural deformities and body image and self-esteem in adolescents: the mediating role of physical activity. *Int. J. Sport Psychol.* 27:183–196, 1996.

16. Desharnais, R., J. Jobin, C. Cote, L. Levesque, and G. Godin. Aerobic exercise and the placebo effect: a controlled study. *Psychosom. Med.* 55:149–155, 1993.

17. Dishman, R.K. Aerobic power, estimation of physical ability, and attraction to physical activity. *Res. Q. Exerc. Sport.* 49:285–292, 1978.

18. Dishman, R.K. Biologic influences on exercise adherence. *Res. Q. Exerc. Sport.* 52:237–267, 1981.

19. Ehrenberg, M.F., D.N. Cox, and R.F. Koopman. The relationship between self-efficacy and depression in adolescents. *Adol.* 26:361–374, 1991.

20. Eitzen, D.S. Athletics in the status system of male adolescents. A.Yiannikis, T.McIntyre, M.Melnich, and D.Hart (eds.). *Sport Sociology: Contemporary Themes.* Dubuque, IA: Kendall/Hunt, 1976, pp.114–119.

21. Evans, J., and G.C. Roberts. Physical competence and the development of children's peer relationships. *Quest.* 39:23–35, 1987.

22. Feltz, D.L. Self-confidence and sports performance. *Exercise Sport Sciences Reviews (Vol.12).* New York: Macmillan, 1988, pp.423–457.

23. Feltz, D.L., and E.W., Brown. Perceived competence in soccer skills among young soccer players. *J. Sport Psychol.* 6:385–394, 1984.

24. Feltz, D.L., and L.Petchlikoff. Perceived competence among interscholastic sport participants and dropouts. *J. Sport Psychol.* 5:231–235, 1983.

25. Finkenberg, M.E. Effect of participation in taekwando on college women's self-concept. *Percept. Mot. Skills.* 71 898–894, 1990.

26. Finkenberg, M.E., D. Shows, and J.M. DiNucci. Participation in adventure-based activities and self-concepts of college men and women. *Percept. Mot. Skills.* 78:1119–1122, 1994.

27. Fisher, S., and S. Cleveland. *Body Image and Personality.* New York: Van Nostrand, 1958.

28. Fitts, W.H. *Tennessee Self-Concept Scale Manual.* Nashville, TN: Counsellor Recordings and Tests, 1965.

29. Fleming, J.S., and B.E. Courtney. The dimensionality of self-esteem II: hierarchical facet model for revised measurement scales. *J. Pers. Soc. Psychol.* 46:404–421, 1984.

30. Fox, K.H. The self-esteem complex and youth fitness. *Quest* 40:230–246, 1988.

31. Fox, K.H. *The Physical Self-Perception Profile Manual.* DeKalb, IL: Northern Illinois University, Office for Health Promotion, 1990.

32. Fox, K.H. *The Physical Self: From Motivation to Well-Being.* Champaigne, IL: Human Kinetics, 1997.

33. Fox, K.H., and C.B. Corbin. The physical self-perception profile: development and preliminary validation. *J. Sport Exerc. Psychol.* 11:408–430, 1989.

34. Fox,K.H., C.B. Corbin, and W.H. Couldry. Female physical estimation and attraction to physical activity. *J. Sport Exerc. Psychol.* 7:125–136, 1985.

35. Franzoi, S.I. Further evidence of the reliability and validity of the Body Esteem Scale. *J. Clin. Psychol.* 50:237–239, 1994.

36. Franzoi, S.I., and M.E. Herzog. The body esteem scale: a convergent and discriminant validity study. *J. Pers. Assess.* 48:173–178, 1986.

37. Franzoi, S.I., and S.A. Shields. The body esteem scale: multidimensional structure and sex differences in a college population. *J. Pers. Assess.* 48:173–178, 1984.

38. Freud, S. *Ego and The Id.* London: Institute of Psychoanalysis and the Hogarth Press, 1927.

39. Gayton, W.F., G.R. Mathews, and G.N. Burchstead. An investigation of the validity of the physical self-efficacy scale in predicting marathon performance. *Percept. & Mot. Sk.* 63: 752–754, 1986.

40. Gayton, W.F., K. Skelton, M. Waichunas, and J.F. Hearns. Validities of the physical estimation scale in predicting running times. *Percept. & Mot. Sk.* 68:252–254, 1989.

41. Godin, G., and R.J. Shephard. Gender differences in perceived physical self-efficacy among older individuals. *Percept. & Mot. Sk.* 60:599–602, 1985.

42. Gruber, J.J. Physical activity and self-esteem development in children: a meta-analysis. *Am. Acad. Phys. Educ. Paper* 19:30–48, 1985.

43. Hall, G.S. Some aspects of the early sense of self. *Am. J. Psychol.* 9:351–395, 1898.

44. Hansford, B.C., and J.A. Hattie. The relationship between self and achievement/performance measures. *Rev. Ed. Res.* 52:123–142, 1982.

45. Harter, S. The perceived competence scale for children. *Child Develop.* 53:87–97, 1982.

46. Harter, S. Developmental perspectives on the self-system. *Handbook of Child Psychology: Socialization, Personality and Social Development Vol.4.* E.M. Hetherington (ed.) New York: Wiley, 1983. pp., 275–375.

47. Harter, S. *Manual for the Self-Perception Profile for Children.* Denver: University of Denver, 1985.

48. Harter, S. Causes, correlates, and the functional role of global self-worth. R.J. Sternberg and J.J. Kolligian (eds.). *Competence Considered.* New Haven, CT: Yale University Press, 1990.

49. Hattie, J. *Self-Concept.* Hillsdale, NJ: Lawrence Erlbaum, 1992.

50. Hilyer, J.C., and W. Mitchell. Effect of physical fitness training combined with counseling on the self-concept of college students. *J. Couns. Psychol.* 26:427–436, 1979.

51. Holmes, T., P. Chamberlin, and M. Young. Relations of exercise to body image and sexual desirability among a sample of university students. *Psychol. Rep.* 74:920–922, 1994.

52. Hopper, C, G.D. Guthrie, and T. Kelly. Self-concept and skill development in youth soccer players. *Percept. Mot. Skills.* 72:275–285, 1991.

53. Horn, T.S., and C.A. Hasbrook. Psychological characteristics and the criteria children use for self-evaluation. *J. Sport Psychol.* 9:208–223, 1987.

54. Horn, T.S., and C. Lox. The self-fulfilling prophecy theory: when coaches' expectations become reality. J.M. Williams (ed.). *Applied Sport Psychology: Personal Growth to Peak Performance.* Mountain View, CA: Mayfield, 1993, pp. 68–81.

55. Jackson, L.A., C.N. Hodge, and J.M. Ingram. Gender and self-concept: a reexamination of stereotypic differences and the role of gender attitudes. *Sex Roles.* 30:615–630, 1994.

56. James, W. *Principles of Psychology (Vol. 1).* New York: Henry Holt and Company, 1890.

57. Kavusama, M., and E. McAuley. Exercise and optimism: are highly active individuals more optimistic? *J. Sport Exer. Psychol.* 17:246–258, 1995.

58. Kentzierski, D. Self-schemata and exercise. *Bas. Appl. Soc. Psychol.* 9:45–61, 1988.

59. King, A.C., C.B. Taylor, W.L. Haskell, and R.F. DeBusk. Influence of regular aerobic exercise on psychological health: a randomized controlled trial of healthy middle-aged adults. *Health Psy.* 8:305–324, 1989.

60. Kleiber, D.A. Sport and human development: a dialectical interpretation. *J. Humanist. Psychol.* 23:76–95, 1983.

61. Klint, K.A., and M.R. Weiss. Perceived competence and motives for participation in youth sports: a test of Harter's competence motivation theory. *J. Sport Psychol.* 9:55–65, 1987.

62. Kolody, B., and J.F. Sallis. A prospective study of ponderosity, body image, self-concept, and psychological variables in children. *J. Dev. Behav. Ped.* 16:1–5, 1995.

63. LaGuardia, R., and E.E. Labbe. Self-efficacy and anxiety and their relationship to training and race performance. *Percept. & Mot. Sk.* 77:27–34, 1993.

64. Lirgg, C.D. Gender differences in self-confidence in physical activity: a meta-analysis of recent studies. *J. Sport Exerc. Psychol.* 13:294–310, 1991.

65. Mahoney, E.R., and M.D. Finch. The dimensionality of body cathexis. *J. Psychol.* 92: 277–279, 1976.

66. Marsh, H.W. Causal ordering of self-concept and achievement: a multiwave, longitudinal panel analysis. *J. Educ. Psychol.* 82:646–656, 1986.

67. Marsh, H.W. The effects of attending single sex and coeducational high schools on achievement, attitudes and behavior and on sex differences. *J. Ed. Psychol.* 81:70–85, 1989.

68. Marsh, H.W. Age and sex effects in multiple dimensions of self-concept: preadolescence to early adulthood. *J. Ed. Psychol.* 81:417–430, 1989.

69. Marsh, H.W. The failure of high ability high schools to deliver academic benefits: the importance of academic self-concept and educational aspirations. *Amer. Ed. Res. J.* 28: 445–480, 1991.

70. Marsh, H.W. *Self-Description Questionnaire II: Manual.* Sydney, Australia: Publication Unit, Faculty of Education, University of Western Sydney, 1992.

71. Marsh, H.W. Physical fitness self-concept: relations to field and technical indicators of physical fitness for boys and girls aged 9–15. *J. Sport Exerc. Psychol.* 15:184–206, 1993.

72. Marsh, H.W. Sport motivation orientations: beware of the jingle-jangle fallacies. *J. Sport Exerc. Psychol.* 16:306–326, 1994.

73. Marsh, H.W. Construct validity of physical self-description questionnaire responses: relations to external criteria. *J. Sport Exerc. Psychol.* 18:111–131, 1996.

74. Marsh, H.W. The measurement of physical self-concept: a construct validation approach. K.R. Fox (ed.). *The Physical Self: From Motivation to Well-Being.* Champaigne, IL: Human Kinetics, 1997.

75. Marsh, H.W., D. Chessor, R. Craven, and L. Roche. The effects of gifted and talented programs on academic self-concept: the big fish strikes again. *Am. Ed. Res. J.* 32:285–319, 1995.

76. Marsh, H.W., and R. O'Niell. Self-description questionnaire III (SDQIII): the construct validity of multidimensional self-concept ratings by late-adolescents. *J. Ed. Meas.* 21: 153–174, 1984.

77. Marsh, H.W., and J.W. Parker. Determinants of student self-concept: is it better to be a relatively large fish in a small pond even if you don't learn to swim as well? *J. Pers. Soc. Psychol.* 47:213–231, 1984.

78. Marsh, H.W., and N.D. Peart. Competitive and cooperative physical fitness training programs for girls: effects of physical fitness and multidimensional self-concepts. *J. Sport Exerc. Psychol.* 10:390–407, 1988.

79. Marsh, H.W., C. Perry, C. Horsely, and L.A. Roche. Multidimensional self-concepts of elite athletes: how do they differ from the general population? *J. Sport Exerc. Psychol.* 17: 70–83, 1995.

80. Marsh, H.W., and G.E. Richards. The Tennessee self-concept scales: reliability, internal structure, and construct validity. *J. Pers. Soc. Psychol.* 55:612–624, 1988.

81. Marsh, H.W., G.E. Richards, and J. Barnes. Multidimensional self-concepts: the effect of participation in an Outward Bound program. *J. Pers. Soc. Psychol.* 45:173–187, 1986.

82. Marsh, H.W., G.E. Richards, and J. Barnes. Multidimensional self-concepts: a long-term follow-up of the effect of participation in an Outward Bound program. *Pers. Soc. Psychol. Bull.* 12:475–492, 1986.

83. Marsh, H.W., G.E. Richards, S. Johnson, I. Roche, and P. Tremayne. Physical self-description questionnaire: psychometric properties and multitrait-multimethod analysis of relationships to existing instruments. *J. Sport Exerc. Psychol.* 16:270–305, 1994.

84. Marsh, H.W., I.D. Smith, and J. Barnes. Multidimensional self-concepts: relationships with inferred self-concepts and academic achievement. *Austr. J. Psychol.* 36:367–386, 1984.

85. Marsh, H.W., and R.J. Sonstroem. Importance rating and specific components of physical self-concept: relevance to predicting global components of self-concept and exercise. *J. Sport Exerc. Psychol.* 17:84–104, 1995.

86. Martinek, T.J. *Pygmalion in the Gym: Causes and Effects of Expectations in Teaching and Coaching.* West Point, NY: Leisure Press, 1982.

87. Mboya, M.M. Gender differences in teachers' behaviors in relation to adolescents' self-concepts. *Psychol. Reports* 77:831–839, 1995.

88. McAuley, E., K.S. Courneya, and J. Lettunich. Effects of acute and long-term exercise on self-efficacy responses in sedentary middle-aged males and females. *Gerontologist* 31: 534–542, 1991.

89. McAuley, E., and D. Gill. Reliability and validity of the physical self-efficacy scale in a competitive sport setting. *J. Sport Psychol.* 5:410–418, 1983.

90. McGue, M., B. Hirsch, and D.T. Lykken. Age and the self-perception of ability: a twin study analysis. *Psychol. Aging* 8:72–80, 1993.

91. McKinmon, A.D., and B.G. Berger. Self-concept and mood changes associated with aerobic dance. *Austr. J. Psychol.* 45:134–140, 1993.

92. Miller, R. Effects of sport instruction on children's self-concept. *Percept. Mot. Skills.* 68: 239–242, 1989.

93. Morgan, W.P. Methodological considerations. W.P. Morgan (ed.). *Physical Activity and Mental Health.* Washington, DC: Taylor & Francis, 1997, pp. 3–32.

94. Netz, Y., G. Tenenbaum, and M. Sagiv. Pattern of psychological fitness as related to pattern of physical fitness among older adults. *Percept. Mot. Skills.* 67:647–655, 1988.

95. Nichols, J.A. Development of perception of attainment and causal attributions for success and failure in reading. *J. Educ. Psychol.* 71:94–99, 1979.

96. O'Connor, P.J., R.D. Lewis, E.M. Kirschner, and D.B. Cook. Eating disorder symptoms in former female college gymnasts: relations with body composition. *Am. J. Clin. Nutr.* 64:840–843, 1996.

97. O'Malley, P.M., and J.C. Bachman. Self-esteem: change and stability between ages 13 and 23. *Dev. Psychol.* 19:257–268, 1983.

98. Ossip-Klein, D.J., E.J. Doyne, E.D. Bowman, K.M. Osborn, L.B. McDougall-Wilson and R.A. Niemeyer. Effects of running or weight lifting on self-concept in clinically depressed women. *J. Consult. Clin. Psychol.* 57:158–161, 1989.

99. Pauly, J.T., J.A. Palmer, C.C, Wright, and G.J. Pfeiffer. The effect of a 14-week employee fitness program on selected physiological and psychological parameters. *J. Occ. Med.* 24: 457–463, 1982.

100. Pino-Graziano, R.D., L.L. Harlow, and R.J. Sonstroem. Inclusion of physical acceptance in tests of the exercise and self-esteem model. *Med. Sci. Sports Exerc.* 28:S136, 1996. (abstract).

101. Plummer, O.K., and Y.O. Koh. Effects of "aerobics" on self-concepts of college women. *Percept. Mot. Skills.* 65:271–275, 1987.

102. Porat, Y., D. Lufi, and G. Tenenbaum. Psychological components contribute to select young female gymnasts. *Int. J. Sport Psychol.* 20:279–286, 1989.

103. Rainey, D., and J. Wigtil. Aerobic running as a counseling technique for undergraduates with low self-esteem. *J. Coll. Stud. Personnel* 16:53–57, 1985.

104. Riley, J.H. The relationship of self-concept with physical estimation and physical performance for preadolescent boys and girls. *J. Early Adol.* 3:327–333, 1983.

105. Roberts, G.C., D.A. Kleiber, and J.L. Duda. An analysis of motivation in children's sport: the role of perceived competence in participation. *J. Sport Psychol.* 3:206–216, 1971.

106. Rodin, J. Cultural and psychosocial determinants of weight concerns. *Ann. Int. Med.* 119: 643–645, 1993.

107. Rogers, C.R. The significance of the self-regarding attitudes and perceptions. M.L. Reymert (ed.). *Feeling and Emotion: The Mooseheart Symposium.* New York: McGraw-Hill, 1950.

108. Roid, G.H., and W.H. Fitts. *Tennessee Self-Concept Scale (Revised Manual).* Los Angeles: Western Psychological Services, 1994.

109. Rosenberg, M. *Society and the Adolescent Self-Image.* Princeton, N.J.:Princeton University Press, 1965.

110. Rosenberg, M. Self-concept and psychological well-being in adolescence. R.L. Leahy (ed.). *The Development of the Self.* New York: Academic Press, 1985.

111. Rosenberg, M., C. Schooler, C. Schoenbach, and F. Rosenberg. Global self-esteem and specific self-esteem: different concepts, different outcomes. *Am. Soc. Rev.* 60: 141–156, 1995.

112. Rosenthal, R.J., and L. Jacobson. *Pygmalion in the Classroom: Teacher Expectation and Pupils' Intellectual Development.* New York: Holt, Rinehart and Winston, 1968.

113. Ryckman, R.M., and J. Hamel. Perceived physical ability differences in the sport participation motives of young athletes. *Int. J. Sport. Psychol.* 24:270–283, 1993.

114. Ryckman, R.M., M.A. Robbins, B. Thornton, and P. Cantrell. Development and validation of a physical self-efficacy scale. *J. Pers. Soc. Psychol.* 42:891–900, 1982.

115. Safrit, M.J., T.M. Wood, and R.K. Dishman. The factorial validity of the physical estimation and attraction scales for adults. *J. Sport Psychol.* 7:166–190, 1985.

116. Scheirer, M.A., and R.E. Kraut. Increasing educational achievement via self-concept change. *Rev. Ed. Res.* 49:131–150, 1979.

117. Secord, P.F., and S.M. Jourard. The appraisal of body cathexis: body cathexis and self. *J. Consult. Psychol.* 17:343–347, 1953.

118. Shavelson, R.J., J.J. Hubner, and G.C. Stanton. Self-concept: validation of construct interpretations. *Rev. Ed. Res.* 46:407–441, 1976.

119. Smoll, F.L., and R.E. Smith. Leadership behaviors in sport: a theoretical model and research paradigm. *J. Appl. Soc. Psychol.* 7:75–91, 1989.

120. Sonstroem, R.J. Attitude testing examining certain psychological correlates of physical activity. *Res. Q. Exerc. Sport* 45:93–103, 1974.

121. Sonstroem, R.J. The validity of self-perceptions regarding physical and athletic ability. *Med. Sci. Sports* 8:126–132, 1976.

122. Sonstroem, R.J. Physical estimation and attraction scales: rationale and research. *Med. Sci. Sports* 10:97–102, 1978.

123. Sonstroem, R.J. Exercise and self-esteem. R.L. Terjung (ed.). *Exercise and Sports Science Reviews (Vol. 12).* Lexington, MA:Collomore Press, 1984, pp. 123–155.

124. Sonstroem, R.J. Exercise and self-esteem. W.P. Morgan (ed.). *Physical Activity and Mental Health.* Washington, DC:Taylor & Francis, 1997, pp. 127–143.

125. Sonstroem, R.J. The physical self-system: a mediator of exercise and self-esteem. K.R. Fox (ed.). *The Physical Self: From Motivation to Well-Being.* Champaigne, IL:Human Kinetics, 1997, pp. 3–26.

126. Sonstroem, R.J., L.L. Harlow, and L. Josephs. Exercise and self-esteem: validity of model expansion and exercise associations. *J. Sport Exerc. Psychol.* 16:29–42, 1994.

127. Sonstroem, R.J., L.L. Harlow, and K.S. Salisbury. Path analysis of a self-esteem model across a competitive swim season. *Res. Q. Exerc. Sport.* 64:335–342, 1993.

128. Sonstroem, R.J., and K.P. Kampper. Prediction of athletic participation on middle school males. *Res. Q. Exerc. Sport.* 51:685–694, 1980.

129. Sonstroem, R.J., and W.P. Morgan. Exercise and self-esteem: rationale and model. *Med. Sci. Sports Exerc.* 21:329–337, 1989.

130. Sonstroem, R.J., and S.A. Potts. Life adjustment correlates of physical self-concepts. *Med. Sci. Sports Exerc.* 28:619–625, 1996.

131. Sonstroem, R.J., E.D. Speliotis, and J.L. Fava. Perceived physical competence in adults: an examination of the Physical Self-Perception Profile. *J. Sport Exerc. Psychol.* 14:207–221, 1992.

132. Stein, P.N., and R.W. Motta. Effects of aerobic and non-aerobic exercise on depression and self-concept. *Percept. Mot. Skills.* 74:79–89, 1992.

133. Summerlin, J.R., S.A. Berretta, G. Privette, and C.M. Bundrick. Subjective biological self and self-actualization. *Percept. Mot. Skills.* 79:1327–1337, 1994.

134. Tafarodi, R.W., and W.B. Swann. Self-liking and self-competence as dimensions of global self-esteem: initial validation of a measure. *J. Pers. Assess.* 65:322–342, 1995.

135. Tappe, M.K., and J.L. Duda. Personal investment predictors of life satisfaction among physically active middle-aged and older adults. *J. Psychol.* 122:557–566, 1988.

136. Thompson, J.K. (ed.). *Body Image, Eating Disorders and Obesity.* Washington, DC:American Psychological Association, 1976.

137. Tucker, L.A. Effects of a weight-training program on the self-concepts of college males. *Percept. Mot. Skills* 54:1055–1061, 1982.

138. Vallerand, R.J., L.G. Pelletier, and F. Gagne. On the multidimensional versus unidimensional perspectives of self-esteem: a test using the group-comparison approach. *Soc. Behav. Personal.* 9:121–132, 1991.

139. Valois, P., R.J. Shephard, and G. Godin. Relationship of habit and perceived physical ability to exercise behavior. *Percept. Mot. Skills* 62:811–816, 1986.

140. Vealey, R.S. Conceptualization of sport-confidence and competitive orientation: preliminary investigation and instrument development. *J. Sport Psychol.* 8:221–246, 1986.

141. Veroff, J. Social comparison and the development of motivation. C. Smith (ed.). *Achievement Related Motives in Children.* New York:Russell Sage Foundation, 1969, pp.46–101.

142. Weiss, M.R., and S.C. Duncan. The relationship between physical competence and peer acceptance in the context of children's sport participation. *J. Sport Exerc. Psychol.* 14: 177–191, 1992.

143. Weiss, M.R., V. Ebbeck, and T.S. Horn. Children's self-perceptions and sources of physical competence information: a cluster analysis. *J. Sport Exerc. Psychol.* 19:52–70, 1997.

144. Weiss, M.R., E. McAuley, V. Ebbeck, and D.M. Wiese. Self-esteem and causal attributions for children's physical and social competence in sport. *J. Sport Exerc. Psychol.* 12:21–36, 1990.

145. Welk, G.J., C.B. Corbin, and L.A. Lewis. Physical self-perceptions of high school athletes. *Ped. Exerc. Sci.* 7:152–161, 1995.

146. Wells, L.E., and G. Marwell. *Self-Esteem: Its Conceptualization and Measurement.* Beverly Hills, CA: Sage, 1976.

147. White, R.W. Motivation reconsidered: the concept of competence. *Psychol. Rev.* 66: 297–333, 1959.

148. Whitehead, J.R. A study of children's physical self-perceptions using an adapted physical self-perception profile questionnaire. *Ped. Exerc. Sc.* 7:132–151, 1995.

149. Wigfield, A., J.S. Eccles, D. MacIver, D.A, Reuman, and C. Midgeley. Transitions during early adolescence: changes in children's domain-specific self-perceptions and general self-esteem across the transition to junior high school. *Dev. Psychol.* 27:552–565, 1991.

150. Wylie, R.C. *The Self-Concept: A Review of Methodological Considerations and Measuring Instruments.* Lincoln, NB: University of Nebraska Press, 1974.

151. Wylie, R.C. *The Self-Concept: Theory and Research in Selected Topics (vol. 2, rev. edit.).* Lincoln, NE: University of Nebraska Press, 1979.

7
Translational Control of Gene Expression in Muscle

DONALD B. THOMASON, PH.D.

Translation is the process of sequentially decoding mRNA codons to condense the appropriate amino acid on a growing polypeptide. It is tightly regulated both temporally and spatially in cells. Increasingly, researchers are learning about the control mechanisms that regulate translation, and recognize that the control process provides a means to modulate gene expression. In this review, these mechanisms as they apply to cardiac and skeletal muscle (SM) will be discussed.

Working muscle provides both unique advantages and disadvantages to the study of translational control. On the one hand, there is usually sufficient mass of striated muscle to allow confident analyses. Furthermore, depending upon the degree to which one wishes to make a distinction, muscle can be very homogenous in terms of cell type—muscle versus nonmuscle. Unique among many tissues, muscle is quite plastic in its gene expression, and exhibits an amazing adaptive response to a change in functional demand. This means that it is quite easy to produce a change in translation and gene expression. One distinct disadvantage of studying muscle is the relative magnitude of protein synthesis. In other words, the rate of protein synthesis tends to be lower as compared to many other tissues and cells. Nonetheless, this disadvantage is often overcome simply by the mass of the tissue available.

The paragraphs that follow discuss the current state of knowledge regarding the control of translation in striated muscle, especially in relation to adaptational responses to functional demand. In some instances, however, tissues other than muscle will be discussed. In particular, the first part of this chapter contains a brief review and update of the translation mechanism, while the second part examines data from experiments that illustrate various control mechanisms in muscle.

Researchers are, by no means, complete in their understanding of translational control mechanisms, as will become evident from the areas in which information is sparse. Much work needs to be done on emerging areas of research on translational control, as well as working to verify and bolster putative mechanisms observed in prokaryotes and lower eukaryotes. In the concluding remarks of his 1874 paper describing the different characteristics of "les muscles rouges" and "les muscles pâles" of the rabbit, Ranvier foresaw the work that lay ahead for physiologists with his statement, "That the research will have to be painstaking"[1] [114]. Indeed, it has been and will continue to be so, as these translational control mechanisms are investigated in greater detail.

THE TRANSLATION PROCESS: TRYING TO KEEP THE TERMINOLOGY STRAIGHT

The terminology associated with the various components of translation is confusing, sometimes appears arbitrary and duplicative, and can be overwhelming in volume. This is not anyone's fault. As with any field that has grown and evolved over several decades, the terminology reflects progress. Throughout this review, factors will be referred to by their generally accepted designation, by their subunits with the α, β, γ, and δ labels, and by their aliases, where applicable.

Translating the codons of a mRNA into a nascent polypeptide is a complex process involving many required steps and components. To simplify the discussion, three sequential phases are usually identified: (1) initiation of the translation complex of ribosome and mRNA, (2) elongation of the polypeptide by condensation of amino acids, and (3) termination by release of the nascent polypeptide and dissociation of the ribosome and mRNA. Each of these phases is in itself a series of complex covalent and noncovalent interactions of the many components. This section provides a succinct background for the remainder of the discussion, with Figure 7.1 listing the key components and their general site of action.

Initiation of protein synthesis begins with the assembly of a preinitiation complex of ribosomal RNA (rRNA) and proteins. It is accepted that for the preinitiation complex to form, the 40S ribosomal subunit (consisting of the 18S rRNA and more than 30 additional proteins) must exist as a separate entity from the 60S ribosomal subunit (consisting of 28S, 5S, and 5.8S rRNAs, and approximately 50 additional proteins). Their association is prevented by the (eukaryotic) initiation factor 3 (eIF-3). (Several comprehensive reviews provide more detail on these and subsequent translational processes [55, 91, 118].) By maintaining the dissociation of the 40S and 60S ribosomal subunits, this initiation factor allows the 40S subunit to accept the ternary complex of eIF-2 (consisting of 3 subunits α, β, and γ) binding an obligatory guanosine-5'-triphosphate (GTP) and the initiator Met-tRNA. Although eIF-1A was once thought to also maintain dissociation of the 40S and 60S ribosomal subunits, recent evidence indicates that binding of the ternary complex to the 40S subunit is catalyzed by eIF-1A [19]. In the pres-

---

[1] "Ces recherches doivent être minutieuses."

FIGURE 7.1.

A schematic representation of translation. The key components discussed in the text and their general site of action are shown in relation to an mRNA (thick solid line) and the protein for which it codes (thick mottled line). Ribosomal components are designated by their sedimentation coefficients (40S, 60S, 80S).

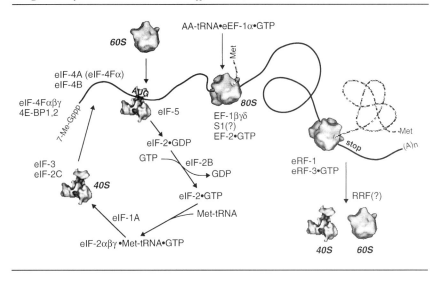

ence of mRNA, however, the ternary complex subsequently lacks stability if another factor, eIF-2C, is not present (referred to by Roy et al. as co-eIF-2A) [120].

Preinitiation complex recognition of an mRNA (actually a ribonucleo-protein complex, or mRNP) requires a number of additional cofactors. Probably the most common mechanism for recognition and binding of the mRNA is the "scanning model." In this model, the preinitiation complex binds to a mRNP that consists of 7-methyl-guanylate capped mRNA and several cofactors, and then "scans" downstream of the cap for the start codon. Like the assembly of the preinitiation complex, assembly of the mRNA ribonucleoprotein complex is also quite ordered. eIF-4F (consisting of 3 subunits α, β, and γ) recognizes the 7-methyl-guanylate cap, binds tightly to the structure, and disrupts secondary structure very near the cap [75]. The β subunit of eIF-4F is also known as eIF-4A and, although considered an eIF-4F subunit, has a somewhat more complicated binding and release pattern [110].[2] The cap-binding activity of eIF-4Fα has its own regu-

---

[2] Worthy of mention at this point is the participation of eIF-4F in an alternative initiation process at an internal ribosome entry site (IRES). Though common for viral mRNAs, it is much less common for eukaryotic mRNAs and requires the binding of the eIF-4F γ subunit to specific mRNA sequences downstream of the 5'–end [111].

latory proteins that bind the eIF-4Fα (also known as eIF-4E), and hence are known as 4E-BP1 and 4E-BP2 (also referred to as phosphorylated heat and acid stable proteins I and II, or PHAS-I and PHAS-II). These regulatory proteins prevent eIF-4Fα from binding the mRNA cap. The activity of the eIF-4Fα binding proteins is regulated by phosphorylation of the binding protein by a mitogen activated protein (MAP) kinase-independent mechanism [5, 128]; phosphorylation enhances the dissociation of the subunit and the binding protein. Interestingly, the α subunit of eIF-4F is also regulated by its phosphorylation state. This phosphorylation occurs via a MAP kinase-dependent mechanism that does not directly promote dissociation of its binding protein [42]. The most notable reason for considering a potential role of the binding proteins is the location of their expression. While expression of 4E-BP2 is ubiquitous, expression of 4E-BP1 is greatest in SM, adipose tissue, and pancreas [140]. These tissues are very sensitive to insulin stimulation of protein synthesis (to be discussed).

Another initiation factor, eIF-4B, has two binding sites, one for the mRNA and another for 18S, thus aiding the association of the mRNA with the preinitiation complex [89, 90, 100]. Researchers often draw mRNA as a linear structure for discussion purposes, but in fact, the molecule has significant secondary and tertiary structure. This structure would tend to retard preinitiation complex scanning were it not for the unwinding (helicase) activity of two of the initiation factors, eIF-4A and eIF-4B. These cofactors help to "melt" the RNA structure in an adenosine tri-phosphate (ATP) dependent manner such that the 40S preinitiation complex is able to scan for the initiator codon [61].

For the 60S ribosomal subunit to bind to form the complete 80S ribosome, the GTP bound to eIF-2 must be hydrolyzed, which causes the release of this cofactor from the initiation complex. Yet another cofactor, eIF-5, participates in this hydrolysis in a mechanism that involves its direct interaction with eIF-2 [18]. Among the initiation factors released from the 40S initiation complex, eIF-2·guanosine-5'-diphosphate (GDP) is notable since eIF-2 cannot participate in ternary complex formation until the exchange of GTP for GDP occurs in a reaction catalyzed by eIF-2B [17]. The 60S subunit binding completes the formation of the fully functional 80S ribosome, and condensation of amino acids begins following the initiator methionine.

One may appreciate the importance of translational control when considering the energy expended for the elongation of a polypeptide. Whereas a single high-energy phosphate bond is consumed for initiation, each amino acid added to the growing polypeptide usually consumes four high-energy phosphate bonds, as follows: (1) Aminoacyl-tRNA acts as the precursor to the polypeptide, providing the classical codon translation. (2) Formation of the charged tRNA itself consumes two high-energy phosphate bonds through the pyrophosphate cleavage of ATP by the specific aminoacyl-tRNA synthetases and subsequent pyrophosphatase action. (3) The aminoacyl-tRNA combines with the α subunit of elongation factor 1 (eEF-1α) bound to a molecule of GTP to form the complex that is capable of binding to the A-site of the ribosome. (4) The transfer of the aminoacyl-tRNA from its synthetase to eEF-1α may occur through the formation of an intermediate complex, such that both eEF-1α and GTP stimulate the rate-limiting dissociation of the aminoacyl-tRNA from its synthetase [101, 119].

eEF-1 itself is an interesting molecule. It consists of four subunits—α, β, γ, and δ. The first subunit, eEF-1α, is involved in transfer of the tRNA to the ribosome binding site where GTP hydrolysis occurs, while the latter three facilitate the exchange of GTP for GDP on eEF-1α, analogous to the exchange factor in initiation. It is unclear to what extent the activity of eEF-1 is modulated in physiological situations, but clearly phosphorylation of the subunits through a protein kinase C-activated mechanism increases the activity of eEF-1 [148, 149]. Intriguingly, phosphorylation of the β and γ subunits by casein kinase II also occurs, and this phosphorylation is stimulated by GDP and dependent upon the presence of the eEF-1α subunit, apparently as eEF-1α·GDP [108]. Although a modulatory role for eEF-1 phosphorylation in muscle *in vivo* has not been directly demonstrated, an emerging body of literature indicates its potential for modulation. Furthermore, the possibility of isoform expression of the subunits also arises. Recent reports indicate the expression of an mRNA (termed S1) with a significant homology to the eEF-1α subunit [77]. Interestingly, expression of this mRNA is developmentally regulated and apparently inversely regulated with eEF-1α [78], a pattern of expression analogous to the differential expression of the skeletal and cardiac α-actin isoforms [86, 104, 143]. Furthermore, S1 expression is greatest in the brain, cardiac muscle, and SM, and is significantly upregulated following myotube formation by myoblasts in culture [78]. However, no evidence exists at this writing that S1 indeed has EF-1α activity.

When the aminoacyl-tRNA is correctly positioned in the ribosome A-site, the peptide bond forms and the ribosome translocates under control of eEF-2. Upon binding eEF-2·GTP, translocation of the peptidyl-tRNA from the A-site to the P-site of the ribosome occurs, followed by hydrolysis of the GTP and release of eEF-2. eEF-2 carries all of its translocation functionality as a monomeric protein, and its regulation is relatively straightforward. Of minor concern for normal physiological regulation is the adenosine diphosphate- (ADP-) ribosylation of the diphthamide residue and inactivation of eEF-2 by *Diphtheria* toxin [23, 59, 144]. Of potential physiological importance is the phosphorylation-dependent inactivation of eEF-2. A specific kinase, the calmodulin-dependent protein kinase III, inactivates eEF-2 translocation activity [98]. Support that this kinase activity has a physiological role is upheld by data that show that the phosphatase blocker okadaic acid increases the level of eEF-2 phosphorylation in reticulocyte lysates

[116], which subsequently indicates the presence of balanced kinase and phosphatase activities. This is further supported by data that indicate that insulin binding to its receptor decreases eEF-2 phosphorylation and that this decrease is associated with a decrease in the kinase activity [115]. The kinase itself is autophosphorylated and its activity increases in a calcium-calmodulin-dependent manner that suggests amplification of the calcium second-messenger signal [117].

By comparison, termination of polypeptide elongation is relatively simple—or is it? It was once thought that when a termination codon appeared in the A-site of the ribosome, a releasing factor (eRF-1) recognized the termination codon in the A-site and hydrolyzed the peptidyl-tRNA in the P-site. In turn, the nascent polypeptide and the tRNA was released. (A brief review of termination was recently published by Nakamura et al. [99].) While this simple mechanism is still considered fundamentally correct, recent evidence complicates the picture and emphasizes a common theme that has also developed in the initiation and elongation phases—GTP hydrolysis. A second releasing factor, eRF-3[3], has GTP binding capabilities but, as a binary complex, no hydrolytic activity [44]. A mechanism has been proposed, however, whereby eRF-3 association with eRF-1 and the ribosome, positions the releasing complex correctly while in the "GTP state," following which cleavage of the peptidyl-tRNA and activation of eRF-3 GTPase activity by eRF-1 and the ribosome forces the complex into the "GDP state" and causes release of the eRFs [44]. Interestingly, eRF-1 may have the additional role of enhancing the association of phosphatase 2A with the ribosome, a mechanism that could enhance dephosphorylation of regulated proteins [2], but certainly its most important role is to recognize the termination codons. Whether eRF-1 recognizes the termination codons appears to depend somewhat on both the base immediately following the termination codon as well as the penultimate and C-terminal amino acids. In mammals, highly expressed genes do not have a purely random distribution of bases following the termination codon, and termination efficiency is much greater if the UGA termination codon is followed by G or A [135]. C or U in this position has relatively weak termination efficiency, which sometimes causes recoding of the termination codon [135]. As shown in bacteria, but not yet in eukaryotes, termination efficiency is also promoted by cooperative effects of basic and hydrophilic amino acids in the penultimate position, as well as the size and structure forming ability of the terminal amino acid [9]. Thus, the emerging picture of termination of translation is one of a process that is just as rich and potentially complicated as the preceding initiation and elongation steps.

---

[3] No known eRF-2 exists. Prokaryotic releasing factors that recognize stop codons are RF-1 and RF-2. RF-3 in prokaryotes is functionally similar to the eukaryotic eRF-3.

Finally, once the nascent protein is released, the ribosome must be disassembled. As one may suspect, this, too, may be an ordered process. Unfortunately, very little is known about the process, especially in eukaryotes. Certainly ionic conditions affect the integrity of the ribosome, but it is difficult to imagine how this determinant could be manipulated in time and space to disassemble only those ribosomes that have completed a protein. More telling is the data from prokaryotes. In bacteria, a ribosome releasing factor (RRF) is essential for cell growth, as demonstrated with mutant *E. coli* that carry a frame-shifted RRF chromosomal gene and a wild-type RRF gene on a temperature-sensitive plasmid [60]. The cells were only capable of growth under temperature permissive conditions. As yet, a comparable gene has not been demonstrated in eukaryotes, but given the conservation of many protein synthesis mechanisms and components from prokaryotes to eukaryotes, it is probable that such a factor(s) will be found in the future.

Thus, a number of points where translation can be controlled are affirmed. Some of these points have been well characterized; others are just being recognized for their potential. In muscle, relatively few have been explored, as will be discussed in the following section.

CONTROL OF TRANSLATION

Protein Synthesis Modulation, In General

Measurement of protein synthesis rate in muscle, without pointing out the particular means of modulation, is a common and easily incorporated technique that usually provides the initial data from which more detailed mechanistic studies are launched. Incorporation of a radiolabeled amino acid over a short time period (relative to protein breakdown and amino acid reuse) provides data that can be expressed both in absolute and relative terms [153]. While methods of delivery (usually either constant infusion or flooding-dose) vary, all methods rely on measuring amino acid precursor levels (either free amino acid or aminoacyl-tRNA) and the extent of incorporation into the protein. The difference between the two types of precursor measurements is in the assumptions inherent in each technique. Both assume that the precursor level measured is the same as that seen by the translation machinery (eEF-1 for all except methionine, which also must initiate protein synthesis). The method of measuring free amino acid levels, while sometimes necessary because of low aminoacyl-tRNA levels, also assumes that the charging rate of the tRNA does not change with the experimental treatment. Unfortunately, this assumption is rarely tested. Nonetheless, both techniques often give comparable data and the assumptions are only a concern with the mechanistic interpretation of these data. Studies that identify general changes in protein synthesis in muscle are discussed next, and Table 7.1 provides a summary of these data.

TABLE 7.1.
Summary of Translation Control Points and Mechanisms

	Model	Effect	Mechanism	References
General Synthesis				
skeletal muscle	acute exercise	short-term ↓ synthesis		[6, 34, 35]
			energy status?	[13, 73, 74, 87, 88, 137]
		long-term ↑ synthesis		[6, 16, 157, 158]
	repeated resistance exercise	↑ synthesis	insulin-dependent	[40, 41]
	repeated endurance exercise	↑ synthesis		[10, 11]
	chronic stimulation	↑ synthesis	post-transcriptional	[129, 150]
	denervation		post-transcriptional	[155]
	immobilization and lack of weightbearing		post-transcriptional	[137, 141]
cardiac muscle	pressure overload	long-term ↑ synthesis	transcriptional	[14, 20, 92, 93, 97)
	hyperthyroidism	long-term ↑ synthesis	transcriptional	[37, 131]
Initiation				
skeletal muscle	diabetes and starvation	↓ synthesis		[21, 45, 107, 124, 156]
			↓ initiation	[27, 38, 52, 62, 66, 67, 71, 113, 156]
	diabetes	↓ initiation	↓ eIF-2B activity in fast-twitch muscle NADPH/NADP⁺?	[65]
			↓ casein kinase II? subunit availability	[3, 4, 146]
	diabetes	↓ cap-binding	↑eIF4-Fα association with 4E-BPI 4E-BPI dephosphorylation	[69, 70, 128]
	diabetes + insulin	prevention of ↓ cap-binding	4E-BP1 phosphorylation	[70, 128]
			↑ MAP kinase-dependent 4E-BP1 phosphorylation	[5]
			↑ association of eIF-4Fα and γ	[70]
			↓ eIF-4Fα phosphorylation	
	sepsis	↓ synthesis	↓ eIF-2B activity	[145]
			↓ eIF-2B subunit ε	[25, 63, 147, 151]
			↑ TNF	
			↑ interleukin-1	
cardiac muscle	volume load	↓ synthesis	↑ eIF-2α phosphorylation HSC 70 translocation energy status	[74, 84, 87, 88, 134, 137]
	pressure load	long-term ↑ synthesis	subunit availability	[14, 20, 154]
		short-term ↓ synthesis	17 kDa inhibitor histone H1?	[53, 103]
		not known	↑ eIF-4Fα phosphorylation	[152]
	cultured myocyte active-tension development	not known	↑ eIF-4Fα phosphorylation	[152]
	hyperthyroidism	long-term ↑ synthesis	subunit availability	[131]

(continued)

TABLE 7.1.
(continued)

	Model	Effect	Mechanism	References
Elongation and Termination				
skeletal muscle	starvation	↓ synthesis	↓ eEF-1 ↓ eEF-2	[64, 146]
	refeeding	↑ synthesis	↑ insulin- and AA-dependent elongation	[163]
			↓ calcium-calmodulin-dependent kinase III?	[115]
	lack of weight bearing	↓ synthesis	↓ HSC 70-dependent elongation energy status	[73, 74, 137]
cardiac muscle	diabetes	↓ synthesis	↓ eEF-2	[146]
	cultured myocyte contractile arrest	↓ synthesis	↓ elongation	[47, 130]
Other Control Points				
cytoskeleton	stretch maturation	↑ MHC expression	localization?	[30, 31]
	volume load	cytoskeleton reorganization		[136]
mRNA binding factors	chronic stimulation	↑ cyt *c* expression	↑ inhibition of mRNA binding protein?	[159]

An acute bout of exercise is a potent modulator of muscle protein synthesis, both during and following the exercise. Modulation of translation on such a rapid time scale is inconsistent with the time necessary for transcription to affect translation to such a magnitude. For example, a single bout of running or swimming exercise by untrained rats immediately decreases protein synthesis in the hindlimb muscles by 35–80% [6, 34, 35], depending upon the method of measurement. These data are consistent with studies that indicate protein synthesis is modulated by contractile state and closely correlated with the energy status of the working muscle [13, 73, 74, 87, 88, 137]. The depressive effects of an acute bout of exercise on protein synthesis are relatively short-lived, however, and protein synthesis rates return to normal or exceed basal levels. In rats, the recovery period is marked by a mild increase in hindlimb muscle protein synthesis rate within an hour [6], followed by subsequent rebound to 40–50% above basal levels within the next 12–17 hours [157, 158], and an apparent return toward basal levels within the next 36–41 hours [157, 158]. In the latter two studies, selected RNA species (actin, cytochrome *c*, 18S, and 28S) did not change within the first day, and it was not until after the second day post-exercise that the rRNA species began to increase. Modulation of protein synthesis in the human vastus lateralis following an acute bout of exercise is similar, exhibiting an increase to 14% above basal levels within 4 hours post-exercise [16].

Clearly, a single exercise bout is sufficient to initiate rapid control of gene expression at the level of translation.

Several repeated exercise bouts maintain the increases in the protein synthesis rate, but there appears to be a strong insulin dependency for this response in the case of resistance exercise [41]. Four bouts of ankle extension resistance exercise by rats over a week's period of time increased the insulin stimulated protein synthesis rate in the gastrocnemius and soleus muscles through an apparent increase in translational efficiency (expressed as protein synthesis per unit of RNA) [40, 41]. The ability of the combination to enhance protein synthesis relative to age-matched non-exercised animals is independent of the age of the animals [40].

Changes in translation (and other post-transcriptional processes) that result from exercise training or other chronic changes in functional demand, are not necessarily tightly linked to transcription. For example, cytochrome c protein content of the red quadriceps of the rat increases during a 4-day running exercise training protocol despite no significant change in cytochrome c mRNA . However, running exercise training has very little effect on the half-life of the cytochrome c protein [11], a parameter determined solely by the degradation rate of the protein [126]. Therefore, because protein expression is the balance between synthesis and degradation, the synthesis rate of cytochrome c protein must have increased as a result of running exercise training despite the absence of a change in the level of cytochrome c mRNA. This is not to say that a transcriptional mechanism will not eventually be manifest, as shown by an intensity-dependent increase in the mRNA levels of actin and cytochrome c, as well as 18S rRNA, following running exercise training [94]. Nevertheless, despite the eventual transcriptional changes that take place with exercise training, as much as a 25–45% increase in the amount of protein synthesized per mg RNA per day occurs within hours of an exercise bout without a corresponding increase in actin mRNA, cytochrome c mRNA, 18S rRNA, or 28S rRNA expression [157, 158]. This dissociation of translation from transcription is also manifest in other models that change the functional demand placed upon SM. Chronic stimulation, well known for producing a fast-to-slow transition of muscle phenotype, causes a rapid increase in citrate synthase activity that precedes changes in its mRNA by 8–10 days [129]. Similarly, transcutaneous stimulation of the quadriceps following surgery decreases muscle atrophy and maintains the pool of polyribosomal mRNA [150]. Analogously, but in the opposite direction, cytochrome c oxidase activity during denervation is uncoupled from its nuclear-derived VIc subunit and mitochondrial-derived subunit III mRNA expression [155]. Decreased activity during immobilization or non-weight bearing also shows a rapid decrease in protein synthesis within 5–6 hours without corresponding decreases in RNA expression [137, 141]. Obviously, the rapid control of protein synthesis in response to altered functional demand is an important factor in control of gene expression that can act independently of transcription, especially within short time periods following a change in functional demand.

The heart, on the other hand, seems to be primarily transcriptionally driven for its changes in protein synthesis. Nevertheless, rapid modulation of protein synthesis does occur, especially during down-regulation of translation (to be discussed in the next section). Numerous authors have extensively reviewed this subject; therefore, only a few of the salient points will be elaborated upon.

One of the most popular models for adaptation of the heart, pressure overload, produces hypertrophy that is caused by an increase in protein synthesis rate accompanied by an increase in RNA expression [14, 20, 92, 93, 97]. Similarly, hyperthyroidism also produces cardiac hypertrophy through an increase in protein synthesis rate, and this, too, is tightly linked to an increase in transcription [37, 131]. α-Adrenoreceptor action may play some part in control of increased translation and transcription, as shown in newborn pigs [8]. Unfortunately, few studies examine the rapid changes in protein synthesis that take place in the variety of cardiac models available, and as discussed in the next section, these changes provide considerable insight into the mechanisms of translational control.

Specific Control Points

INITIATION. As discussed, initiation of translation is a series of complex steps whereby entry of the mRNA into the polypeptide synthesis process is controlled. It is not surprising that there is considerably more data concerning initiation than the other basic steps of elongation and termination.

Perhaps some of the most revealing information about the control of initiation in muscle comes from studies that involve insulin action and starvation. Diabetes and fasting both decrease protein synthesis rates in muscle [21, 45, 107, 124, 156] in a mechanism where efficiency of translation decreases as an apparent result of decreased initiation [27, 38, 52, 66, 67, 113, 156]. There is evidence that the activity of eIF-2 and eIF-2B decrease, the effect of which is decreased formation of the ternary complex. This response, however, is both model and tissue specific, as will be explained. Diabetic animals exhibit a decrease in the activity of eIF-2B in fast-twitch but not slow-twitch or cardiac muscle [65]. Since phosphorylation of the eIF-2α subunit inhibits eIF-2B guanine nucleotide exchange activity, an obvious possibility is that eIF-2α is phosphorylated or itself diminished. According to Karinch et al. however, this does not appear to be the case [65]. Alternative explanations offered by the authors for the diminished eIF-2B activity are based upon the balance of activator and inhibitors of eIF-2B. NADPH is an activator and $NADP^+$ is an inhibitor; therefore, one possible mechanism includes the lack of "protection" against some other inhibitor by an unchanged $NADPH/NADP^+$ ratio in fast-twitch muscle versus protection against inhibition by an increased $NADPH/NADP^+$ ratio in the heart [65]. Along similar lines, a possible activator of eIF-2B, casein kinase II activity, diminishes in diabetic fast-twitch muscle but not the heart, thereby potentially offering protection against inhibition in the heart [65]. Starvation similarly decreases formation of the ternary complex in SM, while extracts of the muscle have diminished nucleotide exchange activity [62]. Measured indirectly by translation efficiency, nutritional status seems to have most of its effect on SM protein synthesis through modulation of initiation rate [71].

The theme of regulation of initiation at the level of ternary complex formation and recycling of eIF-2 for complex formation extends into other models, as well. Most notable is the severe challenge of sepsis, that produces muscle wasting [26, 43, 63]. Recent evidence indicates depressed eIF-2B activity [145] and depressed expression of the eIF-2B subunit ε during sepsis [147, 151]. An interesting insight into the potential mechanisms for the decrease comes from data that implicate cytokine release by macrophages. Amrinone, known as a cardiac glycoside, also inhibits the tumor necrosis factor (TNF) secretion from macrophages. When given during sepsis, the drug prevents the down-regulation of initiation observed with sepsis alone [63], apparently by preventing the decreased expression of eIF-2Bε [151]. An antagonist to interleukin-1 infused during sepsis produces a similar result [25, 147]. Taken together, the above data indicate (perhaps not unexpectedly) significant control of translation in the formation of the ternary structure and recycling of eIF-2 necessary for this structure.

As mentioned previously, the nucleotide exchange function of eIF-2B is directly and efficiently inhibited by phosphorylation of the α subunit of eIF-2 (phosphorylation and translational control are reviewed by Hershey [54]), thus locking eIF-2α into its inactive GDP complex. eIF-2α phosphorylation is an extremely powerful control point for protein synthesis. This is evident when considering yeast. In yeast, amino acid starvation increases eIF-2α phosphorylation through the action of general control of amino acid synthesis, non-derepressible-2, or GCN2, (comparably eIF-2α kinase). This activity sets into motion a series of events in yeast that lead to increased amino acid biosynthesis. Further explanation is necessary at this point. Some eukaryotic genes (~10%) possess upstream open reading frames (uORFs) in their transcripts, such that ribosome recognition of the incorrect initiator codon results in a short protein whose translation blocks both recognition of the correct ORF and may repress synthesis from the correct ORF [15]. In yeast, decreased formation of the ternary complex by eIF-2α phosphorylation relieves the inhibition of GCN4 DNA binding factor expression by the uORF mechanism, which in turn leads to increased transcription of the enzymes responsible for amino acid biosynthesis [29, 58, 160]. Since a small yet significant proportion of eukaryotic mRNAs contain uORFs, the question of how the translation repression by the uORFs can be relieved is raised. The yeast example of GCN4 may be a model by which the general signal of eIF-2α phosphorylation, and the overall diminished protein synthesis that results, produces a specific upregulation of synthesis of a subset of proteins.

The more generalized effect of eIF-2α phosphorylation is decreased formation of the ternary complex. In mammals, the specific kinase requires heme and can be held in an inactive form by complexing with members of the heat-shock protein (HS) family, specifically HSC70 (the constitutive form in normal, unstressed cells) [50, 83, 85]. HSC70 provides a normal chaperone function by associating with nascent polypeptides as elongation proceeds to ensure correct folding, and binds damaged and denatured proteins to prevent incorrect re-folding and direct proteolytic disposal [7, 28, 102]. The sequestration of the eIF-2α kinase by the chaperone molecule provides a unique regulation of the kinase activity by factors that compete with the HSC70 chaperone or otherwise alter the association with the kinase [84, 87]. In cardiac muscle responding to a volume load in the absence of a pressure load, protein synthesis is depressed [134, 137] through an inhibition of initiation [88]. Specifically, eIF-2α is initially phosphorylated by the activated kinase, with activation taking place through an apparent mass action accumulation of HSC70 on nascent polypeptides, possibly as a result of depressed adenosine tri-phosphate (ATP) levels [87]. The HSP70 family possesses ATPase activity, and their association with polypeptides is affected by ATP concentration [49, 74, 109, 127]. Incidentally, a transient inhibition of protein synthesis in the heart that involves induction of a small protein at the onset of an increased pressure load also occurs [53]. It is tempting to speculate that this protein, too, sequesters HSC70, and may be similar to the translational inhibitor histone H1 found in diabetic muscle [103]. Together, these data most likely illustrate that the most probable common form of translational control by eIF-2α phosphorylation is the decrease of initiation through decreased ternary complex formation. One of the interesting features to note is the putative link, though indirect, of the eIF-2α phosphorylation mechanism to muscle ATP nucleotide levels [74, 87, 88]. The link between energy levels in the cell and protein synthesis is a potential broad level of control at the initiation stage, and specifically at ternary complex formation, not only as described previously for adenine nucleotides, but also for the exchange reaction involving the guanine nucleotides. Specifically, data support the possibility that initiation is sensitive to the GDP/GTP ratio, and raising the ratio by raising GDP concentration inhibits initiation [82].

Once again, as indicated from the effects of insulin, the next step of initiation, 7-methyl-guanylate cap-binding, exhibits control. Diabetes also slows SM initiation rate, as noted previously, through the increased association of the cap-binding protein eIF-4Fα subunit (also known as eIF-4E) with its inhibitor 4E-BP1 (also known as PHAS-I) [69]. Treatment with insulin increases the phosphorylation of 4E-BP1, which prevents its association with eIF-4Fα subunit [69, 128]. Insulin-like growth factor I has a similar effect in aortic smooth muscle [48]. The ability of insulin to cause phosphorylation of 4E-BP1 in SM is present even in non-diabetic animals, and presumably enhances protein synthesis by releasing the eIF-4Fα subunit from its inhibitor [70]. The 4E-BP1 phosphorylation (and counteractive dephosphorylation) in response to insulin levels does not depend on insulin only, however, but rather on other events downstream of insulin binding, since modulation of the phosphorylation state of 4E-BP1 occurs in models of both type I and type II diabetes [133]. As mentioned previously, insulin-stimulated phosphorylation of 4E-BP1 occurs through a MAP kinase-independent mechanism [5]. Even so, inhibition of 4E-BP1 activity alone may not be the only effect, as insulin treatment also causes a better than 10-fold increase in the association between the eIF-4Fα and γ subunits (also known as eIF-4G) [70]. In the study by Kimball et al. [70], insulin treatment did not increase the phosphorylation state of the eIF-4Fα subunit, and apparently shifted the phosphorylation state to the unphosphorylated form. Other models increase the phosphorylation state of this subunit. Cardiac myocytes stimulated to contract in culture exhibit a more than 3-fold increase in the phosphorylation state of the eIF-4Fα subunit, a response that is dependent upon active tension development [152]. A similar increase in eIF-4Fα subunit phosphorylation is seen with an *in vivo* model of hemodynamic overload but not volume overload [152]. This phosphorylation apparently occurs through a different mechanism than that produced by insulin treatment *in vitro*. This result is interesting since this subunit has a single phosphorylation at Ser-53. The particular function of this phosphorylation is not clear. While overexpression of the eIF-4Fα subunit seems to improve translation efficiency of mRNAs with "excessive" 5' secondary structure [72], which implicates its cap-binding function as a rate-limiting step for these mRNAs as well as being mitogenic through a *Ras*-activating pathway in overexpressing cells [76], phosphorylation alone does not seem to increase the association of the subunit with the cap structure [12]. The specific phosphorylation observed in these studies is at a threonine residue, however, and thus may have a different functional role than the serine phosphorylation [12]. The eIF-4Fγ subunit, on the other hand, can also be phosphorylated, and this modification does increase its association with the mRNA cap structure [12]. Therefore, a variety of potential control mechanisms extend to the cap-binding stage of initiation. They have a diverse and not yet fully understood set of control points, and at least in some cases, depend upon the contractile state of muscle.

Once cap recognition is complete, ribosomal assembly must take place from the subunits. In muscle, the ribosome pool appears to be quite labile, and thus synthesis can be partly controlled by availability of the subunits, as is the case in diabetes and insulin stimulation [3, 4, 146]. Another metabolic challenge, thyroxine-induced hypertrophy of the heart, produces an increase in protein synthesis rate with no change in efficiency (expressed as amino acid incorporation per μg of RNA) [131]. A concomitant increase in RNA synthesis keeps the translation machinery from being "starved" for the ribosomal subunits. In cardiac muscle, there is a strong mechanical component to the synthesis of ribosomal RNA on a sufficiently rapid time scale to prevent a loss of efficiency of translation. The well-characterized pressure-induced increase in cardiac muscle protein synthesis increases both the synthesis and availability of ribosomal subunits [14, 20, 154]. Conversely, chronically stimulated SM experiences a mobilization of ribosomes into translating polysomes, which precedes ribosome synthesis [129]. Therefore, whether transcription and synthesis of ribosomal RNA keeps pace with other demands affecting translation can be a controlling factor, even if eventually compensated.

Elongation and Termination. Considerably less information regarding control of polypeptide elongation and termination in muscle can be found than is found for initiation. From a teleological point of view, there may simply be less regulation since an unfinished protein may have little, if any, functional value. Furthermore, as previously noted, synthesis of even a short peptide expends a great deal of energy. Nevertheless, regulation does occur.

Once again, hormonal influences have a large effect on elongation and termination. Within the first 3 days of diabetes onset in rats, elongation rate in cardiac muscle decreases 37%, with a coincident 66% decrease in eEF-2 [146]. The reader should recall that eEF-2 can also be inactivated by the action of a specific calcium-calmodulin-dependent protein kinase [121–123]. Because of the balance of kinase and phosphatase activities within cells, one would also expect diabetes to increase the level of phosphorylated eEF-2, since insulin binding to its receptor decreases the activity of the eEF-2 kinase [115]. Circumstantial evidence supports this mechanism. In response to feeding after a period of fast, increased protein synthesis in SM of mice occurs through both increased elongation and initiation rate, but requires plasma insulin as well as the amino acid substrate [163]. Not surprisingly, lack of insulin action has many characteristics of starvation. White muscle of trout exhibit a decrease in both eEF-1 and eEF-2 in response to starvation [64]. As cited above, diabetic rats, too, show depression of eEF-2 levels [146].

It is interesting to note that the response of SM protein synthesis to insulin is primarily through modulation of initiation and limited to muscles that have a predominant fast-twitch characteristic and significant glycolytic metabolism [39, 68]. Elongation rate modulation, on the other hand, has been demonstrated in muscle having slow-twitch, oxidative metabolism. The soleus muscle, an ankle extensor, maintains its muscle mass in response to weight bearing activity, but atrophies rapidly when weight bearing or stretching is absent [138, 139]. An initial response during atrophy is a rapid decrease in protein synthesis [137], apparently due to a defect in elongation rate [73]. Rather than occurring through modulation of an elongation factor, the chaperone HSC70 again seems to play a role in protein synthesis, this time directly. In yeast, variants expressing mutant chaperone proteins grow very slowly because the wild-type chaperone aids in the passage of the nascent polypeptide through the ribosome channel, exerting (for lack of a better analogy) a "tugging" action. Increased expression of an elongation factor overcomes the slow growth of the mutants [102]. In the atrophying soleus muscle, HSC70 dissociates from the growing nascent polypeptide, and therefore, cannot exert the tugging action [74]. In this case, increased ATP levels within the muscle seem to promote the dissociation of the chaperone molecules from the growing proteins [74]. As an interesting corollary, in addition to the constitutive expression of HSC70 (as occurs in most cells), slow-twitch oxidative fibers also constitutively express the inducible form, HSP70 [80, 81]. Therefore, it appears that the slow-twitch fibers not only have the necessary components to deal with their higher metabolism, but also regulate protein synthesis in a manner different from fast-twitch fibers. It is possible, too, that muscle, in general, regulates protein synthesis in a different manner than other tissues. The identification of a statin-like protein possessing homology with eEF-1α in SM, heart, and brain [77] opens the possibility for tissue-specific isoform expression of the components of the protein synthesis apparatus.

The previously mentioned mechanical effect that influences ribosome synthesis also manifests itself at the level of elongation (and probably also initiation). Beating cardiac myocytes whose contractions are arrested show a rapid down-regulation of protein expression [112, 125, 130]. In the case of actin expression, this is in part a result of decreased synthesis [130], and in the case of α-myosin heavy chain, this is a result of a decrease in nascent polypeptide chain elongation with a concomitant stabilization of the mRNA [47]. Cotranslational modification of mRNA stability is an emerging area of interest, pioneered by the early work on tubulin that linked elongation to control of mRNA stability [46, 106, 161, 162]. For example, contrasting with the apparent stabilization of α-myosin heavy chain and β-myosin heavy chain mRNAs with decreased translation [47, 137], differentiation of myoblasts into myotubes decreases the half-life of the mRNA for a polyA-binding protein [1]. The actual mechanism for modification of mRNA half-life, and its relation to translation, may depend on sequences within the RNA, the translated protein itself [161, 162], and other "binding" factors, as will be discussed.

Besides the classical initiation and elongation factors, direct interaction of mRNA with post-transcriptional and translational regulatory factors also regulates translational expression of genes. The particular type of regulation depends on both location and structure of regulatory elements within the mRNA. For example, binding of protein to the 5'-untranslated region (5'-UTR) can sterically hinder translation [132]. Although the 3'-UTR sequence has been reported to increase translational efficiency *in vitro*, in some cases *in vivo* analyses indicate this region may act to stabilize the mRNA [142], perhaps cotranslationally. The most studied regulation of this sort involves the genes associated with iron metabolism. Transferrin receptor and ferritin protein expression are inversely regulated in an iron-dependent manner. Both mRNAs possess specific nucleotide sequences termed iron responsive elements (IRE) that bind an IRE-specific binding protein (IRE-BP). The transferrin receptor has five loosely conservative IREs in its 3'-UTR and transferrin has a single IRE in its 5'-UTR. The IREs compete for the IRE-BP [51, 95], and the competition is the source of the inverse regulation. In the presence of iron, IRE-BP binding to the ferritin 5'-UTR IRE is diminished, relieving steric hindrance, as well as activating the position and flanking region-dependent enhancer properties of the IRE [32, 33]. Conversely, the same action at the 3'-UTR of the transferrin receptor mRNA decreases the stability of the mRNA [95]. Thus, an inverse regulation of expression of the transferrin receptor and ferritin proteins can be found. The extent to which mRNA binding proteins regulate gene expression in muscle will only be judged with time. Intriguing data are beginning to emerge, as in the recent data that indicate a factor that inhibits cytochrome *c* mRNA protein binding during chronic stimulation and whose presence coincides with increased expression of cytochrome *c* [159].

The presence of a mechanical influence on muscle translation is probably to be expected, as many studies have shown an association between the cytoskeleton and myofibrils and the elongation factors, initiation factors, and ribosomes [24, 36, 56, 57, 79, 96, 105]. Rabbit muscles that are stretched for 4 or 6 days show an increase in slow myosin heavy chain expression and a distinct distribution of this mRNA (in polysomes) to the subsarcolemmal region of the fiber [31]. This sarcolemmal distribution pattern of myosin mRNA also manifests itself in developing muscle as it matures from the fetal stage to the more mature (and active) adult stage [30], perhaps to indicate an exclusion of the translating polysomes from the densely packed myofibrils and cytoskeleton association of these complexes.

Termination is seemingly the least economical and kinetically least sensitive control point for influencing gene expression at the level of translation [73], at least at the simplistic yes or no level. This simplistic approach is misleading, however, because when considering the many hundreds of proteins expressed in muscle, the possibility of each carrying gene-specific termination rate control in the C-terminal structure is intriguing [9]. Perhaps, the ultimate synthesis rate of a protein (i.e., the replacement rate at steady-state), is influenced not only in time, but also in space by the termination rate. The observation that the elongation factors are also cytoskeleton-binding proteins may influence location of expression; a slower termination rate results in more ribosomes per mRNA, which means more elongation factors and the possibility of greater cytoskeleton binding. This begins to push into the realm of post-translational and cotranslational control. Indeed, newly synthesized proteins are degraded more quickly than "aged" proteins in cardiac myocytes, indicating kinetic pools and compartmentalization [22].

SUMMARY—WHAT NEXT?

As stated in the beginning of this review, researchers are by no means complete in their understanding of translation in muscle. Many specific mechanisms are yet to be worked out, and many models of muscle use have yet to be investigated. Several topics of considerable interest should be considered in future research.

The first topic for future research is the sensitivity of translation to metabolism. Few tissues expend as much energy as muscle, especially working muscle. Both direct pathways for influence (e.g., guanine and adenine nucleotide levels, and $NADP^+$ and NADPH levels) and indirect pathways (e.g., insulin binding and MAP kinase signaling) exist. Future data from studies in these areas will be, by the ubiquitous and global nature of the signals involved, difficult to interpret and at times circumstantial. Nonetheless, metabolism is probably one of the greatest influences on muscle gene expression, and therefore worth the effort (i.e., Ranvier's comment).

Other emerging topics that should be of interest include compartmentalization and localization of translation in muscle. Evidence was cited indicating that changes in mRNA distribution within muscle cells and association of the translation machinery within structural components of muscle may play a role in controlling expression. Recent evidence from the author's laboratory indicates that the cytoskeleton of cardiac muscle is quite labile, and may explain some long-term changes in translation [136]. Therefore, researchers may begin approaching muscle translation from a subcellular anatomical point of view.

Finally, the rapidly emerging field of mRNA binding proteins, acting in concert with RNA sequences to provide translational repressor or enhancer activity and influence mRNA stability, will no doubt yield much new data with which to struggle and reconcile. This area, too, will be hard to assess since a global view of muscle protein synthesis is no longer considered. In other words, individual proteins and their mRNAs must also be considered. Thus, the data will not be rapidly forthcoming.

REFERENCES

1. Adamou, J., and J. Bag. Alteration of translation and stability of mRNA for the poly(A)-binding protein during myogenesis. *Eur. J. Biochem.* 209:803–812, 1992.

2. Andjelkovic, N., S. Zolnierowicz, C. Van Hoof, J. Goris, and B.A. Hemmings. The catalytic subunit of protein phosphatase 2A associates with the translation termination factor eRF1. *EMBO J.* 15:7156–7167, 1996.

3. Ashford, A.J., and V.M. Pain. Effect of diabetes on the rates of synthesis and degradation of ribosomes in rat muscle and liver in vivo. *J. Biol. Chem.* 261:4059–4065, 1986.

4. Ashford, A.J., and V.M. Pain. Insulin stimulation of growth in diabetic rats. Synthesis and degradation of ribosomes and total tissue protein in skeletal muscle and heart. *J. Biol. Chem.* 261:4066–4070, 1986.

5. Azpiazu, I., A.R. Saltiel, A.A. DePaoli Roach, and J.C. Lawrence. Regulation of both glycogen synthase and PHAS-I by insulin in rat skeletal muscle involves mitogen-activated protein kinase-independent and rapamycin-sensitive pathways. *J. Biol. Chem.* 271: 5033–5039, 1996.

6. Bates, P.C., T. Decoster, G.K. Grimble, J.O. Holloszy, D.J. Millward, and M.J. Rennie. Exercise and muscle protein turnover in the rat. *J. Physiol. Lond.* 303:41P, 1980.

7. Beckmann, R.P., L.E. Mizzen, and W.J. Welch. Interaction of Hsp 70 with newly synthesized proteins: implications for protein folding and assembly. *Science* 248:850–854, 1990.

8. Beinlich, C.J., K.M. Baker, and H.E. Morgan. Alpha-adrenergic receptor agonists stimulate ribosome formation in hearts from enalapril-treated piglets. *J. Mol. Cell. Cardiol.* 25: 395–406, 1993.

9. Björnsson, A., S. Mottagui-Tabar, and L.A. Isaksson. Structure of the C-terminal end of the nascent peptide influences translation termination. *EMBO J.* 15:1696–1704, 1996.

10. Booth, F.W. Cytochrome c protein synthesis rate in rat skeletal muscle. *J. Appl. Physiol.* 71:1225–1230, 1991.

11. Booth, F.W., and J.O. Holloszy. Cytochrome c turnover in rat skeletal muscles. *J. Biol. Chem.* 252:416–419, 1977.

12. Bu, X., D.W. Haas, and C.H. Hagedorn. Novel phosphorylation sites of eukaryotic initiation factor-4F and evidence that phosphorylation stabilizes interactions of the p25 and p220 subunits. *J. Biol. Chem.* 268:4975–4978, 1993.

13. Bylund-Fellenius, A.C., K.M. Ojamaa, K.E. Flaim, J.B. Li, S.J. Wassner, and L.S. Jefferson. Protein synthesis versus energy state in contracting muscles of perfused rat hindlimb. *Am. J. Physiol.* 246:E297–305, 1984.

14. Camacho, J.A., C.J. Peterson, G.J. White, and H.E. Morgan. Accelerated ribosome formation and growth in neonatal pig hearts. *Am. J. Physiol.* 258:C86–C91, 1990.

15. Cao, J., and A.P. Geballe. Inhibition of nascent-peptide release at translation termination. *Mol. Cell. Biol.* 16:7109–7114, 1996.

16. Carraro, F., C.A. Stuart, W.H. Hartl, J. Rosenblatt, and R.R. Wolfe. Effect of exercise and recovery on muscle protein synthesis in human subjects. *Am. J. Physiol.* 259:E470–476, 1990.

17. Chakrabarti, A., and U. Maitra. Release and recycling of eukaryotic initiation factor 2 in the formation of an 80 S ribosomal polypeptide chain initiation complex. *J. Biol. Chem.* 267:12964–12972, 1992.

18. Chaudhuri, J., K. Das, and U. Maitra. Purification and characterization of bacterially expressed mammalian translation initiation factor 5 (eIF-5): demonstration that eIF-5 forms a specific complex with eIF-2. *Biochemistry* 33:4794–4799, 1994.

19. Chaudhuri, J., K. Si, and U. Maitra. Function of eukaryotic translation initiation factor 1A (eIF1A) (formerly called eIF-4C) in initiation of protein synthesis. *J. Biol. Chem.* 272: 7883–7891, 1997.

20. Chua, B.H.L., L.A. Russo, E.E. Gordon, B.J. Kleinhans, and H.E. Morgan. Faster ribosome synthesis induced by elevated aortic pressure in rat heart. *Am. J. Physiol.* 252:C323–C327, 1987.

21. Clark, A.F., and K. Wildenthal. Disproportionate reduction of actin synthesis in hearts of starved rats. *J. Biol. Chem.* 261:13168–13172, 1986.

22. Clark, W.A. Evidence for post-translational kinetic compartmentation of protein turnover pools in isolated adult cardiac myocytes. *J. Biol. Chem.* 268:20243–20251, 1993.

23. Collier, R.J. Effect of Diptheria toxin on protein synthesis: inactivation of one of the transfer factors. *J. Mol. Biol.* 25:83–98, 1967.

24. Condeelis, J. Elongation factor 1 alpha, translation and the cystoskeleton. *Trends Biochem. Sci.* 20:169–170, 1995.

25. Cooney, R., E. Owens, C. Jurasinski, K. Gray, J. Vannice, and T. Vary. Interleukin-1 receptor antagonist prevents sepsis-induced inhibition of protein synthesis. *Am. J. Physiol.* 30:E636–E641, 1994.

26. Cooney, R.N., S.R. Kimball, and T.C. Vary. Regulation of skeletal muscle protein turnover during sepsis: mechanisms and mediators. *Shock* 7:1–16, 1997.

27. Cox, S., N.T. Redpath, and C.G. Proud. Regulation of polypeptide-chain initiation in rat skeletal muscle: starvation does not alter the activity or phosphorylation state of initiation factor eIF-2. *FEBS Lett.* 239:333–338, 1988.

28. Craig, E.A. Chaperones: helpers along the pathways to protein folding. *Science* 260: 1902–1903, 1993.

29. Dever, T.E., L. Feng, R.C. Wek, A.M. Cigan, T.F. Donahue, and A.G. Hinnebusch. Phosphorylation of initiation factor 2 alpha by protein kinase GCN2 mediates gene-specific translational control of GCN4 in yeast. *Cell* 68:585–596, 1992.

30. Dix, D.J., and B.R. Eisenberg. Distribution of myosin mRNA during development and regeneration of skeletal muscle fibers. *Dev. Biol.* 143:422–426, 1991.

31. Dix, D.J., and B.R. Eisenberg, Redistribution of myosin heavy chain mRNA in the mid-region of stretched muscle fibers. *Cell Tissue Res.* 263:61–69, 1991.

32. Dix, D.J., P.N. Lin, Y. Kimata, and E.C. Theil. The iron regulatory region of ferritin mRNA is also a positive control element for iron-independent translation. *Biochemistry* 31:2818–2822, 1992.

33. Dix, D.J., P.N. Lin, A.R. McKenzie, W.E. Walden, and E.C. Theirl. The influence of the base-paired flanking region on structure and function of the ferritin mRNA iron regulatory element. *J. Mol. Biol.* 231:230–240, 1993.

34. Dohm, G.L., G.J. Kasperek, E.B. Tapscott, and G.R. Beecher. Effect of exercise on synthesis and degradation of muscle protein. *Biochem. J.* 188:255–262, 1980.

35. Dohm, G.L., E.B. Tapscott, H.A. Barakat, and G.J. Kasperek. Measurement of *in vivo* protein synthesis in rats during an exercise bout. *Biochem. Med.* 27:367–373, 1982.

36. Durso, N.A., and R.J. Cyr. Beyond translation: elongation factor-1 alpha and the cytoskeleton. *Protoplasma* 180:99–105, 1994.

37. Everett, A.W., A.M. Sinha, P.K. Umeda, S. Jakovcic, M. Rabinowitz, and R. Zak. Regulation of myosin synthesis by thyroid hormone: relative change in the alpha- and beta-myosin heavy chain mRNA levels in rabbit heart. *Biochemistry* 23:1596–1599, 1984.

38. Flaim, K.E., M.E. Copenhaver, and L.S. Jefferson. Effects of diabetes on protein synthesis in fast- and slow-twitch rat skeletal muscle. *Am. J. Physiol.* 239:E88–95, 1980.

39. Flaim, K.E., J.B. Li, and L.S. Jefferson. Protein turnover in rat skeletal muscle: effects of hypophysectomy and growth hormone. *Am. J. Physiol.* 234:E38–43, 1978.

40. Fluckey, J.D., T.C. Vary, L.S. Jefferson, W.J. Evans, and P.A. Farrell. Insulin stimulation of protein synthesis in rat skeletal muscle following resistance exercise is maintained with advancing age. *J. Gerontol. A. Biol. Sci. Med. Sci.* 51:B323–330, 1996.

41. Fluckey, J.D., T.C. Vary, L.S. Jefferson, and P.A. Farrell. Augmented insulin action on rates of protein synthesis after resistance exercise in rats. *Am. J. Physiol.* 270:E313–319, 1996.

42. Flynn, A., and G. Proud. Insulin-stimulated phosphorylation of initiation factor 4E is mediated by the MAP kinase pathway. *FEBS Lett.* 389:162–166, 1996.

43. Freund, H.R., J.H. James, R. LaFrance, et al. The effect of indomethacin on muscle and liver protein synthesis and on whole-body protein degradation during abdominal sepsis in the rat. *Arch. Surg.* 121:1154–1158, 1986.

44. Frolova, L., X. Le Goff, G. Zhouravleva, E. Davydova, M. Philippe, and L. Kisselev. Eukaryotic polypeptide chain release factor eRF3 is an eRF1- and ribosome-dependent guanosine triphosphatase. *RNA* 2:334–341, 1996.

45. Garlick, P.J., D.J. Millward, W.P.T. James, and J.C. Waterlow. The effect of protein deprivation and starvation on the rate of protein synthesis in tissues of the rat. *Biochim. Biophys. Acta* 414:71–84, 1975.

46. Gay, D.A., S.S. Sisodia, and D.W. Cleveland. Autoregulatory control of beta-tubulin mRNA stability is linked to translation elongation. *Proc. Natl. Acad. Sci. USA* 86:5763–5767, 1989.

47. Goldspink, P.H., D.B. Thomason, and B. Russell. Beating affects the posttranscriptional regulation of alpha-myosin mRNA in cardiac cultures. *Am. J. Physiol.* 271:H2584–2590, 1996.

48. Graves, L.M., K.E. Bornfeldt, G.M. Argast, et al. cAMP- and rapamycin-sensitive regulation of the association of eukaryotic initiation factor 4E and the translational regulator PHAS-I in aortic smooth muscle cells. *Proc. Natl. Acad. Sci. USA* 92:7222–7226, 1995.

49. Greene, L.E., R. Zinner, S. Naficy, and E. Eisenberg. Effect of nucleotide on the binding of peptides to 70-kDa heat shock protein. *J. Biol. Chem.* 270:2967–2973, 1995.

50. Gross, M., A. Olin, S. Hessefort, and S. Bender. Control of protein synthesis by hemin: purification of a rabbit reticulocyte hsp 70 and characterization of its regulation of the activation of the hemin-controlled eIF-2(alpha) kinase. *J. Biol. Chem.* 269:22738–22748, 1994.

51. Harford, J.B., and R.D. Klausner. Coordinate post-transcriptional regulation of ferritin and transferrin receptor expression: the role of regulated RNA-protein interaction. *Enzyme* 44:28–41, 1990.

52. Harmon, C.S., C.G. Proud, and V.M. Pain. Effects of starvation, diabetes and acute insulin treatment on the regulation of polypeptide-chain initiation in rat skeletal muscle. *Biochem. J.* 223:687–696, 1984.

53. Havre, P.A., and G.L. Hammond. Isolation of a translation-inhibiting peptide from myocardium. *Am. J. Physiol.* 255:H1024–H1031, 1988.

54. Hershey, J.W. Overview: phosphorylation and translation control. *Enzyme* 44:17–27, 1990.

55. Hershey, J.W. Translational control in mammalian cells. *Ann. Rev. Biochem.* 60:717–755, 1991.

56. Hesketh, J.E., and I.F. Pryme. Interaction between mRNA, ribosomes and the cytoskeleton. *Biochem. J.* 277:1–10, 1991.

57. Heuijerjans, J.H., F.R. Pieper, F.C. Ramaekers, et al. Association of mRNA and eIF-2 alpha with the cytoskeleton in cells lacking vimentin. *Exp. Cell. Res.* 181:317–330, 1989.

58. Hinnebusch, A.G. Translational control of GCN4: gene-specific regulation by phosphorylation of eIF-2. J.W.B. Hershey, M.B. Matthews, and N. Sonenberg (eds.). *Translational Control.* Cold Spring Harbor:Cold Spring Laboratory Harbor Press, 1996, pp. 199–244.

59. Honjo, T., Y. Nishizuka, and O. Hayaishi. Diptheria toxin-dependent adenosine diphosphate ribosylation of aminoacyl transferase II and inhibition of protein synthesis. *J. Biol. Chem.* 243:3553–3555, 1968.

60. Janosi, L., I. Shimizu, and A. Kaji. Ribosome recycling factor (ribosome releasing factor) is essential for bacteral growth. *Proc. Natl. Acad. Sci. USA* 91:4249–4253, 1994.

61. Jaramillo, M., T.E. Dever, W.C. Merrick, and N. Sonenberg. RNA unwinding in translation: assembly of helicase complex intermediates comprising eukaryotic initiation factors eIF-4F and eIF-4B. *Mol. Cell. Biol.* 11:5992–5997, 1991.

62. Jeffrey, I.W., F.J. Kelly, R. Duncan, J.W. Hershey, and V.M. Pain. Effect of starvation and diabetes on the activity of the eukaryotic initiation factor eIF-2 in rat skeletal muscle. *Biochimie* 72:751–757, 1990.

63. Jurasinski, C.V., L. Kilpatrick, and T.C. Vary. Amrinone prevents muscle protein wasting during chronic sepsis. *Am. J. Physiol.* 31:E491–E500, 1995.

64. Jurss, K., I. Junghahn, and R. Bastrop. The role of elongation factors in protein synthesis rate variation in white teleost muscle. *J. Comp. Physiol. B* 162:345–350, 1992.

65. Karinch, A.M., S.R. Kimball, T.C. Vary, and L.S. Jefferson. Regulation of eukaryotic initiation factor-2B activity in muscle of diabetic rats. *Am. J. Physiol.* 264:E101–108, 1993.

66. Kelly, F.J., and L.S. Jefferson. Control of peptide-chain initiation in rat skeletal muscle: development of methods for preparation of native ribosomal subunits and analysis of the effect of insulin on formation of 40 S initiation complexes. *J. Biol. Chem.* 260: 6677–6683, 1985.

67. Kimball, S.R., and L.S. Jefferson. Effect of diabetes on guanine nucleotide exchange factor activity in skeletal muscle and heart. *Biochem. Biophys. Res. Commun.* 156:706–711, 1988.

68. Kimball, S.R., and L.S. Jefferson. Regulation of initiation of protein synthesis by insulin in skeletal muscle. *Acta Diabetol.* 28:134–139, 1991.

69. Kimball, S.R., L.S. Jefferson, P. Fadden, T.A. Haystead, and J.C. Lawrence, Jr. Insulin and diabetes cause reciprocal changes in the association of eIF-4E and PHAS-I in rat skeletal muscle. *Am. J. Physiol.* 270:C705–709, 1996.

70. Kimball, S.R., C.V. Jurasinski, J.C. Lawrence, Jr., and L.S. Jefferson. Insulin stimulates protein synthesis in skeletal muscle by enhancing the association of eIF-4E and eIF-4G. *Am. J. Physiol.* 272:C754–759, 1997.

71. Kita, K., S. Matsunami, and J. Okumura. Relationship of protein synthesis of mRNA levels in the muscle of chicks under various nutritional conditions. *J. Nutr.* 126:1827–1832, 1996.

72. Koromilas, A.E., A. Lazaris-Karatzas, and N. Sonenberg. mRNAs containing extensive secondary structure in their 5′ non-coding region translate efficiently in cells overexpressing initiation factor eIF-4E. *EMBO J.* 4153–4158, 1992.

73. Ku, Z., and D.B. Thomason. Soleus muscle nascent polypeptide chain elongation slows protein synthesis rate during non-weightbearing. *Am. J. Physiol.* C115–126, 1994.

74. Ku, Z., J. Yang, V. Menon, and D.B. Thomason. Decreased polysomal HSP70 may slow nascent polypeptide elongation during skeletal muscle atrophy. *Am. J. Physiol.* 268: C1369–C1374, 1995.

75. Lawson, T.G., K.A. Lee, M.M. Maimone, et al. Dissociation of double-stranded polynucleotide helical structures by eukaryotic initiation factors, as revealed by a novel assay. *Biochemistry* 28:4729–4734, 1989.

76. Lazaris-Karatzas, A., M.R. Smith, R.M. Frederickson, et al. Ras mediates translation initiation factor 4E-induced malignant transformation. *Genes Dev.* 6:1631–1642, 1992.

77. Lee, S., A.M. Francoeur, S. Liu, and E. Wang. Tissue-specific expression in mammalian brain, heart, and muscle of S1, a member of the elongation factor-1 alpha gene family. *J. Biol. Chem.* 267:24064–24068, 1992.

78. Lee, S., L.A. Wolfraim, and E. Wang. Differential expression of S1 and elongation factor-1 alpha during rat development. *J. Biol. Chem.* 268:24453–24459, 1993.

79. Liu, G., J. Tang, B.T. Edmonds, J. Murray, S. Levin, and J. Condeelis. F-actin sequesters elongation factor 1 alpha from interaction with aminoacyl-tRNA in a pH-dependent reaction. *J. Cell. Biol.* 135:953–963, 1996.

80. Locke, M., B.G. Atkinson, R.M. Tanguay, and E.G. Noble. Shifts in type I fiber proportion in rat hindlimb muscle are accompanied by changes in HSP72 content. *Am. J. Physiol.* 266:C1240–C1246, 1994.

81. Locke, M., E.G. Noble, and B.G. Atkinson. Inducible isoform of HSP70 is constitutively expressed in a muscle fiber type specific pattern. *Am. J. Physiol.* 261:C774–C779, 1991.

82. Manchester, K.L. Control of initiation of eukaryotic protein synthesis by guanine nucleotides and methionyl-tRNAi. *Biochem. Int.* 24:475–484, 1991.

83. Matts, R.L., and R. Hurst. The relationship between protein synthesis and heat shock proteins levels in rabbit reticulocyte lysates. *J. Biol. Chem.* 267:18168–18174, 1992.

84. Matts, R.L., R. Hurst, and Z. Xu. Denatured proteins inhibit translation in hemin-supplemented rabbit reticulocyte lysate by inducing the activation of the heme-regulated eIF-2 alpha kinase. *Biochemistry* 7323–7328, 1993.

85. Matts, R.L., Z. Xu, J.K. Pal, and J.J. Chen. Interactions of the heme-regulated eIF-2 alpha kinase with heat shock proteins in rabbit reticulocyte lysates. *J. Biol. Chem.* 267: 18160–18167, 1992.

86. Mayer, Y., H. Czosnek, P.E. Zeelon, D. Yaffe, and U. Nudel. Expression of the genes coding for the skeletal muscle and cardiac actin in the heart. *Nucl. Acids Res.* 12: 1087–1100, 1984.

87. Menon, V., and D.B. Thomason. Head-down tilt increases rat cardiac muscle eIF-2α phosphorylation. *Am. J. Physiol.* 269:C802–C804, 1995.

88. Menon, V., J. Yang, Z. Ku, and D.B. Thomason. Decrease in heart peptide initiation during head-down tilt may be modulated by HSP70. *Am. J. Physiol.* 268:C1375–C1380, 1995.

89. Méthot, N., A. Pause, J.W. Hershey, and N. Sonenberg. The translation initiation factor eIF-4B contains an RNA-binding region that is distincty and independent from its ribo-nucleoprotein consensus sequence. *Mol. Cell. Biol.* 14:2307–2316, 1994.

90. Méthot, N., G. Pickett, J.D. Keene, and N. Sonenberg. In vitro RNA selection identifies RNA ligands that specifically bind to eukaryotic translation initiation factor 4B: the role of the RNA remotif. *RNA* 2:38–50, 1996.

91. Moldave, K. Eukaryotic protein synthesis. *Ann. Rev. Biochem.* 54:1109–1149, 1985.

92. Morgan, H.E., and K.M. Baker. Cardiac hypertrophy: mechanical, neural, and endocrine dependence. *Circulation* 83:13–25, 1991.

93. Morgan, H.E., E.E. Gordon, Y. Kira, D.L. Siehl, P.A. Watson, and B.H.L. Chua. Biochemical correlates of myocardial hypertrophy. *Physiologists* 28:18–27, 1985.

94. Morrison, P.R., R.B. Biggs, and F.W. Booth. Daily running for 2 wk and mRNAs for cytochrome c and alpha-actin in rat skeletal muscle. *Am. J. Physiol.* 257:C939–939, 1989.

95. Mullner, E.W., B. Neupert, and L.C. Kuhn. A specific mRNA binding factor regulates the iron-dependent stability of cytoplasmic transferrin receptor mRNA. *Cell* 58:373–382, 1989.

96. Murray, J.W., B.T. Edmonds, G. Liu, and J. Condeelis. Bundling of actin filaments by elongation factor 1 alpha inhibits polymerization at filament ends. *J. Cell. Biol.* 135: 1309–1321, 1996.

97. Nagai, R., N. Pritzl, R.B. Low, et al. Myosin isozyme synthesis and mRNA levels in pressure-overloaded rabbit hearts. *Circ. Res.* 60:692–699, 1987.

98. Nairn, A.C., and H.C. Palfrey. Identification of the major Mr 100,000 substrate for cal-modulin-dependent protein kinase III in mammalian cells as elongation factor-2. *J. Biol. Chem.* 262:17299–17303, 1987.

99. Nakamura, Y., K. Ito, and L.A. Isaksson. Emerging understanding of translation termination. *Cell* 87:147–150, 1996.

100. Naranda, T., W.B. Strong, J. Menaya, B.J. Fabbri, and J.W. Hershey. Two structural domains of initiation factor eIF-4B are involved in binding to RNA. *J. Biol. Chem.* 269: 14465–14472, 1994.

101. Negrutskii, B.S., T.V. Budkevich, V.F. Shalak, G.V. Turkovskaya, and A.V. El'Skaya. Rabbit translation elongation factor 1 alpha stimulates the activity of homologous aminoacyl-tRNA synthetase. *FEBS Lett.* 382:18–20, 1996.

102. Nelson, R.J., T. Ziegelhoffer, C. Nicolet, M. Werner-Washburne, and E.A. Craig. The translation machinery and 70 kd heat shock protein cooperate in protein synthesis. *Cell* 71:97–105, 1992.

103. O'Leary, N.E., W.B. Mehard, I.R. Cheema, K. Moore, and M.G. Buse. A translational inhibitor from muscles of diabetic rats: identification as histone H1. *Am. J. Physiol.* 253: E81–E89, 1987.

104. Ordahl, C.P. The skeletal and cardiac α-actin genes are coexpressed in early embryonic striated muscle. *Dev. Biol.* 117:488–492, 1986.

105. Owen, C. H., D.J. DeRosier, and J. Condeelis. Actin crosslinking protein EF-1a of Dictyostelium discoideum has a unique bonding rule that allows square-packed bundles. *J. Struct. Biol.* 109:248–254, 1992.

106. Pachter, J.S., T.J. Yen, and D.W. Cleveland. Auto-regulation of tubulin expression is achieved through specific degradation of polysomal tubulin mRNAs. *Cell* 51:283–292, 1987.

107. Pain, V.M., and P.J. Garlick. Effect of streptozotocin diabetes and insulin treatment on the rate of protein synthesis in tissues of the rat in vivo. *J. Biol. Chem.* 249:4510–4514, 1974.

108. Palen, E., R.C. Venema, Y.W. Chang, and J.A. Traugh. GDP as a regulator of phosphorylation of elongation factor 1 by casein kinase II. *Biochemistry* 33:8515–8520, 1994.

109. Palleros, D.R., W.J. Welch, and A.L. Fink. Interaction of hsp70 with unfolded proteins: effects of temperature and nucleotides on the kinetics of binding. *Proc. Natl. Acad. Sci. USA* 88:5719–5723, 1991.

110. Pause, A., N. Méthot, Y. Svitkin, W.C. Merrick, and N. Sonenberg. Dominant negative mutants of mammalian translation initiation factor eIF-4A define a critical role for eIF-4F in cap-dependent and cap-independent initiation of translation. *EMBO J.* 13:1205–1215, 1994.

111. Pestova, T.V., I.N. Shatsky, and C.U. Hellen. Functional dissection of eukaryotic initiation factor 4F: the 4A subunit and the central domain of the 4G subunit are sufficient to mediate internal entry of 43S preinitiation complexes. *Mol. Cell. Biol.* 16:6870–6878, 1996.

112. Qi, M., K. Ojamaa, E.G. Eleftheriades, I. Klein, and A. M. Samarel. Regulation of rat ventricular myosin heavy chain expression by serum and contractile activity. *Am. J. Physiol.* 267:C520–528, 1994.

113. Rannels, D.E., L.S. Jefferson, A.C. Hjalmarson, E.B. Wolpert, and H.E. Morgan. Maintenance of protein synthesis in hearts of diabetic animals. *Biochem. Biophys. Res. Commun.* 40:1110–1116, 1970.

114. Ranvier, L. De quelques fait relatifs à l'histologie et à la physiologie des muscles striés. *Arch. Physiol. Norm. et Path.* 2:Ser. I, 5–15, 1874.

115. Redpath, N.T., E.J. Foulstone, and C.G. Proud. Regulation of translation elongation factor-2 by insulin via a rapamycin-sensitive signalling pathway. *EMBO J.* 15:2291–2297, 1996.

116. Redpath, N.T., and C.G. Proud. The tumour promoter okadaic acid inhibits reticulocytelysate protein synthesis by increasing the net phosphorylation of elongation factor 2. *Biochem. J.* 262:69–75, 1989.

117. Redpath, N.T., and C.G. Proud. Purification and phosphorylation of elongation factor-2 kinase from rabbit reticulocytes. *Eur. J. Biochem.* 212:511–520, 1993.

118. Redpath, N.T., and C.G. Proud. Molecular mechanisms in the control of translation by hormones and growth factors. *Biochim. Biophys. Acta* 1220: 147–162, 1994.

119. Reed, V.S., M.E. Wastney, and D.C. Yang. Mechanisms of the transfer of aminoacyl-tRNA from aminoacyl-tRNA synthetase to the elongation factor 1 alpha. *J. Biol. Chem.* 269: 32932–32936, 1994.

120. Roy, A.L., D. Chakrabarti, B. Datta, R.E. Hileman, and N.K. Gupta. Natural mRNA is required for directing Met-tRNA(f) binding to 40S ribosomal subunits in animal cells: involvement of Co-eIF-2A in natural mRNA-directed initiation complex formation. *Biochemistry* 27:8203–8209, 1988.

121. Ryazanov, A.G. Ca^{2+}/calmodulin-dependent phosphorylation of elongation factor 2. *FEBS Lett.* 214:331–334, 1987.

122. Ryazanov, A.G., B.B. Rudkin, and A.S. Spirin. Regulation of protein synthesis at the elongation stage. New insights into the control of gene expression of eukaryotes. *FEBS Lett.* 285:170–175, 1991.

123. Ryazanov, A.G., and A.S. Spirin. Phosphorylation of elongation factor 2: a key mechanism regulating gene expression in vertebrates. *New Biol.* 2:843–850, 1990.

124. Samarel, A.M., M.S. Parmacek, N.M. Magid, R.S. Decker, and M. Lesch. Protein synthesis and degradation during starvation-induced cardiac atrophy in rabbits. *Circ. Res.* 60: 933–941, 1987.

125. Samarel, A.M., M.L. Spragia, V. Maloney, S.A. Kamal, and G.L. Engelmann. Contractile arrest accelerates myosin heavy chain degradation in neonatal rat heart cells. *Am. J. Physiol.* 263:C642–652, 1992.

126. Schimke, R.T., and D. Doyle. Control of enzyme levels in animal tissues. *Ann. Rev. Biochem.* 39:929–976, 1970.

127. Schumacher, R.J., R. Hurst, W.P. Sullivan, N.J. McMahon, D.O. Toft, and R.L. Matts. ATP-dependent chaperoning activity of reticulocyte lysate. *J. Biol. Chem.* 269:9493–9499, 1994.

128. Scott, P.H., and J.C. Lawrence, Jr. Insulin activates a PD 098059-sensitive kinase that is involved in the regulation of p70S6K and PHAS-I. *FEBS Lett* 409:171–176, 1997.

129. Seedorf, U., E. Leberer, B.J. Kirschbaum, and D. Pette. Neural control of gene expression in skeletal muscle: effects of chronic stimulation on lactate dehydrogenase isoenzymes and citrate synthase. *Biochem. J.* 239:115–120, 1986.

130. Sharp, W.W., L. Terracio, T.K. Borg, and A.M. Samarel. Contractile activity modulates actin synthesis and turnover in cultured neonatal rat heart cells. *Circ. Res.* 73:172–183, 1993.

131. Siehl, D., B.H.L. Chua, N. Lautensack-Belser, and H.E. Morgan. Faster protein and ribosome synthesis in thyroxine-induced hypertrophy of rat heart. *Am. J. Physiol.* 248: C309–C319, 1985.

132. Stripecke, R., C.C. Oliveira, J.E.G. Mccarthy, and M.W. Hentze. Proteins binding to 5′ untranslated region sites: a general mechanism for translational regulation of mRNAs in human and yeast cells. *Mol. Cell. Biol.* 14:5898–5909, 1994.

133. Svanberg, E., L.S. Jefferson, K. Lundholm, and S.R. Kimball. Postprandial stimulation of muscle protein synthesis is independent of changes in insulin. *Am. J. Physiol.* 272: E841–847, 1997.

134. Takala, T. Protein synthesis in the isolated perfused rat heart. *Basic Res. Cardiol.* 76: 44–61, 1981.

135. Tate, W.P., E.S. Poole, J.A. Horsfield, et al. Translational termination efficiency in both bacteria and mammals is regulated by the base following the stop codon. *Biochem. Cell. Biol.* 73:1095–1103, 1995.

136. Thomason, D.B., O. Anderson III, and V. Menon. Fractal analysis of cytoskeleton rearrangement in rat cardiac muscle during head-down tilt. *J. Appl. Physiol.* 81:1522–1527, 1996.

137. Thomason, D.B., R.B. Biggs, and F.W. Booth. Protein metabolism and β-myosin heavy-chain mRNA in unweighted soleus muscle. *Am. J. Physiol.* 257:R300–R305, 1989.

138. Thomason, D.B., and F.W. Booth. Atrophy of the soleus muscle by hindlimb unweighting. *J. Appl. Physiol.* 68:1–12, 1990.

139. Thomason, D.B., R.E. Herrick, D. Surdyka, and K.M. Baldwin. Time course of soleus muscle myosin expression during hindlimb suspension and recovery. *J. Appl. Physiol.* 63: 130–137, 1987.

140. Tsukiyama Kohara, K., S.M. Vidal, A.C. Gingras, et al. Tissue distribution, genomic structure, and chromosome mapping of mouse and human eukaryotic initiation factor 4E-binding proteins 1 and 2. *Genomics* 38:353–363, 1996.

141. Tucker, K.R., M.J. Seider, and F.W. Booth. Protein synthesis rates in atrophied gastrocnemius muscles after limb immobilization. *J. Appl. Physiol.* 51:73–77, 1981.

142. Ueno, S., Y. Kotani, K. Kondoh, A. Sano, Y. Kakimoto, and A.T. Campagnoni. The 3′-untranslated region of mouse myelin basic protein gene increases the amount of mRNA in immortalized mouse oligodendrocytes. *Biochem. Biophys. Res. Commun.* 204:1352–1357, 1994.

143. Vandekerckhove, J., G. Bugaisky, and M. Buckingham. Simultaneous expression of skeletal muscle and heart actin proteins in various striated muscle tissues and cells. *J. Biol. Chem.* 261:1838–1843, 1986.
144. Van Ness, B.G., J.B. Howard, and J.W. Bodley. ADP-ribosylation of elongation factor 2 by diphtheria toxin: isolation and properties of the novel ribosyl-amino acid and its hydrolysis products. *J. Biol. Chem.* 255:10717–10720, 1980.
145. Vary, T.C., C.V. Jurasinski. A.M. Karinch, and S.R. Kimball. Regulation of eukaryotic initiation factor-2 expression during sepsis. *Am. J. Physiol.* 266:E193–201, 1994.
146. Vary, T.C., A. Nairn, and C.J. Lynch. Role of elongation factor 2 in regulating peptide-chain elongation in the heart. *Am. J. Physiol.* 266:E628–E634, 1994.
147. Vary, T.C., L. Voison, and R.N. Cooney. Regulation of peptide-chain initiation in muscle during sepsis by interleukin-1 receptor antagonist. *Am. J. Physiol.* 271:E513–520, 1996.
148. Venema, R.C., H.I. Peters, and J.A. Traugh. Phosphorylation of elongation factor 1 (EF-1) and valyl-tRNA synthetase by protein kinase C and stimulation of EF-1 activity. *J. Biol. Chem.* 266:12574–12580, 1991.
149. Venema, R.C., H.I. Peters, and J.A. Traugh. Phosphorylation of valyl-tRNA synthetase and elongation factor 1 in response to phorbol esters is associated with stimulation of both activities. *J. Biol. Chem.* 266:11993–11998, 1991.
150. Vinge, O., L. Edvardsen, F. Jensen, F.G. Jensen, J. Wernerman, and H. Kehlet. Effect of transcutaneous electrical muscle stimulation on postoperative muscle mass and protein synthesis. *Br. J. Surg.* 83:360–363, 1996.
151. Voisin, L., K. Gray, K.M. Flowers, S.R. Kimball, L.S. Jefferson, and T.C. Vary. Altered expression of eukaryotic initiation factor 2B in skeletal muscle during sepsis. *Am. J. Physiol.* 270:E43–50, 1996.
152. Wada, H., C.T. Ivester, B.A. Carabello, G.T. Cooper, and P.J. McDermott. Translational initiation factor eIF-4E. A link between cardiac load and protein synthesis. *J. Biol. Chem.* 271:8359–8364, 1996.
153. Waterlow, J.C., P.J. Garlick, and D.J. Millward. *Protein Turnover in Mammalian Tissues and in the Whole Body.* Amsterdam:North-Holland, 1978.
154. Watson, P.A., T. Haneda, and H.E. Morgan. Effect of higher aortic pressure on ribosome formation and cAMP content in rat heart. *Am. J. Physiol.* 256:C1257–C1261, 1989.
155. Wicks, K.L., and D.A. Hood. Mitochondrial adaptations in denervated muscle: relationship to muscle performance. *Am. J. Physiol.* 260:C841–850, 1991.
156. Williams, I.H., B.H.L. Chua, R.H. Sahms, D. Siehl, and H.E. Morgan. Effects of diabetes on protein turnover in cardiac muscle. *Am. J. Physiol.* 239:E178–E185, 1980.
157. Wong, T.S., and F.W. Booth. Protein metabolism in rat gastrocnemius muscle after stimulated chronic concentric exercise. *J. Appl. Physiol.* 69:1709–1717, 1990.
158. Wong, T.S., and F.W. Booth. Protein metabolism in rat tibialis anterior muscle after stimulated chronic eccentric exercise. *J. Appl. Physiol.* 69:1718–1724, 1990.
159. Yan, Z., S. Salmons, Y.I. Dang, M.T. Hamilton, and F.W. Booth. Increased contractile activity decreases RNA-protein interaction in the 3'-UTR of cytochrome c mRNA. *Am. J. Physiol.* 271:C1157–1166, 1996.
160. Yang, W., and A.G. Hinnebusch. Identification of a regulatory subcomplex in the guanine nucleotide exchange factor eIF2B that mediates inhibition by phosphorylated eIF2. *Mol. Cell. Biol.* 16:6603–6616, 1996.
161. Yen, T.J., D.A. Gay, J.S. Pachter, and D.W. Cleveland. Autoregulated changes in stability of polyribosome-bound beta-tubulin mRNAs are specified by the first 13 translated nucleotides. *Mol. Cell. Biol.* 8:1224–1235, 1988.
162. Yen, T.J., P.S. Machlin, and D.W. Cleveland. Autoregulated instability of beta-tubulin mRNAs by recognition of the nascent amino terminus of beta-tubulin. *Nature* 334:580–585, 1988.
163. Yoshizawa, F., M. Endo, H. Ide, K. Yagasaki, and R. Funabiki. Translational regulation of protein synthesis in the liver and skeletal muscle of mice in response to refeeding. *J. Nutr. Biochem.* 6:130–136, 1995.

8
Skeletal Muscle Lipoprotein Lipase: Molecular Regulation and Physiological Effects in Relation to Exercise

RICHARD L. SEIP, PH.D.
CLAY F. SEMENKOVICH, M.D.

The mechanisms by which the body adapts to exercise at the cellular level are becoming more clear. In skeletal muscle (SM), the past two decades have seen advances in the understanding of the events of acquisition, utilization, and storage of glucose and fatty acids—the main fuels for muscle contraction. How SM chooses its fuel for oxidation and what signals initiate the uptake and storage of intramuscular fuels remains unclear.

Lipoprotein lipase (LPL) plays a central role in the trafficking of lipoprotein-derived fatty acids. It hydrolyzes circulating lipoprotein triglycerides, liberates fatty acids for tissue uptake, and changes lipoprotein composition in a way that may lower atherosclerotic risk. LPL is most abundant in adipose tissue, heart, and SM, sites where fatty acids are metabolized or re-esterified and stored as triglycerides. Much of the knowledge about synthesis, maturation, packaging, degradation, and release of active LPL has been gained from adipose tissue model systems. Considerable attention has been focused on the differentiation of preadipocytes to adipocytes, which is marked by a large increase in LPL gene expression. Fewer studies of LPL regulation in SM exist.

The *in vivo* activities of LPL in muscle and adipose tissue LPL are often reciprocally regulated. However, while adipose tissue blood flow is relatively constant, muscle blood flow and metabolic rate can increase more than ten- to 20-fold during exercise. Thus, knowledge gained through the study of adipocyte LPL regulation may not be directly relevant to muscle tissue.

In this review we will describe SM LPL regulation under conditions of rest, provide details about mechanisms where possible, and in a few instances, give known details beyond effects on LPL mass and mRNA. Then, we will discuss the regulation of LPL by exercise. In the last section, we will examine the influence of SM LPL activity on circulating triglycerides.

HISTORY OF THE BLOOD "FAT-CLEARING" FACTOR

The first evidence of a blood fat-clearing factor appeared in 1943, when heparinized blood transfused from one dog to a fed, second animal quickly reduced the opacity of the serum of the second dog [53]. The factor responsible was isolated from various tissues [65], although no activity was detected in SM in this early report. The tissue-derived factor was identified as LPL due to its ability to hydrolyze lipoprotein triglycerides [65, 66]. The factor had a pH optimum of 8.1, was inhibited by 0.5 M NaCl or protamine, and required a serum cofactor later identified as apolipoprotein CII [98]. Through the 1970s, LPL activities of heart, SM, and adipose tissue homogenates, or acetone ether powder extracts, were measured chemically as the amount of free fatty acid produced when incubated with a chylomicron or a very low density lipoprotein triglyceride substrate. Later, methods using emulsions radiolabeled with ^{14}C- or ^{3}H-triolein substrate for the assay of LPLA in small tissue homogenate samples were published [74, 75, 141]. All of these methods were used in investigations of tissue specific changes in LPL. Recently, assays that employ fluorescent acyl probes were introduced [36, 150].

The number of published papers quantifying LPL increased with the development of a radiochemical immunoassay in 1983 [97], and an enzyme-linked immunoassay in 1987 [50]. The description of LPL sequence data [63, 151] enabled the measurement of LPL mRNA and the study of LPL gene regulation at the transcriptional level. For studies of regulation of LPL gene expression, simultaneous measurement of LPL mass and activity is critical, since a large proportion of total intracellular LPL can be catalytically inactive [108].

CURRENT UNDERSTANDING OF LPL

LPL Gene

In 1987, a flurry of published reports detailed the cDNA sequence of LPL in various species that included human [151], cow [129], and guinea pig [106]. In 1989, the structure of the human gene was published [62, 32].

The LPL gene has been localized to the short arm of chromosome 8 (8p22) [133]. It spans about 30 kilobases (kb) and includes 10 exons [32]. In humans, exons 1–9 range in length between 105 and 276 base pairs. Exon 10, which codes for all the 3' untranslated region of the mRNA, is 1948 base pairs in length [32]. Exon 1 encodes the 5' untranslated region, the signal peptide [151], and the first two amino acid residues of the mature protein [151]. LPL is a serine hydrolase; exon 4 encodes the catalytic serine at residue 132. High homology between human and other mammalian and avian LPL sequences exists [110]. LPL also has high sequence homology with hepatic lipase but not pancreatic lipase [62]. Over 40 human mutations of LPL have been reported [16]. Dysfunctional LPL leads to chylomicronemia, hypertrigyceridemia, and associated pathologies. The consequences of human LPL mutations and restriction fragment length polymorphisms were recently reviewed [16].

The LPL promoter contains several potential binding sites for known transcription factors. The following regulatory elements, indicated as the nucleotide distance upstream from the start of transcription, exist. There is a putative TATA box at -27, three octamer sites at -580, -186, and -46, two CCAAT boxes at -65 and -506, sequences with partial homology to the glucocorticoid response element at -644, a cAMP responsive element at -306, and HNF-3/fork head family transcription factor binding sites at positions -702 and -468 [32, 44,109]. The CCAAT box at -65 was shown to specifically bind known transcription factors Oct-1 and NF-Y [31,109]. Recently, the binding of nuclear proteins Oct-1 and Oct-2 to the -46 to -39 Oct motif was increased 12-fold with the addition of TFII B, a general transcription factor [88]. Two cis-regulatory regions, LP alpha and LP beta, are important for LPL gene expression during adipogenesis [44]. Several reviews describe agents inducing gene expression and modes of regulation [1, 15, 43].

EXISTENCE OF TWO MESSENGER RNA SPECIES. Adipose tissue expresses two species of LPL mRNA, 3.2 and 3.6 kb in length, but human skeletal and cardiac muscle express predominantly LPL mRNA of 3.6 kb in length. The different lengths are due to polyadenylation at two different sites of the 3' untranslated region [151]. The 3.6 kb form is more efficiently translated [111].

LPL PROTEIN STRUCTURE. Mature, catalytically-active LPL is a dimer, each subunit of which is 448 amino acids with a predicted molecular weight of about 50 kilodaltons. The three dimensional structure of LPL is maintained by disulfide bonding between 5 pairs of cysteines; the 2 subunits of the dimer are linked by hydrophobic bonds. LPL is glycosylated, which is necessary for both activity and secretion. Immature intracellular LPL contains additional mannose residues. Thus, LPL obtained from tissue or cell homogenates can have electrophoretic molecular weights in the 55–70 kd range. The catalytic triad for LPL consists of Ser_{132}, Asp_{156}, and His_{241}. The pentapeptide Gly-Tyr-Ser-Leu-Gly at positions 130–134 is conserved among eight species [110]. LPLA can be blocked by the serine lipase inhibitor tetrahydrolipstatin [153]. LPL contains domains for binding lipid (residues 387 to 394), heparin (229 to 370), apo CII, and apo B [110].

TRANSGENIC MOUSE LINES. Transgenic mice that overexpress human LPL [72, 131] or underexpress native LPL [26] have been developed. One mouse line utilized the chicken beta actin promoter to overexpress LPL in heart, SM, and aorta [131]. This line is resistant to the hyperlipidemic effect of high fat diets [130, 131], as well as the hypertriglyceridemic effect of a high sucrose diet [131]. Using the muscle creatine kinase promoter, another transgenic line overexpresses a human LPL "mini-gene" exclusively in the heart and SM [72]. Muscle mitochondria content is increased in these animals, and animals with extremely high levels of LPL expression develop a myopathy. Mice homozygous for defective LPL [26] die within

12 hours of birth after suckling, probably due to microinfarcts in critical organs caused by chylomicron packing in capillaries. Mice heterozygous for defective LPL may be useful to study the role of hypertriglyceridemia in atherogenesis. Taken together, triglyceride levels in genetically-altered mice vary inversely with LPL gene dosage, (i.e., overexpression of LPL leads to proportionately lower blood triglyceride levels, and inactivation of LPL causes elevated triglycerides) [26]. To date, there are no published reports of exercise effects in any of these genetically-altered mice.

Physiological Functions of LPL

TRAFFICKING OF LIPOPROTEIN-DERIVED FATTY ACIDS. LPL is a multifunctional protein important in triglyceride metabolism. Catalytically-active LPL is found anchored to the luminal side of the capillary endothelium in many tissues, where its main function is to mediate the initial hydrolysis of triglycerides in circulating lipoproteins [37]. In this way, it augments the local tissue supply of fatty acids. The hydrolysis of lipoprotein triglycerides also decreases the triglyceride content of the lipoprotein particles, a process that modifies both the blood lipoprotein lipid profile and the properties of the lipoprotein particles. Tissue sources of significant amounts of LPL mRNA include adipose, heart, SM, and adrenals [61], with lesser amounts found in kidney, lung, intestine, and brain [61]. Macrophages also express LPL [51, 84]. Physiological stimuli in the form of diet, hormonal change, and muscular exercise distribute lipoprotein-derived fatty acids to tissues by altering LPL gene expression in muscle, adipose tissue, and heart.

Tissue Specific Regulation. A striking aspect of LPL regulation, clearly seen with feeding and fasting, is the coordination of LPLA activity between specific tissues. In adipose tissue, food intake raises LPLA, and fasting decreases LPLA [12, 34, 49, 73]. The opposite is true in heart, and to some extent, in SM tissue. Such coordinated, reciprocal regulation of LPL in adipose, as compared to heart or SM in relation to food intake, serves to direct triglyceride fatty acids to adipose tissue for storage in the early postprandial period, and to heart and muscle in the fasting state.

LPL serves other physiologic functions. It acts as a ligand in binding lipoproteins to receptors [7, 25, 93, 136] and cell surfaces [41], and may play a role in atherosclerosis, facilitating the formation of foam cells from macrophages [96, 123].

LPL Metabolism

The rate of whole body production or degradation of LPL in humans has not been studied. Such a study could be undertaken using nonradioactive isotopic amino acid tracers infused intravenously to label the enzyme during its synthesis. In the absence of these data, the rates of LPL production, degradation, and clearance will be described briefly.

LPL PRODUCTION. The processes required for expression of physiologically-effective LPL (i.e., catalytically-active LPL) that is anchored on the capillary luminal endothelium originate in cells of the tissues adjacent to capillaries. These processes include synthesis of the LPL protein, glycosylation in the endoplasmic reticulum, maturation by trimming of high mannose residues, translocation from the endoplasmic reticulum to the Golgi apparatus, inhibition of lysosomal degradation, packaging into vesicles, and the exocytosis of the LPL-containing vesicles. *In vivo*, the subsequent migration and anchoring of LPL via movement from cells of origin along a succession of heparan sulfate binding sites [10] to the capillary endothelium are the final steps required for physiologically-functional LPL. Several reviews describe in detail the overall synthesis and maturation in adipocytes [15, 43, 146].

It is likely that the synthesis and release of LPL by adipose and muscle tissues are similar processes. Synthesis of immunoreactive LPL commences in cultured adipocytes within 1 hour of insulin stimulation, and catalytically-active LPL is measurable within 2 hours [128]. In the rat heart, total protein synthesis and LPLA are related [29]. Inhibition of protein synthesis by cycloheximide rapidly decreases the activity of the enzyme in both adipose tissue and heart [13]. Movement of LPL from sites of synthesis to the plasma membrane in cultured adipocytes occurs within 40 minutes [99]. In the perfused rat heart treated with cycloheximide, the half-life for the decay of heparin nonreleasable fraction is 4 hours, and that of the heparin releasable (HR) fraction about 2 hours [13].

DEGRADATION AND CLEARANCE. After secretion by cells, LPL attaches to the plasma membrane, from which it apparently can move to adjacent heparan sulfate binding sites. In cultured adipocytes, about 25% of the LPL on the surface is internally degraded within 4 hours [95], but in cardiac myocytes, reuptake does not occur [10]. Presumably, the majority of LPL secreted by myocytes becomes functionally active LPL in the capillary lumen. When ^{125}I-labeled bovine LPL is injected intravenously into rats, 50% of the dose is taken up by the liver and the remainder by extrahepatic tissues [145]. One hour after hepatic uptake, a large proportion of the LPL retains active. Thus, LPL taken up by the liver is degraded slowly.

Extrahepatic uptake occurs mostly in tissues which themselves produce LPL [24, 48]. *In vivo*, the extrahepatic uptake of injected LPL depends on the native conformation of LPL, and is inhibited by simultaneous heparin injection [145], which probably competes with vascular endothelial surface heparan sulfate to bind LPL [10]. Heparin given intravenously 1 hour after radiolabeled LPL injection stimulates the reappearance in the circulation of the labeled LPL originally taken up extrahepatically [145]. LPL binding sites on the vascular endothelial surface downstream from capillaries decrease with increasing vessel size [20], so that when LPL is released from a capillary binding site, it distributes to the blood rather than the endothelial surfaces. In summary, LPL is secreted by various tissues, hydrolyzes triglycerides in the vascular space within the tissue of origin, and then moves via the circulation to the liver where uptake and clearance occurs.

REGULATION OF LPL IN RESTING MUSCLE

Regulation of gene expression occurs at several levels [11]. In transcriptional regulation, a change occurs in mRNA quantity due to increased or decreased mRNA synthesis. Once mRNA is synthesized, its stability can be altered through interactions with RNA binding proteins. In translational regulation, increased or decreased utilization of the mRNA makes protein. Posttranslational regulation includes modifications (such as glycosylation) of synthesized protein, leading to altered function. Adipose tissue and heart show large increases in LPL mRNA during development [61], and both have been used to study the induction of LPL gene expression. Multiple forms of regulation were demonstrated for LPL in cultured adipocytes [100, 109, 128]. Some cellular factors and the specific sites at which they act have now been identified [109, 152].

Only one study of LPL regulation using a tissue culture model of SM was performed. This study examined cyclic AMP-increased LPLA in myotubes grown from the L8 rat myoblast cell line [106]. Possible differences between muscle and heart LPL regulation might exist since the same treatment did not increase activity in cardiomyocytes [106]. The 3- to 20-fold higher LPLA in adipose as compared to muscle tissue, plus the interest in understanding the connections between adipose LPL regulation, adipose triglyceride storage, and obesity, has directed research interest toward adipose LPL. The relatively small volume of work with regard to SM LPL regulation in animals and humans will be discussed below, and is limited to non-exercise studies (exercise studies will be reviewed in a subsequent section).

Diet

FEEDING AND FASTING. Feeding and fasting markedly affect LPLA in adipose tissue and moderately influence heart muscle; however, they have a smaller effect on SM. For example, feeding in the rat decreased HR LPLA in heart muscle by 28% (with a range from 2–61%), and markedly increased activity in adipose tissue by 488% (with a range of 470–520%) [49]. Short-term fasting of 24 hours duration in rats decreased total LPLA in acetone ether powders obtained from adipose tissue by 43.1 μmol FFA·g^{-1}·h^{-1} (-72%), decreased LPLA in 10 SMs by an average of only 0.9 μmol FFA·g^{-1}·h^{-1} (-25%) [137], and increased heart muscle LPLA by 15.4 μmol FFA·g^{1}·h^{-1} (+24%). The rat is about 45% SM and 7% fat [23]. Whole body muscle LPLA in the fed rat is two-thirds that of total adipose tissue, while total body muscle LPLA in the fasted rat is about twice that of total body adipose LPLA [137]. Assuming no difference in blood flow, SM in the rat is an important site for triglyceride hydrolysis, especially during fasting.

With long-term fasting (6 days) in male Wistar rats, the diversion of triglyceride-derived fatty acids to muscle is further emphasized. Soleus and deep red quadriceps muscle total LPLA increased by 83–193% vs. baseline (i.e., fed rats), but no change in superficial (white) vastus muscle was noted [68]. Adipose tissue LPLA decreased by 64%.

Lithell et al. [76] showed that 8 hours of normal eating in humans increased adipose HR LPLA by 46%, and decreased SM HR LPLA by 32%. The ratio of SM HR LPLA to adipose tissue LPLA was higher during fasting (with a ratio of SM/AT = 0.31) than with feeding (ratio = 0.15). In contrast, 7 days of caloric restriction (intake = 400 kcal·day^{-1}) decreased both SM HR activity (–40 to –50%) and adipose tissue HR LPLA by 50–80% [138, 140].

Mechanism. To our knowledge, there are no data showing human muscle LPL mass or mRNA effects due to fasting. Using Sprague-Dawley rats, Doolittle et al. [34], reported a 130% rise in heart total LPLA, a 94% rise in LPL mass, and no change in LPL mRNA in response to an overnight fast. In contrast, overnight fasting induced a 50% decrease in LPLA in adipose tissue, no change in LPL mass, and a 70% rise in LPL mRNA. These data indicate posttranslational regulation in both tissues. In a study involving the guinea pig heart, Liu and Olivecrona [82] found no difference between feeding and fasting in total LPLA. However, heparin added to perfused hearts from fasted animals released more LPL in an initial burst than fed animal hearts, suggesting that fasting posttranslationally redistributes heart LPL to favor the HR fraction [82]. Longer term fasting (6 days) increased SM LPL mRNA by 3-fold in the rat, with correlated changes in muscle LPL mRNA and LPLA [68]. Thus, short-term fasting and feeding regulates LPL mostly posttranslationally, but extended fasting shifts regulation to the pretranslational level.

WEIGHT (FAT) LOSS. Both acute caloric deficits and substantial weight loss maintained via isocaloric feeding decrease SM LPLA. In a before-and-after supervised weight loss of 12 kilograms (13% of body weight—BW) over 3 months, 11 obese women were studied after 2 days of isocaloric feeding [40]. Prior to weight loss, SM LPLA was 13% lower as compared to normal weight controls. After weight loss, there was an additional 70% decline in fasting SM HR LPLA. These results are similar to ones reported in heart muscle of obese Zucker rats studied after weight loss under stabilized, reduced-weight conditions [9].

DIETARY CHANGES. In young lean men, raising dietary carbohydrate to 70% of the total caloric intake for 3 days lowered fasting SM HR LPL by 62% and raised fasting insulin by 4.5 mU·L^{-1} (60%) [78]. However, reducing carbohydrate from a typical 48% to 31% of daily caloric intake increased HR SM LPL by 83% without affecting fasting insulin or the insulin response to infused glucose [79]. Thus, elevated insulin levels that accompany carbohydrate ingestion may lower SM LPLA, but another mechanism besides insulin may increase SM LPL during low carbohydrate intake. Roberts et al. [115] found that LPLA in SM tissue homogenates obtained from marathon runners was decreased by 71% in response to a diet of complex, but not simple, carbohydrates (both comprised 70% of the total calories). The LPLA response to the complex carbohydrate diet was particularly strong in runners who were vegetarians. Both diets significantly decreased serum-free fatty acids (10–20%) and led to modest increases in insulin.

In the Sprague-Dawley rat, increased dietary saturated fatty acids substituted for polyunsaturated fatty acids reduced both heart and soleus muscle LPLA [86]. If insulin is an important regulator of muscle LPL and resistance to insulin affects expression of muscle LPLA (to be discussed in the next section), certain dietary fatty acids may indirectly affect SM LPLA by affecting insulin sensitivity. For example, dietary omega 3 fatty acids reverse insulin resistance in rats [135], but not in humans.

Hormones

INSULIN. Eight hours of normal feeding that lowered SM HR LPLA by 32% in healthy, normal weight men and women also caused a 100% increase in insulin [76]. Experimental 3-day diet treatments which increased SM HR LPLA also lowered circulating insulin [78, 115]. While these findings suggest that insulin may decrease SM LPL, in neither study were changes statistically correlated. The failure of insulin or tolbutamide administration alone to lower heart total LPLA in fasted rats, even though both increased adipose LPLA, provides a further argument against an independent effect of insulin [14]. Increased blood glucose appears necessary for the lowering of LPLA by insulin in rat heart [14]; however, glucose infusion that causes a sustained elevation of insulin increases SM HR LPLA in man [140].

Independent of eating, normal SM LPLA may require insulin. For example, newly diagnosed insulin-dependent diabetic patients had 54% lower SM HR LPLA [139] as compared to controls. In rats, pancreatectomy reduced red and white muscle total LPLA by 60–75% [73]. In perfused rat hearts, streptozotocin treatment for 4 days before sacrifice reduced HR LPL by 74% [83]. Further study of cardiomyocytes isolated from streptozotocin-induced diabetic rats showed that LPLA was reduced by 31%, LPL mass was reduced by 22%, but LPL mRNA was not changed [22]. Reduced LPL mass was due to decreased protein synthesis, not degradation, making LPL specific activity slightly lower in diabetic cardiomyocytes.

A number of studies have examined SM LPLA during euglycemic hyperinsulinemic clamps in humans (Table 8.1). In each of these studies, the investigators measured the HR fraction of SM LPL. An early study by Taskinen and Nikkila did not clamp insulin, but assessed the effect of glucose

TABLE 8.1.

Hyperinsulinemic Clamp Studies Showing the Effect of Insulin on Resting Muscle Lipoprotein Lipase Activity

Reference	Type of Subject	Clamp & Insulin Level	SM HR LPLA, % Rise vs. Pre-Clamp Level
Taskinen et al., 1981 [140]	1) Normal 2) Obese normolipidemic 3) Obese hypertriglyceridemic	mean glucose, mean insulin 1) 134 mg·dL^{-1}, 52 μU·mL^{-1} 2) 134 mg·dL^{-1}, 99 μU·mL^{-1} 3) 157 mg·dL^{-1}, 95 μU·mL^{-1}	1) ↑ 162% at 5h 2) ↑ 86% at 5h 3) ↑ 72% at 5 hr
Kiens et al., 1989 [60]	mean BMI = 21.4 Men, bike VO$_2$ max = 48–60 mL O$_2$·kg^{-1}·min^{-1}	euglycemic; [insulin] = 44 μU·mL^{-1}	↓ 33% at 4h
Farese, Yost, and Eckel, 1991 [46]	Within 20% of ideal BW by Life Insurance tables	euglycemic; [insulin] = 68 μU·mL^{-1} (409 pmol)	↓ 14%
Richelsen et al., 1993 [113]	Women, mean BMI = 37.8	euglycemic; [insulin] = 204 μU·mL^{-1}	↓ 22% at 4h
Ferraro, Eckel, et al., 1993 [47]	Insulin resistant	euglycemic; [insulin] = 99 μU·mL^{-1}	↑ 7% at 6h
Eckel, Yost, and Jensen, 1995 [40]	1) Normal weight 2) Obese women (94 kg) before wt loss (BMI 34.3) 3) Obese women after 12 kg wt loss in 3 mo. (BMI = 30)	euglycemic; insulin infusion rate = 40 mU·m^{-2}·min^{-1}	1) ↓ 18% at 6h 2) ↑ 41% at 6h 3) ↑ 67% at 6h

infusion over 5 hours on SM LPLA in normal and obese subjects [140]. In normal subjects given glucose, the average glucose level rose to 134 mg ·dL^{-1}, and the average insulin level was 52μU·mL^{-1}. SM HR LPLA rose by 162%. In obese subjects, both glucose (>150 mg·dL^{-1}) and insulin levels (>95μU·mL^{-1}) were higher compared to the non-obese. SM HR LPLA rose by 86% in the obese subjects with normolipidemia, and rose by 72% in those with hypertriglyceridemia. The results indicate that a simultaneous rise in glucose and insulin upregulates SM LPL.

When euglycemia is maintained and insulin levels are elevated to the range of 44 to 204μU·mL^{-1}, SM LPLA falls in healthy adults [40, 46, 47, 60, 113]. The fall in SM HR LPLA is greater if subjects are leaner and more fit, or if the insulin level is higher [113]. The studies in healthy subjects showed that high insulin downregulates HR SM LPLA. These results complement findings of earlier high carbohydrate diet studies, which showed a rise in HR SM LPLA with a fall in insulin. Hyperinsulinemia induces a rise (not a fall) in SM HR LPLA in subjects who are insulin resistant[40, 113]. This rise has been hypothesized to be part of an adaptive response that inhibits further fat storage in obese persons [38].

Collectively, the hyperinsulinemic clamp studies suggest that SM LPLA is responsive to insulin, but the response is impaired in insulin resistance. A concern with some of these studies is the possible contamination of SM samples with intermyofibral fat. In obese persons, small adipose tissue depots may exist in muscles between fibers. Because the insulin resistant subjects of these studies are also obese, muscle specimens from these subjects may contain some adipose tissue. The reported rise in obese subjects could partly reflect the normal adipose tissue LPLA response to insulin.

CATECHOLAMINES. Data in rats and humans show that catecholamines increase SM and decrease adipocyte LPLA. In rat SM, beta adrenergic stimulation with 10nM epinephrine increased muscle total LPL by 75–102% [87]. Both fasting and exercise increase rat myocardial LPLA and increase norepinephrine content approximately 2-fold in rat myocardium [92]. In addition, rats injected with epinephrine or norepinephrine 1 hour before sacrifice tend to increase LPLA by 20–30% [92]. Chronic (4 days) infusion of isoproterenol (a beta agonist) into rats increased vastus lateralis muscle LPLA 4-fold, did not affect heart LPLA, and lowered white adipose tissue LPLA by 50% [33]. Recently in humans, plasma norepinephrine was positively related (r = 0.83) to SM HR LPLA during a 2-hour saline infusion. Administration of isoproterenol to humans (during a pancreatic clamp to prevent hyperinsulinemia) significantly increased muscle LPLA and mRNA [39]. Reserpine given daily for 2 days blocked accumulation of catecholamines in rats but failed to affect myocardial LPLA [92]. This result is the only example of a lack of an effect of catecholamines on SM LPLA.

In adipocytes, where LPL is usually reciprocally-regulated as compared to muscle, catecholamines inhibit LPLA via a transacting factor that inhibits translation of LPL mRNA by interacting with a specific region of the LPL mRNA [152].

THYROID HORMONE. SM HR LPLA is elevated in hyperthyroidism and depressed in hypothyroidism. SM HR LPLA was 46% higher in thyrotoxic patients, and the rate of fat removal during an intravenous glucose tolerance test (IVGTT) was 23% faster in thyrotoxic patients [81]. In hypothyroid rat heart, LPLA was 2- to 4-fold higher than euthyroid rat heart [83]. There was no difference in LPL mass or LPL mRNA. Also in rat heart, T3 restores some LPLA lost by streptozotocin-induced diabetes, but does not increase LPLA in euthyroid rats [83].

In rat adipose tissue, the absence of thyroid hormone induced a 4.5-fold increase in LPL mass and 3-fold increases in both HR and non-releasable LPLA, but no change in LPL mRNA [121]. This effect of hypothyroidism on LPL translation may be mediated by a cytoplasmic factor that binds to the 3' untranslated region of the LPL mRNA [59].

ESTROGEN. Similar SM LPLA in men and women [92, 141] imply that there is no effect of estrogen on SM LPLA. However, exogenous estrogen given to male Sprague-Dawley rats increased heart and diaphragm HR LPLA [149]. Five days of estrogen injection into male Sprague-Dawley rats increased both fatty acid content and triglyceride stores of red vastus muscle, presumably due in part to increases in total LPLA (42% at rest, 76% post-exercise) [42].

GROWTH HORMONE. Growth hormone (GH) added to preadipocytes (OB1771 cells) in culture increases LPL mRNA, mass, and activity within hours [4]. Calcium ions selectively abolish this differentiation-associated induction at a transcriptional level [5]. In contrast, GH administration to humans decreases adipose tissue LPLA [105] and increases plasma triglycerides. There are no available studies of GH on SM LPL regulation.

Fatty Acids

Fatty acids may be a posttranslational regulator of LPL. Active LPL anchored to the capillary endothelium might be displaced by elevated local arterial concentrations of circulating fatty acids. The correlation between circulating fatty acids and freely circulating LPL following a fat meal supports this idea [58].

In cell culture studies, fatty acids facilitated removal of LPL from endothelial cell binding sites in one study [124] but not in another study [116]. Incubation of cardiac myocytes with oleic acid inhibited HR activity [116], giving rise to the speculation that fatty acids may regulate (i.e., inhibit) the translocation of LPL from its site of synthesis to its functional site at the capillary endothelium.

Intramuscular fatty acid concentrations are low, in the range of 30 $nmol \cdot g^{-1}$ tissue wet weight. [144]. Fatty acids regulate gene expression of various enzymes in several model systems [3, 122, 125, 134, 142]. In muscle, high intracellular fatty acids might block LPL gene expression and low levels might induce LPL gene expression.

Sepsis

Sepsis raises blood triglycerides [71], due at least in part to down-regulation of tissue LPL. In fasted rats, sepsis decreased LPL mRNA by 50%, LPL mass by >50%, and LPLA in soleus muscle by 80% and in adipose tissue by 50% [71].

Summary

Less is known about LPL regulation in SM than adipose tissue. In humans, feeding causes a fall in SM HR LPLA, and a high carbohydrate diet decreases SM LPLA. Insulin is a leading candidate for regulating SM LPL in response to dietary changes. Four to 6 hours of hyperinsulinemia and euglycemia without feeding lowers SM HR LPLA in normal weight persons, but slightly increases SM HR LPLA in obese, insulin-resistant persons. Other hormones, such as catecholamines, thyroid hormone, and estrogen, appear to up-regulate LPL in resting SM. Circulating fatty acids may inhibit HR LPL. The regulatory role of intramuscular fatty acids remains unknown.

REGULATION OF MUSCLE LPL BY EXERCISE

Exercise may affect gene expression in muscle fibers in many ways: (1) through electrical stimulation; (2) through physical deformation; (3) through fluctuations in circulating hormones and energy substrates; and, (4) through intracellular chemical changes that include a fall in the energy state (ATP/ADP and NAD/NADH$^+$ ratios), decreased pH, and increased intracellular calcium ions within muscle fibers [148]. Clearly, cell culture studies cannot completely recapitulate these stimuli, and studies of resting muscle in live animals need to take recent exercise into account. This section summarizes the time course of the LPL response to exercise in rats and humans, and offers speculation on important regulatory factors.

Acute Exercise Increases SM LPL mRNA and Mass

LaDu et al. [69] first reported effects of exercise on SM LPL mRNA. Freely eating male Wistar rats were sacrificed immediately or 24 hours after 2 hours of swimming. Both red (deep) and white (superficial) vastus muscle showed increases in total LPLA up to 30% immediately post-exercise, falling to less than 20% at 24 hours. LPL mRNA in these muscles was 65–100% higher just after exercise but not different from baseline 24 hours later. The changes in LPLA and mRNA in muscle were highly correlated (r = +0.86), leading the authors to conclude that exercise could regulate LPL through pretranslational mechanisms. Regulation of muscle total LPL by exercise differed from regulation by short-term fasting, which was posttranslational [68].

Ong et al. [101] found increased LPL mass and activity in both HR and heparin nonreleasable fractions, but no change in LPL mRNA in SM obtained from rats which were exercise trained up to 2 hours daily for 6 weeks. The rats were fasted, but it was unclear how long post-exercise the samples were obtained. In contrast to LaDu et al. who found increased mRNA immediately post-exercise [69], these data suggest posttranslational regulation of LPLA.

Recently, several studies were performed on humans. Simsolo et al. [132] studied 10 adult male runners before and 10 days after cessation of daily exercise training. In the trained state, vastus lateralis muscle was sampled in the morning 24 hours after the previous day's exercise. HR activity was lower by 45% after detraining, and heparin nonreleasable activity was 75% lower after detraining, but LPL mRNA and mass were not different. Nevertheless, two of the subjects experienced a clear fall in LPL mRNA, which paralleled falls in LPL mass and activity. Individual changes in LPL mRNA and LPL mass were also significantly correlated (r = 0.69). The authors concluded that exercise regulated SM LPL by posttranslational mechanisms, but because several subjects did not follow the group trend, the authors also concluded that pretranslational mechanisms may operate in some subjects [132].

When muscle tissue is sampled soon after exercise, LPL mRNA increases. This is shown by two recent human studies [126, 127]. In the first study, daily leg cycling was performed for 5 to 13 days by men ages 20–72 [126]. The intensity was equivalent to 55–70% of cycling VO_2 max, and the total exercise energy expenditure was estimated at 3500–5800 kcal. Both the vastus lateralis muscle and thigh subcutaneous adipose tissues were sampled when the men were in the fasted state 14–18 hours following the previous day's endurance exercise. Because muscle HR LPLA is unchanged or even reduced due to a heparin-like effect of exercise [104] in the early post-exercise condition, both the HR and nonreleasable pools of LPLA were analyzed. LPLA in the SM heparin nonreleasable pool was elevated compared to pretraining, but there was no change in HR LPLA. Exercise significantly increased LPL mRNA by 117%. In adipose tissue, LPLA, mass, and mRNA did not change. The study provided evidence of pretranslational regulation of human muscle LPL by short-term exercise.

To determine if LPL mRNA might be more elevated in humans earlier in the post-exercise period, vastus lateralis muscle was sampled in five women and four men soon after exercise [127]. Four days of daily exercise consisting of 60–90 minutes of continuous cycling per day did not increase LPL mRNA in samples taken on the morning of the 5th day, exactly 20 hours after the 4th exercise bout. On the 5th day, a 90-minute exercise bout at a workload equivalent to 63% of VO_2 max failed to affect LPL mRNA immediately following the bout. However at 4 hours post-exercise, LPL mRNA rose, and peaked at 282% of the pretraining level and 215% of pre-acute exercise level. At 8 hours post-acute exercise, LPL mRNA was still elevated (208% of pretraining), but had begun to fall, as compared to 4 hours post-exercise. The results confirmed the pretranslational effect of LPL observed earlier [126] and also suggested the following: (1) the greatest rise in LPL mRNA occurs between 0 and 8 hours post-exercise, and (2) the pretranslational regulation was a transient effect primarily due to the most recent bout of exercise. Total LPL immunoreactive mass rose by 93% at 8 hours post-exercise, closely following the LPL mRNA rise, to suggest that increased LPL mRNA led to increased LPL synthesis.

Figures 8.1 and 8.2 combine the LPL mRNA and LPL mass data from the three human studies [126, 127, 132] to describe a post-exercise time course for their responses. In both figures, the 24-hr post-exercise data point from Simsolo et al. [132] is the LPL variable in the trained state expressed as a percent of the detrained value. The rise and then fall in LPL mRNA are consistent with a model proposed by Williams and Neufer [148] who predicted that an intermittent exercise stimulus delivered for only a fraction of each day is sufficient to temporarily increase the mRNA of SM genes. If repeated frequently, the exercise stimulus may increase mRNA to a new baseline between bouts that is higher than resting untrained baseline levels [148]. However, runners training >20 km week [132] did

FIGURE 8.1.

Muscle LPL mRNA response to acute exercise in humans. The letters B and E label arrows that indicate the beginning and end of acute exercise, respectively. Third order regression was used to fit the data, including times -2 h and 0.2–24 h post-exercise. Numbers in parentheses are the numbers of subjects. Data points labeled "9" were taken from ref. 127, datum labeled "23" was taken from ref. 126, and datum labeled "14" was taken from ref. 132. The 24-hr post-exercise data point from ref. 132 actually represents the LPL mRNA of runners in the trained state, 24 hours after their most recent training run, expressed as a percent of the detrained value.

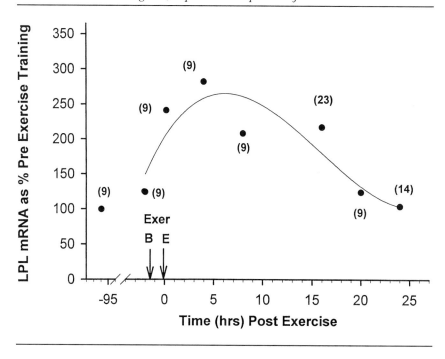

not show significantly elevated levels compared to the detrained state. More training may be necessary to maintain elevated mRNA for 24 hours post-bout.

The lack of data in the 8- to 16–hour post-exercise window make it difficult to conclude when the LPL mass peak occurs. However, the high levels at both 8 and 16 hours post-exercise vs. pretraining are compatible with elevated muscle LPLA. Elevated muscle LPLA may explain the rise in post-heparin plasma LPLA that occurs 24 hours following acute exercise in young adult men [56, 57] and the concomitant decrease in plasma triglycerides (to be discussed below). In response to a single endurance exercise bout of 1–3 hours in normal healthy adults, the fasting blood triglyceride

FIGURE 8.2.

Muscle LPL mass response to acute exercise in humans. Third order regression was used to fit the data, including times 0.2–24 h post-exercise. Numbers in parentheses are the numbers of subjects. Data points labeled "9" were taken from ref. 127, datum labeled "23" was taken from ref. 126, and datum labeled "14" was taken from ref. 132.

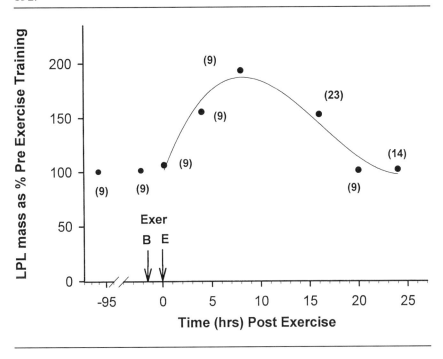

level falls to its lowest level (17–33%) 18–24 hours later [28, 30, 35]. After 24 hours, blood triglycerides begin to return to prebout levels, completing a return to normal levels within 3–5 days [35].

The muscle LPL response to acute exercise is similar to the transient post-exercise responses of GLUT4 [89, 112] and hexokinase II [94], proteins vital to the acquisition of glucose. GLUT4 expression in rats increases within 3 hours following exercise and returns to baseline by 24 hours post-exercise [89]. Hexokinase II is also induced by a single bout of exercise, and mRNA levels increase within 8 hours and return to baseline by 24 hours post-exercise [94]. If most of the exercise-induced increase in these messages is due to increased transcription, it is likely that a common muscle transcription factor coordinates gene expression of the proteins responsible for replenishing fuels used by vigorous exercise.

Potential Regulators of Exercise-Associated Increase in Muscle LPL Gene Expression

Insulin, catecholamines, fatty acids, and electrochemical events associated with contraction are the candidates most likely to affect LPL gene expression in muscle. Each of these are discussed in this section.

INSULIN. Insulin levels fall with acute exercise, remain attenuated after a bout, and are low following chronic training. SM LPLA is elevated post-acute and post-chronic exercise, suggesting an inverse relationship between insulin and muscle LPL. Euglycemic hyperinsulinemia in rested, normal-weight humans decreases muscle HR LPLA [40, 46, 60]. It appears that low insulin increases SM LPL, while high insulin decreases SM LPL. No studies have examined the effect of exercise simultaneous with elevated insulin levels on muscle LPL. Feeding can blunt the increase in LPLA normally seen in trained animals after exercise, presumably by increasing insulin [17, 101].

CATECHOLAMINES. Evidence in both rats [87] and humans [39] shows that catecholamines raise resting SM LPLA. During cycle exercise, catecholamines rise when intensity reaches 40–70% of VO_2 max [67]. Muscle HR LPLA elevated in the morning following a previous day's military maneuvers was significantly correlated with 24–hour urinary catecholamine excretion ($r = 0.8$) [77]. In young adult men and women during acute exercise, we observed 9-fold and 5-fold increases in plasma norepinephrine and epinephrine, respectively, both of which returned to baseline within 1 hour post-exercise [127]. These changes preceded the peaks for LPL mRNA and mass shown in Figures 8.1 and 8.2. Catecholamines increase intracellular cAMP; the LPL promoter has a cAMP responsive element [32].

FATTY ACIDS. During exercise, circulating non-esterified fatty acids increase several-fold from 300μM at rest to 800–1000μM [55, 64]. However, intramyofibral concentrations of fatty acids may fall during exercise due to increased beta oxidation. Although no data address this issue, it is possible that a fall in intracellular fatty acids signals the induction of LPL gene expression.

MUSCLE CONTRACTIONS. LPL mass and mRNA in the vastus lateralis muscle rose following a leg cycling exercise bout of 90-minute duration, during which subjects pedaled 60–90 times·min^{-1}. The total number of vastus muscle contractions ranged from 3600–9000 [127]. Many studies now show increased mRNAs for proteins induced by contractile activity [148]. The electrochemical events characteristic of contraction are unique to SM and may represent a proximal regulator of LPL gene expression.

PHYSIOLOGICAL RELEVANCE OF EXERCISE-INDUCED MUSCLE LPLA

The main utility of elevated LPLA due to exercise in muscle of healthy persons is to replenish intramyofibrillar triglyceride stores depleted by exercise. An important outcome of elevated muscle LPLA is the reduction of circulating triglycerides.

Muscle utilizes circulating free fatty acids, fatty acids from intramuscular triglycerides, fatty acids derived from LPL-catalyzed hydrolysis of lipoproteins, circulating glucose, and glucose from intramuscular glycogen for energy. In young healthy adults, the maximal rate of lipid oxidation occurs during work intensity of about 65% [119], and at this intensity, utilization of intramuscular triglyceride is also maximal [119]. At higher work intensities (80–90% of VO_2 max), lipid substrate utilization is decreased [119] and carbohydrate is the dominant fuel. Endurance training in young adults increases submaximal lipid utilization [55].

In muscle fibers of endurance trained humans, triglyceride droplets are visible microscopically. After competitive cross-country skiing lasting 8 hours, intramuscular triglyceride content decreased by 65% in slow twitch fibers, and by 35% in fast twitch fibers [80]. When endurance exercise in the range of 55–70% of VO_2 max was performed for several hours, intramuscular triglyceride content decreased by 30–41% [45, 85]. Thus, high volume exercise depletes intramuscular lipid stores.

During exercise in animals, muscle LPLA may increase [18] but this is rarely observed in humans [80]. Increases in LPL expression in humans are detected following exercise. The contribution of lipoprotein derived fatty acids to muscle total lipid energy utilization during exercise has been estimated at no more than 3–10% [90, 102, 143]. Thus, non-lipoprotein derived lipid sources contribute 90% of the total lipid energy. In turn, muscle lipid utilization may comprise 60% of the total energy usage at 65% of VO_2 max [119]. Intramyofibral lipid droplets may contribute up to 20–25% of the total energy required for exercise at 65% of VO_2 max [119]. It is likely that the increase in muscle LPL following exercise serves to replenish intramuscular triglyceride depleted by exercise [90].

Relevance to Blood Triglyceride Levels in Normolipidemia

SM LPL is an important determinant of blood triglyceride levels. In the cross-sectional study of Nikkila and Taskinen [91], athletes demonstrated 75% higher HR LPLA in SM, and 250% higher activity in adipose tissue vs. controls. The muscle LPL activities in athletic and control women were similar to their male counterparts. However, the ratio of adipose to muscle activity in women was greater (ratio of 8–9) than in men due to increased adipose tissue LPLA. Adipose tissue HR LPLA was only 4 times greater than muscle tissue LPLA in male athletes, and adipose tissue was 2.6 times greater than muscle LPLA in male controls. Thus, athletes actually had higher adipose LPLA compared to muscle, and adipose tissue LPL was thought to contribute more than muscle to whole body LPLA. Triglycerides were lower in the athletes compared to controls. However, this study most likely overestimated fat mass, and also did not take into account tissue blood flow, a factor that determines the volume of lipoprotein triglyceride substrate presented to tissues.

Longitudinal studies consistently show a decrease in fasting blood triglyceride level in response to exercise training ranging from 1 week or less [21, 52, 103, 117, 126, 127] to 6 months or more [54]. Acute exercise bouts of 1 to 3 hours can decrease triglycerides by 20–30%, and triathlon competitors may decrease plasma triglycerides by up to 70% [70].

Adipose tissue has higher LPLA and protein than SM. However, SM, by virtue of its mass and capacity to increase blood flow with modest activity, clears a significant portion of circulating triglycerides. SM is probably the major site of triglyceride clearance in aerobically fit persons. In young healthy men, approximately 50% of the clearance of infused triglyceride emulsion was attributed to muscle LPL [118]. Following a marathon run (42 km), a time when SM LPLA is elevated, there was faster clearance of blood triglycerides after Intralipid infusion[1] [120], with the rate of clearance in runners 92% higher as compared to sedentary men.

Healthy men were used exclusively in human studies that showed an important contribution of muscle LPL to triglyceride clearance. In some cases, endurance-trained subjects with low adiposity, high muscle mass, and high beta oxidative potential were used. These factors may prevent generalizing results to other groups.

We have examined the impact of specific tissues on plasma triglycerides by calculating triglyceride clearance using whole body muscle and adipose tissue mass, LPLA, resting blood flow, and assumed plasma triglyceride concentrations (Table 8.2). Behnke and Wilmore [6] used a 70 kg. man with 44.7% muscle mass and 15% fat mass as a reference [6]. Multiplying a representative muscle LPLA of 0.84 μmol FFA $\cdot g^{-1} \cdot h^{-1}$ from the reference [140] by the calculated SM mass (0.447×70 kg $= 31.3$ kg.) gives an estimate of the whole body, fasting muscle HR LPLA of 438 μmol FFA$\cdot min^{-1}$. With 20% of a resting cardiac output of 5.0 L min^{-1} distributed to the muscles, muscles receive 1000 mL per minute, or roughly 550 mL plasma $\cdot min^{-1}$. For adipose tissue, resting subcutaneous abdominal adipose tissue blood flow has been measured at 14 to 30 mL $\cdot min^{-1} \cdot kg^{-1}$ [19, 27], and for perirenal adipose tissue, 23 mL $\cdot min^{-1} \cdot kg^{-1}$ [19]. If an average flow of 23 mL$\cdot min^{-1} \cdot kg^{-1}$ fat mass is assumed for a total fat mass of 10.5 kg., then blood flow to the whole body adipose tissue depot is estimated at 242 mL$\cdot min^{-1}$. The smaller blood flow to the adipose depot limits its contribution to triglyceride clearance. Thus, in the average man during fasted rest, the 3.5-fold higher HR LPLA in adipose vs. muscle is more than

---

[1] The infusion of Intralipid, a triglyceride-rich emulsion which lacks apolipoproteins, differs from the ingestion of a fat meal. Gut responses to food intake and carbohydrate stimulation of pancreatic insulin release are absent. The absence of an increase in circulating insulin preserves the fasting ratio of muscle:adipose LPLA.

TABLE 8.2.

Contributions of Skeletal Muscle and Adipose Tissue LPL Activities Toward Triglyceride Clearance, Estimated for the Reference Man and Woman [6], During Fasting

Variable	Reference Man (BW = 70 kg)		Reference Woman (BW = 56.7 kg)	
	Muscle	Adipose	Muscle	Adipose
Tissue mass	31.3 kg (44.7% BW)	10.5 kg (15% BW)	20.4 kg (30.6% BW)	15.3 kg (27% BW)
Lipoprotein lipase activity,[a] (heparin releasable)	14 $\mu mol \cdot kg^{-1} \cdot min^{-1}$	51 $\mu mol \cdot kg^{-1} \cdot min^{-1}$	14 $\mu mol \cdot kg^{-1} \cdot min^{-1}$	83 $\mu mol \cdot kg^{-1} \cdot min^{-1}$
Tissue LPL activity, whole body	14 $\mu mol \cdot kg^{-1} \cdot min^{-1}$ × 31.3 kg = 438 $\mu mol \cdot min^{-1}$	51 $\mu mol \cdot kg^{-1} \cdot min^{-1}$ × 10.5 kg = 536 $\mu mol \cdot min^{-1}$	14 $\mu mol \cdot kg^{-1} \cdot min^{-1}$ × 20.4 kg = 286 $\mu mol \cdot min^{-1}$	83 $\mu mol \cdot kg^{-1} \cdot min^{-1}$ × 15.3 kg = 1270 $\mu mol \cdot min^{-1}$
Tissue blood flow, whole body, resting	1000 mL·min^{-1}[b]	242 mL·min^{-1}[d]	900 mL·min^{-1}[c]	352 mL·min^{-1}[d]
Tissue plasma flow,[e] whole body, resting	550 mL·min^{-1}	133 mL·min^{-1}	540 mL·min^{-1}	211 mL·min^{-1}
Arterial plasma triglyceride conc.[f]	1300 $\mu mol \cdot L^{-1}$	1300 $\mu mol \cdot L^{-1}$	1010 $\mu mol \cdot L^{-1}$	1010 $\mu mol \cdot L^{-1}$
Substrate per minute presented to tissue	1300 $\mu mol \cdot L^{-1}$ × 550 mL·min^{-1} = 715 $\mu mol \cdot min^{-1}$	1300 $\mu mol \cdot L^{-1}$ × 133 mL·min^{-1} = 173 $\mu mol \cdot min^{-1}$	1010 $\mu mol \cdot L^{-1}$ × 540 mL·min^{-1} = 545 $\mu mol \cdot min^{-1}$	1010 $\mu mol \cdot L^{-1}$ × 211 mL·min^{-1} = 213 $\mu mol \cdot min^{-1}$
Fractional TG clearance, across tissue bed	438 $\mu mol \cdot min^{-1}$ ÷ 715 $\mu mol \cdot min^{-1}$ = 0.61	536 $\mu mol \cdot min^{-1}$ ÷ 173 $\mu mol \cdot min^{-1}$ >1.0	286 $\mu mol \cdot min^{-1}$ ÷ 545 $\mu mol \cdot min^{-1}$ = 0.52	1270 $\mu mol \cdot min^{-1}$ ÷ 213 $\mu mol \cdot min^{-1}$ >1.0
Plasma total triglyceride content[g]	3900 μmol	3900 μmol	2525 μmol	2525 μmol
Fractional TG clearance, whole body	438 $\mu mol \cdot min^{-1}$ ÷ 3900 $\mu mol \cdot min^{-1}$ = 0.11	173 $\mu mol \cdot min^{-1}$ ÷ 3900 $\mu mol \cdot min^{-1}$ = 0.044	286 $\mu mol \cdot min^{-1}$ ÷ 2525 $\mu mol \cdot min^{-1}$ = 0.11	213 $\mu mol \cdot min^{-1}$ ÷ 2525 $\mu mol \cdot min^{-1}$ = 0.084

[a] heparin releasable LPL activities for vastus lateralis muscle reported by Taskinen and Nikkila, 1981; ref [140].
[b] taken from Berne and Levy, 1997; ref [8].
[c] assumes 20% of the resting cardiac output of 4.5 L·min^{-1}.
[d] calculated by multiplying whole body adipose tissue mass in kg × 23 mL·kg^{-1}·min^{-1}, which is the mean plasma flow through abdominal and perirenal adipose tissue measured during fasting conditions; ref [107].
[e] assumes hematocrit = 45% for men and 40% for women.
[f] fasting plasma triglyceride concentration corresponding to 50th percentile for men ages 25–29 (115 mg·dL^{-1}) and women ages 20–34 (90 mg·dL^{-1}); ref. [114].
[g] assumes plasma volume of 3 L for men and 2.5 L for women.

compensated by a 3-fold greater mass of muscle vs. adipose, and a 3-fold greater blood flow in muscle vs. adipose tissue.

Under the conditions of eating, altered tissue blood flow due to physical activity, and altered body composition, the contribution of muscle LPL to triglyceride clearance will differ.

EATING. SM from fed rats holds about two-thirds the amount of the total body adipose tissue functional LPLA, but in the fasting rat, SM holds about twice the activity of whole body adipose tissue HR LPLA [137]. Eating in humans increases adipose tissue HR LPLA by 46% and decreases muscle HR LPLA by 32%. In addition, eating increases adipose tissue blood flow by 2- to 3-fold in normal weight persons [107]. These two changes increase adipose tissue clearance of tissue delivered plasma triglycerides by 4.5-fold, diverting more dietary fatty acids toward adipose tissue for storage. Exercise training lowers the plasma triglyceride and chylomicron responses to a high fat meal [147] with no change in body weight. Elevated basal LPL may mediate this change.

ALTERED TISSUE BLOOD FLOW DUE TO PHYSICAL ACTIVITY. Submaximal activity increases blood flow to both muscle [97] and adipose tissue [19]. In SM, blood flow increases in proportion to the intensity of the exercise. Maximal blood flow through a muscle bed has been measured at 2.47 $L \cdot kg^{-1}$, or about 75 times the resting flow of 33 $mL \cdot kg^{-1} \cdot min^{-1}$ [2]. Adipose tissue blood flow data during exercise are sparse. While one study reported that exercise can increase adipose tissue blood flow by 2.5- to 6.8-fold [19], work intensities were not available. It is likely that exercise increases muscle blood flow to a greater extent than it does adipose tissue flow. A disproportionate increase in muscle vs. adipose tissue would increase muscle clearance of triglycerides.

ALTERED BODY COMPOSITION. For subjects with muscle and adipose tissue masses different from Behnke and Wilmore's reference adults, the importance of each tissue as an organ that reduces blood triglycerides changes in proportion to the change in mass.

SUMMARY

LPL directs the body wide distribution of fatty acids derived from circulating triglycerides. This is accomplished by tissue-specific regulation. In adipose tissue, LPLA per gram is higher than in muscle tissue. Eating increases adipose tissue LPLA and may increase blood flow. Exercise greatly increases SM blood flow and LPLA over a longer time frame as compared to the effect of eating on adipose tissue LPLA. The regulation of LPLA occurs at several levels and is better understood in adipose tissue models. In muscle, the study of regulation has been neglected. LPL expression in muscle may be more complex than in adipose tissue owing to the changes in blood flow and metabolism associated with contractile activity, as well as to other factors intrinsic to contraction, such as electrical events and cellular deformation.

Sixty to 90 minutes of continuous leg exercise at 60% of VO_2 max induces muscle LPL expression, increases LPL mRNA in humans within 4 hours of exercise, and raises immunoreactive mass by 8 hours post-exercise. Within 24 hours, both LPL mRNA and mass have returned to normal levels. Increased muscle LPL mass following exercise may serve to replenish intramyofibral stores of triglyceride, which are depleted with endurance exercise and are greater in aerobically-trained individuals as compared to untrained individuals. The post-exercise increase in muscle LPL mass coincides with the post-exercise acute fall in circulating triglycerides typically observed in subjects capable of exercising for 60–90 minutes at 60% of VO_2 max. The low fasting triglyceride levels often seen in highly trained individuals are due in part to their high levels of muscle LPLA.

Both the physiological mediator and the molecular mediator of the exercised-induced induction of muscle LPL expression are unknown. Hopefully, the next decade will see careful studies aimed at better defining the molecular physiology of LPL expression in muscle.

REFERENCES

1. Ailhaud, G. Cellular and secreted lipoprotein lipase revisited. *Clin. Biochem.* 23:343–347, 1990.
2. Andersen, P., and B. Saltin. Maximal perfusion of skeletal muscle in man. *J. Physiol.* (London) 366:233–249, 1985.
3. Assimacopoulos-Jeannet, F., S. Thumelin, E. Roche, V. Esser, J.D. McGarry and M. Prentki. Fatty acids rapidly induce the carnitine palmitoyltransferase I gene in the pancreatic beta-cell line INS-1. *J. Biol. Chem.* 272:1659–1664, 1997.
4. Barcellini-Couget, S., A. Pradines-Figueres, P. Roux, C. Dani and G. Ailhaud. The regulation by growth hormone of lipoprotein lipase gene expression is mediated by c-fos protooncogene. *Endocrinology* 132:53–60, 1993.
5. Barcellini-Couget, S., G. Vassaux, R. Negrel and G. Ailhaud. Rise in cytosolic Ca^{++} abolishes in preadipose cells the expression of lipoprotein lipase stimulated by growth hormone. *Biochem. Biophys. Res. Commun.* 199:136–143, 1994.
6. Behnke, A.R., and J.H. Wilmore. *Evaluation and Regulation of Body Build and Composition.* Englewood Cliffs, N.J.:Prentice-Hall, 1974.
7. Beisiegel, U., W. Weber, and G. Bengtsson-Olivecrona. Lipoprotein lipase enhances the binding of chylomicrons to low density lipoprotein recepor-related protein. *Proc. Nat. Acad. Sci.* 88:8342–8346, 1991.
8. Berne, R.M., and M.N. Levy. *Cardiovascular Physiology*, Ed. 7th. St. Louis:Mosby-Year Book, Inc., 1997. pp. 269–270.
9. Bessesen, D.H., A.D. Robertson, and R.H. Eckel. Weight reduction increases adipose but decreases cardiac LPL in reduced-obese Zucker rats. *Am. J. Physiol.* 261:E246–E251, 1991.
10. Blanchette-Mackie, E.J., H. Masuno, N.K. Dwyer, T. Olivecrona, and R.O. Scow. Lipoprotein lipase in myocytes and capillary endothelium of heart: immunocytochemical study. *Endocrin. Metabol.* 19:E818–E828, 1989.
11. Booth, F.W., and D.B. Thomason. Molecular and cellular adaptation of muscle in response to exercise: perspectives of various models. *Physiol. Rev.* 71:541–585, 1991.
12. Borensztajn, J., M.S. Rone, S.P. Babirak, J.A. McGarr, and L.B. Oscai. Effect of exercise on lipoprotein lipase activity in rat heart and skeletal muscle. *Am. J. Physiol.* 229:394–397. 1975.
13. Borensztajn, J., M.S. Rone, and T. Sandros. Effects of colchicine and cycloheximide on the functional and non-functional lipoprotein lipase reactions of rat heart. *Biochem. Biophys. Acta* 398:394–400, 1975.
14. Borensztajn, J., D.R. Samols, and A.H. Rubenstein. Effects of insulin on lipoprotein lipase activity in the rat heart and adipose tissue. *Am. J. Physiol.* 223:1271–1275, 1972.
15. Braun, J.E., and D.L. Severson. Regulation of the synthesis, processing and translocation of lipoprotein lipase. *Biochem. J.* 287:337–347, 1992.
16. Brunzell, J.D. Familial lipoprotein lipase deficiency and other causes of the chylomicronemia syndrome. C.R. Scriver, A.L. Beaudet, W.S. Sly, and D. Valle, D. (eds.). *The Metabolic and Molecular Bases of Inherited Disease.* New York:McGraw-Hill, 1995, pp. 1913–1932.
17. Budahoski, S., S.T. Kozlowski, R.L. Terjung, H. Kaciuba-Uscilko, K. Nazar, and I. Falecka-Wieczorak. Changes in muscle lipoprotein lipase activity during exercise in dogs fed on a mixed fat-rich meal. *Pflugers Archiv.* 394:191–193, 1982.
18. Budohoski, L. Exercise-induced changes in lipoprotein lipase activity (LPLA) in skeletal muscles of dogs. *Pflugers Archiv.* 405:188–192, 1997.

19. Bulow, J. Adipose tissue blood flow during exercise. *Danish Medical Bulletin.* 30:85–100, 1983.

20. Camps, L., M. Reina, M. Llobera, S. Vilaro, and T. Olivecrona. Lipoprotein lipase: cellular origin and functional distribution. *Cell. Physiol.* 27:C673–C681, 1990.

21. Carlson, L.A., and F. Mossfeldt. Acute effect of prolonged heavy exercise on the concentration of plasma lipids and lipoproteins in man. *Acta Physiol. Scand.* 61:51-59, 1964.

22. Carroll, R., L. Liu, and D.L. Severson. Post-transcriptional mechanisms are responsible for the reduction in lipoprotein lipase activity in cardiomyocytes from diabetic rat hearts. *Biochem. J.* 310:67–72, 1995.

23. Caster, W.O., J. Poncelet, A.B. Simon, and W.D. Armstrong. Tissue weights of the rat. I. Normal values determined by dissection and chemical methods. *Proc. Soc. Exp. Biol. Med.* 91:122–126, 1956.

24. Chajek-Shaul, T., G. Bengtsson-Olivecrona, J. Peterson, and T. Olivecrona. Metabolic fate of rat heart endothelial lipoprotein lipase. *Am. J. Physiol.* 255:E247–E254, 1988.

25. Chappell, D.A., G.L. Fry, M.A. Waknitz, et al. Lipoprotein lipase induces catabolism of normal triglyceride-rich lipoproteins via the low density lipoprotein receptor-related protein/α2-macroglobulin receptor in vitro. *J. Biol. Chem.* 268:14168–14175, 1993.

26. Coleman, T., R.L. Seip, J.M. Gimble, D. Lee, N. Maeda, and C.F. Semenkovich. COOH-terminal disruption of lipoprotein lipase in mice is lethal in homozygotes, but heterozygotes have elevated triglycerides and impaired enzyme activity. *J. Biol. Chem.* 270: 12518–12525, 1995.

27. Coppack, S.W., R.D. Evans, R.M. Fisher, et al. Adipose tissue metabolism in obesity: lipase action in vivo before and after a mixed meal. *Metabolism* 41:264–272, 1992.

28. Crouse, S.F., B.C. O'Brien, J.J. Rohack et al. Changes in serum lipids and apolipoproteins after exercise in men with high cholesterol: influence of intensity. *J. Appl. Physiol.* 79: 279–286, 1995.

29. Cryer, A. Comparative biochemistry and physiology of lipoprotein lipase. J. Borensztajn (ed.). *Lipoprotein Lipase.* Chicago: Evener, 1987, pp. 277–327.

30. Cullinane, E.M., S. Siconolfi, A. Saritelli, and P.D. Thompson. Acute decrease in serum triglycerides with exercise: is there a threshold for an exercise effect? *Metabolism* 31: 844–847, 1982.

31. Currie, R.A., and R. H. Eckel. Characterization of a high affinity octamer transcription factor binding site in the human lipoprotein promoter. *Arch. Biochem. Biophys.* 298: 630–639, 1992.

32. Deeb, S.S., and R. Peng. Structure of the human lipoprotein lipase gene. *Biochemistry* 28:4131–4135, 1989.

33. Deshaies, Y., A. Geloen, A. Paulin, A. Marette, and L.J. Bukowiecki. Tissue-specific alterations in lipoprotein lipase activity in the rat after chronic infusion with isoproterenol. *Horm. Metab. Res.* 25:13–16, 1993.

34. Doolittle, M.H., O. Ben-Zeev, J. Elovson, D. Martin, and T.G. Kirchgessner. The response of lipoprotein lipase to feeding and fasting. *J. Biol. Chem.* 265:4570–4577, 1990.

35. Dufaux, B., G. Assman, U. Order, A. Hoederath, and W. Hollman. Plasma lipoproteins, hormones, and energy substrate during the first days after prolonged exercise. *Int. J. Sports. Med.* 2:256–260, 1981.

36. Duque, M., M. Graupner, H. Stutz, et al. New fluorogenic tiacylglycerol analogs as substrates for the determination and chiral discrimination of lipase activities. *J. Lipid Res.* 37:868–876, 1996.

37. Eckel, R.H. Lipoprotein lipase. A multifunctional enzyme relevant to common metabolic diseases. *N. Engl. J. Med.* 320:1060–1067, 1989.

38. Eckel, R.H. Insulin resistance: an adaptation for weight maintenance. *Lancet* 340: 1452–1453, 1992.

39. Eckel, R.H., D.R. Jensen, I.R. Schlaepfer, and T.J. Yost. Tissue specific regulation of lipoprotein lipase by isoproterenol in normal-weight humans. *Am. J. Physiol.* 271: R1280–R1286, 1996.

40. Eckel, R.H., T.J. Yost, and D.R. Jensen. Sustained weight reduction in moderately obese women results in decreased activity of skeletal muscle lipoprotein lipase. *Eur. J. Clin. Invest.* 25:396–402, 1995.

41. Eisenberg, S., E. Sehayek, T. Olivecrona, and I. Vlodavsky. Lipoprotein lipase enhances binding of lipoproteins to heparan sulfate on cell surfaces and extracellular matrix. *J. Clin. Invest.* 90:2013–2021, 1992.

42. Ellis, G.S., S. Lanza-Jacoby, A. Gow, and Z.V. Kendrick. Effects of estradiol on lipoprotein lipase activity and lipid availability in exercised male rats. *J. Appl. Physiol.* 77(1):209–215, 1994.

43. Enerback, S., and J.M. Gimble. Lipoprotein lipase gene expression: physiological regulators at the transcriptional and post-transcriptional level. *Biochim. Biophys. Acta* 1169: 107–125, 1993.

44. Enerback, S., B.G. Ohlsson, L. Samuelsson, and G. Bjursell. Characterization of the human lipoprotein lipase (LPL) promoter: evidence of two cis-regulatory regions, LP-A and LP-B, of importance for the differentiation-linked induction of the LPL gene during adipogenesis. *Mol. Cell. Biol.* 12:4622–4633, 1992.

45. Essen, B. Intramuscular substrate utilization during prolonged exercise. *Ann. New York Acad. Sci.* 301:30–44, 1977.

46. Farese, R.V., T.J. Yost, and R.H. Eckel. Tissue-specific regulation of lipoprotein lipase activity by insulin/glucose in normal-weight humans. *Metabolism* 40:214–216, 1991.

47. Ferraro, R.H., R.H. Eckel, D.E. Larson, et al. Relationship between skeletal muscle lipoprotein lipase activity and 24-hour macronutrient oxidation. *J. Clin. Invest.* 92:441–445, 1993.

48. Friedman, G., T. Chajek-Shaul, T. Olivecrona, O. Stein, and Y. Stein. Fate of milk 125-I-labeled lipoprotein lipase in cells in culture: comparison of lipoprotein lipase- and non-lipoprotein lipase synthesizing cells. *Biochem. Biophys. Acta* 711:114–122, 1982.

49. Galan, X., M. Llobera, and I. Ramirez. Lipoprotein lipase and hepatic lipase in Wistar and Sprague-Dawley rat tissues: differences in the effects of gender and fasting. *Lipids* 29:333–336, 1994.

50. Goers, J.W.F., M.E. Pedersen, P.A. Kern, J. Ong, and M.C. Schotz. An enzyme-linked immunoassay for lipoprotein lipase. *Anal. Biochem.* 166:27–35, 1987.

51. Goldman, R., and O. Sopher. Control of lipoprotein lipase secretion by macrophages: effect of macrophage differentiation agents. *J. Leukocyte Biol.* 47:79–86, 1990.

52. Gyntelberg, F., R. Brennan, J.O. Holloszy, G. Schonfeld, M.J. Rennie and S. W. Weidman. Plasma triglyceride lowering by exercise despite increased food intake in patients with type IV hyperlipoproteinemia. *Am. J. Clin. Nutr.* 30:716–720. 1977.

53. Hahn, P.F. Abolishment of alimentary lipemia following injection of heparin. *Science* 98: 19–20, 1943.

54. Holloszy, J.O., J.S. Skinner, G. Toro, and T.K. Cureton. Effects of a six month program of endurance exercise on the serum lipids of middle-aged men. *Am. J. Cardiol.* 14: 753–760, 1964.

55. Hurley B.F., P.M. Nemeth, W.H. Martin, III, J.M. Hagberg, G.P. Dalskey, and J. O. Holloszy. Muscle triglyceride utilization during exercise: effect of training. *J. Appl. Physiol.* 60:562–567, 1986.

56. Kantor, M.A., E.M. Cullinane, P.N. Herbert, and P.D. Thompson. Acute increase in lipoprotein lipase following prolonged exercise. *Metabolism* 33:454–457, 1984.

57. Kantor, M.A., E.M. Cullinane, S.P. Sady, P.N. Herbert, and P.D. Thompson. Exercise acutely increases high density lipoprotein-cholesterol and lipoprotein lipase activity in trained and untrained men. *Metabolism* 36:188–192, 1987.

58. Karpe, F., T. Olivecrona, G. Walldius, and A. Hamsten. Lipoprotein lipase in plasma after an oral fat load: relation to free fatty acids. *J. Lipid Res.* 33:975–984, 1992.

59. Kern, P.A., G. Ranganathan, A. Yukht, J.M. Ong, and R.C. Davis. Translational regulation of lipoprotein lipase by thyroid hormone is via a cytoplasmic repressor that interacts with the 3' untranslated region. *J. Lipid Res.* 37:2332–2340, 1996.

60. Kiens, B., H. Lithell, K.J. Mikines, and E.A. Richter. Effects of insulin and exercise on muscle lipoprotein lipase activity in man and its relation to insulin action. *J. Clin. Invest.* 84:1124–1129, 1989.

61. Kirchgessner, T.G., R.C. BeBoeuf, C.A. Langner, et al. Genetic and developmental regulation of the lipoprotein lipase gene: loci both distal and proximal to the lipoprotein lipase structural gene control enzyme expression. *J. Biol. Chem.* 264:1473–1482, 1989.

62. Kirchgessner, T.G., J.C. Chuat, C. Heinzmann, et al. Organization of the human lipoprotein lipase gene and evolution of the lipase gene family. *Proc. Natl. Acad. Sci. USA* 86: 9647–9651, 1989.

63. Kirchgessner, T.G., K.L. Svenson, A.J. Lusis, and M.C. Schotz. The sequence of cDNA encoding lipoprotein lipase. *J .Biol. Chem.* 262:8463–8466, 1987.

64. Klein, S., E.F. Coyle, and R.R. Wolfe. Fat metabolism during low-intensity exercise in endurance-trained and untrained men. *Am. J. Physiol.* 267:E934–E940, 1994.

65. Korn, E.D. Clearing factor, a heparin-activated lipoprotein lipase. *J. Biol. Chem.* 215: 1–14, 1954.

66. Korn, E.D. Clearing factor, a heparin-activated lipoprotein lipase. II. Substrate specificity and activation by coconut oil. *J. Biol. Chem.* 215:15–26, 1954.

67. Kotchen, T., L.H. Hartley, T.W. Rice, E.H. Mougey, L.G. Jones, and J.W. Mason. Renin, norepinephrine, and epinephrine responses to graded exercise. *J. Appl. Physiol.* 31: 178–184, 1971.

68. LaDu, M.J., H. Kapsas, and W.K. Palmer. Regulation of lipoprotein lipase in adipose and muscle tissues during fasting. *Am. J. Physiol.* 260:R953–R960, 1991.

69. LaDu, M.J., H. Kapsas, and W.K. Palmer. Regulation of lipoprotein lipase in adipose and muscle tissues during exercise. *J. Appl. Physiol.* 71:404–409, 1991.

70. Lamon-Fava, S., J.R. McNamara, H.W. Farber, N.S. Hill, and E.J. Schaefer. Acute changes in lipid, lipoprotein, apolipoprotein, and low-density lipoprotein particle size after an endurance triathlon. *Metabolism* 38:921–925, 1989.

71. Lanza-Jacoby, S., N. Sedkova, H. Phetteplace, and D. Perrotti. Sepsis-induced regulation of lipoprotein lipase expression in rat adipose tissue and soleus muscle. *J. Lipid Res.* 701: 710, 1997.

72. Levak-Frank, S., H. Radner, A. Walsh, R. Stollberger, G. Knipping, G. Hoefler, W. Sattler, et al. Muscle-specific overexpression of lipoprotein lipase causes a severe myopathy characterized by proliferation of mitochondria and peroxisomes in transgenic mice. *J. Clin. Invest.* 96:976–986, 1995.

73. Linder, C., S.S. Chernick, T.R. Fleck, and R.O. Scow. Lipoprotein lipase and uptake of chylomicron triglyceride by skeletal muscle of rats. *Am. J. Physiol.* 231:860–864, 1976.

74. Lithell, H., and J. Boberg. A method of determining lipoprotein-lipase activity in human adipose tissue. *Scand. J. Clin. Lab. Invest.* 37:551–561, 1977.

75. Lithell, H., and J. Boberg. Determination of lipoprotein-lipase activity in human skeletal muscle tissue. *Biochem. Biophy. Acta* 528:58–68, 1978.

76. Lithell, H., J. Boberg, K. Hellsing, G. Lundqvist, and B. Vessby. Lipoprotein-lipase activity in human skeletal muscle and adipose tissue in the fasting and the fed states. *Atherosclerosis* 30:89–94, 1978.

77. Lithell, H., M. Cedermark, J. Froberg, P. Tesch. and J. Karlsson. Increase of lipoprotein lipase activity in skeletal muscle during heavy exercise: relation to epinephrine excretion. *Metabolism* 30:1130–1133, 1981.

78. Lithell, H., I. Jacobs, B. Vessby, K. Hellsing, and J. Karisson. Decrease of lipoprotein lipase activity in skeletal muscle in man during a short-term carbohydrate-rich dietary regime. With special reference to HDL-cholesterol, apolipoprotein and insulin concentrations. *Metabolism* 31:994–998, 1982.

79. Lithell, H., B. Karistrom, I. Selinus, B. Vessby, and B. Fellstrom. Is muscle lipoprotein lipase inactivated by ordinary amounts of dietary carbohydrates? *Hum. Nutr. Clin. Nutr.* 39C:289–295, 1985.

80. Lithell, H., J. Orlander, R. Schele, B. Sjodin, and J. Karlsson. Changes in lipoprotein-lipase activity and lipid stores in human skeletal muscle with prolonged heavy exercise. *Acta. Physiol. Scand.* 107:257–261, 1979.

81. Lithell, H., B. Vessby, I. Selinus, and P.A. Dahlberg. High muscle lipoprotein lipase activity in thyrotoxic patients. *Acta Endocrinol.* 109:227–231, 1985.

82. Liu, G., and T. Olivecrona. Synthesis and transport of lipoprotein lipase in perfused guinea pig hearts. *Am. J. Physiol.* 263:H438–H446, 1992.

83. Liu, L., and D.L. Severson. Regulation of myocardial lipoprotein lipase activity by diabetes and thyroid hormones. *Can. J. Physiol. Pharmacol.* 72:1259–1264, 1994.

84. Mahoney, E.M., J.C. Khoo. and D. Steinberg. Lipoprotein lipase secretion by human monocyte and rabbit alveolar macrophages in culture. *Proc. Natl. Acad. Sci.* 79:1639–1642, 1982.

85. Martin, W.H., III. Effect of endurance training on fatty acid metabolism during whole body exercise. *Med. Sci. Sports Exerc.* 29:635–639, 1997.

86. Matsuo, T., H. Sumida, and M. Suzuki. Effects of chemical sympathectomy on lipoprotein lipase activities in peripheral tissues of rats fed high fat diets consisting of different fats. *J. Nutr. Sci. Vitaminol.* 41:377–386, 1995.

87. Miller, W.C., J. Gorski, L.B. Oscai, and W.K. Palmer. Epinephrine activation of heparin-nonreleasable lipoprotein lipase in 3 skeletal muscle fiber types of the rat. *Biochem. Biophys. Res. Comm.* 164:615–619, 1989.

88. Nakshatri, H., P. Nakshatri, and R.A. Currie. Interaction of Oct-1 with TFIIB. *J. Biol. Chem.* 270:19613–19623, 1995.

89. Neufer, P.D., and G. L. Dohm. Exercise induces a transient increase in transcription of the GLUT-4 gene in skeletal muscle. *Am. J. Physiol.* 265:C1597–C1603, 1993.

90. Nikkila, E.A. Role of lipoprotein lipase in metabolic adaptation to exercise and training. J. Borensztajn (ed.). *Lipoprotein Lipase.* Chicago: Evener Publishers, Inc., 1987, pp. 187–199.

91. Nikkila, E.A., M.R. Taskinen, S. Rehunen, and M. Harkonen. Lipoprotein lipase activity in adipose tissue and skeletal muscle of runners: relation to serum lipoproteins. *Metabolism* 27:1661–1671, 1978.

92. Nikkila, E.A., P. Torsti, and O. Penttila. Effects of fasting, exercise, and reserpine on catecholamine content and lipoprotein lipase activity of rat heart and adipose tissues. *Life Sciences* 4:27–35, 1965.

93. Nykjaer, A., G. Bengtsson-Olivecrona, A. Lookene, et al. The alpha2-macroglobulin receptor/low density lipoprotein receptor-related protein binds lipoprotein lipase and beta-migrating very low density lipoprotein associated with the lipase. *J. Biol. Chem.* 268:15048–15055, 1993.

94. O'Doherty, R.M., D.P. Bracy, D.H. Osawa, D.H. Wasserman, and D.K. Granner. Rat skeletal muscle hexokinase II mRNA and activity are increased by a single bout of acute exercise. *Am. J. Physiol.* 266:E171–E178, 1994.

95. Obunike, J.C., P. Sivaram, L. Paka, M.G. Low, and I.J. Goldberg. Lipoprotein lipase degradation by adipocytes: receptor-associated protein (RAP)-sensitive and proteoglycan-mediated pathways. *J. Lipid Res.* 37:2439–2449, 1996.

96. Olivecrona, G., and T. Olivecrona. Triglyceride lipases and atherosclerosis. *Curr. Opin. Lipidol.* 6:291–305, 1995.

97. Olivecrona, T., and G. Bengtsson. Immunochemical properties of lipoprotein lipase: development of an immunoassay procedure applicable to several mammalian species. *Biochem. Biophys. Acta* 752:38–45, 1983.

98. Olivecrona, T., and Bengtsson-Olivecrona, G. Lipoprotein lipase from milk- the model enzyme in lipoprotein lipase research. Borensztajn, J. (ed.). *Lipoprotein Lipase.* Chicago: Evener Press, 1987, pp. 15–58.

99. Olivecrona, T., S.S. Chernick, G. Bengtsson-Olivecrona, M. Garrison, and R.O. Scow. Synthesis and secretion of lipoprotein lipase in 3T3-L1 adipocytes: demonstration of inactive forms of lipase in cells. *J. Biol. Chem.* 262:10748–10759, 1987.

100. Ong, J.M., T.G. Kirchgessner, M.C. Schotz, and P.A. Kern. Insulin increases the synthetic rate and messenger RNA level of lipoprotein lipase in isolated rat adipocytes. *J. Biol. Chem.* 263:12933–12938, 1988.

101. Ong, J.M., R.B. Simsolo, M. Saghizadeh, J.W. Goers, and P.A. Kern. Effects of exercise training and feeding on lipoprotein lipase gene expression in adipose tissue, heart, and skeletal muscle of the rat. *Metabolism* 44:1596–1605, 1995.

102. Oscai, L.B., D.A. Essig, and W.A. Palmer. Lipase regulation of muscle triglyceride hydrolysis. *J. Appl. Physiol.* 69:1571–1577, 1990.

103. Oscai, L.B., J.A. Patterson, D.L. Bogard, R.J. Beck, and B.L. Rothermel. Normalization of serum triglycerides and lipoprotein electrophoretic patterns by exercise. *Am. J. Cardiol.* 30:775–780, 1972.

104. Oscai, L.B., R.W. Tsika, and D.A. Essig. Exercise training has a heparin-like effect on lipoprotein lipase activity in muscle. *Can. J. Physiol. Pharmacol.* 70:905–909, 1992.

105. Oscarsson, J., M. Ottosson, J.O. Johansson, et al. Two weeks of daily injections and continuous infusion of recombinant human growth hormone (gh) in GH-deficient adults: effects on serum lipoproteins and lipoprotein and hepatic lipase activity. *Metabolism* 5: 370–377, 1996.

106. Palmer, W.K., and L.B. Oscai. Dibutyryl cAMP-induced increases in triacylglyceryl lipase activity in developing L8 myotube cultures. *Can. J. Physiol. Pharmacol.* 68:689–693, 1990.

107. Potts, J.L., S.W. Coppack, R.M. Fisher, S.M. Humphreys, G.F. Gibbons, and K. N. Frayn. Impaired postprandial clearance of triacylglycerol-rich lipoproteins in adipose tissue in obese subjects. *Am. J. Physiol.* 268:E588–E594, 1995.

108. Pradines-Figueres, A., C. Vannier, and G. Ailhaud. Lipoprotein lipase stored in adipocytes and muscle cells is a cryptic enzyme. *J. Lipid Res.* 31:1467–1476, 1990.

109. Previato, L., C.L. Parrott, S. Santamarina-Fojo, and H.B. Brewer, Jr. Transcriptional regulation of the human lipoprotein lipase gene in 3T3-L1 adipocytes. *J. Biol. Chem.* 266: 18958–18963, 1991.

110. Raisonnier, A., J. Etienne, F. Arnault, et al. Comparison of the cDNA and amino acid sequences of lipoprotein lipase in eight species. *Comp. Biochem. Physiol.* 111B:385–398, 1995.

111. Ranganathan, G., J.M. Ong, A. Yukht, et al. Tissue-specific regulation of human lipoprotein lipase. *J. Biol. Chem.* 270:7149–7155, 1995.

112. Ren, J.M., C.F. Semenkovich, E.A. Gulve, J. Gao. and J.O. Holloszy. Exercise induces rapid increases in GLUT4 expression, glucose transport capacity, and insulin-stimulated glycogen storage in muscle. *J. Biol. Chem.* 269:14396–14401, 1994.

113. Richelsen, B., S.B. Pedersen, T. Moller-Pedersen, O. Schmitz, N. Moller, and J.D. Borglum. Lipoprotein lipase activity in muscle tissue influenced by fatness, fat distribution, and insulin in obese females. *Eur. J. Clin. Invest.* 23:226–233, 1993.

114. Rifkind, B.M., and P. Segal. Lipid research clinics program reference values for hyperlipidemia and hypolipidemia. *JAMA* 250:1869–1872, 1983.

115. Roberts, K.M., E.G. Noble, D.B. Hayden, and A.W. Taylor. Lipoprotein lipase activity in skeletal muscle and adipose tissue of marathon runners after simple and complex carbohydrate-rich diets. *Eur. J. Appl. Physiol.* 57:75–80, 1988.

116. Rodrigues, B., M. Spooner, and D.L. Severson. Free fatty acids do not release lipoprotein lipase from isolated cardiac myocytes or perfused hearts. *Am. J. Physiol.* 262:E216–E223, 1992.

117. Rogers, M.A., C. Yamamoto, D.S. King, J.M. Hagberg, A.A. Ehsani, and J.O. Holloszy. Improvement in glucose tolerance after one week of exercise in patients with mild NIDDM. *Diabetes Care* 11:613–618, 1988.

118. Rogol, A.D. Drugs to enhance athletic performance in the adolescent. *Seminars Adoles. Med.* 1:317–324, 1985.

119. Romijn, J.A., E.F. Coyle, S. Sidossis, et al. Regulation of endogenous fat and carbohydrate metabolism in relation to exercise intensity and duration. *Am. J. Physiol.* 28:E380–E391, 1993.

120. Sady, S.P., P.D. Thompson, E.M. Cullinance, M.A. Kantor, E. Domagala, and P.N. Herbert. Prolonged exercise augments plasma triglyceride clearance. *JAMA* 256: 2552–2555, 1986.

121. Saffari, B., J.M. Ong, and P A. Kern. Regulation of adipose tissue lipoprotein lipase gene expression by thyroid hormone in rats. *J. Lipid Res.* 33:241–249, 1992.

122. Safonova, I., J. Aubert, R. Negrel, and G. Ailhaud. Regulation by fatty acids of angioten-sinogen gene expression in preadipose cells. *Biochem. J.* 322:235–239, 1997.

123. Santamarino-Fojo, S., and K.A. Dugi. Structure, function and role of lipoprotein lipase in lipoprotein metabolism. *Curr. Opin. Lipidol.* 5:117–125, 1994.

124. Saxena, U., L.D. Witte, and I.J. Goldberg. Release of endothelial cell lipoprotein lipase by plasma lipoproteins and free fatty acids. *J. Biol. Chem.* 264:4349–4355, 1989.

125. Schoonjans, K., M. Watanabe, H. Suzuki, et al. Induction of the acyl-coenzyme A synthe-tase gene by fibrates and fatty acids is mediated by a peroxisome proliferator response element in the C promoter. *J. Biol. Chem.* 270:19269–19276, 1995.

126. Seip, R.L., T.J. Angelopoulos, and C.F. Semenkovich. Exercise induces human lipopro-tein lipase gene expression in skeletal muscle but not adipose tissue. *Am. J. Physiol.* 268: E229–236, 1995.

127. Seip, R.L., K. Mair, T.G. Cole, and C.F. Semenkovich. Induction of human skeletal muscle lipoprotein lipase gene expression by short-term exercise is transient. *Am. J. Physiol.* 272: E255–E261, 1997.

128. Semenkovich, C.F., M. Wims, L. Noe, J. Etienne, and L. Chan. Insulin regulation of lipoprotein lipase activity in 3T3-L1 adipocytes is mediated at posttranscriptional and posttranslational levels. *J. Biol. Chem.* 264:9030–9038, 1989.

129. Senda, M., K. Oka, W.V. Brown, and P. K. Qasba. Molecular cloning and sequence of a cDNA coding for bovine lipoprotein lipase. *Proc. Natl. Acad. Sci.* 84:4369–4373, 1987.

130. Shimada, M., S. Ishibashi, T. Gotoda, et al. Overexpression of human lipoprotein lipase protects diabetic transgenic mice from diet-induced hypertriglyceridemia and hypercholester-olemia. *Arterioscler. Thromb. Vasc. Biol.* 15:1688–1694, 1995.

131. Shimada, M., H. Shimano, T. Gotoda, et al. Overexpression of human lipoprotein lipase in transgenic mice. *J. Biol. Chem.* 268:17924–17929, 1993.

132. Simsolo, R.B., J.M. Ong, and P. A. Kern. The regulation of adipose tissue and muscle lipoprotein lipase in runners by detraining. *J. Clin. Invest.* 92:2124–2130, 1993.

133. Sparks, R.S., S. Zollman, I. Klisak, et al. Human genes involved in lipolysis of plasma lipoproteins: mapping of loci for lipoprotein lipase to 8p22 and hepatic lipase to 15q21. *Genomics* 1:138–144, 1987.

134. Steineger, H.H., H.N. Sorensen, J.D. Tugwood, S. Skrede, O. Spydevold, and K.M. Gautvik. Dexamethasone and insulin demonstrate marked and opposite regulation of the steady-state mRNA level of the peroxisomal proliferator-activated receptor (PPAR) in hepatic cells. Hormonal modulation of fatty acid-induced transcription. *Eur. J. Biochem.* 225:967–974, 1994.

135. Storlien, L.H., A.B. Jenkins, D.J. Chisholm, W.S. Pascoe, S. Khouri, and E. W. Kraegen. Influence of dietary fat composition on development of insulin resistance in rats. *Diabetes* 40:280–289, 1991.

136. Takahashi, S., J. Suzuki, M. Kohno, et al. Enhancement of the binding of triglyceride-rich lipoproteins to the very low density lipoprotein receptor by apolipoprotein E and lipoprotein lipase. *J. Biol. Chem.* 270:15747–15754, 1995.

137. Tan, M.H., T. Sata, and R.J. Havel. The significance of lipoprotein lipase in rat skeletal muscle. *J. Lipid Res.* 18:363–370, 1977.

138. Taskinen, M.R., and E.A. Nikkila. Effect of caloric restriction on lipid metabolism in man. *Atherosclerosis* 32:289–299, 1979.

139. Taskinen, M.R., and E.A. Nikkila. Lipoprotein lipase activity of adipose tissue and skeletal muscle in insulin-deficient diabetes. *Diabetologia* 17:351–356, 1979.

140. Taskinen, M.R., and E.A. Nikkila. Lipoprotein lipase of adipose tissue and skeletal muscle in human obesity: response to glucose and to semistarvation. *Metabolism* 30:810–817, 1981.

141. Taskinen, M.R., E.A. Nikkila, J.K. Huttunen, and H. Hilden. A micromethod for assay of lipoprotein lipase activity in needle biopsy samples of human adipose tissue and skeletal muscle. *Clinica Chimica Acta* 104:107–117, 1980.

142. Tollet, P., M. Stromstedt, L. Fryland, R.K. Berge, and J.A. Gustafsson. Pretranslational regulation of cytochrome P450A1 by free fatty acids in primary cultures of rat hepatocytes. *J. Lipid Res.* 35:248–254, 1994.

143. Van der Husse, G.J., and R.S. Reneman. Lipid metabolism in muscle. L.B. Rowell, J.T. Shepherd (eds.). *Exercise: Regulation and Integration of Multiple Systems. Handbook of Physiology: Section 12.* New York: Oxford University Press, 1996, pp. 952–994.

144. Van Der Vusse, G.J. and T.H.M. Roemen. Gradient of fatty acids from blood plasma to skeletal muscle in dogs. *J. Appl. Physiol.* 78:1839–1843, 1995.

145. Wallinder, L., J. Peterson, T. Olivecrona, and G. Bengtsson-Olivecrona. Hepatic and extrahepatic uptake of intravenously injected lipoprotein lipase. *Biochem. Biophys. Acta* 795:513–524, 1984.

146. Wang, C.S., J. Hartsuck, and W.J. McConathy. Structure and functional properties of lipoprotein lipase. *Biochem. Biophys. Acta* 1132:1–17, 1992.

147. Weintraub, M.S., Y. Rosen, R. Otto, S. Eisenberg, and J.L. Breslow. Physical exercise conditioning in the absence of weight loss reduces fasting and postprandial triglyceride-rich lipoprotein levels. *Circulation* 79:1007–1014, 1989.

148. Williams, R.S., and Neufer, P.D. Regulation of gene expression in skeletal muscle by contractile activity. L.B. Rowell, and J.T. Shepherd (eds.). *Exercise: Regulation and Integration of Multiple Systems. Handbook of Physiology, Section 12,* New York: Oxford University Press, 1996, pp. 1124–1150.

149. Wilson, D.E., C.M. Flowers, S.I. Carlile, and K.S. Udall. Estrogen treatment and gonadal function in the regulation of lipoprotein lipase. *Atherosclerosis* 24:491–499, 1976.

150. Wilton, D.C. A continuous fluorescence displacement assay for the measurement of phospholipase A2 and other lipases that release long-chain fatty acids. *Biochem. J.* 266:435–439, 1990.

151. Wion, K.L., T.G. Kirchgessner, A.J. Lusis, M.C. Schotz, and R.M. Lawn. Human lipoprotein lipase complementary DNA sequence. *Science* 235:1638–1640, 1987.

152. Yukht, A., R.C. Davis, J.M. Ong, G. Ranganathan, and P.A. Kern. Regulation of lipoprotein lipase translation by epinephrine in 3T3-L1 cells: importance of the 3' untranslated region. *J. Clin. Invest.* 96:2438–2444, 1995.

153. Zambon, A., I. Schmidt, U. Beisiegel, and J.D. Brunzell. Dimeric lipoprotein lipase is bound to triglyceride-rich plasma lipoproteins. *J. Lipid Res.* 37:2394–2404, 1996.

9
Ubiquitin-Proteasome Pathway of Intracellular Protein Degradation: Implications for Muscle Atrophy During Unloading

GEORGE N. DEMARTINO, PH.D.
GEORGE A. ORDWAY, PH.D.

Nearly all proteins in mammalian cells undergo a continuous cycle of turnover consisting of synthesis and degradation. Under steady-state conditions, where levels of total cellular protein or levels of individual proteins do not change, rates of synthesis and degradation are exactly matched. However, under a variety of physiological and pathological conditions, rates of either synthesis or degradation can be altered differentially. Such alterations can occur for individual or limited groups of proteins, leading to changes in their cellular concentrations and concomitant functional capacities. Alternatively, global alteration in relative rates of protein synthesis and protein degradation brings about the net growth or atrophy of tissues. Although changes in rates of protein synthesis by transcriptional or translational control mechanisms are commonly recognized as important means for modifying the level or content of cellular proteins, regulation of protein degradation as a means to this end remains less appreciated by many scientists. Nevertheless, changes in rates of protein degradation rather than changes in rates of protein synthesis are the principal means for altering protein levels under many physiological and pathological conditions.

This article will review the rapidly growing information about the ubiquitin-proteasome system pathway of intracellular protein degradation. This proteolytic system has received increasingly wide attention as a consequence of its demonstrated involvement in a surprisingly large and diverse number of cellular processes where protein degradation is a key regulatory or adaptive event [18, 20, 79, 81]. The review will consider: (1) the structure and function of the ubiquitin-proteasome system's multiple protein components, where extraordinarily significant and rapid progress has been achieved in recent years; (2) the evidence for a major role of the ubiquitin-proteasome pathway in intracellular protein degradation; (3) the recent identification of specific physiological substrates for the ubiquitin-proteasome pathway; and (4) the emerging data regarding the regulation of the ubiquitin-proteasome pathway under physiological and pathological conditions, and the consequences of this regulation for growth and atrophy of tissues, such as skeletal muscle (SM). Although the review will focus on the ubiquitin-proteasome system, it will also briefly consider other proteolytic pathways and emphasize the general importance of protein degradation, regardless of the specific pathway by which it occurs, as a mechanism for the control of cellular metabolism and function.

PHYSIOLOGICAL IMPORTANCE AND ROLES OF INTRACELLULAR PROTEIN DEGRADATION

Protein degradation plays a number of diverse and essential roles in cellular function. Most of these roles are regulatory in nature and allow the organism to assume new physiological states, either in response to changing physiological demands or as part of normally programmed events. For example, protein degradation is a mechanism for rapidly altering the content of cellular proteins, including proteins that control critical cellular processes. As noted by Schimke almost 30 years ago, proteins with constitutively short half-lives are able to change their cellular concentrations much more quickly than proteins with constitutively long half-lives, when rates of protein synthesis are changed comparably [140]. Changes in degradative rates can magnify these effects on protein content. Therefore, short-lived proteins are particularly well suited to mediate the response of a cell or organism to changing physiological demands. In fact, proteins that function as rate-limiting enzymes in metabolic pathways whose product flux changes under different physiological conditions invariably have short-half-lives, and are subject to changes in concentration in response to these conditions [60, 61]. Thus, rapid turnover, a seemingly wasteful process for proteins in the steady state, is a "price" that the cell pays for the ability to rapidly change the level of regulatory proteins at a later time.

In addition to controlling levels of individual proteins, protein degradation determines the total protein content of cells and tissues, and is responsible for global alterations of tissue protein in response to changing physiological demands. Thus, tissues atrophy when overall rates of protein degradation exceed overall rates of protein synthesis, whereas tissues grow when overall rates of protein degradation fall below those of protein synthesis. As will be discussed, regulation of overall rates of protein degradation represents a principal basis for growth or atrophy characteristic of many physiological or pathological states, especially in SM [52, 111]. Protein degradation also brings about qualitative as well as quantitative changes in cellular proteins. For example, entire complements of proteins are removed by degradation in response to temporally controlled regulatory programs, such as cellular remodeling during differentiation.

Protein degradation serves other important adaptive functions for the organism. Under certain conditions, such as starvation, increased protein degradation in SM functions as an important adaptive mechanism for the organism by providing amino acids for the maintenance of energy metabolism [60, 61]. Some amino acids derived from proteolysis can be used directly as energy sources, while others are utilized by the liver as substrates for gluconeogenesis. It is possible that increased protein degradation characteristic of various disease states occurs for the same reason. Finally, protein degradation serves an important quality control function in the cell by selectively removing mutated, damaged, or otherwise abnormally-structured proteins, whose accumulation might be deleterious to cellular function.

PATHWAYS OF INTRACELLULAR PROTEIN DEGRADATION

Most cells, including SM fibers, contain multiple pathways for the degradation of their constituent proteins [39, 60, 77, 79]. The relative physiological roles and importance of these pathways are difficult to access for a variety of technical reasons that will not be discussed here, but were reviewed in detail elsewhere [60, 152, 181]. Nevertheless, the existence of multiple pathways has greatly complicated the study of the mechanisms and regulation of intracellular protein degradation in intact cells and tissues. Although this article focuses mainly on the ubiquitin-proteasome pathway, it is appropriate to briefly review the other systems that may contribute in important ways to intracellular protein degradation in mammalian cells.

Lysosomal Mechanisms of Intracellular Protein Degradation

Nearly all mammalian cells contain lysosomes. These organelles have high concentrations of various endoproteases (including cathepsins D, B, L, and H) and exoproteases (including numerous lysosomal carboxypeptidases and aminopeptidases), whose combined action can extensively hydrolyze substrate proteins. Since their discovery in the 1950s, lysosomes have been intensively studied with regard to their role in intracellular protein degradation. Lysosomes degrade intracellular proteins by several different mechanisms [39]. For example, many membrane-bound proteins, such as cell surface receptors, are degraded in lysosomes after endocytosis. Soluble intracellular proteins and some organellar proteins are also degraded in lysosomes by an analogous non-selective process, macroautophagy, whereby cellular contents are engulfed and sequestered within membrane-bound structures that ultimately fuse with lysosomes. This process is induced during certain catabolic states and is particularly active in tissues such as liver and kidney [36]. Withdrawal of serum from cultured cells promotes the selective lysosomal degradation of proteins bearing a specific sequence motif, "KFERQ" [40]. Such proteins, which represent 20–35% of total soluble cellular proteins, are translocated across lysosomal membranes by an adenosine triphosphate- (ATP) dependent mechanism involving their interaction with a specific cytoplasmic hsc70-like protein and a resident lysosomal membrane protein, LGP96 [16, 17, 28]. A role for this latter mechanism in increased proteolysis associated with physiological or pathological conditions other than serum withdrawal has not yet been defined, but seems probable. Despite the clearly demonstrated occurrence of lysosomal proteolysis by these various mechanisms, the overall quantitative importance of protein degradation in lysosomes remains uncertain. Lysosomal mechanisms may contribute significantly to overall rates of cellular protein degradation only under certain highly catabolic conditions, and/or in specific cells and tissues. Furthermore, many cellular proteins may be excluded from lysosomal proteolysis. For example, inhibition of lysosomal function does not affect degradation of many specific proteins, including contractile proteins of muscle, regardless of the physiological state of the cell [176]. Such results indicate that non-lysosomal pathways contribute importantly to many aspects of intracellular protein degradation.

The Calpain System

Most mammalian cells contain at least two isozymes of calpains (calcium-dependent neutral protease). These cytoplasmic proteases are completely dependent on calcium for activity, and their structures represent chimeras of a papain-like protease and a calmodulin-like calcium-binding protein. They are part of a larger calcium-dependent protease system consisting of an endogenous protein calpain inhibitor, calpastatin, and an endogenous protein activator [27, 117]. Some tissues such as muscle, contain at least one additional form of calpain, which is more poorly characterized biochemically but has been identified as the gene product responsible for limb girdle muscular dystrophy [133, 149, 150]. Calpains are very attractive candidates for catalysts of intracellular protein degradation because calcium ions regulate aspects of intracellular protein degradation in many cells, including skeletal and cardiac muscle fibers [169]. The mechanistic basis for this effect is unclear, however, and in our opinion there is no definitive evidence that calpains play a role in catalyzing overall rates of intracellular protein degradation. On the other hand, considerable evidence has been presented supporting a role for calpains in the limited proteolysis of selected proteins during calcium-mediated signal transduction pathways [27]. In general, however, the exact physiological roles of calpains remain uncertain and require considerable additional investigation.

THE UBIQUITIN-PROTEASOME PATHWAY FOR PROTEIN DEGRADATION

Substantial and growing evidence indicates that the ubiquitin-proteasome pathway catalyzes most non-lysosomal protein degradation in eukaryotic cells. This pathway, first identified and characterized in pioneering studies by Hershko and Ciechanover almost 20 years ago, represents a elegantly complex, multicomponent system that selectively targets proteins for destruction. Although many aspects of the molecular basis for the selection process are not understood, much detailed information is available regarding the identities and general functions of the essential protein components of the pathway. As the name implies, ubiquitin-proteasome pathways consist of two major components that represent the pathway's functionally distinct portions. The first portion utilizes ubiquitin as a covalent tag for proteins destined for degradation. The second portion features degradation of the ubiquitin-tagged proteins by a large protease complex, the 26S proteasome (the term "26S" refers to the protein's approximate sedimentation coefficient). As will be described in detail in this review, each portion of the pathway consists of additional proteins and utilizes ATP to accomplish these general functions.

Ubiquitin Marks Proteins for Degradation

Ubiquitin is an 8,500-dalton protein that is widely distributed and highly conserved in eukaryotes. Yeast and human ubiquitin differ by only 2 of 76 amino acids [78]. Ubiquitin probably has multiple cellular functions, but is best characterized in its role as a destruction signal for proteins. For this role, ubiquitin must be covalently attached to proteins by the concerted action of three conjugating enzymes, termed E1, E2, and E3 [75, 77, 79] (Figure 9.1). Proteins tagged with multiple molecules of ubiquitin then are recognized and degraded by the 26S proteasome. Conjugation begins with the "activation" of ubiquitin by E1. E1 couples ATP hydrolysis to the formation of a high-energy thiolester linkage between itself (via a specific cysteine residue of the E1 enzyme) and the carboxyterminal glycine of ubiquitin [76, 81]. Most, if not all, ubiquitin activation is probably catalyzed by a single E1 enzyme. The ubiquitin is transferred from E1 to E2 (also called ubiquitin conjugating or ubiquitin carrier enzyme), where it forms another thiolester linkage with a specific E2 cysteine residue. Finally, the ubiquitin is covalently conjugated (via its activated carboxyterminus) to an amino group (usually the free ϵ-amino group of a lysine residue) on the target substrate protein by the action of E3 (also called ubiquitin-protein ligase). The mechanism of action of E3 enzymes is not well defined but may involve formation of a ternary complex among E2-ubiquitin, E3, and the substrate. In some instances, ubiquitin may be transferred covalently to E3 prior to substrate ubiquitination, but this feature does not appear to be part of the conjugation mechanism for all proteins [81]. In any case, the resulting linkage between ubiquitin and the target protein is in the form of an isopeptide bond and results in a branched protein structure. The covalent attachment of a single ubiquitin to a target protein is not a strong signal for degradation. The conjugation process, however, appears to be highly pro-

FIGURE 9.1.

Ubiquitination of cellular proteins. Cellular proteins are selected for degradation by the covalent attachment of a polyubiquitin chain. The chain is built by repeated cycles of conjugation via the action of E1, E2, and E3 conjugating enzymes. Conjugation may be determined by specific sequences present in the substrate protein (denoted by the hatched area).

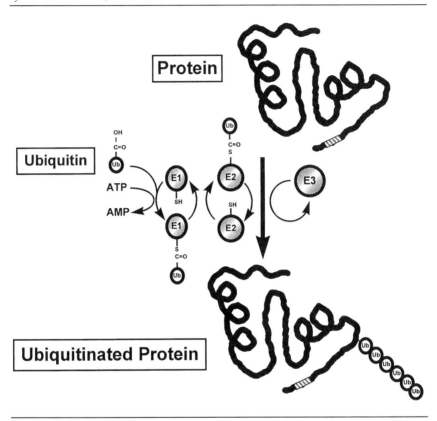

cessive; the reactions are repeated such that additional ubiquitin molecules are linked to ϵ-amino groups of the previously conjugated ubiquitin (usually to lysine 48) via additional isopeptide bonds [14]. This process results in a branched polyubiquitin chain of regularly repeating structure. Specific, but as yet incompletely defined, structural features of the polyubiquitin chain are recognized by the 26S proteasome, thereby targeting the ubiquitinated protein for destruction (to be discussed).

The molecular basis for the selection of proteins for ubiquitination is not well understood, but probably involves recognition of specific structural features of the substrate protein by components of the proteolytic pathway.

What are these structural features and which proteins of the system recognize them? Current evidence indicates that there is not a single or perhaps even a limited number of structures common to proteins degraded by the ubiquitin pathway. Rather, individual proteins may contain relatively unique structural features that dictate their ubiquitination and subsequent degradation. For example, specific amino acid sequences obligatory for degradation have been identified in cyclins MATα2 regulator, c-Jun, and p53. Mutations in or deletions of these structures can often stabilize the proteins in question. For example, c-Jun contains a 27 amino acid sequence required for its ubiquitination and degradation. However, v-Jun, the transforming variant of this transcription factor, lacks this sequence and is not degraded. This phenomenon may be the basis for the transforming activity of v-Jun [165]. In other instances, sequences have been fused experimentally to other proteins where they promote ubiquitination and degradation of proteins otherwise refractory to this process. "Degradation sequences" are not necessarily the sites of ubiquitination, but might represent binding domains for ubiquitin-conjugating enzymes or for other enzymes that modify the protein as required for the degradative process (to be discussed).

The question arises how diverse structures can be recognized by the ubiquitin conjugating machinery. Part of the answer may lie in the existence of large families of E2 and E3 enzymes, whose combinatorial pairing produces specificities appropriate for given structural features of the target protein [21, 88]. Although such specificity has been demonstrated in certain instances, details of this important aspect of molecular recognition remain to be elucidated. Interestingly, phosphorylation of substrate proteins is emerging as an important determinant of ubiquitination and subsequent degradation [15, 113]. Perhaps this modification induces conformational changes in proteins that expose otherwise cryptic recognition and binding sites for the conjugating machinery. The generality and regulatory significance of a phosphorylation-dephosphorylation mechanism in the control of protein ubiquitination is currently unknown, but the preliminary evidence for its importance provides an indication of the complexity of the recognition process. Numerous proteins degraded by the ubiquitin-proteasome pathway contain "PEST" sequences, structural motifs rich in *p*roline, glutama*te*, *s*erine, and *t*hreonine, found in many constitutively short-lived proteins [121]. It is possible that PEST sequences could specify the interaction of substrate proteins with either E2/E3 conjugating enzymes or protein kinases. Recent reports have shown that Hsc70 is required for the ubiquitin-dependent degradation of certain substrates *in vitro,* and it is possible that this chaperone may function to unfold these substrates as a requirement for ubiquitination and/or degradation [11].

Although the number of identified "degradation sequences" is limited at present, it seems likely to grow significantly as more physiological substrates of the ubiquitin pathway are found. This information should help to determine whether degradation signals contain common structural features and/or whether multiple proteins utilize specific signals. In any case, the identification of "degradation sequences" indicates that there was pressure for proteins to evolve with structures that dictate their own destruction, just as there was pressure for them to evolve with structures that dictate their specific functions. Such results further highlight the importance of regulated protein degradation as a mechanism in the control of cellular function.

UBIQUITINATED PROTEINS ARE DEGRADED BY THE 26S PROTEASOME

After a protein is modified by attachment of a polyubiquitin chain, its likely fate is degradation by the 26S proteasome. (As will be discussed, however, some proteins can escape degradation by mechanisms that remove the chain.) The 26S proteasome is a large protease complex that discriminates between ubiquitinated and non-ubiquitinated forms of most proteins, rapidly degrading the former but not the latter [25]. The molecular basis for this selectivity is not known in detail, but current evidence suggests that the polyubiquitin chain, rather than the protein to which it is attached, first binds to the 26S proteasome. Thus, the polyubiquitin chain serves a targeting function for the substrate, probably by increasing affinity of the protein for the 26S proteasome [38]. As described below, this function may allow other regions of the protease complex to bind to and/or modify the substrate in a manner necessary for degradation.

The 26S proteasome is an extraordinarily complicated protein. It has a molecular weight of about 2,100,000 and consists of approximately 48 subunits representing 35 distinct gene products [25, 125, 132]. Current evidence indicates that the 26S proteasome is the only protease that degrades ubiquitinated proteins. As described in the next section, the 26S proteasome is composed of at least two large multisubunit subcomplexes: A core protease subcomplex, the 20S proteasome, and a regulatory module, proteasome activator 700 (PA700).

The 20S Proteasome is the Proteolytic Core of the 26S Proteasome

The 20S proteasome is a large protease complex found in certain bacteria [155] and archaebacteria [29], and in all examined eukaryotes [25, 158]. It was identified independently in multiple laboratories in diverse experimental contexts during the 1970s, and was first purified and biochemically characterized in the early 1980s. The proteasome has a number of very unusual and complicated structural and functional properties that distinguish it from other well-studied intracellular and extracellular proteases. These features confused and retarded some aspects of the early molecular characterization of the enzyme. Nevertheless, recent work, culminated by determination of the crystal structures of the archaebacterial and yeast proteasomes, has proceeded with remarkable rapidity [25].

The proteasome has a native molecular weight of 700,000 and is composed of 28 subunits [67, 125]. The subunits are arranged in four heptameric rings that are stacked on top of one another to form a cylindrical particle [80]. In eukaryotes, the 28 subunits represent the products of 14 genes, none of which are related to the primary sequence of any known protease [74, 157]. This finding is highly unusual since most proteases in nature are members of one of four large protease superfamilies. All proteasome subunits, however, are homologous to one another and thereby comprise a novel gene family [157]. These homologous polypeptides can be subdivided into two sets of seven subunits (termed α and β) whose members are more closely related to one another [182]. The α-type subunits and β-type subunits appear to have evolved from two respective ancestral proteins that compose the proteasome found in the archaebacterium *Thermoplasma acidophilum*. Regardless of the source, however, the overall morphology of proteasomes is remarkably similar; the two outer or terminal rings are composed exclusively of α subunits, whereas the two inner rings are composed of exclusively of β subunits [94, 129]. In eukaryotes, each outer ring contains all seven α-type subunits and each inner ring contains all seven β-type subunits. Thus, the proteasome is an extended multisubunit dimer with C2 symmetry about planar axis through the two inner rings (Figure 9.2).

FIGURE 9.2.
Structure of the 20S proteasome from archaebacteria and eukaryotes.

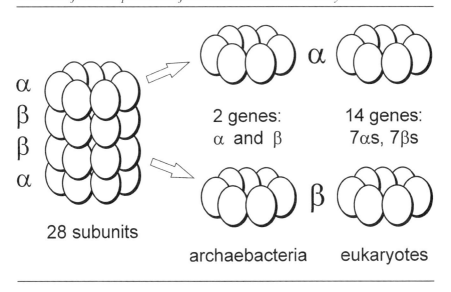

Early biochemical work indicated that the eukaryotic proteasome is a multicatalytic protease, containing three or more active sites with distinct catalytic specificities. The activities have been defined by their hydrolysis of small synthetic peptides and have been termed "trypsin-like" (cleavage after a basic amino acid residue), "chymotrypsin-like" (cleavage after a hydrolphobic residue), and "peptidyl-glutamylpeptide hydrolyzing" (cleavage after an acid residue) [123, 135]. These activities also are differentially affected by various protease inhibitors, but cannot be classified easily according to inhibitor profiles of known proteases. Furthermore, the specificities observed with small synthetic peptides are not achieved with larger peptides (e.g., the trypsin-like activity does not always cleave after basic residues), indicating that catalytic specificity for a given substrate can be dictated by properties of the proteasome other than a given active site [42]. The multiple catalytic sites of the proteasome function in a coordinated fashion, such that polypeptide substrates are channeled from one site to another. In other words, substrates undergo multiple cleavages prior to their release from the enzyme [42]. Until the recent determination of proteasome crystal structures, the identities of catalytic subunits were not established because of the lack of structural similarity with known proteases, and since no proteasome subunit functions in isolation.

The recently determined crystal structures of archaebacterial and yeast proteasomes have confirmed, clarified, and greatly extended many structural and functional features of the proteasome obtained by biochemical and molecular studies [66, 101]. For example, crystal structures obtained in the presence of low molecular weight active-site inhibitors indicate that the active sites are located on β subunits. Thus, in the archaebacterial proteasome, all 14 copies of the β subunit are catalytically active. Furthermore, the proteasome has a novel catalytic mechanism in which an amino-terminal threonine residue functions as the catalytic nucleophile [101, 141]. In eukaryotes, six subunits representing three distinct β-type polypeptides (i.e., three different subunits present in each of the two inner rings) are likely catalysts based on the existence of amino-terminal threonine residues for these subunits. These findings provide a structural basis for the multicatalytic model of the proteasome, cast doubt on the existence of additional catalytic sites as proposed by some kinetic studies, and explain the failure of previous kinetic studies to classify the enzyme within known protease families. The crystal structures, however, have not revealed exactly how these different catalytic sites achieve their specificities or how they function coordinately. Nevertheless, the crystal structures have shown that the active sites are sequestered from potential substrates present in bulk solution because they face the interior of a central chamber formed by the centers of the abutting β rings [66, 101]. This topology may have evolved as a mechanism to prevent the inappropriate degradation of cellular proteins by the proteasome. Access of proteins to the proteolytic sites is further impeded by two constrictions at the ends of the proteasome. These 13 Å-diameter openings are formed by the centers of the outer α rings and restrict passage of potential substrates to small peptides and unfolded proteins. Although these openings are assumed to be the sites of entry of substrates to the central interior chamber, the yeast crystal structure shows that a channel between the openings and the active sites is blocked by aminoterminal portions of the α subunits [66]. Such findings imply the existence of regulatory mechanisms that "open" the proteasome structure at the terminal rings to allow access of substrates to the active sites. As will be described, it is possible that specific proteasome regulatory proteins that bind to the terminal rings of the proteasome mediate regulation of substrate access.

The 20S proteasome has been identified and purified from a large number of tissues and species. It is unclear, however, whether it ever functions in intact cells as an isolated particle. For example, the 20S proteasome degrades small peptides only at very slow rates and is incapable of degrading larger polypeptides unless they have been highly denatured [175]. Even in the latter case, only certain forms of the 20S proteasome, those "activated" *in vitro* by exposure to low concentrations of SDS, certain polycations, heat, or extremes in ionic strength, can degrade proteins at appreciable rates [25, 109]. The exact molecular bases for the effects of these disparate treatments are unclear, but are likely related to conformational changes in the proteasome that "open" the structure sufficiently to allow substrates access to the active sites. Thus, these *in vitro* treatments may mimic the effects of specific regulatory proteins in control of proteasome function.

26S Proteasome is Composed of the 20S Proteasome and a Regulatory Module, PA700

The 20S proteasome is unable to degrade ubiquitinated proteins, and its catalytic activities are unaffected by ATP. These features cast early doubt on its role in ubiquitin-dependent protein degradation. In contrast, studies by Rechsteiner and colleagues and by Goldberg and colleagues identified a much larger protease (Mr >1,500,000), the "26S protease" that selectively degrades ubiquitinated proteins in an ATP-dependent fashion [86, 174]. Although some early studies emphasized distinctions between the 20S proteasome and the "26S protease," the structural and functional relationships between the two proteases were established by two independent kinds of experiments. First, further purification and characterization of the 26S protease showed that it contained proteasome subunits as constituent polypeptides, suggesting that the proteasome was a component of the larger complex [83, 132, 171, 180]. Second, immunoprecipitation and reconstitution experiments of the proteasome in cell-free extracts capable of catalyzing ATP/ ubiquitin-dependent protein degradation showed that the 20S proteasome was obligatory for function of the pathway, but that its activity in this process was mediated by other proteins [32, 44, 107, 108, 156]. Subse-

TABLE 9.1.

Subunits of PA700, The Regulatory Complex of the 26S Proteasome

Subunits of PA700 (Homo sapiens)		Also Identified As	Yeast Homolog	Comments/References
ATPase Subunits				
a	b			
p56	S4		MTS2/YTA5	Putative ATPase [45]
p50		TBP1	YTA1	Putative ATPase [34, 120]
p48	S6	TBP7	YTA2	Putative ATPase [33, 46, 121]
p47	S7	MSS1	CIM5	Putative ATPase [57, 114, 146]
p45	S8		SUG1/CIM3	Putative ATPase [5, 57, 153]
p42			SUG2	Putative ATPase [34]
Non-ATPase Subunits				
P112	S1	TAP2/55.1	SEN3	Identified as TNF-receptor interacting protein [13, 31, 137, 179]
p97	S2		NAS1/HRD2	Identified as gene required for HMG-COA reductase degradation [70, 168]
p58	S3	P91A	SUN2	Identified as suppressor of nin1 mutation [55, 102]
p55				
p50.5	S5b			[37]
p44.5	S5a		SUN1	Polyubiquitin chain binding protein [38, 50, 93]
p44	S10			
p40	S12	MOV34		Embryonic lethal mutation in mouse [137, 167]
p39				Isopeptidase? [95]
p37				Isopeptidase? [95]
p31	S14		NIN1	Identified as cell cycle mutant [92]
p28	S15			

[a] nomenclature of DeMartino, Slaughter, Tanaka, et al. [131]
[b] nomenclature of Rechsteiner, et al. [71]

quent studies have definitively demonstrated that the 26S protease (now called the 26S proteasome) is composed of a complex between the 20S proteasome and a second multisubunit regulatory protein, PA700 (also known as 19S cap or ATPase regulator), that mediates its role in the ATP-dependent degradation of ubiquitinated proteins.

PA700 is a 700,000-dalton protein composed of about 20 subunits, all of which are distinct gene products (Table 9.1). PA700 binds to one or both of the proteasome's terminal rings to form a complex that is structurally and functionally equivalent to the 26S proteasome [1]. Therefore, PA700 acts as a regulator of the 20S proteasome. What properties of PA700 are required for this role? From known features of the degradation of ubiquitinated proteins, PA700 must (1) confer ATP-dependence to proteolysis, (2) selectively recognize polyubiquitinated proteins, and (3) remove and/or disassemble the polyubiquitin chain from the protein substrate. Two additional functions of PA700 can be inferred from the structure of the 20S proteasome. First, PA700 should promote the unfolding of substrate proteins necessary for their entry to the central channel of the proteasome. Second, PA700 may participate in translocation of the polypeptide chain from its initial binding site on the complex to catalytic sites in the interior of the proteasome. Recent analysis of the structure and function of PA700 has provided considerable insight about its role in many of these functions [138] (Figure 9.3).

Purified PA700 is an ATPase. This activity is required for both assembly of the proteasome-PA700 complex (i.e., the 26S proteasome) and the degradation of ubiquitinated proteins [83, 105, 126, 170]. Six subunits of PA700's 20 component subunits are members of a large protein family characterized by a 200 amino acid domain containing a conserved ATP-binding motif [23,

FIGURE 9.3.

Structure and function of the 26S proteasome in the degradation of ubiquitinated proteins. Ubiquitinated proteins are selectively degraded by the 26S proteasome, a 2,100—kDa protein protease complex composed of two multiprotein subcomplexes, the 20S proteasome and PA700. The 20S proteasome is the protease core. It contains multiple catalytic sites within a central channel (represented here in cross-section). PA700 binds on each end of the proteasome cylinder (shown on only one end here for clarity). PA700 is an ATPase that may use this activity to unfold and/or translocate proteins, targeted to the complex via polyubiquitin chains, to the active sites. PA700 also disassembles the polyubiquitin chain.

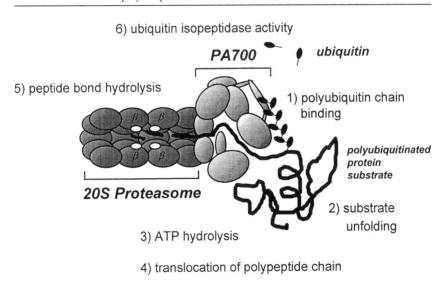

6) ubiquitin isopeptidase activity

PA700 • **ubiquitin**

5) peptide bond hydrolysis

1) polyubiquitin chain binding

polyubiquitinated protein substrate

20S Proteasome

2) substrate unfolding

3) ATP hydrolysis

4) translocation of polypeptide chain

33-35, 45, 47, 84]. One or more of these subunits presumably participates in the ATP-dependent functions of the complex. It is unclear why six different ATPase subunits are present in the complex, but it is reasonable to speculate that they have distinct functions. Interestingly, many of these ATPase subunits were identified originally in yeast and/or humans as putative transcriptional regulatory proteins [45, 90, 120, 121, 146]. It now seems likely, however, that the observed phenotypes or biochemical properties can be explained by proteasome-dependent degradation of proteins required for transcription.

The question arises as to how ATPase activity is mechanistically linked to the function of the 26S proteasome. Unfortunately little information is available regarding the mechanism by which ATP hydrolysis participates in either assembly of the proteasome-PA700 complex or degradation of ubiquitinated proteins. It is reasonable to speculate that ATP hydrolysis is involved in substrate unfolding and/or translocation, perhaps by analogy to the role of ATP hydrolysis in chaperone function and in translocation of proteins across cellular compartments, respectively [7, 42]. These topics represent important areas for future investigation.

At least one subunit of PA700 (designated S5a, SUN1, MCB1, or MBP1) can bind polyubiquitin chains [38, 50, 93, 172]. The subunit interacts with a series of hydrophobic patches on the surface of ubiquitin molecules in the chain. Mutations in these regions disrupt polyubiquitin chain binding and prevent degradation of model substrates to which the chain is attached [10]. Interestingly, yeast mutants lacking this subunit fail to degrade some but not all polyubiquitinated proteins, and such mutants are viable [172]. These results indicate that PA700 contains additional subunits that recognize and bind to polyubiquitin chains. In any case, these studies strongly support the idea that substrates are targeted to the proteasome because PA700 recognizes and interacts with the polyubiquitin chain that modifies the protein substrate.

Early studies of ubiquitin-dependent protein degradation demonstrated that the polyubiquitin chain was disassembled to ubiquitin monomers during proteolysis of the substrate. This so-called "isopeptidase" activity may be required to allow hydrolysis of the protein to proceed after it binds to the 26S proteasome, or may serve an editing function by releasing poorly ubiquitinated proteins before they can be degraded. However, the exact role of the 26S proteasome in this process has been unclear, because cells contain a variety of enzymes with isopeptidase activity called *ubiquitin-specific *processing *proteases (Ubps). These proteins may be required for multiple cellular functions, including the cleavage of at least two forms of ubiquitin fusion proteins produced during ubiquitin synthesis [81]. Recently, isopeptidase activity was demonstrated as an inherent property of highly purified PA700 [95]. The activity removes ubiquitin monomers from the distal end of the polyubiquitin chain by an ATP-independent mechanism.

Work in progress has tentatively identified a PA700 subunit responsible for isopeptidase activity (unpublished data). Additional work will be required to learn how this activity is coordinated with degradation of the protein portion of the ubiquitinated substrate.

Although the primary structures of nearly all other PA700 subunits are known, their individual functions are not. Homologs of many of the mammalian subunits have been identified in yeast, where corresponding mutants display a variety of phenotypes that include defects in cell cycle progression. Some mammalian PA700 subunits were identified initially as proteins with functions apparently unrelated to proteasome-dependent proteolysis. Although such findings have implicated the proteasome in these respective functions, little is known about the possible mechanistic basis for such relationships. Obviously, a major challenge of future work will be to define the roles of all subunits of the 26S proteasome in degradation of proteins.

26S Proteasome Can Degrade Some Non-Ubiquitinated Proteins

The previous discussion has focused on the role of the 26S proteasome in degradation of ubiquitinated proteins, its best-studied function. However, it is clear that at least some nonubiquitinated proteins can be degraded by the 26S proteasome in an ATP-dependent fashion. The best example is that of ornithine decarboxylase (ODC). ODC is the rate-limiting enzyme in polyamine synthesis and has one of the shortest constitutive half-lives of any known protein [72]. Cellular levels and activity of ODC levels are highly regulated. When cellular polyamine concentrations are high, the rate of ODC synthesis is decreased, and ODC activity is inhibited by a specific protein inhibitor, antizyme, whose production is up-regulated under these conditions [72]. ODC is degraded by the 26S proteasome in an ATP-dependent but ubiquitin-independent fashion. Interestingly, degradation occurs only when ODC is bound to antizyme [164]. Thus, antizyme may act to target ODC to the 26S proteasome in a manner analogous to that in which polyubiquitin chains target other proteins. This view was confirmed in studies that showed that fusion of the amino-terminus of antizyme to other proteins can promote degradation of the fusion protein by the 26S proteasome [98, 100]. It is unclear whether antizyme interacts only with ODC or whether it directs the degradation of other cellular proteins. In either case, an important area of future investigation will be to determine the quantitative contribution of ubiquitin-independent degradation of proteins by either the 26S or 20S proteasomes, as well as determine the possible requirement of associated proteins to target these proteins to the protease. ODC contains a PEST sequence, thereby suggesting that this signal does not operate exclusively in the ubiquitin-dependent pathway.

Other Protein Regulators of the Proteasome.

PA700 is only one of several protein regulators of the 20S proteasome. Eukaryotic cells contain a number of other proteins that activate or inhibit various activities of the proteasome. Compared to PA700, much less is known about the cellular roles of these proteins, but their existence indicates that proteasome activity is under complex control in intact cells.

One such protein, PA28, is a 180,000-dalton protein composed of two subunits, α and β, that are about 50% identical in primary structure [2, 48, 103, 116]. These subunits are arranged in alternating fashion in a ring-shaped hexamer with a $(\alpha\beta)_3$ stoichiometry [4, 147]. Like PA700, PA28 binds to one or both of the proteasome's terminal rings [62]. Unlike, PA700, however, PA28 binds without a requirement for ATP or other cofactors. It also activates the proteasome's hydrolysis of small non-ubiquitinated peptides. PA28 does not activate the proteasome's degradation of large proteins regardless of whether they are ubiquitinated. Structure/function studies of PA28 demonstrate that binding depends on the carboxyterminus of the α subunit [106, 147]. The isolated recombinant α subunit, but not the β subunit, can activate the proteasome [148].

Various physiological roles of PA28 exist. Several lines of evidence indicate that PA28 plays a role in proteasome-dependent processing of antigens for presentation by the class I major histocompatibility complex. First, both PA28 subunits are up-regulated by treatment of cells with γ-interferon [2, 85, 130]. Second, PA28 alters the cleavage specificity of the proteasome in a manner that favors production of antigenic peptides [64]. Third, transfection of the gene for PA28α into fibroblasts expressing a viral antigen increases cellular levels of the subunit and increases the recognition of these target cells by cytotoxic T lymphocytes [65]. A role for the proteasome in antigen processing has strong independent experimental support. Inhibitors of the proteasome block antigen processing in intact cells, while three proteasome subunits are up-regulated by interferon-γ treatment [6, 55, 63, 136, 178]. These subunits, two of which are encoded in the major histocompatibility complex, replace three other subunits in the proteasome and seem to alter proteasome specificity [43]. Ubiquitination also has been implicated in this process, although its role is poorly defined. Despite these findings, the manner in which PA28 functions in intact cells is unclear. Although cells contain a population of proteasomes bound to PA28, it not known whether these complexes act in coordination with or independently of proteasome-PA700 complexes. Because both PA700 and PA28 bind to terminal proteasome rings, it is possible that a given proteasome molecule contains PA700 on one end and PA28 on the other; however, no published evidence for this possibility exists. Furthermore, it is unclear whether PA28's role is limited to antigen presentation or whether it plays a wider role in protein degradation. A structural homolog of PA28 is not present in *Saccharomyces cerevisiae*. Obviously, additional work will be required to determine the physiological role of PA28.

Other protein inhibitors of the proteasome have been identified, including several proteins that inhibit the activity of the 20S proteasome. One inhibitor, PI31, is a homodimer of a 31,000-dalton polypeptide [104]. This protein is a novel proline-rich protein which binds to the 20S proteasome in a 2:1 molar ratio, and inhibits both peptidase and protease activities [104]. Two other proteasome inhibitors were identified by Etlinger and colleagues. One proteasome has a native Mr = 240,000 and is composed of a 40,000-dalton polypeptide [118]. The other has a native Mr = 200,000 and is composed of a 50,000-dalton polypeptide [99]. The former protein was identified as δ-aminolevulinic acid dehydratase, an enzyme involved in heme biosynthesis [68]. The significance of this finding is unclear. Finally, Hsp90 and β-amyloid protein were shown to inhibit several peptidase activities of the proteasome [166]. The physiological roles of all these inhibitory proteins are poorly defined, and additional work will be required to determine whether they play significant roles in regulation of proteasome function, either as part of or independently from the proteasome's role in ubiquitin-dependent protein degradation.

ROLE OF THE UBIQUITIN-PROTEASOME PATHWAY FOR PROTEIN DEGRADATION

Much of the early progress on the ubiquitin-proteasome pathway involved detailed biochemical and mechanistic studies on protein components of the pathway. Moreover, most of the characterization of substrate ubiquitination and degradation was carried out on model protein substrates of unknown physiological relevance. Therefore, until recently, both the qualitative and quantitative significance of the ubiquitin-proteasome pathway in intracellular protein degradation was uncertain. During the past several years, however, significant progress was achieved in assessing the physiological roles of the pathway. These rapidly accumulating data demonstrate that the system is responsible for the normal turnover of most cellular proteins, and through identification of specific substrates, have revealed unexpected examples of control of cellular processes by protein degradation.

Mutational Analysis of the Ubiquitin-Proteasome Pathway

Considerable insight into cellular functions of the ubiquitin-proteasome pathway has been achieved by analysis of cells harboring mutations of various components of the system. One of the earliest demonstrations of the physiological importance of the ubiquitin pathway for protein degradation involved the use of a mouse cell line, ts85, which contains a temperature sensitive E1 conjugating enzyme [19]. These cells fail to ubiquitinate endogenous cellular proteins at the non-permissive temperature, a defect that results in a large reduction (>90%) of degradation of normal short-lived proteins, as well as abnormal proteins synthesized in the presence of puromycin or amino acid analogs [19, 51]. A similar inhibition of protein degradation is demonstrated in *Saccharomyces cerevisiae,* from which three E2 conjugating enzymes (Ubc1, Ubc4 and, Ubc5) were deleted [143, 144]. These and related studies demonstrate that ubiquitination of certain proteins or classes of proteins is obligatory for their degradation. Analogous studies have been conducted with cells containing mutations of certain subunits of the 20S or 26S proteasome. Deletions of genes for individual proteasome or PA700 subunits are, with a few exceptions, lethal, thereby highlighting the essential nature of proteasome-catalyzed proteolysis in cellular function [53, 73]. However, yeast that expressed mutant proteasome subunits was identified and analyzed. These cells display markedly reduced rates of degradation of normal short-lived proteins, N-end rule proteins, abnormal proteins containing amino acid analogs, and possible accumulation of abnormally high levels of polyubiquitinated proteins [73, 134, 142]. These important early experiments established an essential cellular role for ubiquitin-dependent protein degradation in intact cells, but left unresolved questions regarding its quantitative significance, since short-lived and N-end rule proteins represent only a small subset of all cellular proteins.

Inhibitors of the Proteasome Reduce Overall Rates of Intracellular Protein Degradation in Intact Cells

In addition to the genetic analysis described previously, the cellular role of the proteasome has been advanced significantly by the recent identification and analysis of low molecular weight cell-permeant inhibitors of the proteasome. Many of these inhibitors are peptide aldehydes (e.g., acetyl-leu-leu-norleucinal, CBZ-leu-leu-leucinal, CBZ-leu-leu-norvalinal, etc.) that inhibit both 20S and 26S forms of the proteasome. Some, however, also inhibit calpains and some inhibit lysosomal cathepsins [136]. These compounds greatly reduce rates of intracellular degradation of several classes of proteins, including normal short-lived and long-lived proteins, as well as proteins synthesized in the presence of amino acid analogs. These effects were attributed to inhibition of the proteasome rather than to calpains or lysosomal proteases, since their rank order of inhibitory potency was the same in intact cells as with purified proteases [136]. Recently, a natural compound, lactacystin, was identified as a proteasome inhibitor that covalently binds to catalytic β subunits [26, 41, 49]. This compound and a derivative, β-lactone, appear to be completely specific for the proteasome. Treatment of mammalian cells with these agents greatly inhibits the degradation of both short- and long-lived proteins, indicating that the proteasome plays an important role in the degradation of most cellular proteins [26]. β-Lactone also appears to inhibit short-lived proteins but not long-lived proteins in yeast [96]. In total, these various results indicate that the proteasome is responsible for degradation of most cellular proteins in mammalian cells and many proteins in yeast. Emerging studies with these inhibitors have and should continue to define the role of the proteasome in the degradation of specific individual cellular proteins. It is important to

TABLE 9.2.
Some Substrates of the Ubiquitin Proteasome
Pathway in Intact Cells

	Reference
MATα repressor	[82]
Phytochrome	[145]
Cyclin	[58, 91, 119]
p53	[139]
c-Jun	[165]
CFTR	[173]
HMG CoA reductase	[70]
NFκB	[122, 124]
IκB	[113, 124]

reemphasize that an effect of proteasome inhibitors on protein degradation does not provide direct evidence for the involvement of ubiquitination because of the possibility of ubiquitin-independent mechanisms for the proteasome. Indeed, these inhibitors should be useful tools in defining such distinctions.

PHYSIOLOGICAL SUBSTRATES OF THE UBIQUITIN-PROTEASOME PATHWAY

Studies of intracellular protein degradation are often conducted by measuring overall rates of the process. Thus, experiments of the type described above provide little information about the identity of individual proteins that contribute to the observed effects. During the past several years, however, substantial progress has been made in identification of specific cellular substrates of the ubiquitin-proteasome pathway [18, 131]. In addition to the growing number of these protein substrates, it is striking that they include some of the most important regulatory proteins of various cellular processes, thereby specifying ubiquitin-proteasome mediated proteolysis as a critical mechanism for cellular control. It is beyond the scope of this review to extensively discuss each of these examples in detail; however, Table 9.2 lists some identified cellular substrates of the pathway. The list does not include other proteins shown to be degraded by the proteasome, but not formally demonstrated to be degraded after ubiquitination. We believe that the list of physiological substrates for the ubiquitin-proteasome system will grow rapidly.

REGULATION OF INTRACELLULAR PROTEIN DEGRADATION BY THE UBIQUITIN-PROTEASOME PATHWAY

Identification of the biochemical pathways responsible for increased protein degradation associated with various physiological and pathological states has been a topic of active investigation for many years. However, surprisingly few firm conclusions have resulted from these experiments. Many early studies examined the role of lysosomes or calpains in altered protein metabolism, but were conducted before the ubiquitin-proteasome pathway had been identified or characterized. Thus, the relative contribution of the ubiquitin-proteasome pathway in these conditions was not considered. Furthermore, until recently, the biochemical complexity of the ubiquitin-proteasome system precluded analysis of some aspects of its regulation, including changes in function of the system under different physiological conditions. However, identification of the system's specific protein components and a general understanding of their functions provide the rationale and requisite molecular reagents for initial examination of such alterations.

Emerging evidence, while incomplete, suggests that the ubiquitin-proteasome pathway is the principal means by which overall rates of protein degradation are modified under numerous conditions. This evidence comes from quantification of changes in levels or activities of one or more components of the pathway that includes: (1) measurement of ATP-dependent proteolysis in both intact tissues and cell-free extracts; (2) measurement of enzymatic activity of individual components of the pathway; (3) measurement of mRNA and protein levels of components of the pathway; and (4) assessment of the level of ubiquitination of endogenous proteins. The results from this kind of analysis show that the overall function of the pathway changes under many conditions (to be discussed), and that such changes generally correlate with alterations in the protein content of pathway components. Although the very large numbers of pathway components have prevented a complete or systematic examination of their levels in any one experimental model, analysis of representative components indicates that many are regulated coordinately. This result is surprising since many components of the pathway (e.g., ubiquitin and the proteasome) are very abundant proteins under normal conditions, and therefore seem unlikely targets for regulation (especially for further increases in content). Thus, these findings suggest that proteins, such as ubiquitin and the proteasome, are among the rate-limiting components for protein degradation. In regards to the proteasome, this conclusion is very different from early views of pathway control that held that regulation would be confined to the ubiquitination portion of the pathway. Obviously, more work will be required to learn about the general features of the physiological control of the ubiquitin-proteasome pathway in intact cells and tissues.

Current evidence regarding alteration and regulation of the function of the ubiquitin-proteasome pathway was obtained mainly in SM, a plastic tissue that exhibits remarkable adaptation in protein composition in response to physiological and pathological states [52, 89, 111, 152]. Muscle protein degradation is altered by many factors or conditions, including

TABLE 9.3.
Physiological Regulators of Protein Degradation in Skeletal Muscle

Factors	Effect of Protein Degradation	Ubiquitin-Proteasome Pathway	Representative References
Insulin	decrease	yes	[54, 59, 87, 115, 127]
Glucocorticoids	increase	yes	[128, 177]
Thyroid hormones	increase	yes	[111]
β_2-Adrenergic agonists	decrease	yes	[54, 59, 87]
Branched chain amino acids	decrease	?	[54]
Glucose	decrease	?	[54, 87]
Conditions			
Fasting	increase	yes	[110, 177]
Infection	increase	yes	[162]
Tumor	increase	yes	[8, 24]
Hindlimb suspension	increase	yes	[154, 161, 163]
Microgravity	increase	probable	[151]
Protein deficiency	decrease	yes	[89, 159]
Acidosis	increase	yes	[112, 128]
Denervation	increase	yes	[110, 163]
Burns	increase	yes	[111]

hormones, nutritional status, injuries (such as burns and trauma), infection, programs of development and differentiation, neural input, and mechanical activity that includes both passive stretch and active contraction. The details of all experimental models in which changes in the ubiquitin-proteasome pathway have been studied cannot be fully discussed here. However, several examples will be used for illustrative purpose, and a summary list of others is provided in Table 9.3.

Insulin and glucocorticoids represent two hormones that play a dominant and interconnected role in the regulation of protein degradation in SM [89, 152]. Each hormone also controls muscle protein synthesis, and these combined effects are responsible for the major aspects of control of SM protein balance under many conditions, especially feeding and fasting. Insulin fosters positive nitrogen balance by promoting protein synthesis and repressing protein degradation [52, 54]. Thus, when circulating levels of insulin decline during fasting or under pathological conditions, such as uncontrolled diabetes, SM loses protein as a consequence of decreased rates of synthesis and increased rates of degradation. During these same conditions, lucocorticoids also promote muscle wasting by exactly the opposite effect, (i.e., by decreasing rates of protein synthesis and increasing rates of protein degradation). Although lack of insulin promotes enhanced protein degradation in isolated muscles, in intact animals, the absence of insulin may allow glucocorticoids to actively accelerate protein degradation. The effects of glucocorticoids on muscle protein synthesis and degradation have produced conflicting reports, and these discrepancies may result from the critical interplay between insulin and glucocorticoids [152]. For example, glucocorticoids increase protein degradation in muscles from fasted but not from fed animals. In addition, direct effects of glucocorticoids on protein degradation in isolated muscles are not observed in the presence of insulin. These results indicate that glucocorticoids are essential for the ability of muscles to increase protein degradation during the fasting state. In fact, glucocorticoid levels rise during starvation. Adrenalectomized animals cannot increase muscle proteolysis during fasting, an effect which is lethal, partly because the inability to increase muscle protein degradation impairs the organism's ability to maintain blood glucose levels.

Although the intracellular signaling mechanisms responsible for the regulation of protein degradation by insulin and glucocorticoids are unclear, the effects of these agents on muscle protein degradation are mediated by the ubiquitin-proteasome pathway [110, 111, 127]. For example, intact SM from insulinopenic rats experiences greatly increased rates of protein degradation, as compared to muscles from normal rats. The excess proteolysis can be eliminated by proteasome inhibitors or by decreasing cellular ATP levels, but not by inhibitors of either lysosomal function or calpains [127]. Ubiquitin transcription and mRNA levels (of both ubiquitin and selectively examined proteasome subunits) are also increased in muscles from insulinopenic rats. These and other results indicate that the ubiquitin-proteasome system plays a key role in increased muscle protein degradation when insulin levels are low.

It is important to note that the effects of various physiological regulators such as insulin and glucocorticoids may be tissue specific in terms of the direction of their effects on protein degradation and the specific proteolytic system that they regulate. For example, in liver as in SM, insulin promotes positive nitrogen balance by suppressing overall rates of protein degradation [79, 116]. In liver, however, the lack of insulin elevates lysosomal autophagy, which may account for most of the increased proteolysis associated with this condition [125]. Furthermore, glucagon, whose levels increase under conditions of low insulin, directly activates liver protein degradation by autophagy, but has little effect on muscle protein degradation. In contrast to their catabolic effects in SM, glucocorticoids have anabolic effects in the heart. These effects, however, occur principally by increased rates of protein synthesis [22]. These results are only some examples of the complex regulatory features involved in the control of protein metabolism in intact animals and indicate the challenge for future work in this area.

Regulation of the function of the ubiquitin-proteasome pathway probably occurs by qualitative changes of the system's protein components as well as by quantitative alterations of their cellular content. Several examples of qualitative changes have been identified. The best-studied example is the change in the proteasome subunit composition promoted by γ-interferon.

This cytokine selectively up-regulates expression of three proteasome subunits that are then incorporated into proteasomes in place of three respective "basal" counterparts [6, 12, 43, 55, 56]. It is unclear whether incorporation is restricted to newly synthesized proteasomes or whether newly synthesized subunits can exchange with previously assembled proteasomes. In any case, the altered proteasomes show substrate specificities and other kinetic properties that differ appreciably from proteasomes of untreated cells, and seem to favor the production of antigenic peptides for presentation by class I molecules [12, 55]. Interestingly, γ-interferon also up-regulates the synthesis of each component subunit of PA28 [2, 130]. PA28 alters the proteasome's cleavage specificity of some peptides [43]. Thus, γ-interferon may regulate both the total activity and the cleavage specificity of the proteasome.

Qualitative changes in the proteins of the ubiquitin-proteasome pathway also may be important in protein degradation required for regulated programs of cellular or organismic development. For example, the subunit composition of the 20S proteasome changes in certain cells during *Drosophila* development [69] and during development of embryonic chick muscle [3]. Other reports have described changes in the subunit composition of PA700 during programmed cell death in insect muscles [30]. During erythroid differentiation, a specific program of proteolysis eliminates many cellular proteins. A novel E2 conjugating enzyme, E2-230K, is up-regulated during this program, and it is attractive to speculate that this enzyme targets selectively those proteins whose elimination is required for the differentiation process [81]. We believe that these examples only represent early reports of the regulation of protein degradation by qualitative alterations in components of the ubiquitin-proteasome pathway. Such a feature further highlights the complexity of the physiological regulation of this system. Learning the features and details of this complexity represents a major challenge for future research.

ROLE OF PROTEIN DEGRADATION AND THE UBIQUITIN-PROTEASOME SYSTEM IN MUSCLE ATROPHY DURING UNLOADING

A large number of studies in experimental animals and in humans demonstrated that passive mechanical stretch or increased mechanical work promotes positive nitrogen balance in skeletal muscles [9, 59]. In contrast, unloading or mechanical inactivity leads to SM wasting. These effects have significant, practical, and clinical consequences in diverse situations that include: (1) muscle performance for athletes; (2) the well-being of patients with spinal cord injuries; (3) casted limbs; (4) illnesses that confine patients to bed for long intervals; and (5) astronauts exposed to microgravity during space travel. Each of these conditions is characterized by increased protein degradation, which contributes importantly to resulting decreases in muscle mass.

A specialized instance of muscle atrophy occurs under conditions of microgravity. Humans and animals exposed to microgravity experience significant muscle wasting, presumably as an adaptive response to decreased mechanical load [151]. Although there are conflicting reports in regards to the basis of this effect, most evidence indicates that an increase in muscle protein degradation, rather than a decrease in muscle protein synthesis, accounts for the loss of muscle protein during weightlessness. The effect is most prominent in slow-twitch muscles and has been observed during space-flight and in earth-based model systems, such as hindlimb suspension of rodents [151, 161]. Recently, strong evidence was obtained for a prominent role of the ubiquitin-proteasome pathway in the mediation of this response. For example, several studies have examined relative contributions of various proteolytic pathways to increased muscle proteolysis in the hindlimb suspension model. Soleus muscles of rats suspended for 3–9 days lose significant tissue protein and have greatly increased rates of protein degradation [154, 161, 163]. Although lysosomal and calpain-dependent proteolytic pathways are up-regulated in these muscles, most of the large increases of protein degradation are a consequence of the increased function of the ubiquitin-proteasome pathway [154, 160, 163]. The latter response also includes large increases in mRNA levels of ubiquitin, an E2 conjugating enzyme, and two representative subunits of the 20S proteasome. These data are in accord with previous studies showing increased ubiquitination of contractile proteins of rats sent into space [32, 42, 97].

CONCLUSIONS AND PERSPECTIVE

Historically, the regulation of intracellular protein degradation as a principal means of controlling the levels of individual proteins or the global protein content of tissues has been poorly appreciated by most scientists. This situation may have resulted from the lack of striking examples of how protein degradation could regulate a critical cellular process, and/or from the lack of details regarding the biochemical mechanisms of the degradative process. This situation has changed dramatically during the past several years, mostly due to studies of the ubiquitin-proteasome pathway. As previously described, not only does the pathway seem to be involved in a large proportion of bulk intracellular protein turnover, but also seems to be involved in a surprising number of processes that utilize selective proteolysis as a regulatory strategy. Thus, the ubiquitin-proteasome system is proving to be as physiologically important as it has been biochemically fascinating.

Despite rapid and extensive progress in this area, we believe that the future holds very significant promise for continued advancement and expansion of important knowledge. Many critical and fundamental questions remain to be answered regarding the biochemical mechanisms and operation of the pathway. Furthermore, it seems likely that additional pathway components, as well as functional interactions among both known and as yet unidentified components, will be identified. However, we also believe that future advances will occur increasingly through studies of the cellular regulation and physiology of the ubiquitin-proteasome pathway. Such advances should be of considerable interest to scientists and of practical benefit to clinicians. For example, it is not unreasonable to expect that the pathway's function will become subject to pharmacological intervention at one of its many possible target sites. This prospect could provide a means of controlling many conditions that include inflammation (via regulation of NFkB activation), cancer (via regulation of cell cycle control), and muscle wasting during disease and space flight (via regulation of bulk protein degradation). Although our optimistic view will require much additional work, the remarkable advances achieved in the 20 years since the discovery of the pathway lead us to believe that this optimism is well founded.

REFERENCES

1. Adams, G.M., S. Falke, A.L. Goldberg, C.A. Slaughter, G.N. DeMartino, and E.P. Gogol. Structural and functional effects of PA700 and modulator protein on proteasomes. *J. Mol. Biol.* In Press, 1997.
2. Ahn, J., N. Tanahashi, K. Akiyama et al. Primary structures of two homologous subunits of PA28, a τ-interferon-inducible protein activator of the 20S proteasome. *FEBS Lett.* 366: 37–42, 1995.
3. Ahn, J.Y., S.O. Hong, K.B. Kwak, et al. Developmental regulation of proteolytic activities and subunit pattern of 20S proteasome in chick embryonic muscle. *J. Biol. Chem.* 266: 15746–15749, 1991.
4. Ahn, K., M. Erlander, D. Letureq, P.A. Peterson, K. Fruh, and Y. Yang. *In vivo* characterization of proteasome regulator PA28. *J. Biol. Chem.* 271:18237–18242, 1996.
5. Akiyama, K., K. Yokota, S. Kagawa, et al. cDNA cloning of a new putative ATPase subunit p45 of the human 26S proteasome, a homolog of yeast transcriptional factor Sug1p. *FEBS Lett.* 363:151–156, 1995.
6. Akiyama, K., K. Yokota, S. Kagawa, et al. cDNA cloning and interferon τ down-regulation of proteasomal subunits X and Y. *Science* 265:1231–1234, 1994.
7. Balzi, E., W. Chen, E. Capieaux, J.H. McCusker, J. E. Haber, and A. Coffeau. The suppressor gene sc11+ of Saccharomyces cerevisuae is essential for growth. *Gene* 83:271–279, 1989.
8. Baracos, V.E., C. DeVito, D.H.R. Hoyle, and A.L. Goldberg. Activation of the ATP-ubiquitin-proteasome pathway in skeletal muscle of cachectic rats bearing a hepatoma. *Am. J. Physiol.* 268:E996–E1006, 1995.
9. Baracos, V.E., and A.L. Goldberg. Maintenance of normal length improves protein balance and energy status in isolated rat skeletal muscles. *Am. J. Physiol.* 251:C588–C596, 1986.
10. Beal, R., Q. Deveraux, G. Xia, M. Rechsteiner, and C. Pickart. Surface hydrophobic residues of multiubiquitin chains essential for proteolytic targeting. *Proc. Natl. Acad. Sci. USA* 93:861–866, 1996.
11. Bercovich, B., I. Stancovski, A. Mayer, et al. Ubiquitin-dependent degradation of certain

protein substrates *in vitro* requires the molecular chaperone Hsc70. *J. Biol. Chem.* 272: 9002–9010, 1997.

12. Boes, B., H. Hengel, T. Ruppert, G. Multhaup, U.H. Koszinowski, and P. Kloetzel. Interferon ᴛ stimulation modulates the proteolytic activity and cleavage site preference of 20S mouse proteasomes. *J. Exp. Med.* 179:901–909, 1994.

13. Boldin, M.P., I.L. Mett, and D. Wallach. A protein related to a proteasomal subunit binds to the intracellular domain of the p55 TNF receptor upstream of its "death domain." *FEBS Lett.* 367:39–44, 1995.

14. Chau, V., J.W. Tobias, A. Bachmair, et al. A multiubiquitin chain is confined to specific lysine in a targeted short-lived protein. *Science* 243:1576–1583, 1989.

15. Chen, A.J., L. Parent, and T. Maniatis. Site-specific phosphorylation of IkB α by a novel ubiquitination-dependent protein kinase activity. *Cell* 84:853-862, 1996.

16. Chiang, H., and J.F. Dice. Peptide sequences that target proteins for enhanced degradation during serum withdrawal. *J. Biol. Chem.* 263:6797–6805, 1988.

17. Chiang, H., S.R. Terlecky, C.P. Plant, and J.F. Dice. A role for a 70-kilodalton heat shock protein in lysosomal degradation of intracellular proteins. *Science* 246:382–385, 1989.

18. Ciechanover, A. The ubiquitin-proteasome proteolytic pathway. *Cell* 79:13–21, 1994.

19. Ciechanover, A., D. Finley, and A. Varshavsky. Ubiquitin dependence of selective protein degradation demonstrated in the mammalian cell cycle mutant ts85. *Cell* 37:57–66, 1984.

20. Ciechanover, A., H. Gonen, S. Elias, and M. Mayer. Degradation of proteins by the ubiquitin-mediated proteolytic pathway. *New Biol.* 2:227–234, 1990.

21. Ciechanover, A., and A.L. Schwartz. How are substrates recognized by the ubiquitin-mediated proteolytic system? *Trends Biochem. Sci.* 14:483–488, 1989.

22. Clark, A.F., G.N. DeMartino, and K. Wildenthal. Effects of glucocorticoid treatment on cardiac protein synthesis and degradation. *Am. J. Physiol.* 19:C821–C827, 1986.

23. Confalonieri, F., and M. Duguet. A 200-amino acid ATPase module in search of a basic function. *Bioessays* 17:639–650, 1995.

24. Costelli, P., C. Garcia-Martinez, M. Liovera, et al. Muscle protein waste in tumor-bearing rats is effectively antagonized by a β_2-adrenergic agonist (clenbuterol). *J. Clin. Invest.* 95: 2367–2372, 1995.

25. Coux, O., K. Tanaka, and A.L. Goldberg. Structure and functions of the 20S and 26S proteasomes. *Ann. Rev. Biochem.* 65:801–847, 1996.

26. Craiu, A., M. Gaczynska, T. Akapian, et al. Lactacystin and *clasto*-lactacystin β-lactone modify multiple proteasome β-subunits and inhibit intracellular protein degradation and major histocompatibility complex class I antigen presentation. *J. Biol. Chem.* 272: 13437–13445, 1997.

27. Croall, D.E., and G.N. DeMartino. Calcium-activated neutral protease (calpain) system: structure, function, and regulation. *Physiol. Rev.* 71:813–847, 1991.

28. Cuervo, A.M., and J.F. Dice. A receptor for the selective uptake and degradation of proteins by lysosomes. *Science* 273:501–503, 1996.

29. Dahlmann, B., F. Kopp, L. Kuehn, et al. The multicatalytic proteinase (prosome) is ubiquitous from eukaryotes to archaebacteria. *FEBS Lett.* 251:125–131, 1989.

30. Dawson, S.P., J.E. Arnold, N.J. Mayer, et al. Developmental changes of the 26S proteasome in abdominal intersegmental muscles of *Manduca sexta* during programmed cell death. *J. Biol. Chem.* 270:1850–1858, 1995.

31. DeMarini, D.J., F.R. Papa, S. Swaminathan, et al. The yeast SEN3 gene encodes a regulatory subunit of the 26S proteasome complex required for ubiquitin-dependent protein degradation in vivo. *Mol. Cell. Biol.* 15:6311–6321, 1995.

32. DeMartino, G.N., M.L. McCullough, J.F. Reckelhoff, D.E. Croall, A. Ciechanover, and M.J. McGuire. ATP-stimulated degradation of endogenous proteins in cell-free extracts of BHK 21/C13 fibroblasts: a key role for the proteinase, macropain, in the ubiquitin-dependent degradation of short-lived proteins. *Biochim. Biophys. Acta* 1073:299–308, 1991.

33. DeMartino, G.N., C.R. Moomaw, O.P. Zagnitko, et al. PA700, an ATP-dependent activator of the 20S proteasome, is an ATPase containing multiple members of a nucleotide-binding protein family. *J. Biol. Chem.* 269:20878–20884, 1994.

34. DeMartino, G.N., R.J. Proske, C.R. Moomaw, et al. Identification, purification, and characterization of a PA700-dependent activator of the proteasome. *J. Biol. Chem.* 271: 3112–3118, 1996.

35. DeMartino, G.N., and C. A. Slaughter. Regulatory proteins of the proteasome. *Enzyme Protein* 47:314–324, 1993.

36. Deter, R., and C. de Duve. Influence of glucagon, an inducer of cellular autophagy, on some physical properties of rat liver lysosomes. *J. Cell. Biol.* 33:437–449, 1967.

37. Deveraux, Q., C. Jensen, and M. Rechsteiner. Molecular cloning and expression of a 26S protease subunit enriched in dileucine repeats. *J. Biol. Chem.* 270:23726–23729, 1995.

38. Deveraux, Q., V. Ustrell, C. Pickart, and M. Rechsteiner. A 26S protease subunit that binds ubiquitin conjugates. *J. Biol. Chem.* 269:7059–7061, 1994.

39. Dice, J.F. Molecular determinants of protein half-lives in eukaryotic cells. *FASEB J.* 1: 349–357, 1987.

40. Dice, J.F. Peptide sequences that target cytosolic proteins for lysosomal proteolysis. *Trends Biochem. Sci.* 15:305–309, 1990.

41. Dick, L.R., A.A. Cruikshank, L. Grenier, F.D. Melandri, S.L. Nunes, and R.L. Stein. Mechanistic studies on the inactivation of the proteasome by lactacystin. *J. Biol. Chem.* 271: 7273–7226, 1996.

42. Dick, L.R., C.R. Moomaw, G.N. DeMartino, and C.A. Slaughter. Degradation of oxidized insulin B chain by the multiproteinase complex macropain (proteasome). *Biochemistry* 30:2725–2734, 1991.

43. Dick, T., T. Ruppert, M. Groettrup, et al. Coordinated dual cleavages induced by the proteasome regulator PA28 lead to dominant MHC ligands. *Cell* 86:253–262, 1996.

44. Driscoll, J.D., and A.L. Goldberg. The proteasome (multicatalytic protease) is a component of the 1500-kDa proteolytic complex which degrades ubiquitin-conjugated proteins. *J. Biol. Chem.* 265:4789–4792, 1990.

45. Dubiel, W., K. Ferrell, G. Pratt, and M. Rechsteiner. Subunit 4 of the 26S protease is a member of a novel eukaryotic ATPase family. *J. Biol. Chem.* 267:22699–22702, 1992.

46. Dubiel, W., K. Ferrell, and M. Rechsteiner. Tat-binding protein 7 is a subunit of the 26S protease. *Biol. Chem. Hoppe-Seyler* 375:237–240, 1994.

47. Dubiel, W., K. Ferrell, and M. Rechsteiner. Subunits of the regulatory complex of the 26S protease. *Mol. Biol. Rep.* 21:27–34, 1995.

48. Dubiel, W., G. Pratt, K. Ferrell, and M. Rechsteiner. Purification of an 11S regulator of the multicatalytic protease. *J. Biol. Chem.* 267:22369–22377, 1992.

49. Fenteany, G., R.F. Standaert, W.S. Lane, S. Choi, E.J. Corey, and S.L. Schreiber. Inhibition of proteasome activities and subunit-specific amino-terminal threonine modification by lactacystin. *Science* 268:726–731, 1995.

50. Ferrell, K., Q. Deveraux, S. van Nocker, and M. Rechsteiner. Molecular cloning and expression of a multiubiquitin chain binding subunit of the human 26S protease. *FEBS Lett.* 381:143–148, 1996.

51. Finley, D., A. Ciechanover, and A. Varshavsky. Thermolability of ubiquitin-activating enzyme from the mammalian cell-cycle mutant ts85. *Cell* 37:43–55, 1984.

52. Florini, J.R. Hormonal control of muscle growth. *Nerve Muscle* 10:577–598, 1987.

53. Fujiwara, T., K. Tanaka, E. Orino, et al. Proteasomes are essential for yeast proliferation. *J. Biol. Chem.* 260:16604–16613, 1990.

54. Fulks, R.M., J.B. Li, and A.L. Goldberg. Effects of insulin, glucose, and amino acids on protein turnover in rat diaphragm. *J. Biol. Chem.* 250:290–298, 1997.

55. Gaczynska, M., A.L. Goldberg, K. Tanaka, K.B. Hendil, and K.L. Rock. Proteasome subunits X and Y alter peptidase activities in opposite ways to the interferon-gamma-induced subunits LMP2 and LMP7. *J. Biol. Chem.* 271:17275–17280, 1996.

56. Gaczynska, M., K.L. Rock, and A.L. Goldberg. τ-Interferon and expression of MHC genes regulate peptide hydrolysis by proteasomes. *Nature* 365:264–267, 1993.

57. Ghisiain, M., A. Udvardy, and C. Mann. S. cerevisiae 26S protease mutants arrest cell division in G2/metaphase. *Nature* 366:358–362, 1993.

58. Glotzer, M., A.W. Murray, and M.W. Kirschner. Cyclin is degraded by the ubiquitin pathway. *Nature* 349:132–138, 1991.

59. Goldberg, A.L. Influence of insulin and contractile activity on muscle size and protein balance. *Diabetes Suppl.t* 28:18–24, 1979.

60. Goldberg, A.L., and J.F. Dice. Intracellular protein degradation in mammalian and bacterial cells. *Ann. Rev. Biochem.* 43:835–869, 1975.

61. Goldberg, A.L., and A.C. St. John. Intracellular protein degradation in mammalian and bacterial cells: part 2. *Ann. Rev. Biochem.* 45:747–803, 1976.

62. Gray, C.W., C.A. Slaughter, and G.N. DeMartino. PA28 activator protein forms regulatory caps on proteasome stacked rings. *J. Mol. Biol.* 236:7–15, 1994.

63. Groettrup, M., R. Kraft, S. Kostka, S. Standera, R. Stohwasser, and P. Kloetzel. A third interferon τ induced subunit exchange in the 20S proteasome. *Science* 274:1385–1389, 1996.

64. Groettrup, M., T. Ruppert, L. Kuehn, et al. The interferon-τ-inducible 11S regulator (PA28) and the LMP2/LMP7 subunits govern the peptide production by the 20S proteasome in vitro. *J. Biol. Chem.* 270:23808–23815, 1995.

65. Groettrup, M., A. Soza, M. Eggers, et al. A role for the proteasome regulator PA28a in antigen presentation. *Nature* 381:166–168, 1996.

66. Groll, M., L. Ditzel, J. Lowe, et al. Strucutre of the 20S proteasome from yeast at 2.4A resolution. *Nature* 386:463–471, 1997.

67. Grziwa, A., W. Baumeister, B. Dahlmann, and F. Kopp. Localization of subunits in proteasomes from Termoplasma acidophium by immunoelectron microscopy. *FEBS Lett.* 290: 186–190, 1991.

68. Guo, G.G., M. Gu, and J.D. Etlinger. 240-kDa proteasome inhibitor (CF-2) is identical to σ-aminolevulinic acid dehydratase. *J. Biol. Chem.* 269:12399–12402, 1994.

69. Haass, C., and P.M. Kloetzel. The Drosophila proteasome undergoes changes in its subunit pattern during development. *Exp. Cell. Res.* 180:243–252, 1989.

70. Hampton, R.Y., R.G. Gardner, and J. Rine. Role of the 26S proteasome and *HRD* genes in the degradation of 3-hydroxy-3methylglutaryl-CoA reductase, an integral endoplasmic reticulum membrane protein. *Mol. Bio. Cell* 7:2029–2044, 1996.

71. Hayashi, M., M. Inomata, Y. Saito, H. Ito, and S. Kawashima. Activation of intracellular calcium-activated neutral proteinase in erythrocytes and its inhibition by exogenously added inhibiors. *Biochim. Biophys. Acta* 1094:249–256, 1991.

72. Hayashi, S., Y. Murakami, and S. Matsufuji. Ornithine decarboxylase antizyme: a novel type of regulatory protein. *Trends Biochem. Sci.* 21:27–30, 1996.

73. Heinemeyer, W., J.A. Kleinschmidt, J. Saidowsky, C. Escher, and D.H. Wolf. Proteinase yscE, the yeast proteasome/multicatalytic-multifunctional proteinase: mutants unravel its function in stress induced proteolysis and uncover its necessity for cell survival. *EMBO J.* 10:555–562, 1991.

74. Heinemeyer, W., N. Trondle, G. Albrecht, and D.H. Wolf. PRE5 and PRE6, the last missing genes encoding 20S proteasome subunits from yeast? Indication for a set of 14 different subunits in the eukaryotic proteasome core. *Biochemistry* 33:12229–12237, 1994.

75. Hershko, A. Ubiquitin-mediated protein degradation. *J. Biol. Chem.* 263:15237–15240, 1988.

76. Hershko, A. The ubiquitin pathway for protein degradation. *Trends Biochem. Sci.* 16: 265–268, 1991.

77. Hershko, A., and A. Ciechanover. Mechanisms of intracellular protein breakdown. *Ann. Rev. Biochem.* 51:335–364, 1982.

78. Hershko, A., and A. Ciechanover. The ubiquitin pathway for the degradation of intracellular proteins. *Prog. Nuc. Acid Res. Mol. Biol.* 33:19–56, 1986.

79. Hershko, A., and A. Ciechanover. The ubiquitin system for protein degradation. *Ann. Rev. Biochem.* 61:761–807, 1992.

80. Hochstrasser, M. Ubiquitin, proteasomes, and the regulation of intracellular protein degradation. *Curr. Opin. Cell Biol.* 7:215–223, 1995.

81. Hochstrasser, M. Ubiquitin-dependent protein degradation. *Ann. Rev. Genet.* 30:405–439, 1996.

82. Hochstrasser, M., M.J. Ellison, V. Chau, and A. Varshavsky. The short-lived MATα2 transcriptional regulator is ubiquitinated in vivo. *Proc. Natl. Acad. Sci USA* 88:4606–4610, 1991.

83. Hoffman, L., G. Pratt, and M. Rechsteiner. Multiple forms of the 20S multicatalytic and the 26S ubiquitin-ATP-dependent proteases from rabbit reticulocyte lysate. *J. Biol. Chem.* 267:22362–22368, 1992.

84. Hoffman, L., and M. Rechsteiner. Nucleotidase activities of the 26S proteasome and its regulatory complex. *J. Biol. Chem.* 271:32538–32545, 1996.

85. Honoré, B., H. Leffers, P. Madsen, and J.E. Celis. Interferon-gamma up-regulates a unique set of proteins in human keratinocytes. Molecular cloning and expression of the cDNA encoding the RGD-containing protein IGUP I-5111. *Eur. J. Biochem.* 218:421–430, 1993.

86. Hough, R., G. Pratt, and M. Rechsteiner. Purification of two high molecular weight proteases from rabbit reticulocyte lysate. *J. Biol. Chem.* 262:8303–8313, 1987.

87. Jefferson, L.S., J.B. Li, and S.R. Rannels. Regulation by insulin of amino acid release and protein turnover in the perfused rat hemicorpus. *J. Biol. Chem.* 252:1476–1483, 1977.

88. Jentsch, S., W. Seufert, T. Sommer, and H. Reins. Ubiquitin-conjugating enzymes: novel regulators of eukaryotic cells. *Trends Biochem. Sci.* 15:105–108, 1990.

89. Kettelhut, I.C., S.S. Wing, and A.L. Goldberg. Endocrine regulation of protein breakdown in skeletal muscle. *Diabet./ Metab. Rev.* 4:751–772, 1988.

90. Kim, Y., S. Björklund, Y. Li, M.H. Sayre, and R.D. Kornberg. A multiprotein mediator of transcriptional activation and its interaction with the C-terminal repeat domain of RNA polymerase II. *Cell* 77:599–608, 1994.

91. King, R.W., R.J. Deshaies, J. Peters, and M.W. Kirschner. How proteolysis drives the cell cycle. *Science* 274:1652–1658, 1996.

92. Kominami, K., G.N. DeMartino, C.R. Moomaw, et al. Nin1p, a regulatory subunit of the 26S proteasome, is necessary for activation of Cdc28p kinase of Saccharomyces cerevisiae. *EMBO J.* 14:3105–3115, 1995.

93. Kominami, K., N. Okura, M. Kawamura, et al. Yeast counterparts of subunits S5a and p58 (S3) of the human 26S proteasome are encoded by two multicopy suppressors of *nin1-1*. *Molecular Biol. Cell* 8:171–187, 1997.

94. Kopp, F., B. Dahlmann, and K.B. Hendil. Evidence indicating that the human proteasome is a complex dimer. *J. Mol. Biol.* 229:14–19, 1993.

95. Lam, Y.A., W. Xu, G.N. DeMartino, and R.E. Cohen. Editing of ubiquitin conjugates by an isopeptidase in the 26S proteasome. *Nature* 385:737–740, 1997.

96. Lee, D.H.L., and A.L. Goldberg. Selective inhibitors of the proteasome-dependent and vacuolar pathways of protein degradation in *Saccharomyces cerevisiae*. *J. Biol. Chem.* 271: 27280–27284, 1996.

97. Lee, L.W., C.R. Moomaw, K. Orth, M.J. McGuire, G.N. DeMartino, and C.A. Slaughter. Relationships among the subunits of the high molecular weight proteinase, macropain (proteasome). *Biochim. Biophys. Acta* 1037:178–185, 1990.

98. Li, X., and P. Coffino. Identification of a region of p53 that confers lability. *J. Biol. Chem.* 271:4447–4451, 1996.

99. Li, X., M. Gu, and J.D. Etlinger. Isolation and characterization of a novel endogenous inhibitor of the proteasome. *Biochemistry* 30:9709–9715, 1991.

100. Li, X., B. Stebbens, L. Hoffman, G. Pratt, M. Rechsteiner, and P. Coffino. The N Terminus of antizyme promotes degradation of heterologous proteins. *J. Biol. Chem.* 271: 4441–4466, 1996.

101. Löwe, J., D. Stock, B. Jap, P. Zwickl, W. Baumeister, and R. Huber. Crystal structure of the 20S proteasome from the archaeon T. acidophilum at 3.4 Å resolution. *Science* 268: 533–539, 1995.

102. Lurquin, C., A. Van Pel, B. Mariamé, et al. Structure of the gene of tum-transplantation antigen P91A :the mutated exon encodes a peptide recognized with Ld by cytolytic T cells. *Cell* 58:293–303, 1989.

103. Ma, C., C.A. Slaughter, and G.N. DeMartino. Identification, purification, and characterization of a protein activator (PA28) of the 20S proteasome. *J. Biol. Chem.* 267: 10515–10523, 1992.

104. Ma, C., C.A. Slaughter, and G.N. DeMartino. Purification and characterization of a protein inhibitor of the 20S proteasome (macropain). *Biochim. Biophys. Acta* 1119:303–311, 1992.

105. Ma, C., J.H. Vu, R.J. Proske, C.A. Slaughter, and G.N. DeMartino. Identification, purification, and characterization of a high-molecular weight, ATP-dependent activator (PA700) of the 20S proteasome. *J. Biol. Chem.* 269:3539–3547, 1994.

106. Ma, C., P.J. Willy, C.A. Slaughter, and G.N. DeMartino. PA28, an activator of the 20S proteasome, is inactivated by proteolytic modification at its carboxyl terminus. *J. Biol. Chem.* 268:22514–22519, 1993.

107. McGuire, M.J., D.E. Croall, and G.N. DeMartino. ATP-stimulated proteolysis in soluble extracts of BHK 21/C13 cells. Evidence for multiple pathways and a role for an enzyme related to the high-molecular-weight protease, macropain. *Arch. Biochem. Biophys.* 262: 273–285, 1988.

108. McGuire, M.J., and G.N. DeMartino. The latent form of macropain (high molecular weight multicatalytic protease) restores ATP-dependent proteolysis to cell-free extracts of BHK fibroblasts pretreated with antimacropain antibodies. *Biochem. Biophys. Res. Commun.* 160:911–916, 1989.

109. McGuire, M.J., M.L. McCullough, D.E. Croall, and G.N. DeMartino. The high molecular weight multicatalytic proteinase, macropain, exists in a latent form in human erythrocytes. *Biochim. Biophys. Acta* 995:181–186, 1989.

110. Medina, R., S.S. Wing, and A.L. Goldberg. Increase in levels of polyubiquitin and proteasome mRNA in skeletal muscle during starvation and denervation atrophy. *Biochem. J.* 307:631–637, 1995.

111. Mitch, W.E., and A.L. Goldberg. Mechanisms of muscle wasting: the role of the ubiquitin-proteasome pathway. *New Eng. J.f Med.* 335:1897–1905, 1996.

112. Mitch, W.E., R. Medina, S. Grieber, et al. Metabolic acidosis stimulates muscle protein degradation by activating the adenosine triphosphate-dependent pathway involving ubiquitin and proteasomes. *J. Clin. Invest.* 93:2127–2133, 1994.

113. Miyamoto, S., M. Maki, M.J. Schmitt, M. Hatanaka, and I.M. Verma. Tumor necrosis factor α-induced phosphorylation of IkBα is a signal for its degradation but not dissociation from NF-kB. *Proc. Natl. Acad. Sci. USA* 91:12740–12744, 1994.

114. Monacco, J.J. Pathways of antigen processing. *Immunol. Today* 13:173–179, 1992.

115. Mortimore, G.E., and C.E. Mondon. Inhibition by insulin of valine turnover in liver: evidence for a general control of proteolysis. *J. Biol. Chem.* 245:2375–2383, 1970.

116. Mott, J.D., B.C. Pramanik, C.R. Moomaw, S.J. Afendis, G.N. DeMartino, and C.A. Slaughter. PA28, an activator of the 20S proteasome, is composed of two nonidentical buy homologous subunits. *J. Biol. Chem.* 269:31466–31471, 1994.

117. Murachi, T. Intracellular regulatory system involving calpain and calpastatin. *Biochem. Int.* 18:263–294, 1989.

118. Murakami, K., and J.D. Etlinger. Endogenous inhibitor of nonlysosomal high molecular

weight protease and calcium-dependent protease. *Proc. Natl. Acad. Sci. USA* 83:7588–7592, 1986.

119. Murray, A. Cyclin ubiquitination :the destructive end of mitosis. *Cell* 81:149–152, 1995.
120. Nelbock, P., P.J. Dillion, A. Perkins, and C.A. Rosen. A cDNA for a protein that interacts with the human immunodeficiency virus Tat transactivator. *Science* 248:1650–1653, 1990.
121. Ohana, B., P.A. Moore, S.M. Ruben, C.D. Southgate, M.R. Green, and C.A. Rosen. The type 1 human immunodeficiency virus Tat binding protein is a transcriptional activator belonging to an additional family of evolutionarily conserved genes. *Proc. Natl. Acad. Sci. USA* 90:138–142, 1993.
122. Orian, A., S. Whiteside, A. Israël, I. Stancovski, A.L. Schwartz, and A. Ciechanover. Ubiquitin-mediated processing of NF-kB transcriptional activator precursor p105. *J. Biol. Chem.* 270:21707–21714, 1995.
123. Orlowski, M. The multicatalytic proteinase complex, a major extralysosomal proteolytic system. *Biochemistry* 29:10289–10297, 1990.
124. Palombella, V.J., O.J. Rando, A.L. Goldberg, and T. Maniatis. The ubiquitin-proteasome pathway is required for processing the NF-kB1 precursor protein and the activation of NF-kB. *Cell* 78:773–785, 1994.
125. Peters, J. Proteasomes: protein degradation machines of the cell. *Trends Biochem. Sci.* 19: 377–382, 1994.
126. Peters, J., W.W. Franke, and J.A. Kleinschmidt. Distinct 19S and 20S subcomplexes of the 26S proteasome and their distribution in the nucleus and the cytoplasm. *J. Biol. Chem.* 269:7709–7718, 1994.
127. Price, S.R., J.L. Bailey, X. Wang, et al. Muscle wasting in insulinpenic rats results from activation of the ATP-dependent, ubiquitin-proteasome proteolytic pathway by a mechanism including gene transcription. *J. Clin. Invest.* 98:1703–1708, 1996.
128. Price, S.R., B.K. England, J.L. Bailey, K. Van Vreede, and W.E. Mitch. Acidosis and glucocorticoids concomitantly increase ubiquitin and proteasome subunit mRNAs in rat muscle. *Am. J. Physiol.* 267:C955–C960, 1994.
129. Pühler, G., S. Weinkauf, L. Bachmann, et al. Subunit stoichiometry and three-dimensional arrangement in proteasomes from Thermoplasma acidophilum. *EMBO J.* 11: 1607–1616, 1992.
130. Realini, C., W. Dubiel, G. Pratt, K. Ferrell, and M. Rechsteiner. Molecular cloning and expression of a т-interferon-inducible activator of the multicatalytic protease. *J. Biol. Chem.* 269:20727–20732, 1994.
131. Rechsteiner, M. Natural substrates of the ubiquitin proteolytic pathway. *Cell* 66:615–618, 1991.
132. Rechsteiner, M., L. Hoffman, and W. Dubiel. The multicatalytic and 26S proteases. *J. Biol. Chem.* 268:6065–6068, 1993.
133. Richard, I., O. Broux, V. Allamand, et al. Mutations in the proteolytic enzyme calpain 3 cause Limb-Girdle Muscular Dystrophy Type 2A. *Cell* 81:27–40, 1995.
134. Richter-Ruoff, B., W. Heinemeyer, and D.H. Wolf. The proteasome/multicatalytic-multifunctional proteinase: in vivo function in the ubiquitin-dependent N-end rule pathway of protein degradation in eukaryotes. *FEBS Lett.* 302:192–196, 1992.
135. Rivett, A.J. The multicatalytic proteinase of mammalian cells. *Arch. Biochem. Biophys.* 268: 1–8, 1989.
136. Rock, K.L., C. Gramm, L. Rothstein, et al. Inhibitors of the proteasome block the degradation of most cell proteins and the generation of peptides presented on MHC class I molecules. *Cell* 78:761–771, 1994.
137. Rothe, M., S.C. Wong, W.J. Henzel, and D.V. Goeddel. A novel family of putative signal transducers associated with the cytoplasmic domain of the 75 kDa tumor necrosis factor receptor. *Cell* 78:681–692, 1994.
138. Rubin, D.M., and D. Finley. The proteasome :a protein-degrading organellee? *Curr. Biol.* 5:854–858, 1995.

139. Scheffner, M., B.A. Werness, J.M. Huibregtse, A.J. Levine, and P.M. Howley. The E6 oncoprotein encoded by human papilomavirus types 16 and 18 promotes the degradation of p53. *Cell* 63:1129–1136, 1990.

140. Schimke, R.T. Regulation of protein degradation in mammalian tissues. H.N. Munro (ed.). *Mammalian Protein Metabolism.* New York:Academic Press, 1970, pp. 177-228.

141. Seemüller, E., A. Lupas, D. Stock, J. Löwe, R. Huber, and W. Baumeister. Proteasome from Thermoplasma acidophilum: a threonine protease. *Science* 268:579–582, 1995.

142. Seufert, W., and S. Jentsch. In vitro function of the proteasome in the ubiquitin pathway. *EMBO J.* 11:3077–3080, 1992.

143. Seufert, W., and S. Jentsch. Ubiquitin-conjugating enzymes UBC4 and UBC5 mediate selective degradation of short-lived and abnormal proteins. *EMBO J.* 9:543–550, 1997.

144. Seufert, W., J. McGrath, and S. Jentsch. UBC1 encodes a novel member of an essential subfamily of yeast ubiquitin-conjugating enzymes involved in protein degradation. *EMBO J.* 9:4535–4541, 1990.

145. Shanklin, J., M. Jabben, and R.D. Vierstra. Red light-induced formation of ubiquitin-phytochrome conjugates: identification of possible intermediates of phytochrome degradation. *Proc. Natl. Acad. Sci. USA* 84:359–363, 1987.

146. Shibuya, H., K. Irie, J. Ninomiya-Tsuji, M. Goebll, T. Taniguchi, and K. Matsumoto. New human gene encoding a positive modulator of HIV tat-mediated transactivation. *Nature* 357:700–702, 1992.

147. Song, X., J.D. Mott, J. von Kampen,et al. A model for the quaternary structure of the proteasome activator PA28. *J. Biol. Chem.* 271:26410–26417, 1996.

148. Song, X., J. von Kampen, C.A. Slaughter, and G.N. DeMartino. Relative functions of the α and β subunits of the proteasome activator, PA28. *J. Biol. Chem.* 272:In Press, 1997.

149. Sorimachi, H., S. Imajoh-Ohmi, Y. Emori, et al. Molecular cloning of a novel mammalian calcium-dependent protease distinct from both m-and μ-types. *J. Biol. Chem.* 264: 20106–20111, 1989.

150. Sorimachi, H., T. Toyama-Sorimachi, T. Saido, et al. Muscle-specific calpain, p94, is degraded by autolysis immediately after translation, resulting in disappearance from muscle. *J. Biol. Chem.* 268:10593–10605, 1993.

151. Stein, T.P., and T. Gaprindashvili. Spaceflight and protein metabolism, with special reference to humans. *Am. J. Clin. Nutr.* 60:806S–819S, 1994.

152. Sugden, P.H., and S.J. Fuller. Regulation of protein turnover in skeletal and cardiac muscle. *Biochem. J.* 273:21–37, 1991.

153. Swaffield, J.C., J.F. Bromber, and S.A. Johnston. Alterations in a yeast protein resembling HIV Tat-binding protein relieve requirement for an acidic activation domain in GAL4. *Nature* 357:698–700, 1992.

154. Taillandier, D., E. Aurousseau, D. Meynial-Denis,et al. Coordinate activation of lysosomal, Ca^{2+}-activated and ATP-ubiquitin-dependent proteinases in the unweighted rat soleus muscle. *Biochem. J.* 316:65–72, 1996.

155. Tamura, T., I. Nagy, A. Lupas, et al. The first characterization of a eubacterial proteasome: the 20S complex of Rodococcus. *Curr. Biol.* 5:766–774, 1995.

156. Tanaka, K., and A. Ichihara. Involvement of proteasomes (multicatalytic proteinase) in ATP-dependent proteolysis in rat reticulocyte extracts. *FEBS Lett.* 236:159–162, 1988.

157. Tanaka, K., T. Tamura, T. Yoshimura, and A. Ichihara. Proteasomes: protein and gene structures. *New Biol.* 4:173–187, 1992.

158. Tanaka, K., T. Yoshimura, A. Kumatori, et al. Proteasomes: multi-protease complexes) as 20 S ring-shaped particles in a variety of eukaryotic cells. *J. Biol. Chem.* 263: 16209–16217, 1988.

159. Tawa, N.E., I.C. Kettelhut, and A.L. Goldberg. Dietary protein deficiency reduces lysosomal and nonlysosomal ATP-dependent proteolysis in muscle. *Am. J. Physiol.* 263: E326–E334, 1992.

160. Templeton, G.H., M. Padalino, J. Manton, et al. The influence of suspension-hypokinesia on the rat soleus muscle. *J. Appl. Physiol.* 56:278–286, 1984.

161. Thomason, D.B., and F.W. Booth. Atrophy of the soleus muscle by hindlimb unweighting. *J. Appl. Physiol.* 68:1–12, 1990.

162. Tiao, G., J.M. Fagan, N. Samuels, et al. Sepsis stimulates nonlysosomal, energy-dependent proteolysis and increases ubiquitin mRNA levels in rat skeletal muscle. *J. Clin. Invest.* 94: 2255–2264, 1994.

163. Tischler, M.E., S. Rosenberg, S. Satarug, et al. Different mechanisms of increased proteolysis in atrophy induced by denervation of unweighting of rat soleus muscle. *Metabolism* 39:756–763, 1990.

164. Tokunaga, F., T. Goto, T. Koide, et al. ATP- and antizyme-dependent endoproteolysis of ornithine decarboxylase to oligopeptides by the 26S proteasome. *J. Biol. Chem.* 269: 17382–17385, 1994.

165. Treier, M., L.M. Staszewski, and D. Bohmann. Ubiquitin-dependent c-jun degradation in vivo is mediated by the δ domain. *Cell* 78:787–798, 1194.

166. Tsubuki, S., Y. Saito, and S. Kawashima. Purification and characterization of an endogenous inhibitor specific to the Z-Leu-Leu-Leu-MCA degrading activity in proteasome and its identification as heat-shock protein 90. *FEBS Lett.* 344:229–233, 1994.

167. Tsurumi, C., G.N. DeMartino, C.A. Slaughter, N. Shimbara, and K. Tanaka. cDNA cloning of p40, a regulatory subunit of the human 26S proteasome, and a homolog of the Mov-34 gene product. *Biochem. Biophys. Res. Commun.* 210:600–608, 1995.

168. Tsurumi, C., Y. Shimizu, M. Saeki, et al. cDNA cloning and functional analysis of the p97 subunit of the 26S proteasome, a polypeptide identical to the type-1 tumor-necrosis-factor-associated protein-2/55.11. *Eur. J. Biochem.* 239:912–921, 1996.

169. Turner, P.R., T. Westwood, C.M. Regen, and R.A. Steinhardt. Increased protein degradation results from elevated free calcium levels found in muscle from mdx mice. *Nature* 335:735–738, 1988.

170. Udvardy, A. Purification and characterization of a multiprotein component of the Drosophila 26S (1500 kDa) proteolytic complex. *J. Biol. Chem.* 268:9055–9062, 1993.

171. Ugai, S., T. Tamura, N. Tanahashi, et al. Purification and characterization of the 26S proteasome complex catalyzing ATP-dependent breakdown of ubiquitin-ligated proteins from rat liver. *J. Biochem.* 113:754–768, 1993.

172. van Nocker, S., S. Sadis, D.M. Rubin, et al. The multiubiquitin-chain-binding protein Mcb1 is a component of the 26S proteasome in *Saccharomyces cerevisiae* and plays a nonessential, substrate-specific role in protein turnover. *Mol. Cell. Biol.* 16:6020–6028, 1996.

173. Ward, C.L., S. Omura, and R.R. Kopito. Degradation of CFTR by the ubiquitin-proteasome pathway. *Cell* 83:121–127, 1995.

174. Waxman, L., J.M. Fagan, and A.L. Goldberg. Demonstration of two distinct high molecular weight proteases in rabbit reticulocytes, one of which degrades ubiquitin conjugates. *J. Biol. Chem.* 262:2451–2457, 1987.

175. Wenzel, T., and W. Baumeister. Conformational constraints in protein degradation by the 20S proteasome. *Struct. Biol.* 2:199–204, 1995.

176. Wildenthal, K., J.R. Wakeland, J.M. Ord, and J.T. Stull. Interference with lysosomal proteolysis fails to reduce cardiac myosin degradation. *Biochem. Biophys. Res. Commun.* 96: 793–798, 1980.

177. Wing, S.S., and A.L. Goldberg. Glucocorticoids activate the ATP-ubiquitin-dependent proteolytic system in skeletal muscle during fasting. *Am. J. Physiol.* 264:E668–E676, 1993.

178. Yang, Y., J.B. Waters, K. Früh, and P.A. Peterson. Proteasomes are regulated by interferon τ: implications for antigen processing. *Proc. Natl. Acad. Sci. USA* 89:4928–4932, 1992.

179. Yokota, K., S. Kagawa, Y. Shimizu, et al. cDNA cloning of p112, the largest regulatory subunit of the human 26S proteasome, and functional analysis of its yeast homogue, Sen3p. *Mol. Biol. Cell* 7:853–870, 1996.

180. Yoshimura, T., K. Kameyama, T. Takagi, et al. Molecular characterization of the ''26S'' proteasome complex from rat liver. *J. Struct. Biol.* 111:200–211, 1993.
181. Zak, R., A.F. Martin, and R. Blough. Assessment of protein turnover by use of radioisotopic tracers. *Physiol. Rev.* 59:407–447, 1979.
182. Zwickl, P., A. Grziwa, G. Pühler, B. Dahlmann, F. Lottspeich, and W. Baumeister. Primary structure of the Thermoplasma proteasome and its implications for the structure, function, and evolution of the multicatalytic proteinase. *Biochemistry* 31:964–972, 1992.

10
Biomechanics of Walking and Running: Center of Mass Movements to Muscle Action

CLAIRE T. FARLEY, PH.D.
DANIEL P. FERRIS, M.S.

"Locomotion is a particularly richly studied but frustrating aspect of biology," according to Loeb [91]. This is especially true when one attempts to understand how the numerous subdivisions of the neuromuscular and musculoskeletal systems interact to produce locomotion. At lower levels of organization, the structure and function of the system components become progressively more complex, making it difficult to discern general principles. One way of approaching the study of locomotion is to sequentially progress from a level of whole body dynamics toward a level of muscle-tendon dynamics. We believe this approach can be particularly useful in that information from the higher levels of organization can guide the quest to understand fundamental mechanisms of locomotion at increasingly complex lower levels of organization. Thus, we will first examine the pattern of center of mass movements during locomotion in humans and other legged animals. Next, we will consider how joint mechanics during locomotion are affected by both center of mass dynamics and leg posture. After concentrating on the joint level, we will move to the level of muscle-tendon mechanics by examining the techniques that have been used to investigate muscle-tendon function during locomotion and the conclusions that have been reached to date.

Throughout this review, the locomotion of humans will be compared to the locomotion of other animals. A wealth of information shows that human locomotion is not unique. Indeed, at the level of the center of mass, the dynamics of walking and running are similar in all legged animals that have been studied. The similarities in the dynamics of locomotion among diverse animals, including humans, suggest that there may also be similarities in the mechanisms by which locomotion is produced at other levels of organization within the neuromuscular system. Thus, by comparing diverse species, we can uncover common rules governing locomotion, and we can assess the applicability of data from animal models to biomedical issues in humans.

CENTER OF MASS MECHANICS

Our discussion of center of mass mechanics will be divided into four parts. First, we will discuss the pattern of ground reaction force that occurs during locomotion. Ground reaction force is the force exerted by the ground on the feet. It reflects the acceleration of the body's center of mass during locomotion. Second, the movements and mechanical energy fluctuations of the center of mass that occur as a result of ground reaction force will be discussed. Third, we will discuss the transition from a walking gait to a running gait, an event that is marked by a sudden and distinct change in the pattern of movement of the center of mass. By understanding the reasons for the transition from one gait to another, we can gain insight into the key factors that shape locomotion. Fourth, we will describe behavioral models for locomotion that give insight into how the musculoskeletal system produces the distinctly different ground reaction force and center of mass movements in walking as compared to running.

Ground Reaction Force

The distinct difference between walking and running gaits is apparent in the ground reaction force patterns for the two gaits (Figures 10.1 and 10.2) [26, 27, 29, 34, 35]. In human walking, there is always at least one foot in contact with the ground, and there are short phases of "double support" when both feet are in contact with the ground (Figure 10.1). In contrast, running is a series of bouncing impacts with the ground that are usually alternated with aerial phases when neither foot is in contact with the ground (Figure 10.2). This difference leads to a substantially higher magnitude vertical component of the ground reaction force for running as compared to walking. The pattern of the horizontal component of the ground reaction force is similar, however, for both walking and running (Figures 10.1 and 10.2). In the first half of the stance phase, the horizontal ground reaction force is negative, indicating that it is pushing backwards on the person. In the second half of the stance phase, the horizontal ground reaction force is positive, pushing forward on the person. The ground reaction force pattern for walking and running gaits is similar in humans and in a wide variety of other animals with a range of body shapes, body masses, and numbers of legs [14, 22, 40, 50, 64].

Mechanical Energy Fluctuations of the Center of Mass

The difference in the ground reaction force pattern between walking and running translates into dramatically different patterns of mechanical energy fluctuations for the center of mass during the two gaits [25-28]. During walking, the body vaults over a relatively stiff stance limb and the center of mass reaches its highest point at the middle of the stance phase. As a result, the gravitational potential energy of the center of mass is maximized at the

FIGURE 10.1.

Representative ground reaction force as a function of time for walking (1.25 m/s) in a human. The dashed line represents the stance phase of the right foot, and the solid line represents the stance phase of the left foot. (A) vertical component. (B) horizontal component. In both parts, the ground reaction force is expressed as a multiple of body weight.

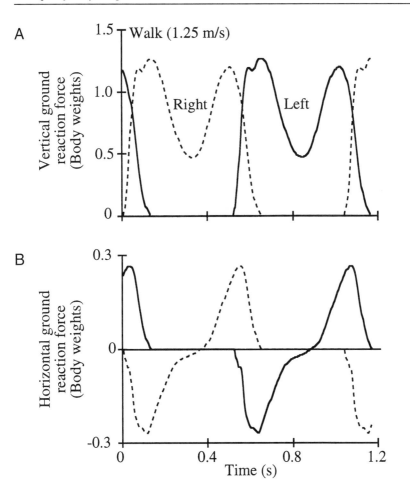

FIGURE 10.2.

Representative ground reaction force as a function of time for running (3.8 m/s) in a human. The dashed line represents the stance phase of the right foot, and the solid line represents the stance phase of the left foot. (A) vertical component. (B) horizontal component. In both parts, the ground reaction force is expressed as a multiple of body weight.

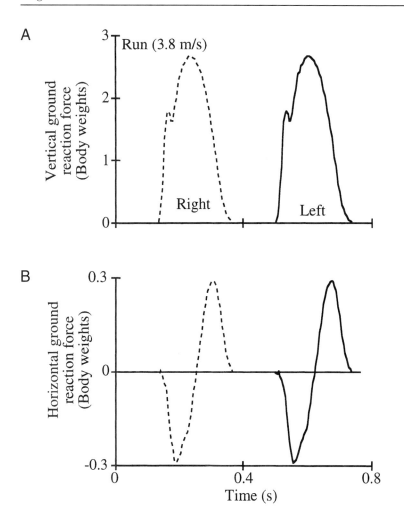

FIGURE 10.3.
An inverted pendulum model and a stick figure representation of a single stance phase of human walking. The model consists of a mass and a rigid strut that connects the point of foot-ground contact and the center of mass of the human. This figure depicts the stick figure and the model at the beginning of the stance phase (left-most position), the middle of the stance phase (center position), and the end of the stance phase (right-most position).

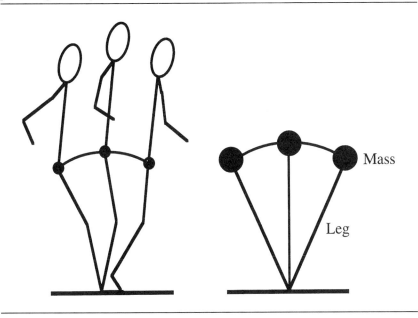

middle of the stance phase (Figure 10.3 and 10.5). In contrast, the stance limb is compliant in running so that the joints undergo substantial flexion during the first half of stance and extension during the second half of stance. This compliance causes the vertical displacement and gravitational potential energy of the center of mass to reach their minimum values at mid-stance in running (Figures 10.4 and 10.6). The pattern of movement of the center of mass has been proposed as the defining difference between a walking gait and a running gait [101].

Unlike the gravitational potential energy fluctuations, the pattern of kinetic energy fluctuations is similar for walking and running. In both gaits, the kinetic energy of the center of mass reaches its minimum value at mid-stance (Figures 10.5 and 10.6) since the horizontal ground reaction force tends to decelerate the body during the first half of the stance phase (Figures 10.1 and 10.2). During the second half of stance, the kinetic energy of the center of mass increases due to the accelerating effect of the horizontal

FIGURE 10.4.

A spring-mass model and a stick figure representation of a single stance phase of human running. The model consists of a linear spring representing the leg and a point mass equivalent to body mass. This figure depicts the model at the beginning of the stance phase (left-most position), at the middle of the stance phase (leg spring is oriented vertically), and at the end of the stance phase (right-most position).

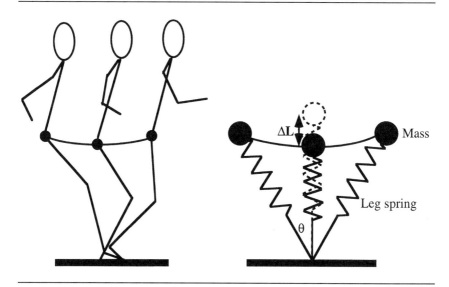

ground reaction force. Although the pattern of kinetic energy fluctuations is similar, the magnitude is much larger for running than for walking (Figures 10.5 and 10.6).

The kinetic energy and gravitational potential energy of the center of mass are approximately 180^0 out of phase in walking. At mid-stance in walking, the gravitational potential energy is at its maximum and the kinetic energy is at its minimum (Figure 10.5). Because these energies are approximately a half-cycle out of phase with each other and their fluctuations are similar in magnitude, substantial pendulum-like exchange occurs between them [25, 26]. During the first half of the stance phase of walking, the center of mass loses kinetic energy but gains gravitational potential energy. In this phase, kinetic energy can be converted to gravitational potential energy. During the second half of the stance phase, the center of mass loses gravitational potential energy but gains kinetic energy. Thus, during this phase, gravitational potential energy can be converted to kinetic energy. A similar energy transfer mechanism occurs as a pendulum swings or as an egg rolls across the ground. As a result, the energy transfer mechanism used in walking is often referred to as the "inverted pendulum mechanism"

FIGURE 10.5.
During moderate speed walking (1.25 m/s), the kinetic energy fluctuations of the center of mass are approximately 180° out of phase with the gravitational potential energy fluctuations, allowing substantial pendulum-like energy exchange. The thick horizontal line at the bottom of the group represents the phases when both feet are in contact with the ground ("double support" phases), and the thin horizontal line represents the phases when only a single foot is in contact with the ground ("single support" phases).

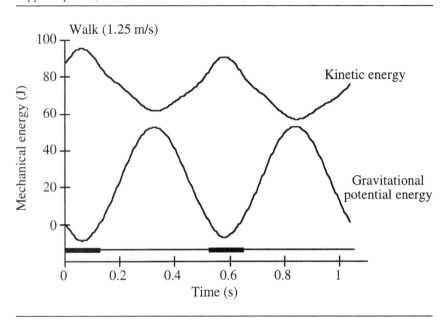

or the "rolling egg mechanism." The pattern of mechanical energy fluctuations is similar in other walking animals as it is in humans [14, 22, 40, 50, 64, 107]. As a result, many other animals, including mammals, birds, reptiles, and arthropods, also conserve substantial mechanical energy by the inverted pendulum mechanism during walking.

In human walking, as much as 60–70% of the mechanical energy required to lift and accelerate the center of mass is conserved by this energy transfer mechanism [28]. Mechanical energy savings are maximized at moderate walking speeds, and fall toward zero at very low and very high walking speeds [28]. At the walking speed where energy conservation is maximized, the magnitudes of the fluctuations in kinetic energy and gravitational potential energy are similar. Nevertheless, the maximum energy recovery by the inverted pendulum mechanism is approximately 70%, substantially less than the theoretical maximum of 100%. At the speed where energy transfer

FIGURE 10.6.

During running (3.8 m/s), the kinetic energy fluctuations of the center of mass are approximately in phase with the gravitational potential energy fluctuations. The stance phases for each limb are noted at the bottom of the graph.

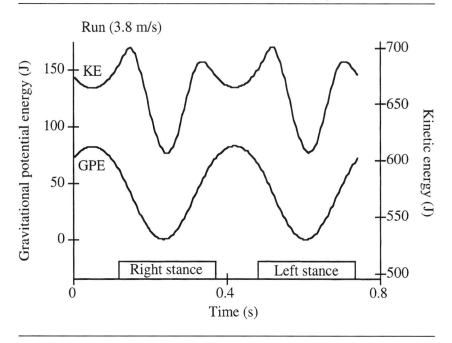

is maximized, the metabolic energy cost per unit distance (i.e., the cost of transport) is lower than at any other walking speed [23]. It has been suggested that metabolic energy cost is minimized because the muscles have to do the least mechanical work at the speed where energy transfer is optimal [23].

The speed at which energy transfer is maximized during walking depends on body size. The optimum speed for energy transfer is lower for a small child than for an adult [21]. While a two-year-old child's optimum speed is about 0.6 m/s, an adult's optimum speed is about 1.6 m/s. A similar difference in optimum speed occurs among animal species due to their different body sizes. For example, a small lizard maximizes energy recovery at a much lower absolute speed than a sheep [22, 40]. In spite of this difference in optimum walking speed, energy transfer by the inverted pendulum mechanism reduces the mechanical work required for lifting and accelerating the center of mass by a similar fraction in animals of all body sizes. A 0.005 kg lizard or a 70 kg sheep reduce the mechanical work required to lift and accelerate the center of mass by about 50% through the inverted pendulum mechanism of energy exchange [22, 40]. Similarly, the mechanical work required to lift and accelerate the center of mass is reduced by about 60–70% for a two-year-old child or an adult human [21]. Thus, body size has a profound effect on the optimum walking speed but has little effect on energy conservation by the inverted pendulum mechanism.

In running, there cannot be substantial pendulum-like exchange between kinetic energy and gravitational potential energy since their fluctuations are nearly in phase with each other (Figure 10.6) [27]. Both kinetic energy and gravitational potential energy reach their minimum values at approximately the middle of the ground contact phase. As a result, the exchange of kinetic energy and gravitational potential energy conserves less than 5% of the mechanical work required to lift and accelerate the center of mass during running. Substantial mechanical energy, however, is conserved through the storage and return of energy in elastic tissues (to be discussed). Because the movements of the center of mass during running are similar to a bouncing ball [27], running is often referred to as a ''bouncing gait.'' A similar pattern of mechanical energy fluctuations occurs during fast gaits used by other animals [14, 22, 40, 51, 52, 64]. For example, trotting dogs, hopping kangaroos, running quail, and trotting cockroaches all have a similar pattern of mechanical energy fluctuations as running humans. Although the pattern of limb movements and gaits varies among these animals, all show the characteristic pattern of kinetic energy and gravitational potential energy being nearly exactly in phase with each other. All of these gaits are referred to as bouncing gaits.

Gait Transitions

It is clear that walking and running are distinctly different in terms of their patterns of ground reaction force and patterns of mechanical energy fluctuations. Indeed, simply watching a person gradually increase her forward speed and break from a walk to a run makes it obvious that there are distinct differences between walking and running. What determines the speed range where each of these distinctly different gaits is used? It is likely that by understanding the triggers for the gait transition, we will reach a better understanding of how the neuromuscular system and the physical characteristics of the body shape locomotion.

The transition from walking to running is not a smooth and continuous event. Rather, there is a distinct transition from one gait to the other that can be observed in both the kinematic and kinetic patterns [75, 77, 139]. For example, the transition from walking to running involves sudden changes in ground contact time, duty factor, ground reaction force, and movements of the center of mass. It is not yet clear exactly what triggers the transition from walking to running or vice-versa in humans or other animals [9, 33, 75-78, 86, 102, 103].

It was long believed that humans and other animals choose their gait transition speed based on minimization of the metabolic energy cost of locomotion [73]. In humans, the most economical gait at low speeds is a walk. As walking speed is increased, a speed is eventually reached where running requires less metabolic energy than walking [95, 96]. A similar pattern exists for quadrupedal animals [73]. Walking is most economical at low speeds, trotting is most economical at moderate speeds, and galloping is most economical at the highest speeds. However, the speed where an animal prefers to switch gaits is not the speed that would minimize metabolic energy cost. Horses switch from a trot to a gallop at a speed substantially below the optimal speed for minimizing metabolic energy cost. Thus, galloping actually requires more metabolic energy than trotting at the speed where a horse chooses to switch from a trot to a gallop [41]. Similarly, humans switch from a walk to a run at a speed that is not energetically optimal [76, 103]. These findings suggest that another factor, perhaps biomechanical, actually triggers gait transitions.

Based on the inverted pendulum mechanics of walking, it is reasonable to think that gravity is an important factor in determining the speed where the walk-run transition occurs. In walking, the gravitational force on the center of mass must be at least equal to the centripetal force needed to keep the center of mass moving in a circular arc as it vaults over the stance limb (Figure 3). The required centripetal force is equal to mv^2/L, where m = body mass, v = forward velocity, and L = leg length. The ratio between the centripetal force and the gravitational force $(mv^2/L)/(mg)$ is the Froude number (v^2/gL). Based on the mechanics of an inverted pendulum system, it has been predicted that humans and other animals should be able to use a walking gait only at speeds where the Froude number is less than or equal to 1 [1, 2]. This is so because the gravitational force is sufficient to keep the center of mass moving in a circular arc when the Froude number is less than or equal to 1. Experimental evidence has shown that humans and other bipeds (e.g., birds) with a large range of leg lengths prefer to switch from a walk to a run at a similar Froude number but at different absolute speeds [1, 4, 53, 78, 139]. Furthermore, when humans walk at different levels of simulated reduced gravity, they switch from a walk to a run at a similar Froude number (approximately 0.5) but at very different absolute speeds [86]. These observations suggest that the ratio of centripetal force to gravitational force is important in determining the gait transition speed. Nonetheless, it is puzzling that the gait transition occurs at a substantially lower Froude number than the theoretically predicted Froude number of 1.

Most gait transition studies to date have examined gait choice when humans or other animals move steadily at speeds near the transition speed. However, neither humans nor other animals naturally choose to move in this way in their every day lives. Generally, humans and other animals prefer to use speeds near the middle of each gait and rarely will choose other speeds for an extended period of time [73, 118]. Thus, they tend to make rapid transitions from one gait to another, which occur in concert with abrupt changes in speed [103]. In the extreme case of accelerating from a standstill, humans and other animals seem to immediately choose the appropriate gait for the speed to which they are accelerating. For example, a human sprinter runs, not walks, out of the blocks [24]. Similarly, a dog immediately gallops at the beginning of a sprint regardless of its starting speed. These observations suggest that in the future it will be important to examine gait choices in more natural locomotor patterns, including acceleration and deceleration.

Behavioral Models for Walking and Running

One way to gain insight into the behavior of the overall musculoskeletal system during locomotion is to employ simple mechanical models of walking and running. These behavioral models simulate the movements of the center of mass during locomotion by modeling the output of the integrated musculoskeletal system using mechanical elements. These models can provide a guide for studies of lower levels of organization within the musculoskeletal and neuromuscular systems. They are particularly valuable in delimiting the potential strategies that the neuromuscular system could use to produce walking and running.

WALKING BEHAVIORAL MODELS. The simplest behavioral model for walking is an inverted pendulum. This model consists of a rigid strut that represents the leg and a point mass equal to body mass (Figure 10.3) [1]. In this model, the mass vaults over a rigid leg during the stance phase, and the center of mass reaches its highest point at mid-stance. In the inverted pendulum model, like in a standard pendulum, the gravitational potential energy of the mass is exactly 180^0 out of phase with the kinetic energy. As a result, at mid-stance, the gravitational potential energy is maximized and the kinetic energy is minimized. This pattern of mechanical energy fluctuations is qualitatively similar to the pattern observed during walking in humans (Figure 10.5) and other animals. In bipedal animals, including humans, it is easy to visualize that the rigid strut in the inverted pendulum model corresponds to the stance limb. For animals with four or more legs (e.g., a dog or a ghost crab), all of the legs in contact with the ground cooperate to produce movements of the center of mass similar to those of a mass vaulting over a single rigid limb.

In an idealized inverted pendulum model, 100% recovery of mechanical energy occurs due to the exchange between gravitational potential energy and kinetic energy. As previously discussed, a walking human has a maximum recovery of mechanical energy of about 60–70% [28]. Clearly, part of the reason why human walkers do not achieve 100% recovery is that their legs do not behave exactly like rigid struts. The functional leg length (i.e., distance from point of foot-ground contact to the center of mass) changes to some extent during the stance phase [134]. This is different from the behavior of the rigid strut that represents the leg in the idealized inverted pendulum model. In fact, sensitivity analyses on mechanical models suggest that leg compression is an important parameter in determining the pattern of ground reaction force and center of mass movements during walking [109–111]. Although an inverted pendulum model with a rigid leg does a good job of predicting the mechanical energy fluctuations of the center of mass, it does not accurately predict the ground reaction force pattern [109]. Adding compliance to the leg model greatly improves the prediction of the ground reaction force pattern [5, 109–111, 134, 144].

Leg geometry at the beginning of the stance phase also plays an important role in determining the pattern of ground reaction force and the pendulum-like exchange of mechanical energies during walking. When humans are asked to walk while using exaggerated leg joint flexion during stance, the peak ground reaction force decreases [156] and the pendulum-like exchange of center of mass energy decreases [88]. Chimpanzees, animals that naturally walk with flexed limbs, have similar patterns of ground reaction force and energy exchange as humans walking with exaggerated limb flexion [88]. The role of leg geometry in determining the dynamics of walking is further emphasized by the observation that the peak ground reaction force and loading rate increase when humans walk with stiffer and straighter limbs than usual [31]. These studies suggest that one role of normal joint flexion during the stance phase is to reduce the ground reaction force and the vertical movements of the center of mass. Pelvic tilt and pelvic rotation also serve to reduce the vertical movements of the center of mass during walking [79, 132].

In spite of these deviations from the simple inverted pendulum model for walking, anthropomorphic passive walking machines with rigid stance legs demonstrate walking mechanics very similar to that of humans [98, 99]. These machines take advantage of pendulum-like energy exchange by the center of mass of the body and also by the swinging leg. The idea of having the swing limb move passively via pendulum-like energy exchange is based on mathematical models and observations of humans walking at moderate speeds [53, 97–99, 104, 105]. Electromyographic measurements show that nearly no muscle activity is present in the swing limb at some walking speeds [8]. It is thought that the limb swings forward passively after the muscles start the limb into motion during the period of double support. Because of the energy exchanged by the swing limb and the center of mass, anthropomorphic passive walking machines only need the added energy input of moving down a slight hill to counteract the small energy losses that occur with each stride. It is interesting to note that although passive walking machines do not have any control systems, they are capable of walking in a stable and predictable pattern [98, 99]. Their dynamics are determined by the physical structure of the walker, demonstrating that inherent mechanical properties of the body can greatly simplify the control of locomotion.

RUNNING BEHAVIORAL MODELS. Because the movements of the center of mass during running are similar to those of a bouncing ball, it is not surprising that running models rely upon springs. Running is often modeled as a simple spring-mass model that consists of a single linear "leg spring" and a point mass that is equivalent to body mass (Figure 4) [3, 13, 100]. The leg spring stiffness represents the overall stiffness of the integrated musculoskeletal system. In bouncing gaits, the leg spring compresses during the first half of the ground contact phase and lengthens during the second half of the ground contact phase. These changes in leg length result from flexion and extension of leg joints. In spite of its apparent simplicity, this spring-mass model describes and predicts the dynamics of running gaits in humans and numerous other species remarkably well [15, 37–39, 42, 43, 63].

Leg stiffness plays an important role in determining the dynamics of the interaction between the stance leg and the ground. Many aspects of running depend on a runner's leg stiffness, including the time of foot-ground contact, the vertical excursion of the body's center of mass during the ground contact phase, and the ground reaction force [39, 100]. Leg stiffness is defined as the ratio of the ground reaction force to the compression of the leg spring ($\triangle L$) at the instant at mid-stance when the leg is maximally compressed (Figure 4). In a running human, the leg stiffness represents the average stiffness of the stance limb. In animals with more than one limb simultaneously in contact with the ground, the leg stiffness in the spring-mass model represents the average combined stiffness of all of the limbs in contact with the ground [15, 38].

Leg stiffness remains the same at all forward speeds in running humans (Figure 10.7) [63]. They are able to run at higher speeds, and with shorter ground contact times, by increasing the angle swept by the leg during the stance phase (Figure 10.8). A variety of hopping, trotting, and running animals keep leg stiffness the same at all speeds (Figure 7) and alter the angle swept by the leg to adjust for different speeds [38]. Although the stiffness of the leg remains the same at all speeds of running, humans are capable of altering their leg stiffness during bouncing gaits. Humans change their leg stiffness in order to alter stride frequency during hopping in place or forward running [37, 39]. In addition, recent findings show that humans adjust the stiffness of their legs to offset changes in surface stiffness [42, 43]. If leg stiffness were not adjusted to accommodate surface stiffness, then many aspects of the dynamics of running would vary depending on surface stiffness. By adjusting leg stiffness, humans are able to have the same the peak ground reaction force, ground contact time, and vertical displacement of the center of mass regardless of surface stiffness [42, 43].

FIGURE 10.7.

Leg stiffness versus speed for running humans and trotting dogs. For the dogs, the leg stiffness represents the total stiffness of the two limbs on the ground during each ground contact phase.

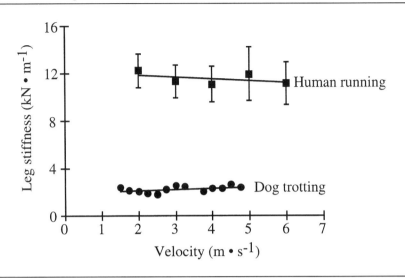

FIGURE 10.8.

The spring-mass model representing low speed running and high speed running. The leg stiffness and leg compression are the same in both models. The only difference is that the angle swept by the leg spring (θ) is greater in the model representing high speed running. Because of the greater angle swept by the leg at the higher speed, the vertical displacement of the mass during the ground contact phase is smaller at the higher speed.

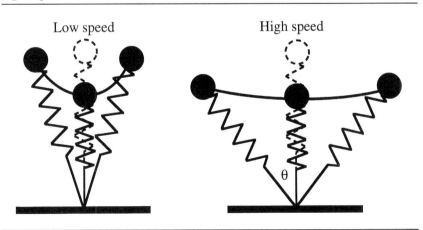

Just as human legs behave like springs during running, the fastest robots also have spring-based legs [126–129]. We can gain insight into the control strategies that are possible in animal bouncing gaits by exploring the range of workable strategies in these robots. These robots use either compressed air or metal springs in their legs to store and return elastic energy with each step as they run, hop, or trot. There are many similarities between bouncing gaits in these robots and in animals. Both these robots and animals run at different speeds by altering the angle swept by their legs while keeping their leg stiffness the same [38, 63, 129]. In addition, altering the robot's leg stiffness leads to changes in stride frequency at the same speed [129], as is observed in humans [37, 39]. The control of these robots is greatly simplified by relying on the passive dynamics of spring-mass system of the robot's body. The robot's movements are largely determined by physical parameters including the stiffness of the leg spring, the angle at which the leg spring is set down, and the mass of the robot [126]. The control algorithms work in concert with the physical properties of the robot's body to produce stable locomotion. It seems logical to suggest that animals rely on the spring-mass dynamics of their bodies in a similar manner, thus simplifying the neural control of locomotion.

JOINT MOMENTS, WORK AND POWER

So far, we have discussed the mechanics of locomotion at the whole body level, including the ground reaction force, mechanical energy of the center of mass, and the behavior of the overall leg. During locomotion, muscles generate moments and perform mechanical work at the joints, producing the ground reaction force and the movements of the body. The next section will concentrate on the current understanding of joint dynamics during walking and running. The focus of this section will be the moments and mechanical work produced by muscles at each joint. Understanding locomotion at the level of muscle action at each joint provides a bridge for understanding the link between the movements of the center of mass and the actions of individual muscle-tendon units. Little published information is available about muscle moments and mechanical work at each joint during locomotion in diverse animal species [44, 94, 136]. Thus, it is difficult to assess the similarities and differences between humans and other animals at this level of organization.

Net Muscle Moments

The muscles of the body operate by exerting moments about joints. To begin to understand how the neuromuscular system produces walking and running, researchers often examine the "net muscle moment" or "generalized muscle moment" about a joint [149, 163]. A net muscle moment includes the moments produced by all of the muscles, tendons, ligaments, and contact forces at the joint. The moment produced by muscle-tendon forces is thought to be much higher than the moment produced by the ligaments or other joint forces over the range of joint angles that occur during locomotion [149, 154]. As a result, the net muscle moment gives a reasonable approximation of the net moment produced by all the muscles at a joint [12, 46]. An inverse dynamics approach can be used to determine the net muscle moments during locomotion. This involves using force platform, kinematic, and anthropomorphic measurements in concert with a rigid linked segment model. The Newtonian equations of angular and translational motion are applied to each segment starting distally and moving proximally [34, 149, 163].

This type of approach has revealed that the net muscle moment during the ground contact phase of walking is the largest at the ankle and is substantially lower at the knee and hip [18, 19, 32, 34, 115, 135, 143, 146, 148, 162]. At the ankle, the net muscle moment tends to extend (equivalent to "plantarflex") the joint throughout the ground contact phase. Electromyographic (EMG) measurements have revealed that both extensor muscles (e.g., gastrocnemius) and flexor muscles (e.g., tibialis anterior) are active during the ground contact phase, occasionally simultaneously [32]. The observation that the net muscle moment tends to extend the ankle shows that the ankle extensor muscles are creating a larger moment than the ankle flexor muscles. The net muscle moment about the ankle is very small during the swing phase.

The net muscle moments at the knee and hip during the ground contact phase of walking are much smaller and more variable than at the ankle [18, 19, 34, 115, 116, 135, 143, 146, 148, 162]. The ground reaction force vector is closely aligned with the knee and hip. As a result, small net muscle moments at the knee and hip are required in order to exert a given force on the ground [135, 143]. The exact pattern of net muscle moment at the knee and hip varies between subjects and is matched by variation in the EMG patterns of the major limb muscles [115]. This observation has led to the proposal that different individuals use different motor strategies for walking [116, 117]. It has been suggested that these individual patterns are consistent with a strategy that minimizes the total muscle effort for each individual [117].

Walking kinematics are far less variable than the net muscle moments or the muscle activation patterns at the knee and hip [148, 151]. A comparison of strides that have dramatically different net muscle moment patterns at the knee and hip shows that the limb kinematics are remarkably similar. This observation led Winter [146] to propose the idea of a "support moment" equal to the sum of the net muscle moments at the ankle, knee, and hip. Data on walking humans show that the support moment is substantially less variable than the net muscle moment at each individual joint. Thus, it seems that changes in muscle activation and net muscle moment at one joint are offset by changes at another joint. This conclusion is further supported by the observation that humans with various injuries can still walk in a kinematically normal manner by changing the pattern of muscle activation [150].

As one would expect, the peak magnitude of the net muscle moment at each joint is higher during running than during walking [32, 92, 93, 147]. The leg is compliant during running, and the major leg joints undergo substantial flexion and extension during the ground contact phase. In contrast, during walking, the limb behaves more like a stiff strut, and the joints undergo smaller angular displacements, remaining relatively extended throughout the ground contact phase. As a result of the postural difference, the muscles must generate larger joint moments in order to exert a given force on the ground during running than during walking. The net muscle moment tends to extend the joint at the ankle, knee, and hip during running (Figure 10.9) [32, 92, 93, 147]. The peak net muscle moment is larger at the knee than at the other joints. Indeed, this is a major difference between running and walking. The magnitude of the peak net muscle moment at the knee is much larger during running than walking. The knee is substantially more flexed at the middle of the ground contact phase of running, and as a result, a higher net muscle moment is required in order to exert a given ground force during running compared to walking.

In contrast to walking, running involves little variability in the pattern and magnitude of the ground reaction force or the net muscle moments [147]. It has been speculated that the net muscle moments are less variable in running than in walking because the muscles are operating closer to their force limits [147].

Joint Power and Work

The net power output at a joint can be calculated from the product of the net muscle moment and the joint angular velocity. When the net muscle moment and the angular velocity are both in the same direction, there is net power production at the joint. Conversely, when the net muscle moment and the joint angular velocity are in opposite directions, there is net power absorption at the joint. The net muscle mechanical work can be calculated from the integral of the power with respect to time.

It is important to realize that the net power output measured at a joint is not necessarily produced by muscles that cross that particular joint. This is because there are many muscles in the body that cross more than one joint. These muscles can transport power produced by muscles acting across one joint and allow them to contribute to the power output at another joint [140]. The extent to which this transfer occurs during human walking or running is not clear [80, 122], but there is evidence that energy transfer by biarticular muscles is substantial during cat locomotion [123].

The net power and net work output are substantially lower at all the joints during walking than during running [131, 162]. During walking, both

FIGURE 10.9.

(A) Net muscle moment at the ankle, knee, and hip during running at 2.5 m/s. A positive net muscle moment indicates that it tends to extend the joint. (B) Net muscle power output at the ankle, knee, and hip during running. Positive values indicate that power is produced, and negative values indicate that power is absorbed.

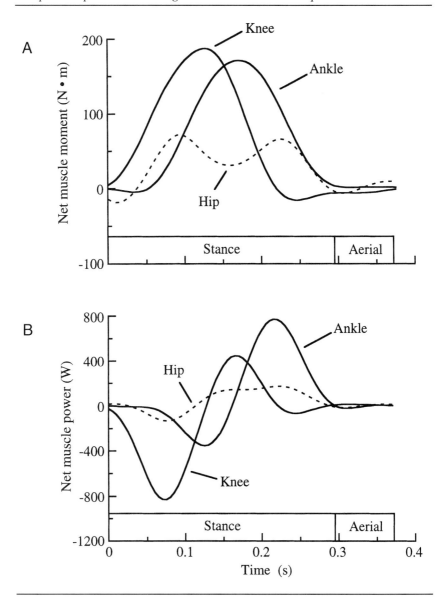

the net muscle moments and the joint angular velocities are lower than in running. The low net power and work outputs at the major limb joints observed during walking would be expected for a limb that is behaving like a stiff strut.

The net power output and work output are much higher during running than walking. The net power outputs for slow jogging have been described extensively [147]. At the ankle and knee, an extensor net muscle moment throughout the ground contact phase exists (Figure 10.9). Meanwhile, the ankle and knee both flex and absorb mechanical energy during the first part of the ground contact phase. Later in the ground contact phase, the ankle and knee both extend and produce mechanical power. The net power output is small and unpredictable at the hip. During low speed jogging, the ankle produces more mechanical energy than it absorbs. In contrast, the knee absorbs more mechanical energy than it produces.

MUSCLE-TENDON MECHANICS

Examining the net muscle action at joints provides a link between whole body dynamics and muscle-tendon dynamics during locomotion. This section will discuss muscle-tendon action during locomotion. Unfortunately, it has been difficult to quantify muscle-tendon forces and length changes during locomotion, although recent technological advances have yielded new and exciting findings. In addition, the incredible complexity and apparent redundancy of the musculoskeletal system has made discerning general principles about muscle-tendon action during locomotion extremely challenging. In this section, we will examine information about muscle-tendon forces and muscle-tendon length changes during locomotion. We will then discuss how this information can be incorporated into forward dynamics and inverse dynamics approaches in order to uncover fundamental rules about how the neuromuscular system produces locomotion.

Muscle-Tendon Force During Locomotion

While center of mass movements and net muscle moments at joints can be calculated relatively easily from force platform and video data using an inverse dynamics approach, muscle-tendon forces during locomotion are much more difficult to determine. Each leg joint has multiple muscle-tendon units that span it, and each muscle-tendon has its own unique force-generating capabilities. Thus, the contribution of each muscle-tendon unit acting about a joint to the net muscle moment is not easily determined. It may seem reasonable to use simplifying assumptions to partition the net muscle moment among different muscles that have a given action (e.g., all synergists experience equal stresses), but direct measurements *in vivo* have shown that the distribution of muscle force is not so simple. In fact, the contribution of each synergist changes for different locomotion speeds, different gaits, and even during the course of a single stance phase [10, 44, 68, 70, 145].

One way researchers have attempted to solve this problem is by employing inverse optimization techniques. Inverse optimization (sometimes called static optimization [161]) uses a model of the musculoskeletal system and requires it to produce specified movement dynamics while optimizing a given cost function (e.g., minimization of the sum of muscle forces) [152]. Although numerous optimization criteria have been suggested for use in the cost function (e.g., minimal muscle force, minimal muscle stress, minimal energy expenditure, minimal ligament force, minimal intra-articular contact force, minimal instantaneous muscle power, and minimal muscle fatigue), no single "best" parameter has been found. In fact, when several of the most commonly used criteria were compared, they predicted remarkably similar patterns of muscle activation, but none demonstrated a close match to the actual EMG patterns over a complete stride cycle [30]. At present, we do not yet sufficiently understand the distribution of forces among synergists to identify any general rules [65].

Muscle-tendon force calculations from an inverse dynamics approach are also complicated by the possibility of coactivation of antagonistic muscle groups. When antagonistic muscle groups are simultaneously active, a higher agonist force is required to exert a given net muscle moment. For example, during the ground contact phase of running, there is an extensor net muscle moment at the knee. EMG studies have shown that knee extensor (e.g., vasti muscles) and knee flexor muscles (e.g., gastrocnemius) are active simultaneously. As a result of this coactivation, a higher force is required from the knee extensors than if there were no coactivation. The coactivation makes it impossible to determine the force in either muscle group from an inverse dynamics approach, since there are an infinite number of combinations of extensor and flexor forces that could produce the same net muscle moment. It is interesting to note, however, that there is little coactivation of extensor and flexor muscles at the ankle during bouncing gaits. Thus, an inverse dynamics approach to calculating ankle extensor force yields reasonably similar values as a direct measurement of the muscle-tendon force [11, 12, 46]. There is substantial antagonist coactivation at the knee and the hip during locomotion, and as a result, an inverse dynamics approach is less likely to yield accurate muscle force values at those joints.

Forces in muscle-tendon units are measured *in vivo* through the use of force transducers on tendons (recently reviewed by Gregor and Abelew [57]). In a few cases, a buckle transducer was placed on the Achilles' tendon of humans [46, 47, 58, 59, 82, 84]. The results from these studies show that the peak Achilles' tendon force slightly decreases or remains about the same (~2.6 kN or 3.6 bodyweights) as humans increase walking speed from

FIGURE 10.10.
Horizontal ground reaction force, vertical ground reaction force, and Achilles tendon force (measured with a tendon buckle) for a human walking at different speeds. Reprinted with permission from Komi et al. [84].

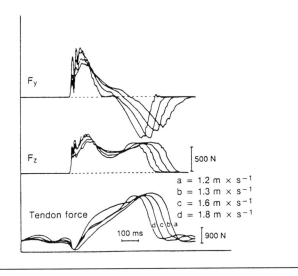

1.2 to 1.8 m/s (Figure 10.10) [84]. As they increase speed further and begin running, the peak tendon force increases to a maximum (~9 kN or 12.5 bodyweights) at a speed of approximately 6 m/s and then changes very little at higher running speeds [84]. Interestingly, both walking and running involve greater peak Achilles' tendon forces than maximal height squat jumps or countermovement jumps [84]. While these studies have provided rare *in vivo* muscle-tendon data for human locomotion, the invasiveness of the technique limits the possibilities for human studies.

Alternatively, the use of force transducers on the tendons of animals has enabled researchers to investigate numerous different research questions [10, 57, 69, 121, 122, 125, 130]. With animals, tendons can be surgically separated so that force data can be collected from individual muscle-tendon units. Unfortunately, current buckle-type transducers may affect the muscle's force generation since they sometimes damage the tendon, causing it to fray and break [57]. However, new types of force transducers that are actually inserted within a tendon or ligament are being developed that should correct this problem [55, 66, 67, 71, 72, 83, 85].

Muscle-Tendon Length Changes During Locomotion

Perhaps surprisingly, the calculation of muscle and tendon length changes during locomotion is even more complicated than the determination of muscle-tendon forces. The most common method for calculating muscle-tendon length change has been to use a combination of kinematic and anatomical data. In this approach, the instantaneous muscle-tendon length is estimated from the approximate origin and insertion sites for a given muscle-tendon unit, and from joint kinematic data [6, 45, 56, 60, 106, 120]. However, this technique does not partition the total displacement of the muscle-tendon unit into the length changes due to muscle fiber displacement, muscle fiber pennation angle change, or tendon strain. Each of these factors can substantially affect the total muscle-tendon length, and each has different implications for muscle-tendon function [48, 49, 62, 108, 130].

The relevance of partitioning muscle-tendon displacements into respective components becomes evident during "isometric" contractions in which isolated muscle-tendon units are held at a constant total length. When electrically stimulated, the fibers of muscles with long compliant tendons can shorten considerably as the tendon is stretched [36, 62]. Even though the whole muscle-tendon length remains unchanged, each component of the unit changes length substantially. Thus, although it is possible to estimate the length changes of the overall muscle-tendon unit during locomotion, this information tells us little about the relative length changes of the different components of the muscle-tendon unit.

A recent technological innovation is the use of sonomicrometry to measure muscle fiber displacements and velocities *in vivo* [20, 61]. By suturing piezoelectric crystals into a muscle fiber bundle, the time required for ultrasound pulses to travel from one crystal to another can be measured. The transit time can then be used to calculate the instantaneous muscle fiber length. Studies on walking cats and running turkeys have shown that the muscle fiber does not always follow the same displacement pattern as the whole muscle-tendon unit [62, 130]. In walking cats, the medial gastrocnemius muscle fibers shorten at the beginning of the ground contact phase, even though the overall muscle-tendon unit lengthens during this phase [62]. As a result, the tendon is stretched more and stores more elastic energy than would be predicted based on the overall muscle-tendon unit length change. Similarly, when turkeys run on level ground, the gastrocnemius muscle fibers remain nearly isometric during the stance phase while the tendon undergoes substantial length change (Figure 10.11) [130]. The tendon performs the majority of the combined muscle-tendon work while the muscle does very little work. Thus, during level locomotion in both cats and turkeys, the work done by some muscles is greatly reduced by the storage and return of elastic energy in tendons.

Elastic energy storage in tendons is particularly important for bouncing gaits [3]. The ankle extensor tendons have been studied most often, and the results have shown that they play a key role in the storage of elastic energy. In a running human, these tendons can store and return up to 35% of the mechanical energy needed to lift and accelerate the center of

FIGURE 10.11.

Lateral gastrocnemius muscle fiber length, EMG, and force in a turkey during running at 3 m/s on level ground. Muscle fiber length was measured using sonomicrometry, and muscle force was measured using a strain gauge attached to a calcified portion of the tendon. Reprinted with permission from Roberts, T.J., R.L. Marsh, P.G. Weyand, and C.R. Taylor. Muscular force in running turkeys: the economy of minimizing work. Science 275:1113–1115, 1997. Copyright 1997, American Association for the Advancement of Science.

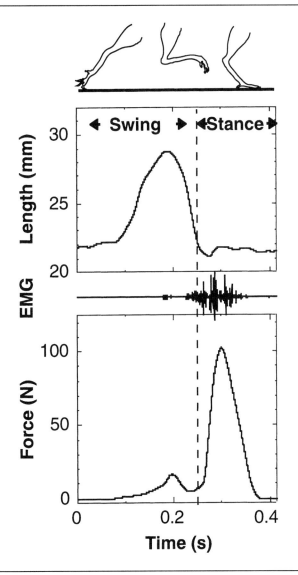

mass during a stride [81]. Tendon buckle studies on hopping wallabies have revealed that the ankle extensor tendons store and return enough elastic energy to reduce the metabolic cost of locomotion by about 50% [10]. It is important to realize that tendon can be divided into two components—the external free tendon and the aponeurosis [159]. A number of recent studies have examined the relative compliance of these two portions of the tendon and have come to different conclusions [36, 89, 124, 125, 133, 137, 164]. As a result, it is not clear which part of the tendon is most important in elastic energy storage during locomotion.

Role of Forward Dynamics Simulations in Understanding Muscle-Tendon Function During Locomotion

A promising alternative to invasive *in vivo* muscle-tendon measurements in human locomotion is forward dynamics computer simulations of human locomotion [160]. Instead of calculating net muscle moments from the ground reaction force and kinematic data (i.e., inverse dynamics), forward dynamics simulations rely on musculoskeletal models and computer software to predict the muscle activation patterns and muscle-tendon dynamics during normal locomotion. The difficulties with this approach, however, are that the results from detailed musculoskeletal models can be extremely sensitive to the specifics of the model [87, 155], and experimental validation of the muscle-tendon mechanics is difficult to obtain. Nonetheless, this approach has been used to simulate human walking with some success [119, 157, 158].

Forward dynamics simulations have also been used in conjunction with sensitivity analyses to determine which aspects of musculoskeletal design are most important in dictating the mechanics of locomotion [54]. In the future, this combination of forward dynamics simulations and sensitivity analyses should prove valuable in providing insight into how muscle-tendon properties and activation patterns can affect joint dynamics and center of mass movements during locomotion.

When forward dynamics simulations are employed in conjunction with optimization techniques, they allow the researcher to probe the link between muscle-tendon properties and muscle activation patterns based on possible goals of the central nervous system (called "dynamic optimization" by Zajac [160] and "forward dynamic optimization" by Winters [152]. In this approach, a parameter or function is assumed to be optimized by the neuromuscular system, and the pattern of muscle activation that optimizes that parameter or function is identified. This approach is used most often to study movements in which an optimality criterion is obvious, such as a single maximum height vertical jump [7, 16, 17, 112-114, 140-142]. For locomotion, it is difficult to determine which parameter or function should be optimized. One possibility is that the minimization of metabolic energy cost is the most important factor in determining which neuromuscular strategy is used in sustained locomotion [4, 138]. However, controlling the level of musculoskeletal forces and stresses can also play an important role [41, 118]. Indeed, it seems most likely that multiple factors work in concert to shape locomotion, suggesting that multiple optimization criteria should be used [153].

Data from experiments on equine locomotion support the idea that multiple factors work in concert to shape locomotion, and thus, that multiple optimization criteria should be used. Experiments have revealed that there are at least two factors involved in the choice of locomotor speed and gait in horses—metabolic energy cost minimization and musculoskeletal force minimization. During unrestrained overground locomotion, horses only use a small range of speeds within each gait, and within this range of speeds, the metabolic energy cost is lower than at any other speed within the gait [74]. This observation suggests that metabolic energy cost is an important factor that influences the choice of speed during locomotion [73]. Nevertheless, when the mechanics and energetics of the transition from trotting to galloping are examined more closely, it is clear that horses do not choose to switch from one gait to another at the speed that would minimize the metabolic energetic cost of locomotion [41]. Rather, the choice of gait transition speed seems to be most influenced by the level of musculoskeletal force [41]. Thus, at least two factors are important in shaping locomotion in horses, emphasizing the need to consider multiple optimization criteria in forward dynamics simulations of locomotion.

Role of an Inverse Dynamics Approach in Understanding Muscle-Tendon Function During Locomotion

The complexity of the neuromuscular system has hindered progress in gaining a fundamental understanding of how locomotion is produced. This complexity has made it difficult to reach a synthesized understanding of locomotion. As a result, it may be helpful to pursue an alternative to a reductionist approach that begins with detailed descriptions of individual muscles and their neural control. This possibility may have been best expressed by Loeb who asked whether "it is useful to collect yet more inexplicable data," and suggested that "it may be useful to consider the performance goals of the whole behavior" [90]. Given the tremendous complexity of the nervous system and the musculoskeletal system, we can imagine a seemingly infinite number of possible neuromuscular strategies that could produce the locomotion of humans and other animals. Indeed, numerous different patterns of joint moments and muscle activation can produce normal walking [115, 116, 148]. By reaching an understanding of overriding performance goals (e.g., the need for a given "support moment" during walking, [146], we can focus in on a more limited range of potential strategies that will produce normal locomotion. An inverse dynamics approach that begins with defined performance goals at the whole organism level allows us to do this.

Simple behavioral models play an important role in an inverse dynamics approach to understanding locomotion. They provide a mechanical description of the overall behavior (or "performance goals") of the musculoskeletal system during locomotion. Behavioral models represent the behavior but not the structure of the musculoskeletal system during locomotion. For example, as described previously, a simple spring-mass system provides a reasonably accurate model of running. This model works because the human leg behaves much like a spring during running. However, we are all well aware that the human leg is not actually a spring. Rather, it is made up of multiple muscles, tendons, and ligaments that span several joints. Thus, after identifying an appropriate behavioral model, we must begin to consider how the real musculoskeletal system produces the observed behavior.

In the example case of running, the observation that the overall leg behaves like a spring suggests that the production of spring-like behavior may be an important organizing principle for the actions of multiple muscle-tendon units. The goal of producing spring-like behavior limits the number of potential solutions for the behavior of individual joints, interactions between multiple joints, and actions of individual muscle-tendon units that span each joint. It also makes it clear that an important next step is to examine the spring-like properties of individual joints and muscle-tendon units during running. At this point in the progression, a combination of information from behavioral models and realistic musculoskeletal models is likely to be most powerful in dissecting the roles of individual joints and muscle-tendon units in determining leg stiffness, and thus, the mechanics of running.

CONCLUSIONS

Humans use the same basic mechanisms to walk and run as other legged animals. Walking gaits rely on a transfer of kinetic and gravitational potential energies with each step similar to an inverted pendulum. Running gaits, on the other hand, can be characterized as bouncing gaits and modeled with a simple spring-mass system. These two behavioral models, the inverted pendulum and the spring-mass system, provide researchers with simple descriptions of overall limb behavior and center of mass movements during walking and running. This information can provide guidance in attempts to discern general rules by which the neuromuscular system produces locomotion at the increasingly complex lower levels of organization.

ACKNOWLEDGMENTS

This work was supported in part by the National Institutes of Health (R29 AR44008) and the National Aeronautics and Space Administration (NGT-51416).

REFERENCES

1. Alexander, R.M. Mechanics and scaling of terrestrial locomotion. T.J. Pedley (ed.). *Scale Effects in Animal Locomotion.* New York: Academic Press, 1977, pp. 93–110.
2. Alexander, R.M. Terrestrial Locomotion. R.M. Alexander and G. Goldspink (eds.). *Mechanics and Energetics of Animal Locomotion.* London: Chapman & Hall, 1977, pp. 168–203.
3. Alexander, R.M. Elastic Mechanisms in Animal Movement. Cambridge: Cambridge University Press, 1988.
4. Alexander, R.M. Optimization and gaits in the locomotion of vertebrates. *Physiol. Rev.* 69:1199–1227, 1989.
5. Alexander, R.M. A model of bipedal locomotion on compliant legs. *Philos. Trans. R. Soc. Lond. Biol. Sci.* B338:189–198, 1992.
6. Alexander, R.M., and A. Vernon. Mechanics of hopping by kangaroos (Macropodidae). *J. Zool. (London)* 177:265–303, 1975.
7. Anderson, F.C., and M.G. Pandy. Storage and utilization of elastic strain energy during jumping. *J. Biomech.* 26:1413–1427, 1993.
8. Basmajian, J.V., and C. De Luca. *Muscles Alive: Their Function Revealed by Electromyography.* Baltimore: Williams & Wilkins, 1985.
9. Beuter, A., and F. Lalonde. Analysis of a phase transition in human locomotion using singularity theory. *Neurosci. Res. Comm.* 3:127–132, 1988.
10. Biewener, A.A., and R.V. Baudinette. In vivo muscle force and elastic energy storage during steady-speed hopping of tammar wallabies, (Macropus eugenii). *J. Exp. Biol.* 198: 1829–1841, 1995.
11. Biewener, A.A., and R. Blickhan. Kangaroo rat locomotion: design for elastic energy storage or acceleration? *J. Exp. Biol.* 140:243–255, 1988.
12. Biewener, A.A., R. Blickhan, A.K. Perry, N.C. Heglund, and C.R. Taylor. Muscle forces during locomotion in kangaroo rats: force platform and tendon buckle measurements compared. *J. Exp. Biol.* 137:191–205, 1988.
13. Blickhan, R. The spring-mass model for running and hopping. *J. Biomech.* 22:1217–1227, 1989.
14. Blickhan, R., and R.J. Full. Locomotion energetics of ghost crab. II. Mechanics of the center of mass during walking and running. *J. Exp. Biol.* 130:155–174, 1987.
15. Blickhan, R., and R.J. Full. Similarity in multilegged locomotion: bouncing like a monopode. *J. Comp. Physiol.* A173:509–517, 1993.
16. Bobbert, M.F., and A.J. Van Soest. Effects of muscle strengthening on vertical jump height: a simulation study. *Med. Sci. Sports Exerc.* 26:1012–1020, 1994.
17. Bobbert, M.F., and J.P.Van Zandwijk. Dependence of human maximum jump height on moment arms of the bi-articular m. gastrocnemius: a simulation study. *Hum. Mov. Sci.* 13:697–716, 1994.
18. Bresler, B., and J.P. Frankel. The forces and moments in the leg during level walking. *J. Appl. Mech.* 72:27–36, 1950.
19. Cappozzo, A., F. Figura, and M. Marchetti. The interplay of muscular and external forces in human ambulation. *J. Biomech.* 9:35–43, 1976.
20. Caputi, A.A., J.A. Hoffer, and I.E. Pose. Velocity of ultrasound in active and passive cat medial gastrocnemius muscle. *J. Biomech.* 25:1067–1074, 1992.
21. Cavagna, G.A., P. Franzetti, and T. Fuchimoto. The mechanics of walking in children. *J. Physiol. (London)* 343:323–339, 1983.
22. Cavagna, G.A., N.C. Heglund, and C.R. Taylor. Mechanical work in terrestrial locomotion: two basic mechanisms for minimizing energy expenditure. *Am. J. Physiol.* 233: R243–R261, 1977.
23. Cavagna, G.A., and M. Kaneko. Mechanical work and efficiency in level walking and running. *J. Physiol. (London)* 268:647–681, 1977.
24. Cavagna, G.A., L. Komarek, and S. Mazzoleni. The mechanics of sprint running. *J. Physiol. (London)* 217:709–721, 1971.

25. Cavagna, G.A., and R. Margaria. Mechanics of walking. *J. Appl. Physiol.* 21:271–278, 1966.
26. Cavagna, G.A., F. P. Saibene, and R. Margaria. External work in walking. *J. Appl. Physiol.* 18:1–9, 1963.
27. Cavagna, G.A., F.P. Saibene, and R. Margaria. Mechanical work in running. *J. Appl. Physiol.* 19:249–256, 1964.
28. Cavagna, G.A., H. Thys, and A. Zamboni. The sources of external work in level walking and running. *J. Physiol. (London)* 262:639–657, 1976.
29. Cavanagh, P.R., and M.A. Lafortune. Ground reaction forces in distance running. *J. Biomech.* 13:397–406, 1980.
30. Collins, J.J. The redundant nature of locomotor optimization laws. *J. Biomech.* 28:251–267, 1995.
31. Cook, T.M., K.P. Farrell, I.A. Carey, J.M. Gibbs, and G.E. Wiger. Effects of restricted knee flexion and walking speed on the vertical ground reaction force during gait. *J. Orthop. Sports Phys. Ther.* 25:236–244, 1997.
32. DeVita, P. The selection of a standard convention for analyzing gait data based on the analysis of relevant biomechanical factors. *J. Biomech.* 27:501–508, 1994.
33. Diedrich, F.J., and W.H. Warren, Jr. Why change gaits? Dynamics of the walk-run transition. *J. Exp. Psychol. Hum. Percept. Perform.* 21:183–202, 1995.
34. Elftman, H. Forces and energy changes in the leg during walking. *Am. J. Physiol.* 124:339–356, 1939.
35. Elftman, H. The work done by muscles in running. *Am. J. Physiol.* 129:672–684, 1940.
36. Ettema, G.J., and P.A. Huijing. Properties of the tendinous structures and series elastic component of EDL muscle-tendon complex of the rat. *J. Biomech.* 22:1209–1215, 1989.
37. Farley, C.T., R. Blickhan, J. Saito, and C.R. Taylor. Hopping frequency in humans: a test of how springs set stride frequency in bouncing gaits. *J. Appl. Physiol.* 71:2127–2132, 1991.
38. Farley, C.T., J. Glasheen, and T.A. McMahon. Running springs: speed and animal size. *J. Exp. Biol.* 185:71–86, 1993.
39. Farley, C.T., and O. Gonzalez. Leg stiffness and stride frequency in human running. *J. Biomech.* 29:181–186, 1996.
40. Farley, C.T., and T.C. Ko. Two basic mechanisms in lizard locomotion. *J. Exp. Biol.* 200:2177–2188, 1997.
41. Farley, C.T., and C.R. Taylor. A mechanical trigger for the trot-gallop transition in horses. *Science* 253:306–308, 1991.
42. Ferris, D.P., and C.T. Farley. Interaction of leg stiffness and surface stiffness during human hopping. *J. Appl. Physiol.* 82:15–22, 1997.
43. Ferris, D.P., M. Louie, and C.T. Farley. Adjustments in running mechanics to accommodate different surface stiffnesses. *Physiologist* 39:A59, 1996.
44. Fowler, E.G., R.J. Gregor, J.A. Hodgson, and R.R. Roy. Relationship between ankle muscle and joint kinetics during the stance phase of locomotion in the cat. *J. Biomech.* 26:465–483, 1993.
45. Frigo, C. Determination of the muscle length during locomotion. E. Asmussen and K. Jorgensen (eds.). *Biomechanics VI-A.* Baltimore, MD: University Park Press, 1978, pp. 355–360.
46. Fukashiro, S., P.V. Komi, M. Jarvinen, and M. Miyashita. Comparison between the directly measured Achilles tendon force and the tendon force calculated from the ankle joint moment during vertical jumps. *Clin. Biomech.* 8:25–30, 1993.
47. Fukashiro, S., P.V. Komi, M. Jarvinen, and M. Miyashita. In vivo Achilles tendon loading during jumping in humans. *Eur. J. Appl. Physiol.* 71:453–458, 1995.
48. Fukunaga, T., Y. Ichinose, M. Ito, Y. Kawakami, and S. Fukashiro. Determination of fascicle length and pennation in a contracting human muscle in vivo. *J. Appl. Physiol.* 82:354–358, 1997.
49. Fukunaga, T., Y. Kawakami, S. Kuno, K. Funato, and S. Fukashiro. Muscle architecture and function in humans. *J. Biomech.* 30:457–463, 1997.
50. Full, R.J. Mechanics and energetics of terrestrial locomotion: bipeds to polypeds. W. Wieser and E. Gnaiger (eds.). *Energy Transformations in Cells and Animals.* Stuttgart: Thieme, 1989, pp. 175–182.

51. Full, R.J., and M.S. Tu. Mechanics of six-legged runners. *J. Exp. Biol.* 148:129–146, 1990.
52. Full, R.J., and M.S. Tu. Mechanics of a rapid running insect: two-, four- and six-legged locomotion. *J. Exp. Biol.* 156:215–231, 1991.
53. Garcia, M., A. Chatterjee, A. Ruina, and M. Coleman. The simplest walking model: stability, complexity, and scaling. *J. Biomech. Eng.* In Press.
54. Gerritsen, K.G., A.J. van den Bogert, and B.M. Nigg. Direct dynamics simulation of the impact phase in heel-toe running. *J. Biomech.* 28:661–668, 1995.
55. Glos, D.L., D.L. Butler, E.S. Grood, and M.S. Levy. In vitro evaluation of an implantable force transducer (IFT) in a patellar tendon model. *J. Biomech. Eng.* 115:335–343, 1993.
56. Goslow, G.E., Jr., R.M. Reinking, and D.G. Stuart. The cat step cycle: hind limb joint angles and muscle lengths during unrestrained locomotion. *J. Morph.* 141:1–41, 1973.
57. Gregor, R.J., and T.A. Abelew. Tendon force measurements and movement control: a review. *Med. Sci. Sports Exerc.* 26:1359–1372, 1994.
58. Gregor, R.J., P.V. Komi, R.C. Browning, and M. Jarvinen. A comparison of the triceps surae and residual muscle moments at the ankle during cycling. *J. Biomech.* 24:287–297, 1991.
59. Gregor, R.J., P.V. Komi, and M. Jarvinen. Achilles tendon forces during cycling. *Int. J. Sports Med.* 8(Suppl. 1):9–14, 1987.
60. Grieve, D.W., S. Pheasant, and P.R. Cavanagh. Prediction of gastrocnemius length from knee and ankle posture. E. Asmussen and K. Jorgensen (eds.). *Biomechanics VI-A.* Baltimore, MD: University Park Press, 1978, pp. 405–412.
61. Griffiths, R.I. Ultrasound transit time gives direct measurement of muscle fiber length in vivo. *J. Neurosci. Methods* 21:159–165, 1987.
62. Griffiths, R.I. Shortening of muscle fibers during stretch of the active cat medial gastrocnemius muscle: the role of tendon compliance. *J. Physiol. (London)* 436:219–236, 1991.
63. He, J.P., R. Kram, and T.A. McMahon. Mechanics of running under simulated low gravity. *J. Appl. Physiol.* 71:863–870, 1991.
64. Heglund, N.C., G.A. Cavagna, and C.R. Taylor. Energetics and mechanics of terrestrial locomotion. III. Energy changes of the centre of mass as a function of speed and body size in birds and mammals. *J. Exp. Biol.* 97:41–56, 1982.
65. Herzog, W. Force-sharing among synergistic muscles: theoretical considerations and experimental approaches. *Exerc. Sport Sci. Rev.* 24:173–202, 1996.
66. Herzog, W., J.M. Archambault, T.R. Leonard, and H.K. Nguyen. Evaluation of the implantable force transducer for chronic tendon-force recordings. *J. Biomech.* 29:103–109, 1996.
67. Herzog, W., E.M. Hasler, and T.R. Leonard. In-situ calibration of the implantable force transducer. *J. Biomech.* 29:1649–1652, 1996.
68. Herzog, W., and T.R. Leonard. Validation of optimization models that estimate the forces exerted by synergistic muscles. *J. Biomech.* 24(Suppl 1):31–39, 1991.
69. Herzog, W., and T.R. Leonard. Soleus forces and soleus force potential during unrestrained cat locomotion. *J. Biomech.* 29:271–279, 1996.
70. Hodgson, J.A. The relationship between soleus and gastrocnemius muscle activity in conscious cats: a model for motor unit recruitment? *J. Physiol. (London)* 337:553–562, 1983.
71. Holden, J.P., E.S. Grood, and J.F. Cummings. Factors affecting sensitivity of a transducer for measuring anterior cruciate ligament force. *J. Biomech.* 28:99–102, 1995.
72. Holden, J.P., E.S. Grood, D.L. Korvick, J.F. Cummings, D.L. Butler, and D.I. Bylski-Austrow. In vivo forces in the anterior cruciate ligament: direct measurements during walking and trotting in a quadruped. *J. Biomech.* 27:517–526, 1994.
73. Hoyt, D.F., and C.R. Taylor. Gait and energetics of locomotion in horses. *Nature* 292:239–240, 1981.
74. Hoyt, R.W., J.J. Knapik, J F. Lanza, B.H. Jones, and J.S. Staab. Ambulatory foot contact monitor to estimate metabolic cost of human locomotion. *J. Appl. Physiol.* 76:1818–1822, 1994.

75. Hreljac, A. Determinants of the gait transition speed during human locomotion: kinetic factors. *Gait Post.* 1:217–223, 1993.

76. Hreljac, A. Preferred and energetically optimal gait transition speeds in human locomotion. *Med. Sci. Sports Exerc.* 25:1158–1162, 1993.

77. Hreljac, A. Determinants of the gait transition speed during human locomotion: kinematic factors. *J. Biomech.* 28:669–677, 1995.

78. Hreljac, A. Effects of physical characteristics on the gait transition speed during human locomotion. *Hum. Mov. Sci.* 14:205–216, 1995.

79. Inman, V.T., H.J. Ralston, and F. Todd. Human locomotion. J. Rose and J. G. Gamble (eds.). *Human Walking (2nd ed.).* Baltimore, MD: Williams & Wilkins, 1994, pp. 2–22.

80. Jacobs, R., M.F. Bobbert, and G.J. van Ingen Schenau. Function of mono- and biarticular muscles in running. *Med. Sci. Sports Exerc.* 25:1163–1173, 1993.

81. Ker, R.F., M.B. Bennett, S.R. Bibby, R.C. Kester, and R.M. Alexander. The spring in the arch of the human foot. *Nature* 325:147–149, 1987.

82. Komi, P.V. Relevance of in vivo force measurements to human biomechanics. *J. Biomech.* 23(Suppl 1):23–34, 1990.

83. Komi, P.V., A. Belli, V. Huttunen, R. Bonnefoy, A. Geyssant, and J.R. Lacour. Optic fibre as a transducer of tendomuscular forces. *Eur. J. Appl. Physiol.* 72:278–280, 1996.

84. Komi, P.V., S. Fukashiro, and M. Jarvinen. Biomechanical loading of Achilles tendon during normal locomotion. *Clin. Sports Med.* 11:521–531, 1992.

85. Korvick, D.L., J.F. Cummings, E.S. Grood, J.P. Holden, S.M. Feder, and D.L. Butler. The use of an implantable force transducer to measure patellar tendon forces in goats. *J. Biomech.* 29:557–561, 1996.

86. Kram, R., A. Domingo, and D.P. Ferris. Effect of reduced gravity on the preferred walk-run transition speed. *J. Exp. Biol.* 200:821–826, 1997.

87. Lehman, S.L. Input identification depends on model complexity. J.M. Winters and S.L.Y. Woo (eds.). *Multiple Muscle Systems: Biomechanics and Movement Organization.* New York: Springer-Verlag, 1990, pp. 94–100.

88. Li, Y., R.H. Crompton, R.M. Alexander, M.M. Gunther, and W.J. Wang. Characteristics of ground reaction forces in normal and chimpanzee-like bipedal walking by humans. *Folia Primatologica* 66:137–159, 1996.

89. Lieber, R.L., M.E. Leonard, C.G. Brown, and C.L. Trestik. Frog semitendinosis tendon load-strain and stress-strain properties during passive loading. *Am. J. Physiol.* 261: C86–C92, 1991.

90. Loeb, G.E. Hard lessons in motor control from the mammalian spinal cord. *Trends Neurosci.* 10:108–113, 1987.

91. Loeb, G.E. Neural control of locomotion: how do all the data fit together? *Bioscience* 39: 800–804, 1989.

92. Mann, R., and P. Sprague. A kinetic analysis of the ground leg during sprint running. *Res. Quart. Exerc. Sport* 51:334–348, 1980.

93. Mann, R.V. A kinetic analysis of sprinting. *Med. Sci. Sports Exerc.* 13:325–328, 1981.

94. Manter, J. The dynamics of quadrupedal walking. *J. Exp. Biol.* 15:522–540, 1938.

95. Margaria, R. Sulla fisiologia e specialmente sul consumo energetico della marcia e della corsa a varie velocita ed inclinazioni del terreno. *Atti Accad. Naz. Lincei Memorie* 7:299–368, 1938.

96. Margaria, R. *Biomechanics and Energetics of Muscular Exercise.* Oxford: Clarendon Press, 1976.

97. McGeer, T. Passive dynamic walking. *Int. J. Robotics. Res.* 9:62–82, 1990.

98. McGeer, T. Principles of walking and running. R.M. Alexander (ed.). *Mechanics of Animal Locomotion.* Berlin: Springer-Verlag, 1992, pp. 113–139.

99. McGeer, T. Dynamics and control of bipedal locomotion. *J. Theor. Biol.* 163:277–314, 1993.

100. McMahon, T.A., and G.C. Cheng. The mechanics of running: how does stiffness couple with speed? *J. Biomech.* 23(suppl. 1):65–78, 1990.

101. McMahon, T.A., G. Valiant, and E.C. Frederick. Groucho running. *J. Appl. Physiol.* 62: 2326–2337, 1987.

102. Mercier, J., D. Le Gallais, M. Durand, C. Goudal, J.P. Micallef, and C. Prefaut. Energy expenditure and cardiorespiratory responses at the transition between walking and running. *Eur. J. Appl. Physiol.* 69:525–529, 1994.

103. Minetti, A.E., L.P. Ardigo, and F. Saibene. The transition between walking and running in humans: metabolic and mechanical aspects at different gradients. *Acta. Physiol. Scand.* 150:315–323, 1994.

104. Mochon, S., and T.A. McMahon. Ballistic walking. *J. Biomech.* 13:49–57, 1980.

105. Mochon, S., and T.A. McMahon. Ballistic walking: an improved model. *Math. Biosci.* 52: 241–260, 1980.

106. Morrison, J.B. The mechanics of muscle function in locomotion. *J. Biomech.* 3:431–451, 1970.

107. Muir, G.D., J.M. Gosline, and J.D. Steeves. Ontogeny of bipedal locomotion: walking and running in the chick. *J. Physiol. (London)* 493:589–601, 1996.

108. Narici, M.V., T. Binzoni, E. Hiltbrand, J. Fasel, F. Terrier, and P. Cerretelli. In vivo human gastrocnemius architecture with changing joint angle at rest and during graded isometric contraction. *J. Physiol. (London)* 496:287–297, 1996.

109. Pandy, M.G., and N. Berme. Synthesis of human walking: a planar model for single support. *J. Biomech.* 21:1053–1060, 1988.

110. Pandy, M.G., and N. Berme. Quantitative assessment of gait determinants during single stance via a three-dimensional model-Part 1: normal gait. *J. Biomech.* 22:717–724, 1989.

111. Pandy, M.G., and N. Berme. Quantitative assessment of gait determinants during single stance via a three-dimensional model-Part 2: pathological gait. *J. Biomech.* 22:725–733, 1989.

112. Pandy, M.G., and F.E. Zajac. Dependence of jumping performance on muscle strength, muscle-fiber speed, and tendon compliance. J.L. Stein, J.A. Ashton-Miller, and M.G. Pandy (eds.). *Issues in the Modeling and Control of Biomechanical Systems: 1989 ASME Winter Annual Meeting in San Francisco.* New York: The American Society of Mechanical Engineers, 1989, pp. 59–63.

113. Pandy, M.G., and F.E. Zajac. Optimal muscular coordination strategies for jumping. *J. Biomech.* 24:1–10, 1991.

114. Pandy, M.G., F.E. Zajac, E. Sim, and W.S. Levine. An optimal control model for maximum-height human jumping. *J. Biomech.* 23:1185–1198, 1990.

115. Pedotti, A. A study of motor coordination and neuromuscular activities in human locomotion. *Biol. Cyber.* 26:53–62, 1977.

116. Pedotti, A., and P. Crenna. Individual strategies of muscle recruitment in complex natural movements. J.M. Winters and S.L.Y. Woo (eds.). *Multiple Muscle Systems: Biomechanics and Movement Organization.* New York: Springer-Verlag, 1990, pp. 542–549.

117. Pedotti, A., V. Krishnan, and L. Stark. Optimization of muscle-force sequencing in human locomotion. *Math. Biosci.* 38:57–76, 1978.

118. Perry, A.K., R. Blickhan, A.A. Biewener, N.C. Heglund, and C.R. Taylor. Preferred speeds in terrestrial vertebrates: are they equivalent? *J. Exp. Biol.* 137:207–219, 1988.

119. Piazza, S.J., and S.L. Delp. The influence of muscles on knee flexion during the swing phase of gait. *J. Biomech.* 29:723–733, 1996.

120. Pierrynowski, M.R. Analytic representation of muscle line of action and geometry. P. Allard, I.A.F. Stokes, and J.P. Blanchi (eds.). *Three-Dimensional Analysis of Human Movement.* Champaign, IL: Human Kinetics, 1995, pp. 215–256.

121. Prilutsky, B.I., W. Herzog, and T.L. Allinger. Force-sharing between cat soleus and gastrocnemius muscles during walking: explanations based on electrical activity, properties, and kinematics. *J. Biomech.* 27:1223–1235, 1994.

122. Prilutsky, B.I., W. Herzog, and T.L. Allinger. Mechanical power and work of cat soleus, gastrocnemius and plantaris muscles during locomotion: possible functional significance of muscle design and force patterns. *J. Exp. Biol.* 199:801–814, 1996.

123. Prilutsky, B.I., W. Herzog, and T. Leonard. Transfer of mechanical energy between ankle and knee joints by gastrocnemius and plantaris muscles during cat locomotion. *J. Biomech.* 29:391–403, 1996.

124. Prilutsky, B.I., W. Herzog, T. Leonard, and T.L. Allinger. Role of the muscle belly and tendon of soleus, gastrocnemius, and plantaris in mechanical energy absorption and generation during cat locomotion. *J. Biomech.* 29:417–434, 1996.

125. Prilutsky, B.I., W. Herzog, T. Leonard, and T.L. Allinger. Authors' response. *J. Biomech.* 30:309, 1997.

126. Raibert, M.H. *Legged Robots That Balance.* Cambridge, MA: MIT Press, 1986.

127. Raibert, M.H. Trotting, pacing and bounding by a quadruped robot. *J. Biomech.* 23(suppl. 1):79–98, 1990.

128. Raibert, M.H., and J.K. Hodgins. Legged robots. R.D. Beer, R.E. Ritzmann, and T. McKenna (eds.). *Biological Neural Networks in Neuroethology and Robotics.* Boston: Academic Press, 1993, pp. 319–354.

129. Raibert, M.H., R.R. Playter, J.K. Hodgins, et al. *Dynamically Stable Legged Locomotion.* Cambridge, MA: Massachusetts Institute of Technology, 1993.

130. Roberts, T.J., R.L. Marsh, P.G. Weyand, and C.R. Taylor. Muscular force in running turkeys: the economy of minimizing work. *Science* 275:1113–1115, 1997.

131. Robertson, D.G., and D.A. Winter. Mechanical energy generation, absorption and transfer amongst segments during walking. *J. Biomech.* 13:845–854, 1980.

132. Saunders, J.B., V.T. Inman, and H.D. Eberhart. The major determinants in normal and pathological gait. *J. Bone Jt. Surg.* 35:543–558, 1953.

133. Scott, S.H., and G.E. Loeb. Mechanical properties of aponeurosis and tendon of the cat soleus muscle during whole-muscle isometric contractions. *J. Morph.* 224:73–86, 1995.

134. Siegler, S., R. Seliktar, and W. Hyman. Simulation of human gait with the aid of a simple mechanical model. *J. Biomech.* 15:415–425, 1982.

135. Simonsen, E.B., P. Dyhre-Poulsen, M. Voigt, P. Aagaard, and N. Fallentin. Mechanisms contributing to different joint moments observed during human walking. *Scan. J. Med. Sci. Sports* 7:1–13, 1997.

136. Smith, J.L., S.H. Chung, and R.F. Zernicke. Gait-related motor patterns and hindlimb kinetics for the cat trot and gallopp. *Exp. Brain Res.* 94:308–322, 1993.

137. Solomonow, M. Comment on "Role of muscle belly and tendon of soleus gastrocnemius and plantaris in mechanical energy absorbtion and generation during cat locomotion." *J. Biomech.* 30:307–308, 1997.

138. Taylor, C.R. Relating mechanics and energetics during exercise. *Adv. Vet. Sci. Comp. Med.* 38A:181–215, 1994.

139. Thorstensson, A., and H. Roberthson. Adaptations to changing speed in human locomotion: speed of transition between walking and running. *Acta. Physiol. Scand.* 131:211–214, 1987.

140. van Ingen Schenau, G.J., M.F. Bobbert, and A.J. van Soest. The unique action of bi-articular muscles in leg extensions. J.M. Winters and S.L.Y. Woo (eds.). *Multiple Muscle Systems: Biomechanics and Movement Organization.* New York: Springer-Verlag, 1990, pp. 639–652.

141. van Soest, A.J., M.F. Bobbert, and G.J. van Ingen Schenau. A control strategy for the execution of explosive movements from varying starting positions. *J. Neurophysiol.* 71:1390–1402, 1994.

142. van Soest, A.J., A.L. Schwab, M.F. Bobbert, and G.J. van Ingen Schenau. The influence of the biarticularity of the gastrocnemius muscle on vertical-jumping achievement. *J. Biomech.* 26:1–8, 1993.

143. Vaughan, C.L. Are joint torques the Holy Grail of human gait analysis? *Hum. Mov. Sci.* 15:423–443, 1996.

144. Vukobratovic, M., A.A. Frank, and D. Juricic. On the stability of biped locomotion. *IEEE Trans. Biomed. Eng.* 17:25–36, 1970.

145. Walmsley, B., J.A. Hodgson, and R.E. Burke. Forces produced by medial gastrocnemius and soleus muscles during locomotion in freely moving cats. *J. Neurophysiol.* 41:1203–1216, 1978.

146. Winter, D.A. Overall principle of lower limb support during stance phase of gait. *J. Biomech.* 13:923–927, 1980.

147. Winter, D.A. Moments of force and mechanical power in jogging. *J. Biomech.* 16:91–97, 1983.

148. Winter, D.A. Kinematic and kinetic patterns in human gait: variability and compensating effects. *Hum. Mov. Sci.* 3:51–76, 1984.

149. Winter, D.A. *Biomechanics and Motor Control of Human Movement.* New York: Wiley, 1990.

150. Winter, D.A. Human movement: a system-level approach. M.A. Arbib (ed.). *The Handbook of Brain Theory and Neural Networks.* Cambridge, MA: MIT Press, 1995, pp. 472–477.

151. Winter, D.A., G.K. Ruder, and C.D. MacKinnon. Control of balance of upper body during gait. J.M. Winters and S.L.Y. Woo (eds.). *Multiple Muscle Systems: Biomechanics and Movement Organization.* New York: Springer-Verlag, 1990, pp. 534–541.

152. Winters, J.M. Concepts in neuromuscular modeling. P. Allard, I.A.F. Stokes and J.P. Blanchi (eds.). *Three-Dimensional Analysis of Human Movement.* Champaign, IL: Human Kinetics, 1995, pp. 257–292.

153. Winters, J.M. Studying posture/movement selection and synergies via a synthesized neuro-optimization framework. J.M. Winters and P.E. Crago (eds.). *Biomechanics and Neural Control of Movement.* New York: Springer-Verlag, In Press.

154. Winters, J.M., and L. Stark. Analysis of fundamental human movement patterns through the use of in-depth antagonistic muscle models. *IEEE Trans. Biomed. Eng.* 32:826–839, 1985.

155. Winters, J.M., and L. Stark. Muscle models: what is gained and what is lost by varying model complexity. *Biol. Cyber.* 55:403–420, 1987.

156. Yaguramaki, N., S. Nishizawa, K. Adachi, and B. Endo. The relationship between posture and external force in walking. *Anthropological Science* 103:117–139, 1995.

157. Yamaguchi, G.T. Performing whole-body simulations of gait with 3-D, dynamic musculoskeletal models. J.M. Winters and S.L.Y. Woo (eds.). *Multiple Muscle Systems: Biomechanics and Movement Organization.* New York: Springer-Verlag, 1990, pp. 663–679.

158. Yamaguchi, G.T., M.G. Pandy, and F.E. Zajac. Dynamic musculoskeletal modeling of human locomotion: perspectives on model formulation and control. A.E. Patla (ed.). *Adaptability of Human Gait.* Amsterdam: North-Holland, 1991, pp. 205–240.

159. Zajac, F.E. Muscle and tendon: properties, models, scaling, and application to biomechanics and motor control. *Crit. Rev. Biomed. Eng.* 17:359–411, 1989.

160. Zajac, F.E. Muscle coordination of movement: a perspective. *J. Biomech.* 26:109–124, 1993.

161. Zajac, F.E., and M.E. Gordon. Determining muscle's force and action in multi-articular movement. *Exerc. Sport Sci. Rev.* 17:187–230, 1989.

162. Zarrugh, M.Y. Kinematic prediction of intersegment loads and power at the joints of the leg in walking. *J Biomech.* 14:713–725, 1981.

163. Zernicke, R.F., and J.L. Smith. Biomechanical insights into neural control of movement. L.B. Rowell and J.T. Shepherd (eds.). *Handbook of Physiology, Section 12. Exercise: Regulation and Integration of Multiple Systems.* New York: Oxford University Press, 1996, pp. 293–330.

164. Zuurbier, C.J., A.J. Everard, P. van der Wees, and P.A. Huijing. Length-force characteristics of the aponeurosis in the passive and active muscle condition and in the isolated condition. *J. Biomech.* 27:445–453, 1994.

11
Muscle Amino Acid Metabolism at Rest and During Exercise: Role in Human Physiology and Metabolism

ANTON J.M. WAGENMAKERS, PH.D.

Amino acids occur in nature in the form of proteins (amino acid polymers connected by peptide linkages) and free amino acids. There are 20 different amino acids in proteins and a few non-protein amino acids (e.g., taurine). The body of a 70 kg man contains about 12 kg of protein and 200–220 gram (g) of free (protein) amino acids. A continuous exchange of amino acids occurs between these pools as proteins are constantly being synthesized and simultaneously being degraded (protein turnover). Skeletal muscle (SM) accounts for some 40–45% of total body mass and contains some 7 kg of protein, primarily in the form of the contractile (= myofibrillar) proteins. About 120 g of the free amino acids are present intracellularly in SM, while only 5 g of free amino acids are present in the circulation. In the 1840s, the German physiologist Von Liebig hypothesized that muscle protein was the main fuel used to achieve muscular contraction. After this view was invalidated, around 1870, by experimental data [36], many exercise physiologists took the opposite stand and disregarded the amino acid pool in muscle as playing any role of significance in exercise and energy metabolism. For over a century, the amino acid pool in SM has been considered an inert reservoir from which the building blocks for the synthesis of contractile proteins and enzymes are obtained.

In this review, we will show that resting SM actively participates in the handling and metabolism of amino acids in the overnight fasted state and following ingestion of a protein-containing meal, and that muscle actively collaborates and exchanges amino acids with other tissues. Major and rapid changes occur in the muscle free amino acid pool during exercise. Evidence will be presented to indicate that changes in the size of the muscle pool of some amino acids play an important role in the establishment and maintenance of a high concentration of tricarboxylic acid- (TCA) cycle intermediates. This mechanism then allows for the maintenance of a high TCA-cycle flux and aerobic oxidation rate during prolonged exercise. Amino acids also seem to play a role in the failure to maintain high concentrations of TCA-cycle intermediates during prolonged exercise, an event that potentially plays a role in the development of fatigue in glycogen depleted muscles. This chapter will conclude that muscle amino acid metabolism occupies a central place in energy metabolism during exercise, not as a direct fuel competing with fatty acids, blood glucose and muscle glycogen, but as a precursor for the synthesis of TCA-cycle intermediates. It will also be shown that muscle is the main site for conversion of amino acid-derived carbon into glutamine, an amino acid with an important function in other tissues of the human body [49, 50].

MUSCLE AMINO ACID METABOLISM AT REST

As an introduction to the changes that occur during exercise, the resting state will be discussed first. In contrast to the liver, which is able to oxidize most of the 20 amino acids that are present in proteins, rat and human SM when incubated *in vitro* can oxidize only six amino acids [15, 16, 93]. These six are the branched-chain amino acids (BCAA) leucine, isoleucine, and valine, and glutamate, aspartate, and asparagine (Figure 11.1).

Rat muscles incubated *in vitro* are in net protein breakdown (protein synthesis < protein degradation) and release amounts of glutamine and alanine in excess by far of the relative occurrence of these amino acids in muscle protein. This suggests that *de novo* synthesis of these amino acids occurs [39]. In 1972, Ruderman and Lund [71] were the first to observe that addition of BCAA to the perfusion medium of rat hindquarters increased the release of alanine and glutamine. The relationship between the metabolism of BCAA on the one hand and the release of alanine and glutamine on the other hand has since been the subject of many studies [39, 94]. Today, most of this relationship has been firmly established. In the BCAA aminotransferase reaction, the amino group is donated to α-ketoglutarate to form glutamate and a branched-chain α-keto acid. In the reaction catalysed by glutamine synthase, glutamate reacts with ammonia to form glutamine. Alternatively, glutamate may donate the amino group to pyruvate to form alanine and regenerate α-ketoglutarate. These reactions provide a mechanism for the elimination of amino groups from muscle in the form of the non-toxic nitrogen carriers, alanine and glutamine (Figure 11.1).

Muscle amino acid metabolism has also been investigated in man *in vivo* in the resting state and during exercise by measuring the exchange of amino acids across a forearm or a leg (arteriovenous difference multiplied by blood flow gives the net exchange of amino acids) [30, 33, 56, 82, 85, 98]. As muscle is the largest and most active tissue in the limbs, the assumption that limb exchange primarily reflects muscle metabolism seems reasonable. After overnight fasting, there is net breakdown of muscle proteins as protein synthesis is slightly lower than protein degradation [17, 63, 69]. This implies that those amino acids that are not metabolized in muscle will be released

FIGURE 11.1.

Schematic presentation of muscle amino acid metabolism—general overview.

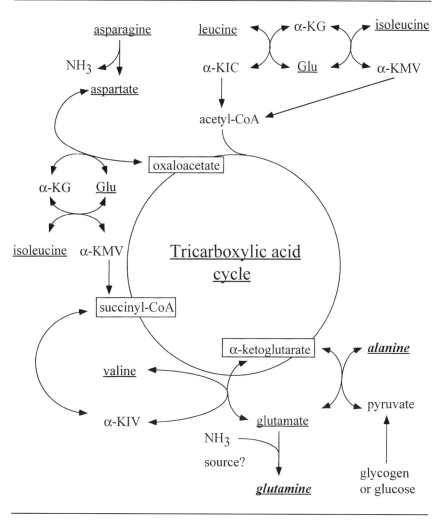

in proportion to their relative occurrence in muscle protein, while a discrepancy will be found when amino acids are transaminated, oxidized, or synthesized. Human limbs release much more glutamine (up to 48% of total amino acid release) and alanine (up to 32%) [56, 82, 85] than would be anticipated from the relative occurrence in muscle protein (glutamine 7% and alanine 9%) [19]. Therefore, glutamine, with two nitrogen (N) atoms per molecule, is dominant for the amino acid N-release from human muscle. On the other hand, the BCAA (19% relative occurrence in muscle protein), glutamate (7%), aspartate and asparagine (together 9%) are not released or are in lower amounts than their relative occurrence. Glutamate, in fact, is constantly taken up from the circulation by SM. This suggests that the BCAA, glutamate, aspartate, and asparagine originating from net breakdown of muscle proteins, and the glutamate taken up from the circulation, are metabolized in muscle and are used for *de novo* synthesis of glutamine and alanine after overnight starvation (Figure 11.2). All other amino acids are released in proportion to their relative occurrence in muscle protein, implying that little or no metabolism occurs.

FIGURE 11.2.

Six amino acids are metabolized in muscle and generate the carbon and nitrogen for synthesis of glutamine. The carbon of alanine originates from blood glucose and muscle glycogen. The α-amino group of alanine is donated by the six amino acids again. Part of the alanine and glutamine are directly generated by net breakdown of muscle proteins. Protein and amino acid-derived carbon primarily are exported from muscle in the form of glutamine and not as previously suggested in the form of alanine (the glucose-alanine cycle)[32]. This implies that glutamine, from a quantitative point of view, is more important than alanine as a precursor for gluconeogenesis in postabsorptive and fasted humans.

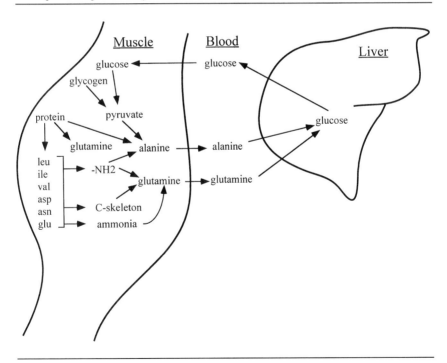

THE ROLE OF AMINO ACID TRANSPORTERS IN RESTING MUSCLE METABOLISM

Amino acid transporters are present not only in the intestine for absorption of nutrition-derived amino acids into the blood (portal vein), but also are present in most tissues [18]. The amino acid transporters are essential for uphill absorption into the tissue against a concentration gradient, as well as for maintenance of these gradients [18]. Rennie [67] has published a state-of-the-art review of the five amino acid transporter systems that presently have been identified in the plasma membrane of SM. Only a brief summary is presented here.

System-A (A stands for alanine) was the first transporter system to be discovered and identified [2]. It transports small, neutral amino acids, particularly alanine and glycine, and is a high-affinity, low-capacity transporter that is sodium dependent. A substantial part of the exchange of alanine between blood and muscle also appears to occur via Systems-ASC (sodium-dependent) and -L (sodium-independent), which are unresponsive to insulin in SM. The combined action of these transporters, in combination with the high intramuscular production rate of alanine, leads to a substantial concentration gradient between muscle and blood, with the muscle concentration being 6- to 10-fold higher [8]. System-ASC is a medium-affinity, medium-capacity, sodium-dependent transporter. Alanine (A), serine (S) and cysteine (C) have been identified as main substrates. System-L (L stands for leucine) in muscle is a low-affinity, high-capacity transporter [18, 47] which handles the BCAA and aromatic amino acids. System-L is not sensitive to insulin, is sodium-independent, and effectively acts as a means of equalizing concentrations of its substrates across the muscle membrane. The distribution ratio between muscle and the extracellular space for the BCAA and aromatic amino acids is about 1.2:1 [8] due to a coupling of this system with the alanine gradient (inward transport of BCAA is coupled to outward transport of alanine).

System-N^m (N stands for nitrogen) is the muscle variant of the System-N transporter, which was first discovered in hepatocytes. It is unusual in muscle since it is a high-capacity, low-affinity, sodium-dependent transporter taking only glutamine, asparagine, and histidine as major substrates [46]. System-N^m is responsible for the large (30- to 40-fold) concentration difference for glutamine between muscle and blood [8], and appears to play a marked role in the controlled release of glutamine from muscle into the circulation (to be discussed). Its activity has been shown to be elevated under conditions of acidosis, corticosteroid treatment, trauma, burns, and sepsis by mechanisms that presently are not understood but may involve the elevation of intracellular sodium concentration [68]. Glutamate, which is taken up by muscle for glutamine synthesis (to be discussed), and aspartate are transported by System-X_{ag}^- (X stands for exchanger). In rat (and probably human) SM, the glutamate transporter has a high-affinity and a low-capacity, and is sodium-independent but H^+-dependent. In terms of the characteristics of this transporter, it is not understood why a >50-fold concentration gradient is maintained between muscle and blood [8], and why muscle, despite this gradient, is able to extract substantial amounts of glutamate from the blood 24 hours (h) a day (to be discussed).

THE SOURCE OF THE CARBON AND NITROGEN USED FOR ALANINE AND GLUTAMINE SYNTHESIS

The question arises whether or not the carbon and nitrogen atoms of these six amino acids that can be degraded in muscle (Figure 11.1) can be used for complete synthesis of both glutamine and alanine. Studies with [^{15}N]-leucine have shown that the amino group of the BCAA is indeed incorporated in humans *in vivo* in the α-amino nitrogen of alanine [44] and of glutamine [22]. As glutamate is central in all aminotransferase reactions in muscle (Figure 11.1), this implies that the amino group of all six amino acids is interchangeable and can be incorporated in the α-amino nitrogen of alanine and of glutamine (Figure 11.2). The source of ammonia in glutamine synthesis (incorporated in the amide nitrogen) forms one of today's remaining puzzles in muscle amino acid metabolism. A small part (5–10%) is derived from the uptake of ammonia from the circulation. The positive femoral arteriovenous difference for ammonia in man is between 5–10% of the glutamine release in postabsorptive subjects at rest [30, 85].

Two intracellular enzymatic reactions are main candidates for the production of the remainder of the required ammonia—adenosine monophosphate (AMP) deaminase and glutamate dehydrogenase. AMP deaminase (Figure 11.3) catalyses the deamination of AMP to inosine monophosphate (IMP). As net breakdown of adenine nucleotides to IMP only occurs during high intensity exercise [26, 27, 48, 58-60, 72, 79, 80] and not at rest, participation of AMP deaminase in production of the ammonia needed for glutamine synthesis would require the purine nucleotide cycle to be active under resting conditions. As proposed by Lowenstein and Goodman [53], the IMP formed by deamination of AMP may be reaminated again in the reactions of the purine nucleotide cycle. As the net reaction of the purine nucleotide cycle is deamination of the α-amino group of aspartate (Figure 11.3), and as the α-amino group of all six amino acids that are metabolized in muscle is interchangeable by reversible transamination reactions (Figure 11.1), this also would imply that all six amino acids can be deaminated via the reactions of the purine nucleotide cycle, when the cycle would operate at a sufficiently high rate under resting conditions. A second possible source of ammonia production in muscle is the reversible reaction catalysed by glutamate dehydrogenase:

$$\text{glutamate} + \text{NAD}^+ <-> \alpha\text{-ketoglutarate} + \text{NH}_4^+ + \text{NADH}$$

FIGURE 11.3.

(A) Schematic presentation of the production of ammonia in skeletal muscle by net breakdown of ATP, (B) or by deamination of aspartate in the purine nucleotide cycle.

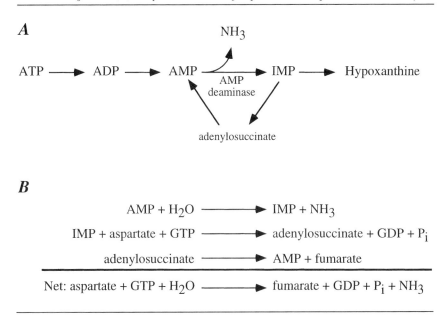

Again, all six amino acids could be deaminated by this reaction after transfer via transamination of the amino group to glutamate, providing that the reaction would be sufficiently active. Early literature suggested, however, that both AMP deaminase and glutamate dehydrogenase have very low activities in muscle both *in vivo* and *in vitro* at the concentrations of the substrates that occur *in vivo* [53]. Nevertheless, estimates of limb production rates in the fed and fasted state indicate that between 20–50 g of glutamine (that is, between 130–325 mmol) are synthesized in the combined human skeletal muscles per 24 h, much more than any other amino acid. This also implies that there must be a corresponding rate of ammonia production in muscle. In more recent literature, IMP reamination rates of 0.05 mmol/kg wet weight per min were observed in resting rat muscles recovering from exercise [78]. Only a fraction of that particular purine nucleotide cycle activity would be required in human muscle in resting conditions to account for the amount of ammonia needed for glutamine synthesis. The V_{max} of glutamate dehydrogenase in human muscle [100] was reported more recently to be between 1–2 mmol/kg wet weight per min and, therefore, can easily account for the observed glutamine production. The complex allosteric control mechanisms of these enzymes [27, 72,

78-80] are not fully understood, however, and we do not know the *in vivo* flux through these pathways both at rest and during exercise.

In vitro muscle incubations and perfusions with [U-^{14}C]-amino acids have led to the general consensus that the carbon skeletons of the six indicated amino acids (Figure 11.1) are used for *de novo* synthesis of glutamine [16, 52, 93]. This was confirmed more recently in rats *in vivo* by Yoshida et al. [104], who showed that leucine C-2 was incorporated into glutamine after giving L-[1,2-^{13}C]leucine. None, or very little, radioactivity was found in lactate, pyruvate, and alanine during incubation of rat diaphragms [93] and perfusion of rat hindquarters [52] with [U-^{14}C]valine. This finding implies that there is no active pathway in muscle for conversion of TCA-cycle intermediates into pyruvate. It also implies that the carbon skeleton of the five amino acids that are converted to TCA-cycle intermediates (Figure 11.1) cannot be used for complete oxidation or for pyruvate and alanine synthesis. Complete oxidation is only possible when carbon enters the TCA-cycle as acetyl-CoA, as is the case for leucine and for part of the isoleucine molecule. Therefore, the only fate of these carbon skeletons is synthesis of TCA-cycle intermediates and glutamine. The next question to be asked concerns the source of the carbon atoms of alanine. The remaining sources of the carbon atoms are muscle glycogen and blood glucose converted by glycolysis into pyruvate (Figure 11.2). In agreement with this conclusion, Chang & Goldberg [15] reported that over 97% of the carbons of the alanine, pyruvate, and lactate released by incubated diaphragms were derived from exogenous glucose. In a recent whole body tracer study in man [64], 42% of the alanine released by muscle was reported to originate from blood glucose.

THE GLUCOSE-ALANINE CYCLE: A CHANGING CONCEPT

The conclusion reached in the previous section slightly changes the concept of the glucose-alanine cycle as proposed by Felig et al. [32] (Figure 11.2), which is now generally accepted textbook knowledge. According to the original formulation of the glucose-alanine cycle, the pyruvate used for alanine production in muscle either was derived from glycolysis of blood glucose or from pyruvate produced by metabolism of other amino acids originating from net protein breakdown. The alanine is then released to the blood and converted to glucose via gluconeogenesis in the liver. In this way, it was believed that carbon derived from muscle protein helped maintain blood glucose concentrations after overnight fasting and during prolonged starvation. The implication, however, of the above conclusions is that all pyruvate is either derived from glycolysis of blood glucose or from breakdown of muscle glycogen followed by glycolysis. In a recent tracer study in man [64], 42% of the alanine released by muscle was reported to originate from blood glucose. This suggests that more than half of the alanine released by muscle is formed from pyruvate derived from muscle glycogen. This route may provide a mechanism to slowly mobilize the sitting muscle glycogen stores during starvation, such that these stores can be used to help maintain the blood glucose concentration (Figure 11.2) and function as fuel in tissues that critically depend on glucose availability, such as brain, red blood cells, and kidney cortex. The amino acids liberated during starvation by increased net rates of protein degradation [17, 63, 69] are instead converted to glutamine, which also is a precursor for gluconeogenesis in the liver in the postabsorptive state [70]. Glutamine also is a precursor for gluconeogenesis in the kidney [103], but renal gluconeogenesis only starts to be significant (>10% of total glucose output) in man after starvation for more than 60 h [9, 62]. Thus, protein-derived amino acids metabolized in muscle still can help maintain blood glucose concentration during starvation but by a different route than was suggested in the original formulation of the glucose-alanine cycle. Indeed, recent tracer studies in man confirmed that glutamine is more important than alanine as a gluconeogenic precursor after overnight starvation [61], and that glutamine is more important than alanine as a vehicle for transport of protein-derived carbon and nitrogen from muscle through plasma to the sites of gluconeogenesis or further metabolism [64].

EFFECT OF INGESTION OF PROTEIN OR A MIXED MEAL

Following ingestion of a mixed protein-containing meal, small amounts of most amino acids are taken up by muscle and most other tissues, as there is net protein deposition in the fed state (protein synthesis > protein degradation), which compensates for the net losses in the overnight fasting period [17, 63, 69]. The increases in the intracellular concentration or availability (arterial blood concentration) of amino acids that are seen in this state have been shown to stimulate protein synthesis and reduce protein degradation, both at whole body level and in SM [7, 63, 99]. An excessively large uptake of BCAA and glutamate is seen in the 4-h period after ingestion of a mixed meal [29] and after ingestion of a large steak [28]. Together, BCAA and glutamate then cover more than 90% of the muscle amino acid uptake. The BCAA originate from dietary protein. After digestion of dietary protein, most of the resulting BCAA escape from uptake and metabolism in gut and liver due to the low BCAA aminotransferase activity in these tissues [45, 94]. Currently, the source of the glutamate is not clear. The diet only seems to deliver a minor proportion as both a [^{15}N]- and [^{13}C]-glutamate tracer were almost quantitatively removed in the first pass through the splanchnic area (gut and liver) [6, 57]. Marliss et al. [56] showed that the splanchnic area in man constantly produces glutamate, after both overnight fasting and after prolonged starvation. This implies that there is a continuous exchange of glutamate between the splanchnic area and the muscle 24 h/day both in the fed and fasted periods. After ingestion of a large steak, the muscle release of glutamine more than doubles, while the alanine release is reduced to 10% of the overnight fasted value. In the 4-h period after ingestion of a mixed meal [29], the dominance of glutamine in carrying N out of SM was even clearer than after overnight fasting. Glutamine then accounted for 71% of the amino acid release and 82% of the N-release from muscle. In summary, these data show that after consumption of protein-containing meals, BCAA and glutamate are taken up by muscle, and their carbon skeletons are used for *de novo* synthesis of glutamine. *De novo* synthesis of glutamine in SM seems to be subject to diurnal cycling, as it is higher in the postprandial period than in the postabsorptive period.

THE FUNCTION OF MUSCLE GLUTAMINE SYNTHESIS AND RELEASE

As discussed in the previous sections, it is clear that glutamine is the main end product of muscle amino acid metabolism, both in the overnight fasted state and during feeding. Alanine only serves to export part of the amino groups. Glutamine is the most abundant amino acid in human plasma ($600-700\mu M$) and in the muscle-free amino acid pool (20 mM; 60% of the intramuscular pool excluding the non-protein amino acid taurine). The synthesis rate of glutamine in muscle is higher than that of any other amino acid. Extrapolations of limb production rates in the fed and fasted state suggest that between 20–50 g of glutamine are synthesized in the combined human skeletal muscles per day. Tracer dilution studies even indicate that > 80 g of glutamine are produced per day [23], but this may be a methodological overestimation due to slow mixing of the glutamine tracer with the large endogenous glutamine pool in muscle [81]. Furthermore, though muscle is the main glutamine producing tissue, other tissues (e.g., adipose tissue, liver, and brain) may also contribute to the rate of appearance of glutamine in the plasma pool that is measured by tracer dilution techniques.

The reason for this high rate of glutamine production in muscle probably is that glutamine plays an important role in human metabolism in other organs. As Sir Hans Krebs [50] already wrote: "Maybe the significance of glutamine synthesis is to be sought in the role of glutamine in other organs, as a precursor of urinary ammonia and as a participant in the biosynthesis of purines, NAD^+, amino sugars and proteins. Glutamine is an important blood constituent, present in higher concentrations than any other amino acid, presumably to serve these various functions. Muscle may play a role in maintaining the high plasma concentration of glutamine." Glutamine is shown to be an important fuel for cells of the immune system [5] and for mucosal cells of the intestine [75, 102]. Low muscle and plasma glutamine concentrations are observed in patients with sepsis and trauma [51, 68, 86], conditions that also are attended by mucosal atrophy, loss of the gut barrier function (bacterial translocation), and a weakened immune response. Though the link between the reduced glutamine concentrations and these functional losses has not been fully underpinned by experimental evidence, the possibility should seriously be considered that it is a causal relationship. Due to its numerous metabolic key functions and a potential shortage in patients with sepsis and trauma, glutamine has recently been proposed to be a conditionally essential amino acid [51] that should especially be added to the nutrition of long-term hospitalized critically-ill and depleted patients. These patients have a reduced muscle mass due to continuous muscle wasting, and therefore, probably also have a reduced capacity for glutamine *de novo* synthesis.

THE GLUTAMINE-GLUTAMATE CYCLE

The existence of the glutamine-glutamate cycle was first demonstrated by Marliss et al. [56]. In muscle, there is a continuous glutamate uptake and glutamine release, with the glutamate uptake accounting for about half of the glutamine release (Figure 11.4). Most of the glutamine produced by muscle is extracted by the splanchnic bed, partly by the gut [75, 102] and partly by the liver [41–43, 70]. This glutamine is converted to glutamate and ammonia by glutaminase. When generated in the gut, the ammonia is transported via the portal vein to the liver and disposed of as urea; the same holds for ammonia directly generated in the liver. In liver, glutaminase is expressed solely in the periportal parenchymal cells (at the inflow site) that also exclusively contain the enzymes necessary for urea synthesis [41–43]. The net splanchnic balance suggests that about half of the glutamate generated by glutaminase action is retained in the splanchnic area and metabolized in gut [75, 102] and liver [41–43, 70]. The other half is released and transported back to the muscle. This glutamine-glutamate cycle provides a means to transport ammonia produced in muscle in the form of a non-toxic carrier (glutamine) through the blood to the splanchnic area where it can be removed as urea (Figure 11.4).

Tracer studies with [15N]- and [13C]-glutamate indicate that close to 100% of the glutamate ingested orally is retained by the splanchnic area [6, 57]. Therefore, it is possible that the glutamine released by muscle is fully metabolized in the splanchnic area, while another endogenous compartment in the splanchnic area releases *de novo* synthesized glutamate that is transported to muscle and used for glutamine synthesis. Windmueller and Spaeth [102] showed that glutamate is not a major end product of gut glutamine metabolism. In perivenous liver cells (situated at liver outflow), a sodium-dependent glutamate transporter (responsible for glutamate uptake against a concentration gradient) [12] and glutamine synthetase are exclusively expressed [41-43]. For this reason, perivenous cells react simi-

FIGURE 11.4.

The glutamine-glutamate cycle operates between muscle and the splanchnic area, and among others functions to transport ammonia in a non-toxic form from the muscle to the liver, where it can be disposed of as urea.

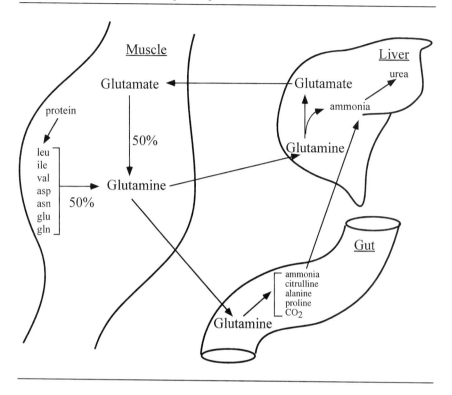

larly to muscle. They extract glutamate and use it for glutamine synthesis [41–43]. The resulting intercellular glutamine cycle in the liver leads to a highly efficient ammonia clearance mechanism by the liver. This process was functionally elucidated by Häussinger [41–43] and others in a series of elegant studies. Therefore, the periportal parenchymal cells, that exclusively express glutaminase and urea cycle activity, are the main candidates for production of the glutamate used by the perivenous cells [43] and by SM. The tracer data [6, 57] also seem to suggest that the glutamate is not formed by the action of glutaminase on blood-derived glutamine, and that the compartments for metabolism of blood-derived glutamine and for *de novo* synthesis of glutamate are fully separated. As indicated, whatever the site and source of the glutamate production, the net end result is a functional glutamine-glutamate cycle between muscle and the splanchnic area.

MUSCLE AMINO ACID METABOLISM DURING PROLONGED EXERCISE LEADING TO GLYCOGEN DEPLETION

During one and two-legged cycling exercise at intensities between 40–70% of W_{max}, only two amino acids change substantially in concentration in the muscle free amino acid pool, glutamate and alanine [8, 48, 73, 74, 85]. Glutamate decreases by 50–70% within 10 min of exercise, while alanine is increased by 50–60% within 10 min of exercise. The low concentration of glutamate is maintained when exercise is continued for periods up to 90 min or until exhaustion, while alanine slowly returns to resting levels. Furthermore, substantial amounts of alanine are released into the circulation during the first 30 min of exercise [74, 85]. Alanine release is reduced again when exercise is continued and the muscle glycogen stores are gradually emptied [85]. Ammonia production by SM gradually increases during these moderate exercise conditions and is minimal only during the first 10 min [74, 85] when the decrease of the muscle glutamate concentration occurs. A completely different situation exists at higher exercise intensities, when activation of AMP deaminase leads to net adenine nucleotide breakdown, accumulation of IMP and ammonia in muscle, and an instantaneous release of ammonia from the muscle [30, 48, 58-60, 72, 79, 80].

THE IMPORTANCE OF TCA-CYCLE ANAPLEROSIS DURING EXERCISE AND THE ROLE OF ALANINE AMINOTRANSFERASE

The functionality of the rapid fall in muscle glutamate concentration during exercise is due most likely to conversion of its carbon skeleton via α-ketoglutarate into other TCA-cycle intermediates. The sum concentration of the most abundant TCA-cycle intermediates in SM has been shown to increase 5-to 10-fold within 5 min after the start of exercise both in rat muscle [4] and in human muscle [31, 38, 73, 74]. The increase, furthermore, is proportional to the exercise intensity in human muscle [73]. This suggests that the increase in concentration of TCA-cycle intermediates may be needed to increase the flux in the TCA-cycle and make adenosine tri-phosphate (ATP) production by aerobic substrate oxidation match the increased ATP demand when going from rest to exercise.

In SM, the rate of aerobic energy production and, therefore, the flux in the TCA-cycle, can increase more than 80-fold going from rest to exercise. The understanding of the mechanisms that lead to this massive increase within minutes after the start of exercise is one of the most interesting and most complex academic challenges of the biochemistry of exercise of the last decades. The substrate of the TCA-cycle is acetyl-CoA, which, after fusion with oxaloacetate, is oxidized to CO_2. Together, the availability of substrate (acetyl-CoA) and cofactors, the inherent enzyme activities, and the concentration of TCA-cycle intermediates determine the flux of the

TCA-cycle. Increases in mitochondrial Ca^{2+}, free adenosine diphosphate (ADP), and $NAD^+/NADH$ are important for allosteric activation of isocitrate dehydrogenase and/or α-ketoglutarate dehydrogenase [40, 101]. Increases in mitochondrial Ca^{2+} and ADP are intimately related to exercise intensity and can thus serve to adjust the flux in the TCA-cycle to the metabolic demands. In addition to allosteric regulation of enzyme activities, the flux of the TCA-cycle also may be increased by increases in the concentration of acetyl-CoA and TCA-cycle intermediates (the substrates of the TCA-cycle enzymes). The concentration of acetyl-CoA increases during incremental exercise and remains more than 2-fold above resting levels at exhaustion [21, 65, 77]. Gibala et al. [38] observed larger increases (5- to 6-fold after 5 min of exercise) for the intermediates that are substrates for the near-equilibrium reactions and that occur at a high resting concentration (malate, fumarate, and succinate) than for the intermediates that are substrates for the three non-equilibrium reactions and that occur at a lower resting concentration (oxaloacetate, isocitrate, and α-ketoglutarate). Oxaloacetate only increased 2-fold after 5 min of exercise, and α-ketoglutarate decreased by 15% after 5 min and continued to decrease, reaching a value of only 35% of the resting concentration at exhaustion [38]. At this moment in time, it is impossible to predict what effect these changes in concentration have on flux through the TCA-cycle, and whether the 2- to 6-fold increase in concentration of all intermediates except α-ketoglutarate is an essential prerequisite for the TCA-cycle flux and ATP production to increase 80-fold. Traditional concepts of metabolic control assumed that one of the enzymes in a metabolic pathway should be rate-limiting [40, 66, 101]. The rate-limiting step should be a non-equilibrium reaction; therefore, in the case of the TCA-cycle citrate synthase, isocitrate dehydrogenase and α-ketoglutarate dehydrogenase were assumed to be main candidates for the overall control of the flux in the cycle [40, 66, 101].

As indicated by Fell [34, 35], more recent mathematical approaches, such as metabolic control analysis, clearly show that control of flux in a multi-enzyme pathway cannot be exerted by one or two enzymes in that pathway when large changes in pathway flux are seen to be associated with much smaller relative changes in metabolite concentrations. The TCA-cycle as such seems a likely candidate for multi-site modulation (i.e., the parallel activation of many or even most of the enzymes of the pathway). Most likely, part of the metabolic control is exerted by the fuel supply (glycolytic enzymes, rate of β-oxidation, and pyruvate dehydrogenase) and allosteric activation of some enzymes in the TCA-cycle; however, the 5- to 6-fold increases in the concentrations of malate, succinate, and fumarate also may turn out to be one of the essential prerequisites for the TCA-cycle flux to increase 80-fold when going from rest to exercise.

The high rate of alanine production during the first 30 min of exercise [74, 85] and the temporary increase in muscle alanine concentration after

FIGURE 11.5.
The alanine aminotransferase reaction feeds carbon into the TCA-cycle during the first minutes of exercise.

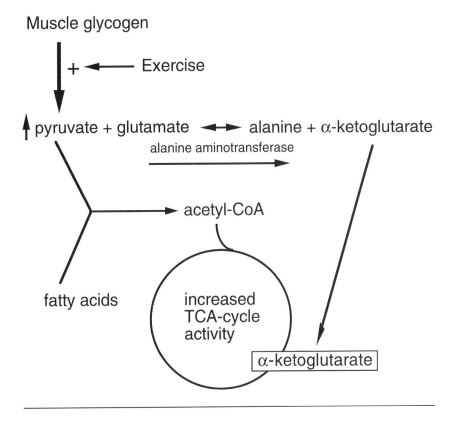

10 min of exercise [73, 74, 85] indicate that the alanine aminotransferase reaction (Figure 11.5) is used for the rapid conversion of glutamate carbon into TCA-cycle intermediates during the first minutes of exercise. Glutamate dehydrogenase can be excluded as a major contributing reaction, as ammonia production rates were very low in the first 10 min of exercise, when the large decrease in muscle glutamate concentration was observed [82, 85]. For the same reason, purine nucleotide cycling, suggested by Aragón and Lowenstein [4] to be the major anaplerotic mechanism during exercise, can be excluded.

The alanine aminotransferase reaction is a near equilibrium reaction. At the start of exercise, the rate of glycolysis and thus of pyruvate formation is high, as indicated by a temporary increase of the muscle pyruvate concentration [25, 31, 74, 76]. The increase in muscle pyruvate concentration automatically forces the alanine aminotransferase reaction towards a new equilibrium, with production of α-ketoglutarate and alanine from pyruvate (continuously supplied by glycolysis) and glutamate (falling in concentration). Felig and Wahren [33] and others [30] showed that the rate of release of alanine from muscle depended on the exercise intensity, and suggested a direct relation between the rate of formation of pyruvate from glucose and alanine release. This led to the suggestion that the glucose-alanine cycle also operated during exercise. In this cycle, glucose taken up by muscle from the blood via glycolysis is converted to pyruvate and then via transamination is converted to alanine. Alanine then subsequently serves as the substrate for gluconeogenesis in the liver and helps to maintain blood glucose concentration during exercise. Instead, we propose that the alanine aminotransferase reaction primarily functions for *de novo* synthesis of α-ketoglutarate and TCA-cycle intermediates at the start of exercise. The augmented glycolysis during exercise thus appears to serve a dual function (Figure 11.5). More pyruvate is generated for the following reasons: (1) to function as a substrate for pyruvate dehydrogenase and subsequent oxidation, and (2) to force the alanine aminotransferase reaction towards production of α-ketoglutarate and TCA-cycle intermediates, and thus to increase TCA-cycle activity and the capacity to oxidize acetyl-CoA derived from pyruvate and fatty acid oxidation. Not only does the alanine release and the rate of glycolysis increase in human SM in proportion to energy demand [31, 33], but the decrease in muscle glutamate and temporary increase in muscle alanine concentration also are in proportion to exercise intensity [73]. Furthermore, most of the decrease in muscle glutamate concentration can be explained by net conversion to TCA-cycle intermediates [73]. This direct coupling of the glycolytic rate via increases in muscle pyruvate concentration to an increased conversion of muscle glutamate to TCA-cycle intermediates seems to provide a powerful mechanism to match the increase in energy demand with the required increase in the concentration of the TCA-cycle intermediates.

Theoretically, pyruvate carboxylase [24], reversal of phosphoenolpyruvate carboxykinase [50], and nicotinamide adenine dinucleotide phosphate- (NADP) dependent malic enzyme also may generate TCA-cycle intermediates in SM. The net flux of these reactions in the direction of TCA-cycle synthesis also depends on a high pyruvate concentration, similar to the alanine aminotransferase reaction. Nonetheless, the observed close-to-equimolar changes in the muscle glutamate concentration and the sum concentration of the TCA-cycle intermediates, as well as the close-to-equimolar alanine formation, seem to point to alanine aminotransferase as the major anaplerotic reaction at the start of exercise. When glycogen depletion occurs during prolonged exercise, then the decrease in muscle pyruvate [74] not only will limit the potential contribution of alanine aminotransferase to TCA-cycle anaplerosis, but also that of pyruvate carboxylase, reversal of phosphoenolpyruvate carboxykinase, and malic enzyme. In other words, it seems unlikely that these other enzymes play a major role in TCA-cycle anaplerosis during brief and prolonged exercise.

THE CARBON DRAIN OF THE BCAA AMINOTRANSFERASE REACTION IN GLYCOGEN-DEPLETED MUSCLES: ITS POTENTIAL ROLE IN FATIGUE MECHANISMS

After the early increase of the concentration of the most abundant TCA-cycle intermediates during prolonged cycling exercise (peak at 5–10 min), a subsequent gradual decrease was observed in human subjects exercising until exhaustion at 70–75% VO_{2max} [38, 74]. Gibala et al. [38] measured all the intermediates except succinyl-CoA. Most intermediates remained 2- to 4-fold higher at exhaustion than at resting conditions. Oxaloacetate returned at exhaustion to the resting concentration and the concentration of α-ketoglutarate decreased continuously immediately after the start of exercise, to a value of only 35% of the resting value at exhaustion. Our group [82, 83, 85, 89, 91, 95] hypothesized that the increased oxidation of the BCAA plays an important role in the decrease of the TCA-cycle intermediates when exercise is continued until exhaustion.

The branched-chain α-keto acid dehydrogenase (BCKADH—the enzyme catalyzing the rate-determining step in the oxidation of BCAA in muscle) is increasingly activated during prolonged exercise, leading to glycogen depletion [83, 89, 90]. After prolonged exercise, the muscle also begins to extract BCAA from the circulation in gradually increasing amounts [1, 83, 85]. Ahlborg et al. [1] suggested that these BCAA were released from the splanchnic bed. By definition, an increase in oxidation of the BCAA will increase the flux through the BCAA aminotransferase step. In the case of leucine, this reaction will put a net carbon drain on the TCA-cycle, as the carbon skeleton of leucine is oxidized to three acetyl-CoA molecules and the aminotransferase step uses α-ketoglutarate as an amino group acceptor (Figure 11.6). Increased oxidation of valine and isoleucine will not lead to net removal of TCA-cycle intermediates, as the carbon skeleton of valine is oxidized to succinyl-CoA and that of isoleucine to both succinyl-CoA and acetyl-CoA (Figure 11.1). Net removal of α-ketoglutarate via leucine transamination (Figure 11.6) can be compensated by regeneration of α-ketoglutarate in the alanine aminotransferase reaction as long as muscle glycogen is available and the muscle pyruvate concentration is kept high (Figure 11.5). Nevertheless, since activation of the BCKADH complex is highest in glycogen-depleted muscle [83], this mechanism eventually is expected to lead to the observed decrease in the concentration of TCA-cycle intermediates. This again may lead to a suboptimal concentration of one or more of the TCA-cycle intermediates and a reduction of the flux in

FIGURE 11.6.

Increased rates of leucine transamination remove α-ketoglutarate from the TCA-cycle during prolonged exercise. The subsequent decrease in the concentration of TCA-cycle intermediates reduces the TCA-cycle flux and limits the maximal rate of fat oxidation in glycogen depleted muscles.

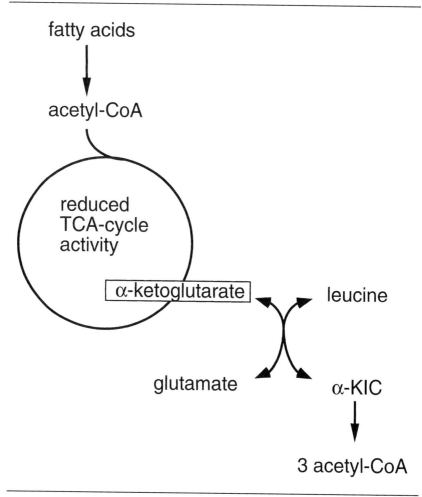

the TCA-cycle, inadequate ATP turnover rates, and via increases in the known cellular mediators to muscle fatigue [37].

BCAA SUPPLEMENTATION AND PERFORMANCE.

After oral ingestion, BCAA escape from hepatic uptake and are rapidly extracted by the leg muscles [3, 54, 83]. This process is accompanied by activation of the BCKADH-complex at rest and increased activation during exercise [83]. This could imply that the indicated carbon-drain on the TCA-cycle is larger after BCAA ingestion, and that BCAA ingestion by this mechanism leads to premature fatigue during prolonged exercise, leading to glycogen depletion. Evidence in support of this hypothesis was obtained [91] in patients with McArdle's disease who have no access to muscle glycogen due to glycogen phosphorylase deficiency. Therefore, these patients can be regarded as an "experiment of nature" from which we can learn what happens during exercise with glycogen-depleted muscles. BCAA supplementation increased heart rate and led to premature fatigue during incremental exercise in these patients. This result could mean that BCAA supplementation has a negative effect on performance by the proposed mechanism in healthy subjects in conditions where the glycogen stores have been completely emptied by highly demanding endurance exercise. With co-ingestion of carbohydrate, however, BCAA ingestion did not change time-to-exhaustion in healthy subjects [10, 55, 84]. (For a review of the performance literature, see [88].) The reason for this lack of a performance effect may be that muscle pyruvate concentrations can be maintained in that case, so that the carbon-drain of the BCAA aminotransferase reaction can be counteracted by the alanine aminotransferase reaction (Figure 11.5). Since BCAA ingestion increases ammonia production by the muscle and plasma ammonia concentration during exercise, both in patients with McArdle's disease [20, 91] and in healthy subjects with and without carbohydrate ingestion [54, 55, 82, 84, 87], and since ammonia may lead to central fatigue and loss of motor coordination, great care seems to be indicated with the use of BCAA supplements during exercise, especially in sports that critically depend on motor coordination. The hypothesis of Blomstrand et al. [11] that BCAA supplements improve endurance performance via a reduction of central fatigue by serotoninergic mechanisms has not been confirmed in recent controlled studies [10, 55, 84]. (For a review of the performance literature, see [88].)

IMPORTANCE OF TCA-CYCLE ANAPLEROSIS FOR THE MAXIMAL RATE OF SUBSTRATE OXIDATION DURING EXERCISE

Muscle glycogen is the primary fuel during prolonged high intensity exercise, such as practiced by elite marathon runners. High running speeds ($\geq$ 20 km per h) are maintained by these athletes for periods of 2 h; however, the runners have to reduce their pace when the muscle glycogen concentration falls and glycolytic rates cannot be maintained. This indicates that either there is a limit in the maximal rate at which fatty acids can be mobilized from adipose tissue and intramuscular stores and subsequently oxidized, or that there is a limitation in the maximal rate of the TCA-cycle when glycolytic rates are falling as a consequence of glycogen depletion. It is proposed here that the decrease in muscle pyruvate concentration that occurs when the glycogen stores are reduced leads to a decrease of the anaplerotic capacity of the alanine aminotransferase reaction, and thus leads to a decrease in the concentration of TCA-cycle intermediates (due to insufficient counterbalance of the carbon-draining effect of the BCAA aminotransferase reaction). This, again, will lead to a reduction of TCA-cycle activity and the need to reduce the pace (fatigue).

The following observations seem to support the previous hypothesis. Patients with McArdle's disease cannot substantially increase the glycolytic rate during exercise due to the glycogen breakdown defect in muscle, and therefore, they do not increase muscle pyruvate. The arterial alanine concentration [91] and the muscle alanine concentration [73] do not increase in these patients during exercise. The muscle glutamate concentration is only about 30% of normal and decreases only a little during incremental exercise [73]. This implies that the anaplerotic capacity of the alanine aminotransferase reaction in these patients is substantially reduced as compared to healthy subjects. Sahlin et al. [73] indeed also observed that two patients with McArdle's disease could only marginally increase the concentration of TCA-cycle intermediates during incremental exercise. The maximal work rate and oxygen consumption of these patients during cycling exercise was between 40–50% of the maximum predicted for their age and build. In ultra-endurance exercise without carbohydrate ingestion, healthy subjects have to reduce the work rate to about the same level when the glycogen stores have been emptied, suggesting that indeed, muscle glycogen is needed to maintain high work rates, potentially by means of its ability to establish and maintain high concentrations of TCA-cycle intermediates.

THE ROLE OF ORALLY-INGESTED CARBOHYDRATE AND BLOOD GLUCOSE IN TCA-CYCLE ANAPLEROSIS

From the previous discussions, it has become clear that the alanine aminotransferase reaction plays an important role in the establishment and maintenance of adequate concentrations of TCA-cycle intermediates during exercise. In the glycogen-depleted state, glucose released from the liver by glycogenolysis and gluconeogenesis, and glucose absorbed from the gut following oral ingestion of carbohydrates, may provide another source of pyruvate to serve as a driving force for synthesis of TCA-cycle intermediates via the alanine aminotransferase reaction. This hypothesis is supported by the finding that oral supplementation with carbohydrates during exercise resulted in higher levels of TCA-cycle intermediates [76]. In fact, this may also explain why higher exercise intensities can be maintained for prolonged periods when athletes ingest carbohydrates during competitive endurance events.

DEAMINATION OF AMINO ACIDS AND GLUTAMINE FORMATION ARE ALTERNATIVE ANAPLEROTIC REACTIONS IN GLYCOGEN-DEPLETED SUBJECTS

Another mechanism that may generate TCA-cycle intermediates is increased deamination rates of amino acids in muscle. Van Hall et al. [85] observed a gradually increasing ammonia production during prolonged one-leg exercise. Since in the study by Van Hall et al. no net breakdown was observed of adenine nucleotides to IMP, the conclusion was drawn that the ammonia production must have originated from the net deamination of amino acids, either via purine nucleotide cycling or via glutamate dehydrogenase. (The exact source of the ammonia production is not known. Refer to the section entitled "Source of the Carbon and Nitrogen Used for Alanine and Glutamine Synthesis.") In contrast to transamination, deamination of the six amino acids that are metabolized in muscle (leucine, valine, isoleucine, aspartate, asparagine, and glutamate) does not use α-ketoglutarate as an amino group acceptor and, therefore, does not lead to a carbon-drain on the TCA-cycle. As TCA-cycle intermediates are formed from five of these six amino acids (only leucine generates acetyl-CoA) (Figure 11.1), deamination also may lead to net synthesis of TCA-cycle intermediates. During prolonged one-leg exercise at 60–65% of the maximal one-leg power output, an excessive net breakdown rate of muscle protein was also observed [96]. During one-leg exercise, the workload per kg muscle in the small muscle group used (maximally 3 kg) was exceedingly high. This may be the reason why one-leg exercise leads to net protein degradation (protein synthesis < protein degradation) in muscle. The amino acid exchange observed under these conditions indicated that BCAA and glutamate released by the net breakdown of muscle protein and taken up from the circulation were used for net synthesis of TCA-cycle intermediates and glutamine.

Removal of amino groups from muscle in the form of glutamine provides another mechanism for net synthesis of TCA-cycle intermediates [97], as illustrated by the following net reactions (see Figure 11.1 for the complete metabolic pathways).

$$2 \text{ glutamate} \rightarrow \text{glutamine} + \alpha\text{-ketoglutarate}$$
$$\text{valine} + \text{isoleucine} \rightarrow \text{succinyl-CoA} + \text{glutamine}$$
$$\text{aspartate} + \text{isoleucine} \rightarrow \text{oxaloacetate} + \text{glutamine}$$

An excessive release of ammonia and glutamine, and an excessive net breakdown of muscle protein (several-fold more than in one-leg exercise in healthy subjects) also was observed during two-legged cycling in patients with McArdle's disease [91], indicating that deamination of amino acids and synthesis of glutamine and TCA-cycle intermediates from glutamate and BCAA provided alternative mechanisms of TCA-cycle anaplerosis in this muscle disease, with zero glycogen availability and low pyruvate concentrations. The fact that high exercise intensities cannot be maintained by these patients as well as in glycogen-depleted muscles seems to indicate that these alternative anaplerotic reactions are not as effective as the alanine aminotransferase reaction and only allow muscular work at 40–50% of W_{max}.

It is far from clear whether dynamic whole body exercise, as practiced by athletes during competition (cycling or running), leads to net protein breakdown in muscle and helps to provide carbon skeletons for synthesis of TCA-cycle intermediates. Different stable isotope tracers used to measure protein synthesis and degradation in laboratory conditions gave different answers. Different answers also were obtained for changes observed at whole body level and at muscle level. (For a detailed review, see Rennie [67].) Whole body measurements with L-[1-^{13}C]leucine suggest that there is increased whole body net protein breakdown during 1–6 h of cycling exercise at intensities of 30-50% VO_{2max}; however, with others tracers (urea and [$^2H_5$-ring]phenylalanine), no such increases were observed [13, 92]. Carraro et al. [14] did not find an effect of cycling exercise at 40% VO_{2max} on muscle protein synthesis measured directly from the incorporation of [^{13}C]-leucine. Furthermore, carbohydrate ingestion, as practiced by endurance athletes during competition, reduces net protein breakdown and amino acid oxidation, and upgrades the relative importance of the alanine aminotransferase reaction for TCA-cycle anaplerosis.

SUMMARY

Six amino acids are metabolized in resting muscle. They are leucine, isoleucine, valine, asparagine, aspartate, and glutamate. These amino acids provide the amino groups and probably the ammonia required for synthesis of glutamine and alanine, which are released in excessive amounts in the postabsorptive state and during ingestion of a protein-containing meal. Only leucine and part of the isoleucine molecule can be oxidized in muscle as they are converted to acetyl-CoA. The other carbon skeletons are used solely for *de novo* synthesis of TCA-cycle intermediates and glutamine. The carbon atoms of the released alanine originate primarily from glycolysis of blood glucose and from muscle glycogen (about half each in resting conditions). After consumption of a protein-containing meal, BCAA and glutamate are taken up by muscle and their carbon skeletons are used for *de novo* synthesis of glutamine. About half of the glutamine released from muscle originates from glutamate taken up from the blood, both after overnight starvation, after prolonged starvation, and after consumption of a mixed meal. Glutamine produced by muscle is an important fuel and regulator of DNA and RNA synthesis in mucosal cells and immune system cells, and fulfils several other important functions in human metabolism.

The alanine aminotransferase reaction functions to establish and maintain high concentrations of TCA-cycle intermediates in muscle during the first 10 min of exercise. The increase in concentration of TCA-cycle interme-diates probably is needed to increase the flux of the TCA-cycle and meet the increased energy demand of exercise. A gradual increase in leucine oxidation subsequently leads to a carbon drain on the TCA-cycle in glyco-gen-depleted muscles, and may thus reduce the maximal flux in the TCA-cycle and lead to fatigue. Deamination of amino acids and glutamine synthe-sis present alternative anaplerotic mechanisms in glycogen-depleted mus-cles, but only allow exercise at 40–50% of W_{max}. One-leg exercise leads to the net breakdown of muscle protein. The liberated amino acids are used for synthesis of TCA-cycle intermediates and glutamine. Today, the impor-tance of this process in endurance exercise in the field (running or cycling) in athletes who ingest carbohydrates is not clear. It is proposed that the maximal flux in the TCA-cycle is reduced in glycogen-depleted muscles due to insufficient TCA-cycle anaplerosis, and that this presents a limitation for the maximal rate of fatty acid oxidation. Interactions between the amino acid pool and the TCA-cycle are suggested to play a central role in the energy metabolism of the exercising muscle.

REFERENCES

1. Ahlborg, G., P. Felig, L. Hagenfeldt, R. Hendler, and J. Wahren. Substrate turnover during prolonged exercise in man: splanchnic and leg metabolism of glucose, free fatty acids, and amino acids. *J. Clin. Invest.* 53:1080–1090, 1974.
2. Akedo, H., and H.N. Christensen. Nature of insulin action on amino acid uptake by isolated diaphragm. *J. Biol. Chem.* 237:118–127, 1962.
3. Aoki , T.T., M.F. Brennan, G.F. Fitzpatrick, and D.C. Knight. Leucine meal increases glutamine and total nitrogen release from forearm muscle. *J. Clin. Invest.* 68:1522–1528, 1991.
4. Aragón, J.J., and J.M. Lowenstein. The purine nucleotide cycle: comparison of the levels of citric acid cycle intermediates with the operation of the purine nucleotide cycle in rat skeletal muscle during exercise and recovery from exercise. *Eur. J. Biochem.* 110: 371–377, 1980.
5. Ardawi, M.S.M., and E.A. Newsholme. Glutamine metabolism in lymphocytes of the rat. *Biochem. J.* 212:835–842, 1983.
6. Battezzati, A., D.J. Brillon, and D.E. Matthews. Oxidation of glutamic acid by the splanch-nic bed in humans. *Am. J. Physiol.* 269:E269–E276, 1995.
7. Bennet, W.M., A.A. Connacher, C.M. Scrimgeour, K. Smith, and M.J. Rennie. Increase in anterior tibialis muscle protein synthesis in healthy man during mixed amino acid infusion: studies of incorporation of [1-13C]leucine. *Clin. Sci.* 76:447–454, 1989.
8. Bergström, J., P. Fürst, and E. Hultman. Free amino acids in muscle tissue and plasma during exercise in man. *Clin. Physiol.* 5:155–160, 1985.
9. Björkman, O., P. Felig, and J. Wahren. The contrasting responses of splanchnic and renal glucose output to gluconeogenic substrates and to hypoglucagonemia in 60h fasted humans. *Diabetes* 29:610–616, 1980.
10. Blomstrand, E., S. Andersson, P. Hassmén, B. Ekblom, and E.A. Newsholme. Effect of branched-chain amino acid and carbohydrate supplementation on the exercise induced change in plasma and muscle concentration of amino acids in human subjects. *Acta Physiol. Scand.* 153:87–96, 1995.
11. Blomstrand, E., P. Hassmén, B. Ekblom, and E.A. Newsholme. Administration of

branched-chain amino acids during sustained exercise-effects on performance and on plasma concentration of some amino acids. *Eur. J. Appl. Physiol. Occup. Physiol.* 63:83–88, 1991.

12. Burger, H.J., R. Gebhart, C. Mayer, and D. Mecke. Different capacities for amino acid transport in periportal and perivenous hepatocytes isolated by digitonin/collagenase perfusion. *Hepatology* 9:22, 1989.

13. Carraro, F., T.D. Kimbrough, and R.R. Wolfe. Urea kinetics in humans at two levels of exercise intensity. *J. Appl. Physiol.* 75:1180–1185, 1993.

14. Carraro, F., C.A. Stuart, W.H. Hartl, J. Rosenblatt, and R.R. Wolfe. Effect of exercise and recovery on muscle protein synthesis in human subjects. *Am. J. Physiol.* 259:E470–E476, 1990.

15. Chang, T.W., and A.L. Goldberg. The origin of alanine produced in skeletal muscle. *J. Biol. Chem.* 253:3677–3684, 1978.

16. Chang, T.W., and A.L. Goldberg. The metabolic fates of amino acids and the formation of glutamine in skeletal muscle. *J. Biol. Chem.* 253:3685–3695, 1978.

17. Cheng, K.N., P.J. Pacy, F. Dworzak, G.C. Ford, and D. Halliday. Influence of fasting on leucine and muscle protein metabolism across the human forearm determined using L-[1-^{13}C,^{15}N]leucine as the tracer. *Clin. Sci.* 73:241–246, 1987.

18. Christensen, H.N. Role of amino acid transport and countertransport in nutrition and metabolism. *Physiol. Rev.* 70:43–77, 1990.

19. Clowes, G.H.A., H.T. Randall, and C.J. Cha. Amino acid and energy metabolism in septic and traumatized patients. *J. Par. Ent. Nutr.* 4:195–205, 1980.

20. Coakley, J.H., A.J.M. Wagenmakers, and R.H.T. Edwards. Relationship between ammonia, heart rate, and exertion in McArdle's disease. *Am. J. Physiol.* 262:E167–E172, 1992.

21. Constantin-Teodosiu, D., J.I. Carlin, G. Cederblad, R.C. Harris, and E. Hultman. Acetyl group accumulation and pyruvate dehydrogenase activity in human muscle during incremental exercise. *Acta Physiol. Scand.* 143:367–372, 1991.

22. Darmaun, D., and P. Déchelotte. Role of leucine as a precursor of glutamine α-amino nitrogen in vivo in humans. *Am. J. Physiol.* 260:E326–E329, 1991.

23. Darmaun, D., D. Matthews, and D. Bier. Glutamine and glutamate kinetics in humans. *Am. J. Physiol.* 251:E117–E126, 1986.

24. Davis, E.J., Ø. Spydevold, and J. Bremer. Pyruvate carboxylase and propionylCoA carboxylase as anaplerotic enzymes in skeletal muscle mitochondria. *Eur. J. Biochem.* 110: 255–262, 1980.

25. Dohm, G.L., V. Patel, and G.J. Kasperek. Regulation of muscle pyruvate metabolism during exercise. *Biochem. Med. Met. Biol.* 35:260–266, 1986.

26. Dudley, G.A., and R.L. Terjung. Influence of aerobic metabolism on IMP accumulation in fast-twitch muscle. *Am. J. Physiol.* 248:C43–C50, 1985.

27. Dudley, G.A., and R.L. Terjung. Influence of acidosis on AMP deaminase activity in contracting fast-twitch muscle. *Am. J. Physiol.* 248:C37–C42, 1985.

28. Elia, M., and G. Livesey. Effects of ingested steak and infused leucine on forearm metabolism in man and the fate of amino acids in healthy subjects. *Clin. Sci.* 64:517–526, 1983.

29. Elia, M., A. Schlatmann, A. Goren, and S. Austin. Amino acid metabolism in muscle and in the whole body of man before and after ingestion of a single mixed meal. *Am. J. Clin. Nutr.* 49:1203–1210, 1989.

30. Eriksson, L.S., S. Broberg, O. Björkman, and J. Wahren. Ammonia metabolism during exercise in man. *Clin. Physiol.* 5:325–336, 1985.

31. Essen, B., and L. Kaijser. Regulation of glycolysis in intermittent exercise in man. *J. Physiol.* 281:499–511, 1978.

32. Felig, P., T. Pozefsky, E. Marliss, and G.F. Cahill. Alanine: a key role in gluconeogenesis. *Science* 167:1003–1004, 1970.

33. Felig, P., and J. Wahren. Amino acid metabolism in exercising man. *J. Clin. Invest.* 50: 2703–2714, 1971.

34. Fell, D.A. The control of flux: 21 years on. *Biochem. Soc. Trans.* 23:341–391, 1995.
35. Fell, D.A. *Understanding the Control of Metabolism.* London: Portland Press, 1997.
36. Fick, A., and J. Wislecenus. On the origin of muscular power. *Philos. Mag.* 31:485–503, 1866.
37. Fitts, R.H. Cellular mechanisms of muscle fatigue. *Physiol. Rev.* 74:49–94, 1994.
38. Gibala, M.J., M.A. Tranapolski, and T.E. Graham. Tricarboxylic acid cycle intermediates in human muscle at rest and during prolonged cycling. *Am. J. Physiol.* 272:E239–E244, 1997.
39. Goldberg, A.L., and T.W. Chang. Regulation and significance of amino acid metabolism in skeletal muscle. *Fed. Proc.* 37:2301–2307, 1978.
40. Hansford, R.G. Control of mitochondrial substrate oxidation. *Curr. Top. Bioenerg.* 10: 217–278, 1980.
41. Häussinger, D. Hepatocyte heterogeneity in glutamine and ammonia metabolism and the role of an intercellular glutamine cycle during ureagenesis in perfused rat liver. *Eur. J. Biochem.* 136:421, 1983.
42. Häussinger, D. Nitrogen metabolism in liver: structural and functional organization and physiological relevance. *Biochem. J.* 267:281, 1990.
43. Häussinger, D., and W. Gerok. Hepatocyte heterogeneity in glutamate metabolism and the role of an intercellular glutamine cycle during ureagenesis in perfused rat liver. *Eur. J. Biochem.* 136:421, 1983.
44. Haymond, M.W., and J.M. Miles. Branched-chain amino acids as a major source of alanine nitrogen in man. *Diabetes* 31:86–89, 1982.
45. Hoerr, R.A., D.E. Matthews, D.M. Bier, and V.R. Young. Leucine kinetics from [^{2}H$_3$]- and [^{13}C]leucine infused simultaneously by gut and vein. *Am. J. Physiol.* 260:E111–E117, 1991.
46. Hundal, H.S., M.J. Rennie, and P.W. Watt. Characteristics of L-glutamine transport in perfused rat hindlimb. *J. Physiol.* 393:283–305, 1987.
47. Hundal, H.S., M.J. Rennie, and P.W. Watt. Characteristics of acidic, basic and neutral amino acid transport in perfused rat hindlimb. *J. Physiol.* 408:93–114, 1989.
48. Katz, A., S. Broberg, K. Sahlin, and J. Wahren. Muscle ammonia and amino acid metabolism during dynamic exercise in man. *Clin. Physiol.* 6:365–379, 1986.
49. Krebs, H.A. Regulation of fuel supply in animals. *Adv. Enzyme Regul.* 10:406–413, 1972.
50. Krebs, H.A. The role of chemical equilibria in organ function. *Adv. Enzyme Regul.* 15: 449–472, 1975.
51. Lacey, J.M., and D.W. Wilmore. Is glutamine a conditionally essential amino acid? *Nutr. Rev.* 48:297–309, 1990.
52. Lee, S.H.C., and E.J. Davis. Amino acid catabolism by perfused rat hindquarter: the metabolic fates of valine. *Biochem. J.* 233:621–630, 1986.
53. Lowenstein, J.M., and M.N. Goodman. The purine nucleotide cycle in skeletal muscle. *Fed. Proc.* 37:2308–2312, 1978.
54. MacLean, D.A., T.E. Graham, and B. Saltin. Stimulation of muscle ammonia production during exercise following branched-chain amino acid supplementation in humans. *J. Physiol.* 493:909–922, 1996.
55. Madsen, K., D.A. MacLean, B. Kiens, and D. Christensen. Effects of glucose, glucose plus branched-chain amino acids or placebo on bike performance over 100 km. *J. Appl. Physiol.* 81:2644–2650, 1996.
56. Marliss, E.B., T.T. Aoki, T. Pozefsky, A.S. Most, and G.F. Cahill. Muscle and splanchnic glutamine and glutamate metabolism in postabsorptive and starved man. *J. Clin. Invest.* 50:814–817, 1971.
57. Matthews, D.E., M.A. Marano, and R.G. Campbell. Splanchnic bed utilization of glutamine and glutamic acid in humans. *Am. J. Physiol.* 264:E848–E854, 1993.
58. Meyer, R.A., and R.L. Terjung. Differences in ammonia and adenylate metabolism in contracting fast and slow muscle. *Am. J. Physiol.* 237: C111–C118, 1979.

59. Meyer, R.A., and R.L. Terjung. AMP deamination and IMP reamination in working skeletal muscle. *Am. J. Physiol.* 239:C32–C38, 1980.

60. Meyer, R.A., G.A. Dudley, and R.L. Terjung. Ammonia and IMP in the different skeletal muscle fibers after exercise in rats. *J. Appl. Physiol.* 49:1037–1041, 1980.

61. Nurjhan, N., A. Bucci, G. Perriello, et al. Glutamine: a major gluconeogenic precursor and vehicle for interorgan carbon transport in man. *J. Clin. Invest.* 95:272–277, 1995.

62. Owen, O.E., P. Felig, A.P. Morgan, J. Wahren, and G.F. Cahill. Liver and kidney metabolism during prolonged starvation. *J. Clin. Invest.* 48:574–583, 1969.

63. Pacy, P.J., G.M. Price, D. Halliday, M.R. Quevedo, and D.J. Millward. Nitrogen homeostasis in man: the diurnal responses of protein synthesis and degradation and amino acid oxidation to diets with increasing protein intakes. *Clin. Sci.* 86:103–118, 1994.

64. Perriello, G., R. Jorde, N. Nurjhan, et al. Estimation of glucose-alanine-lactate-glutamine cycles in postabsorptive humans: role of skeletal muscle. *Am. J. Physiol.* 269:E443–E450, 1995.

65. Putman, C.T., L.L. Spriet, E. Hultman, et al. Pyruvate dehydrogenase activity and acetyl group accumulation during exercise after different diets. *Am . J. Physiol.* 265:E752–E760, 1993.

66. Randle, P.J., P.J. England, and R.M. Denton. Control of the tricarboxylate cycle and its interactions with glycolysis during acetate utilization in rat heart. *Biochem. J.* 117:677–695, 1970.

67. Rennie, M.J. Influence of exercise on protein and amino acid metabolism. L.B. Rowell and J.T. Shepherd (eds.). *Handbook of Physiology, Section 12, Exercise: Regulation and Integration of Multiple Systems.* Oxford, UK: Oxford University Press, 1996, pp. 995–1035.

68. Rennie, M.J., P. Babij, P.M. Taylor, et al. Characteristics of a glutamine carrier in skeletal muscle have important consequences for nitrogen loss in injury, infection and chronic disease. *Lancet* 2:1008–1012, 1986.

69. Rennie, M.J., R.H.T. Edwards, D. Halliday, D.E. Matthews, S.L. Wolman, S.L., and D.J. Millward. Muscle protein synthesis measured by stable isotope techniques in man: the effects of feeding and fasting. *Clin. Sci.* 63:519–523, 1982.

70. Ross, B.D., R. Hems, and H.A. Krebs. The rates of gluconeogenesis from various precursors in the perfused rat liver. *Biochem. J.* 102:942–951, 1967.

71. Ruderman, N.B., and P. Lund. Amino acid metabolism in skeletal muscle: regulation of glutamine and alanine release in the perfused rat hindquarter. *Israel J. Med. Sci.* 8:295–302, 1972.

72. Rundell, K.W., P.C. Tullson, and R.L. Terjung. AMP deaminase binding in contracting rat skeletal muscle. *Am. J. Physiol.* 263:C287–C293, 1992.

73. Sahlin, K., L. Jorfeldt, K.G. Henriksson, S.R. Lewis, and R.G. Haller. Tricarboxylic acid cycle intermediates during incremental exercise in healthy subjects and in patients with McArdle's disease. *Clin. Sci.* 88:687–693, 1995.

74. Sahlin, K., A. Katz, and S. Broberg. Tricarboxylic acid cycle intermediates in human muscle during prolonged exercise. *Am. J. Physiol.* 259:C834–C841, 1990.

75. Souba, W.W. Glutamine: a key substrate for the splanchnic bed. *Ann. Rev. Nutr.* 11:285–308, 1991.

76. Spencer, M.K., Z. Yan, and A. Katz. Effect of glycogen on carbohydrate and energy metabolism in human muscle during exercise. *Am. J. Physiol.* 262, C975–C979, 1992.

77. Spriet, L.L., D.A. MacLean, D.J. Dyck, E. Hultman, G. Cederblad, and T.E. Graham. Caffeine ingestion and muscle metabolism during prolonged exercise in humans. *Am. J. Physiol.* 262:E891–E898, 1992.

78. Tullson, P.C., P.G. Arabadjis, K.W Rundell, and R.L. Terjung. IMP reamination to AMP in rat skeletal muscle fiber types. *Am. J. Physiol.* 270:C1067–C1074, 1996.

79. Tullson, P.C., J. Bangsbo, Y. Hellsten, and E.A. Richter. IMP metabolism in human skeletal muscle after exhaustive exercise. *J. Appl. Physiol.* 78:146–152, 1995.

80. Tullson, P.C., and R.L. Terjung. Adenine nucleotide degradation in striated muscle. *Int. J. Sports Med.* 11:S47–S55, 1990.

81. Van Acker, B.A.C., D.E. Matthews, M. Haisch, et al. Whole body appearance rate of glutamine calculated via the plasma dilution of glutamine tracers: what does it mean? *Clin. Nutr.* 16 (Supplement 2):20, 1997.

82. Van Hall, G. Amino acids, ammonia and exercise in man (Thesis). Maastricht University, The Netherlands, 1996.

83. Van Hall, G., D.A. MacLean, B. Saltin, and A.J.M. Wagenmakers. Mechanisms of activation of muscle branched-chain α-keto acid dehydrogenase during exercise in man. *J. Physiol.* 494:899–905, 1996.

84. Van Hall, G., J.S.H. Raaymakers, W.H.M. Saris, and A.J.M. Wagenmakers. Ingestion of branched-chain amino acids and tryptophan during sustained exercise: failure to affect performance. *J. Physiol.* 486:789–794, 1995.

85. Van Hall, G., B. Saltin, G.J. van der Vusse, K. Söderlund, and A.J.M. Wagenmakers. Deamination of amino acids as a source for ammonia production in human skeletal muscle during prolonged exercise. *J. Physiol.* 489:251–261, 1995.

86. Vinnars, E., J. Bergström, and P. Fürst. Influence of the postoperative state on the intracellular free amino acids in human muscle tissue. *Ann. Surg.* 182:665–671, 1975.

87. Wagenmakers, A.J.M. Role of amino acids and ammonia in mechanisms of fatigue. P. Marconnet, P.V. Komi, B. Saltin, and O.M. Sejersted (eds.). *Muscle Fatigue Mechanisms in Exercise and Training. Med. Sport Sci. Ser. Volume 34.* Basel, Switzerland: Karger, 1992, pp. 69–86.

88. Wagenmakers, A.J.M. Branched-chain amino acids and endurance performance. T. Reilly and M. Orme (eds.). *The Clinical Pharmacology of Sport and Exercise. Excerpta Medica, Int. Congr. Ser. 1125.* Amsterdam, The Netherlands: Elsevier Sci B.V., 1997, pp. 213–221.

89. Wagenmakers, A.J.M., E.J. Beckers, F. Brouns, et al. Carbohydrate supplementation, glycogen depletion, and amino acid metabolism during exercise. *Am. J. Physiol.* 260: E883–E890, 1991.

90. Wagenmakers, A.J.M., J.H. Brookes, J.H. Coakley, T. Reilly, and R.H.T. Edwards. Exercise-induced activation of the branched-chain 2-oxo acid dehydrogenase in human muscle. *Eur. J. Appl. Physiol. Occup. Physiol.* 59:159–167, 1989.

91. Wagenmakers, A.J.M., J.H. Coakley, and R.H.T. Edwards. Metabolism of branched-chain amino acids and ammonia during exercise: clues from McArdle's disease. *Int. J. Sports Med.* 11:S101–S113, 1990.

92. Wagenmakers, A.J.M., D.L.E. Pannemans, A.E. Jeukendrup, et al. Effects of prolonged exercise on protein metabolism in trained men ingesting carbohydrates. *Clin. Nutr.* 16 (Supplement 2):25, 1997.

93. Wagenmakers, A.J.M., H.J.M. Salden, and J.H. Veerkamp. The metabolic fate of branched-chain amino acids and 2-oxo acids in rat muscle homogenates and diaphragms. *Int. J. Biochem.* 17:957–965, 1985.

94. Wagenmakers, A.J.M., and P.B. Soeters. Metabolism of branched-chain amino acids. L.A. Cynober (ed.). *Amino Acid Metabolism and Therapy in Health and Nutritional Disease.* New York: CRC Press Inc., 1995, pp. 67–83.

95. Wagenmakers, A.J.M., and G. Van Hall. Branched-chain amino acids: nutrition and metabolism in exercise. R.J. Maughan and S.M. Shirreffs (eds.). *Biochemistry of Exercise IX.* Champaign, IL: Human Kinetics, 1996, pp. 431–443.

96. Wagenmakers, A.J.M., G. Van Hall, and B. Saltin. Excessive muscle proteolysis during one leg exercise is exclusively attended by increased de novo synthesis of glutamine, not of alanine. *Clin. Nutr.* 15(Supplement):1, 1996.

97. Wagenmakers, A.J.M., G. Van Hall, and B. Saltin. High conversion rates of glutamate and branched-chain amino acids to glutamine during prolonged one leg exercise: an alternative mechanism for synthesis of tricarboxylic acid cycle intermediates. *The Physiologist* 39:A–73, 1996.

98. Wahren, J., P. Felig, and L. Hagenfeldt. Effect of protein ingestion on splanchnic and leg metabolism in normal man and patients with Diabetes Mellitus. *J. Clin. Invest.* 57: 987–999, 1976.

99. Watt, P.W., M.E. Corbett, and M.J. Rennie. Stimulation of protein synthesis in pig skeletal muscle by infusion of amino acids during constant insulin availability. *Am. J. Physiol.* 263: 453–460, 1992.

100. Wibom, R., and E. Hultman. ATP production rate in mitochondria isolated from microsamples of human muscle. *Am. J. Physiol.* 259:E204–E209, 1990.

101. Williamson, J.R., and R.H. Cooper. Regulation of the citric acid cycle in mammalian systems. *FEBS Lett.* 117(Supplement):K73–K85, 1980.

102. Windmueller, H.G., and A.E. Spaeth. Uptake and metabolism of plasma glutamine by the small intestine. *J. Biol. Chem.* 249:5070–5079, 1974.

103. Wirthensohn, G., and W. Guder. Renal substrate metabolism. *Physiol. Rev.* 66:469–497, 1986.

104. Yoshida, S., S. Lanza-Jacoby, and T.P. Stein. Leucine and glutamine metabolism in septic rats. *Biochem. J.* 276:405–409, 1991.

12
Contemporary Exercise Physiology: Fifty Years After the Closure of Harvard Fatigue Laboratory

CHARLES M. TIPTON, PH.D.

INTRODUCTION

In 1947, the Harvard Fatigue Laboratory (Laboratory) was closed [18, 21]. How was it possible that this renowned and revered research laboratory, labeled as a "magnificent anomaly" by Chapman [21], would be disbanded after 2 decades of outstanding productivity [18, 21, 44, 53]? Moreover, what was the Laboratory's impact on the origin, emergence, and establishment of the discipline of exercise physiology in the United States as viewed 5 decades later? Lastly, what heritage from the Laboratory will exercise physiologists carry into the next millennium? These and related questions were presented in the 1997 D.B. Dill Lecture at the annual meeting of the American College of Sports Medicine (ACSM), and will be discussed in subsequent sections.

Because of its importance to exercise physiology, there is no shortage of information on the accomplishments of the Laboratory, either in the research literature [18, 21, 27, 44, 53] or in the introductory pages of contemporary textbooks [15, 24, 51, 62]. In addition, two previous Dill Lectures at ACSM [17, 21] discussed material that pertained to the activities and influences of the Laboratory. While the factors responsible for its closure are complex and difficult to prioritize, the key factors appear to be the following: (1) the aspects related to the death of L.J. Henderson in 1942; (2) the departure of Ancel Keys to the University of Minnesota; (3) the return of Sid Robinson to Indiana University; (4) the dispersion of staff to other laboratories and sites because of World War II; (5) the changing of the presidents (Conant instead of Lowell); (6) the lack of harmony between the deans that replaced Edsall and Donham; (7) the belief of Conant that the Laboratory should decrease its sociological activities and increase its activities in the industrial sector; and, (8) the post-war Harvard University policy that the research endeavors of the Laboratory should not seek governmental funds [17, 18, 20, 21, 27, 43, 44]. It is interesting to note that the Horvaths' text on the history of the Laboratory [44] was the only reference reviewed to mention that the Laboratory's name was changed in 1942 to

315

the Laboratory of Industrial Physiology. This fact indicates the demise of the Harvard Fatigue Laboratory began much sooner than generally believed and reported.

Before examining the relationship between the Laboratory and the emergence of exercise physiology as an academic discipline, it is important to define select terminology that will be used. For example, an exercise physiologist is an individual academically prepared to be a physiologist, by medical, physiological, or biological science departments, who specializes in the discipline of exercise physiology as demonstrated by his/her research, teaching, service, or clinical activities [71]. As will be discussed later, this traditional definition had to be modified because of circumstances that were tangentially associated with the closure of the Laboratory. When the term discipline is used, the definition of Henry [41] is followed. That is, discipline is "... an organized body of knowledge collectively embraced in a formal course of learning. The acquisition of such knowledge is assumed to be an adequate and worthy objective as such, without any demonstration or requirement of practical application."

FIGURE 12.1.
The components of an academic discipline.

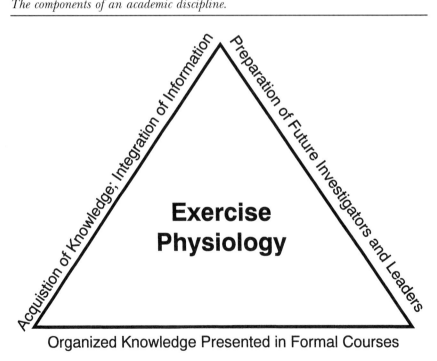

Inherent in the acquisition of knowledge and its organization for dissemination purposes is the specialized academic training of others to continue the process; this relationship is represented in Figure 12.1. Theoretically, an academic discipline is established when the three components form an equilateral triangle. When individuals of a given discipline become sufficiently organized to have meetings, publish research findings, assess dues, and to provide services to its members, the discipline becomes a profession [48, 71] (Figure 12.2). The best known examples are medicine, law, and education.

FIGURE 12.2.
The interrelationships between a discipline and a profession.

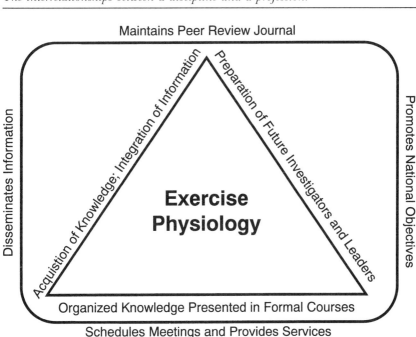

Maintains Peer Review Journal

Preparation of Future Investigators and Leaders

Acquisition of Knowledge; Integration of Information

Disseminates Information

Promotes National Objectives

Exercise Physiology

Organized Knowledge Presented in Formal Courses

Schedules Meetings and Provides Services

TEACHING OF AN ORGANIZED BODY OF KNOWLEDGE: ITS RELATIONSHIPS TO THE ESTABLISHMENT OF THE DISCIPLINE OF EXERCISE PHYSIOLOGY, AND THE TEACHING ACTIVITIES OF THE HARVARD FATIGUE LABORATORY

In the United States, it is unclear which individual(s) in a given educational institution or medical school taught the first course in exercise physiology.

However, before 1900, there were 14 Normal Schools that provided instruction in physical training or physical education for 10 months or longer [48]. In this curriculum were specific courses in exercise physiology, as taught at Harvard University (Sargent and Fitz), Springfield College (Gullick and McCurdy), and Oberlin College (Hanna) [48, 57, 75]. It is noteworthy that at the turn of the century, McCurdy of Springfield College lamented that many of the current instructors of exercise physiology required better academic preparation in the physical and biological sciences [5].

Although Sargent offered summer courses for teachers of physical training at Harvard University during the late 1800s [48, 57], it was the establishment of the Department of Anatomy, Physiology, and Physical Training in 1891 within the Lawrence Scientific School at Harvard University that was an important event for the emergence of exercise physiology as a scientific discipline. At that time, the department implemented a rigorous 4-year science curriculum (which required 2 years of physics, 3 years of chemistry, plus courses in general and medical physiology). The curriculum also included a theory and laboratory course in exercise physiology [48, 57]. According to Kroll [48] and Park [57], this program was the first to require laboratory experiments in exercise physiology, and George W. Fitz, M.D. was responsible for directing and supervising this unique program (graduates were eligible to enter the 2nd year of Harvard Medical School) [48, 57, 72]. Unfortunately, the program was not retained after 1897, and Fitz was not recommended for promotion [48, 57]; hence, the unique model of a rigorous scientific curriculum to prepare students to be instructors of physical training or physicians was lost and/or ignored for numerous decades. As for the establishment of exercise physiology, these losses represented the first funeral at Harvard University.

The elimination of the 4-year curriculum at Harvard University at the beginning of the 20th century did not impede the formal instruction of exercise physiology at other institutions or the coupling of laboratory experiments with the course materials. Two of the many institutions that prepared physical educators in this manner were Springfield College and George Williams College [71]. Known as the "Y" Colleges because of their affiliation with the YMCA, each recruited faculty members who became recognized for their scientific acumen, teaching ability, research publications, and leadership accomplishments, specifically, Peter V. Karpovich, M.D. of Springfield College and Arthur H. Steinhaus, Ph.D. of George Williams College. Both began their respective teaching and related responsibilities in the 1920s and continued them for many decades, and left a legacy that continues today [71].

When the Harvard Fatigue Laboratory was established in 1927 [44], it was organized so that it had no official departmental affiliations [43, 44]. Although the university made arrangements for students to participate in laboratory research projects and to conduct senior theses, the Laboratory did not schedule classes, did not teach formal courses, nor did it give credit or award degrees [27, 31, 43, 44]. Consequently, the establishment and productivity of the Laboratory had a minimal impact on the presentation of organized knowledge in formal classes of instruction (Figure 12.1).

Even though formal instructional and laboratory courses in exercise physiology were available before 1900, this fact is not sufficient evidence that a new academic discipline had been established. Unfortunately, the contents of the courses taught or the texts used at that time (by Gullick, Hanna, Fitz, etc.) are not available today for historians to evaluate the critical mass of information that was presented to students. Although the human physiology textbook written by Flint, Sr. contained numerous undocumented responses to exercise (4th edition in 1896, [29]), and Flint, Jr.'s published material on exercise [30] were available to students, it is unlikely that these materials were the foundations of formal courses in exercise physiology To gain an insight on this issue, citations within relevant texts and manuscripts published by 1900 were examined [19, 36, 47, 49, 50]. Since their documentation was nonexistent or sparse, the citations before 1900 were examined in exercise physiology and related textbooks printed between 1900 and 1935 [7, 11, 25, 34, 42], as well as in the classic paper by Steinhaus [66]. Interestingly, none of the texts contained more than the 28 citations noted by Bainbridge [7], and most had less than 12. From these facts it was concluded that at the turn of the century, exercise physiology in the United States did not have a sufficient critical mass of knowledge to justify being considered as a scientific discipline.

On the other hand, 4 years after the Laboratory was officially established, Bock and Dill listed more than 420 citations [11], approximately 200 more than were used by Bainbridge in 1919 [7]. In fact, Dill was surprised in 1967 they had included this number of citations [27]. One conclusion from this citation approach is that an organized body of knowledge suitable for instruction in formal courses of exercise physiology (Figure 12.1) did exist at the time when Dill was being recognized as being responsible for the activities of the Laboratory [44].

ACQUISITION OF KNOWLEDGE AND THE INTEGRATION OF KNOWLEDGE AT THE HARVARD FATIGUE LABORATORY

Although the name Harvard Fatigue Laboratory infers the muscular exertion of exercise would be the primary intent of its research activities, the Laboratory's primary purpose was to study the physiological, psychological, and sociological responses of workers in industry to stressful stimuli [20, 21, 44]. "Fatigue" was included in the Laboratory's name because the term would help attract the interest and funding of business leaders and because "fatigue" could be understood without being explained or defined [21].

This explanation appears to be correct—in the years between 1927 and its closure, only 16 publications from the Laboratory pertained to fatigue [21].

For the first 7 years of its existence, Henderson directed the activities of the Laboratory, after which Dill (Figure 12.3A) assumed these responsibilities [44]. Using the reference approach described by Chapman [21], the available Laboratory bibliography [53] was examined, which contained 439 separate listings of publications, books, abstracts, papers, and research reports of the Laboratory [53]. This listing is available from the Harvard Medical Library and contains 316 peer reviewed journal articles (Chapman listed 330), three books including those by Bock and Dill [11], one book each by Dill [26] and Henderson [38], and 120 additional items that fall into the remaining categories. Of the material found in the scientific literature, 21% related to hematology, 20% (or 64) pertained to exercise physiology, 11% concerned altitude physiology, 9% were in temperature physiology, and the remaining 39% related to topics associated with comparative physiology, diseases, methodology, clothing, and nutrition. These statistics demonstrate the diverse productivity of the faculty and remind us that research on the effects of muscular activity was but one function of the Laboratory (even though its 7 publications listed as "Studies in Muscular Activity" were seminal in nature) [53]. Despite their content, depth of coverage, and scientific importance, the number of manuscripts published during the Laboratory's 2 decades of existence was not sufficient to justify statements or impressions that the discipline of exercise physiology was established by the accomplishments of the Harvard Fatigue Laboratory.

Following the examples of Chapman [21] and the Horvaths [44], these exercise physiology publications were classified into areas related to cardiovascular, hematological, metabolic, high altitude, environmental, fitness-performance, and sympathetic nervous system physiology. Many of these

FIGURE 12.3.
Individuals associated with the Harvard Fatigue Laboratory who made significant contributions to the discipline of exercise physiology.
(A) David B. Dill (Permission received from Dr. Larry Golding, Executive Director, Southwest Regional Chapter, American College of Sports Medicine.)
(B) Robert E. Johnson (Permission received from Dr. Robert E. Johnson.)
(C) Sid Robinson (Permission received from the Archives of Indiana University.)
(D) Steven M. Horvath (Permission received from Dr. Steven M. Horvath.)
(E) Henry L. Taylor (Permission received from Dr. Arthur Leon of the University of Minnesota.)
(F) Lawrence E. Morehouse (Permission received from Mr. D. Mark Robertson, American College of Sports Medicine.)

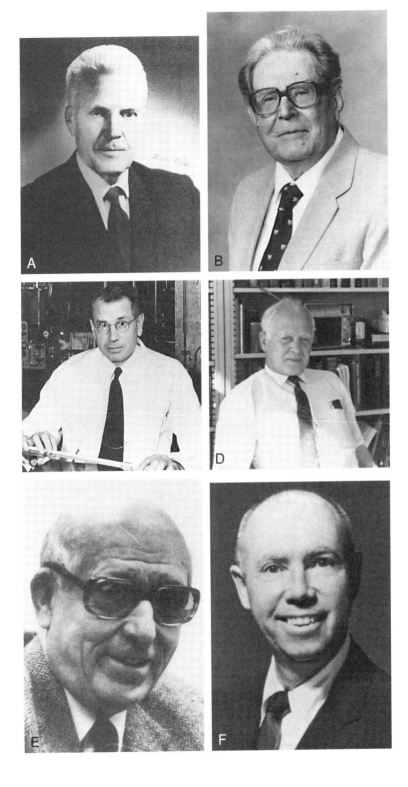

publications contained data collected under field conditions using designs that became models for other laboratories. Although not apparent in Figure 12.1, it is intrinsic in the dissemination of knowledge that scientific rigor be followed in the conduct of any research investigation. Conversations by the author with students of R.E. Johnson (Figure 12.3B), Dill, Robinson, Horvath, and Taylor confirmed the impression that the methodology practiced by the investigators affiliated with the Laboratory was exacting and rigorous, and at the "state of the art" level. Hence, this attribute should always be mentioned when discussing the scientific contributions of the Laboratory.

Scientific productivity from a laboratory represents more than the number of publications or the calculated percentages of these publications in various physiological areas. Specifically, if one examines the different co-authors on the bibliography assembled by McFarland, et al. [53], it is obvious that McArdle and associates [51] were correct when they stated that "many of the great scientist of the 20th century" conducted physiological research at the Harvard Fatigue Laboratory. Using material from the Horvaths [44], that did not include the Harvard staff assigned to the Laboratory, it was evident that 35 of the scientists were from 15 foreign countries (including Asmussen, Brouha, Christensen, Cotton, Hurato, Krogh, Margaria, Missuro, Nielsen, Roughton, and Scholander), and 42 investigators (including Adolph, Cannon, Forbes, Hall, Metheney, Neufeld, Thorndike, and Wald) were affiliated with various academic units at Harvard or elsewhere. In addition, 17 undergraduates (including Barger, Pappenheimer, and Riley) had participated in various research projects. The importance of the listing of these names to the discipline of exercise physiology extends far beyond the research significance of their publications because it demonstrated that the Laboratory had achieved a scientific reputation that could attract talented investigators from the various continents of the world.

Thus, with closure, the activities of the Laboratory became a template in exercise physiology for promoting interdisciplinary investigations, encouraging collaborative research, the training of post-doctoral investigators, attracting foreign scientists, and mentoring the research projects of interested and capable undergraduates.

Select Characteristics of the Exercise Physiology Publications from the Laboratory

Discussed previously were the many exercise physiology topics (cardiovascular, hematological, metabolic, thermal, etc.) that were investigated during the era of the Laboratory. However, as noted by others [21, 44], the physiological changes of humans responding to various stressful stimuli were generally evaluated as a collective response of a single system with minimal regard for the control of the responsible variables. Since physiologists from the time of Claude Bernard have been "trained" to be reductionists and to control as many variables as possible, this characteristic was somewhat unexpected. One explanation, inferred from Chapman [21] and the comments of the Horvaths [44], was that it represented the sociological orientation of Henderson [39, 40], which was to examine the final result and not the sum of the parts. Another possibility to consider was that neither Henderson nor Dill was academically trained as experimental physiologists, and hence their approach was influenced by their interest and preparation in physical chemistry. Perhaps these aspects help to explain why so few of the Laboratory's publications were cellular in nature or concerned with cellular mechanisms [53].

Unexpectedly, only 8% of the total publications from the Laboratory pertained to animals. Most of these studies were comparative in nature and concerned with hematological changes in a variety of species. Although the investigation by Cannon and associates [16, 53] on the changes in the sympathetic nervous system of dogs during exercise were critical studies on autonomic changes, the few animal investigations performed reinforced the concept that human responses were the major focus of the Laboratory during its 20 years of existence. Since the Laboratory exhibited little interest in animal research, it is not surprising that individuals prominent in exercise physiology investigations who left before or after its closure (Keys, Robinson, R.E. Johnson, Horvath, and Dill), did not assume active roles in promoting animal research in their new locations. Another possible factor for the paucity of animal investigations in exercise physiology until several decades later were the convictions of two leaders in physical education research, (Cureton and Karpovich) whom were opposed to the use of animal research to address the issues in humans [71]. Of the physiologists who were interested in exercise, such as Dye, Schneider, Tuttle, or Steinhaus, only the latter extensively used experimental animals to study exercise physiology issues. In fact, Steinhaus performed several studies with dogs that were entitled "Studies in the Physiology of Exercise" [66, 68].

Closure and the Establishment of New Laboratories

As mentioned by the Horvaths [44], the closing of the Laboratory "was a blessing in disguise" because it gave opportunities for many individuals to develop their own laboratories and to achieve their potential as scientific investigators, teachers of graduate courses, and leaders in their chosen discipline. To reinforce their point, the Horvaths listed 17 sites that were classified as 2nd and 3rd generation laboratories. From the standpoint of creating new laboratories and conducting new research in exercise physiology, these number are high because Keys and Robinson had left Harvard University by 1939 [17, 27, 44], and it was many years after the closure that the research laboratories at the University of Illinois (R.E. Johnson), University of California at Santa Barbara (Horvath), and the University of Nevada (Dill) became operational and productive. Although Chapman was not affiliated with Harvard University, he was influenced by Ancel Keys and Henry Taylor during his tenure at the University of Minnesota [17, 27].

Hence, when he established the Weinberger Laboratory at the Texas South-western Medical School in 1965 [20], with Jere Mitchell soon to be its director [71], the Harvard Fatigue Laboratory was Chapman's model..

LABORATORY AND THE PREPARATION AND GRADUATION OF FUTURE INVESTIGATORS WITH AN INTEREST IN EXERCISE PHYSIOLOGY

Physiology has been labeled "the mother of the biological sciences" [4], a distinction that includes exercise physiology as well as cardiovascular, respiratory, comparative, and environmental physiology, to name several. In the United States, the first Ph.D. in physiology was awarded in 1881 [60], with the American Physiological Society (APS) being formed in 1887 [32]. Thus, at the turn of the century, the number of physiologists was low. Since the intent of APS was to recruit experimental physiologists (M.D.s and Ph.D.s) to the organization and not teachers of physiology, many physicians and only a few physiologists taught exercise physiology during the early years. When the Laboratory was established in 1927, APS had approximately 400 members, of which 13 had demonstrated or would exhibit an interest, albeit limited, in the responses to exercise (Adolph, Benedict, Boothby, Cannon, Dawson, Donaldson, Fitz, Forbes, Hatai, Henderson, Lee, Schnei-der, and Tuttle [3]. L.J. Henderson was included in the group although it was known he disliked physical activity other than walking [61]. Flint, Jr. was not listed, even though he conducted exercise related studies, because he allegedly felt the APS should be a society for physicians, and that its membership had too many Ph.D.s [59]. Thus, at that time, exercise physiology lacked a critical mass of investigators and research mentors.

As discussed, the Laboratory was not organized to grant degrees. Even so, it became intimately associated with the preparation and graduation of two Ph.D.s from Harvard University, Sid Robinson of Indiana University (Figure 12.3C) and Steven M. Horvath of the University of California at Santa Barbara (Figure 12.3D). Both were active in the research activities of the Laboratory and become renown for their contributions to exercise physiology[31, 43, 44]. Dill served as the chairman for Robinson but was unable to function in the same capacity for Horvath since Horvath married Dill's daughter [31, 43, 44]. Between 1912 and 1945, universities in the United States and Canada awarded 1274 Ph.D. degrees in physiology [2], with John Hopkins University, Harvard University, and the University of Chicago being the leaders [33]. In retrospect, it was unfortunate for physiology in general, and exercise physiology in particular, that the Laboratory was established and organized so that the training of Ph.D.s was not one of its primary responsibilities.

However, the conditions at Harvard before and during World War II did allow undergraduate, graduate, and postgraduate students to participate in Laboratory projects. One such individual with a B.S. degree, who later was recognized for his achievements in exercise physiology, was Henry L. Taylor (Figure 12.3E). He subsequently was recruited to Minnesota by Ancel Keys [17, 27, 71] Another undergraduate associated with the Laboratory who entered medical school and became known for his accomplishments in respiratory physiology which included exercise, was R.L. Riley of Johns Hopkins University [27, 44]. Lawrence Morehouse was a post-doctoral staff member who participated in the research activities of the Laboratory just prior to its closure [21, 53, 71] (Figure 12.3F). In 1948, he co-authored an exercise physiology textbook [54] that eventually became a required text in many physical education departments. This text underwent numerous revisions over the decades and was a popular choice of many instructors.

In summary, the Laboratory was not a significant factor in the graduation of physiologists or physicians with an interest in exercise physiology. After its closure and relocation of staff, the few laboratories and programs that evolved with an emphasis on exercise physiology did not have an impact on this discipline until later.

CLOSURE AND THE TRANSITION TO THE ERA OF CONTEMPORARY EXERCISE PHYSIOLOGY

Using Figure 12.1 and the equilateral triangle as a model for a discipline, it was evident by 1947 that a sufficient body of knowledge existed in exercise physiology to warrant academic institutions to offer formal instructional courses, and that several peer reviewed journals were publishing data pertaining to exercise responses. Since few university departments with Ph.D. programs in physiology or biology were interested in preparing graduates for a career in exercise physiology, the triangle, as represented in the Figure 12.1 model, was an isosceles triangle rather than an equilateral one. In addition, using the 1947 APS membership as a criteria for identifying potential eligible and qualified physiology mentors for Ph.D. candidates in exercise physiology [28], the number of possible mentors was low (and included Behnke, Cureton, Dill, Dye, Harmon, Horvath, R.E. Johnson, Karpovich, Keys, Morehouse, Robinson, Schneider, Simonson, Steinhaus, Taylor, and Tuttle). From 1947 to 1963, the APS membership list of possible mentors was increased slightly with the addition of Balke, Buskirk, Mitchell, Montoyne, Stainsby, Taylor, and Wasserman. Since few qualified mentors were available, one can conclude that after 1947, departments of physiology and biology had limited influence in increasing the critical mass of individuals interested in or capable of conducting exercise physiology investigations.

After the demise of the Laboratory, the events and circumstances responsible for the emergence and recognition of exercise physiology as an academic discipline did not occur in an orderly, timely, or systematic manner.

Select contributing factors [71] included: (1) the utilization of the "GI Bill of Rights;" (2) the passage of legislation related to funding for health related research, facilities, educational training programs, and NIH study sections, such as the Applied Physiology Study Section; (3) the interest of the APS in applied physiology and its publication of the *Journal of Applied Physiology (JAP)*; (4) the formation of the American College of Sports Medicine (ACSM) in 1954 and its publication of *Medicine and Science in Sports*; (5) the interest in exercise by the general public; and, (6) the epidemiological research that demonstrated that systematic physical activity decreased the morbidity and mortality risks of cardiovascular diseases. Specific details on these factors were discussed previously [71] and will receive cursory mention here.

In general, educational institutions flourished after World War II due to the funding that was available for students, programs, facilities, and research. In addition, the American public increasingly began to believe that a scholastic education was insufficient preparation for one's career or for the resolution of future problems. Since exercise physiology was an integral part of most physical education programs, the number of instructional courses in exercise physiology within physical education departments increased in parallel with the enrollment of undergraduate and graduate students [71]. The same can be stated for textbooks [51, 71]. The first textbook with the scope and depth necessary for graduate students was edited by W.R. Johnson and published in 1960 [45]. However, for advanced courses and better prepared students, the preferred text was published in 1970 by Astrand and Rodahl [6]. When applying the critical mass of information concept, which was described previously, on these and selected contemporary books published after 1996 [15, 51, 62], Johnson's text contained more than 1000 citations, and Astrand and Rodahl's text listed more than 900 references, while the more recent ones had approximately 2100 sources. Although all the texts have some duplications, the percentages are low and indicate the vast amount of information that is associated with the discipline. How authors will handle the current "explosion" of information and its expected acceleration in future decades is a challenge that will be difficult to resolve.

Insights on the subject matter areas within exercise physiology and its changes over the years can be gleaned by inspecting the chapter titles within the various textbooks. For example, in 1893, Kolb [47] discussed forms of fatigue, loss of weight, the circulation of the blood, the work of the heart, cardiac responses, respiration, the heat of the body, analysis of urine, as well as three chapters on how to use boats, statistics of oarsman, and the energy in rowing. In 1931, when Bock and Dill revised Bainbridge's textbook [11], they had 12 chapters on such topics as sources of muscular energy, physicochemical changes in the blood, respiration, the output of the heart, blood supply to tissues, oxygen consumption by tissues, coordination and integration of changes during exercise, the nature of the diet, exercise at high altitude, fatigue, and the benefits of exercise. One year after the closure of the Laboratory, Schneider and Karpovich's 1948 text [64] included 18 chapters that contained essentially the same topics covered by Bock and Dill 17 years earlier, with the addition of the importance of muscles in the contraction process, body types, ergogenic aids, and physical activity for convalescents. In Robergs' and Roberts' text published in 1997 [62], their material is organized into 30 chapters that expand the coverage and details discussed by previous authors to include history, training and adaptations, bone responses, immune functions, measurement of select responses, gender and aging considerations, exercise and disease, clinical exercise physiology, and pediatric exercise science.

When commemorating the 40 years of ACSM existence, Brooks, as well as Costill [14, 23], summarized the major accomplishments in basic and applied exercise physiology since 1954 (Table 12.1). As one would surmise from the chapter listings mentioned previously, the significant investigations were conducted in the same general areas, but were more specific

TABLE 12.1.
Significant Exercise Physicology Subject Matter Areas That Were Investigated Between 1954 and 1994[a]

A. Basic Exercise Physiology
   Exercise Specificity
   Exercise Prescription
   Central and Peripheral Responses and Adaptations
   Responses of Diseased Populations
   Action of Transmitters
   Regulation of Receptors
   Cardiovascular and Metabolic Feed Forward and Feedback Mechanisms
   Substrate Utilization Profiles
   Matching Mechanisms for Oxygen Delivery and Demand
   Mechanisms of Signal Transduction
   Intracellular Lactate Mechanisms
   Plasticity of Muscle Fibers
   Motor Functions of the Spinal Cord
   Hormonal Responses
   The Hypoxemia of Severe Exercise
   Cellular and Molecular Adaptive Responses
B. Applied Exercise Physiology
   Performance of Elite Athletes
   Performance and Heat Stress
   Exercise at Altitude
   Nutritional Aspects of Exercise
   Fluid Balance During Exercise
   Performance and Ergogenic Aids
   Training for Physical Fitness

[a] Information obtained from references [14] and [23] and from unpublished material presented at the 1995 APS Symposium on the History of Exercise Physiology.

concerning the changes in elite performers, select responses of physiological systems, the nature of transmitters and signaling, and the responsible mechanisms at the cellular level. When the next historical listing is published, it will certainly contain more findings related to molecular changes and mechanisms than are currently included in Table 12.1.

Preparation of Exercise Physiologists

As implied earlier, the least developed and most "fragile" component of the discipline of exercise physiology was the preparation of future investigators (Figure 12.1). This situation existed because there were few physiology and biological science departments interested in preparing individuals for such a career, and because there were few qualified investigators who could serve as mentors. Moreover, during its 20 years of existence, the Laboratory, as well as the staff who left for other institutions, had not been overly successful in graduating future researchers. At the same time, Ph.D. programs in physical education were increasing in number and were attracting more students. Consequently, these institutions were graduating individuals to conduct research in physical fitness, exercise physiology, tests and measurements, etc., as well as to instruct undergraduate and graduate students. Fortunately, in the 1960s, various physical education administrators in the Big Ten and Pacific Coast institutions, plus at Pennsylvania State University, recognized the need for qualified faculty who possessed the necessary scientific training to teach and supervise Ph.D. graduate students. Hence, individuals such as Balke and Nagle (Wisconsin), Tipton (Iowa), Gollnick (Washington State), Horvath (University of California at Santa Barbara), and Buskirk (Pennsylvania State University) were recruited to establish specialty programs in exercise physiology within physical education, physiology, applied physiology, biology, and/or interdisciplinary units [71]. Unfortunately, many Ph.D. programs in physical education with an emphasis in exercise physiology lacked faculty who had science backgrounds, rigorous science requirements for doctoral candidates, the requirements of relevant cognate courses, or in-depth preparation in exercise physiology. Consequently, these aspects were severely criticized in the Conant Report of 1963 [22, 71]. In fact, the complete elimination of graduate programs in physical education, including exercise physiology, was suggested in this scathing document. The end result was a "reformation" of graduate programs in physical education, with the "Big Three" serving as models for other institutions to follow [71]. Surprisingly, the concern for rigor in preparing physical education graduate students for a career in exercise physiology was not initially associated with corresponding changes in undergraduate physical education programs, since preparing teachers was the primary function. As a result, many individuals had to complete numerous lower-level science and mathematics courses before being accorded graduate status. When the University of Massachusetts established the Department of Exercise Science in 1971, which was soon followed by the formation of Departments of Kinesiology at the University of California at Los Angles and at the University of Washington, the era was ending when undergraduates had to be academically trained as teachers if they were interested in an exercise physiology career [71]. This trend was confirmed in a l989 survey that indicated that 119 out of 526 institutions offering undergraduate majors in physical education had changed the titles of their departments to reflect the new focus within their academic units [58]. Coupled with these changes were programs of study that included the necessary courses in mathematics, chemistry, and physics to prepare students for graduate school. Since the majority of physiology departments are part of a medical school, few have or will have undergraduate programs. Hence, the preparation of undergraduates for graduate programs in exercise physiology will continue to be the primary responsibility of exercise science and kinesiology-type departments.

Although it is difficult to characterize the "typical" Ph.D. program between the 1960s and the 1980s with an emphasis in exercise physiology, most of the programs contained theory and laboratory courses in systems or medical physiology along with cognate classes, such as biochemistry, pharmacology, neuroanatomy, endocrinology, and histology [71]. When biopsy and analytical procedures were perfected for human tissue investigations [8, 9, 71] and animal exercise experimentation became an accepted and an integral component of exercise physiology research [71], information related to cellular functions and mechanisms began to be included as separate classes or within existing course materials. Unlike basic or biological science departments, which were able to make the necessary changes and transitions to provide instruction and to conduct research in molecular biology, the majority of exercise science, kinesiology, or physical education departments lacked the necessary orientation, faculty, facilities, and/or support funding to incorporate molecular biology training or research in their Ph.D. programs. While Booth is to be commended for his pioneering and dedicated efforts to "up-grade" the molecular biology education and research productivity of exercise physiologists and to encourage exercise science departments to include more molecular biology in the training of their graduates [12, 13], it likely that these changes will occur only in academic units whose deans and heads have the conviction to commit their resources and facilities to recruit exercise-oriented molecular biologists, or who are willing to combine their resources and faculty lines with departments that have molecular biology responsibilities. Of the departments currently preparing exercise physiologists, the ones housed in the basic and biological sciences have the best potential for success. However, there is a notable exception to this perspective; namely, the Department of Kinesiology at the University of Illinois (Chicago), which has recently implemented a Ph.D. program in exercise molecular biology with appropriate courses, with new as well as "re-trained" faculty, with expanded facilities, and with modern equipment [55].

As indicated previously, during the 2 decades of the Laboratory's existence and for at least 3 decades after its closure, a limited number of individuals received Ph.D. or M.D. degrees from basic science departments or medical schools that were interested in exercise physiology as a career [71]. In contrast, the majority of individuals who graduated with specialization or interdisciplinary degrees were from departments of physical education. Therefore, the classic definition of an exercise physiologist was no longer appropriate. In 1976, ACSM changed the physiology membership category to basic and applied science [10]. Two possible reasons for this change were (1) the limited number of graduates from physiology departments who became members of ACSM, and (2) the reluctance of exercise physiologists who had graduated from specialty programs in department of physical education, exercise science, or kinesiology to be classified as physical educators.

When epidemiological evidence indicated that a history of systemic exercise was beneficial in reducing the risks of cardiovascular disease and that exercise stress testing was an integral component of the diagnostic and prescription process in the management of the disease [37, 56, 73], the clinical need arose for qualified individuals with a knowledge of exercise physiology to administer the exercise tests, to assist in the evaluations of the results, and to prescribe the appropriate exercises. Beginning in 1972, ACSM scheduled meetings and a workshop pertaining to guidelines for exercise testing and exercise prescription that resulted in a seminal publication [35] and provided the impetus and foundation for its certification programs [10, 35]. Although ACSM was not the only professional organization to recognize the need to certify individuals to conduct exercise stress tests and to lead exercise classes for preventive and rehabilitative purposes, its programs were the most comprehensive. To date, ACSM has certification programs [10] for program directors (1974), exercise specialists (1975), exercise test technicians (1976), health/fitness instructors (1982), health/fitness directors (1986), and exercise leaders (1986). All the above certification programs require some comprehension of exercise physiology concepts and a good understanding of their "practical" applications for healthy and diseased population. Recently, attempts were initiated to have the College certify individuals as clinical exercise physiologists, which will be discussed in the next section.

EXERCISE PHYSIOLOGY AS A PROFESSION

As noted earlier, a discipline (like medicine) assumes the characteristics of a profession when it organizes itself to specify academic qualifications, charges dues, publishes a journal, schedules meetings and symposia, and renders services to its members and for the general public (Figure 12.2). At the present time, the interests of exercise physiologists are represented, in part, by the activities of the APS and by ACSM. Although APS was instrumental in publishing the *JAP* in 1948 after the report of Simonson [28, 46], the journal was established to serve the scientific needs of other areas of physiology as well. In 1977, APS changed the title to the *Journal of Applied Physiology: Respiratory, Environmental, and Exercise Physiology* to demonstrate its focus (later changed back to *JAP*) and established a membership section entitled environmental, thermal, and exercise physiology (later consolidated to environmental and exercise physiology or EEP) [71]. Since APS had established and had endorsed interest groups beginning in 1928 (that included circulation, gastrointestinal, metabolic, comparative physiology, and temperature regulation, among others) that transformed into membership sections [28], it was evident that the Society had little impetus to promote exercise physiology until the Ph.D. specialization programs had graduated a critical mass of investigators [71]. However, this is no longer an issue between exercise physiologists and APS, as EEP is one of several sections that has a major role in the governance of the Society and in the planning of its activities. At the present time, approximately 3–5% of the APS membership are regarded as exercise physiologists [71].

Beginning in the late 1970s, ACSM became very aggressive in its professional activities and in promoting exercise physiology. In fact, in 1974, R.J. Shepherd wrote an editorial criticizing the excessive "focus" of the College on exercise physiology [65]. There was justification for this perspective because many of the early presidents were exercise physiologist, and because between 1969 and 1976, approximately 60% of the articles published in *Medicine and Science in Sports* were related to exercise physiology [71]. This concern is no longer an issue for ASCM because it has increased the number of exercise physiologists by changing the physiology membership category to basic and applied science, by accepting graduate students in physical education, exercise science, or kinesiology with an interest in exercise physiology, and by promoting activities in regional chapters. At the 1997 ACSM convention, it was reported that approximately 50% of the active members were in the basic and applied science category, indicating that exercise physiologists had become a major constituent of the organization.

Historically, both APS and ACSM have exhibited little leadership or interest in promoting conferences on the content of a curriculum designed to prepare Ph.D.s for a future in exercise physiology, or how the profession could facilitate the development of a discipline. In contrast, during the era of specialization, physical education administrators in the Big Ten Conference scheduled "Body of Knowledge" meetings to discuss general aspects of curriculum content, to promote consensus, and to facilitate implementation of specialization programs. Exercise physiology content was discussed in the 1964, 1965, and 1966 sessions [70], with the results being very helpful to the program administrators [71]. In 1978, several ACSM members (most of whom were APS members as well) with an interest and expertise in exercise physiology (Figure 12.4) felt that ASCM would be interested in an exercise physiology document that addressed the definition of an exercise physiologist, program prerequisites, core and cognate course requirements, in-depth training, post-doctoral experiences, promising areas of research (Table 12.2), and matters of certification. Subsequently, they scheduled a meeting at Pennsylvania State University [71, 74] to discuss these issues. When an oral report was subsequently presented to the ACSM Board of Trustees, it received a "hostile" response because many Board members felt the group was unauthorized and the material inappropriate for discussion purposes. As a result, the report was tabled for eternity. Whether these topics will ever be resumed is unknown; however, the subjects continue

FIGURE 12.4.
Individuals present at the 1978 Pennsylvania State University meeting on exercise physiology. Standing from left to right, Elsworth R. Buskirk, John O. Holloszy, V. Reggie Edgerton, John A. Faulkner, Jack H. Wilmore, Howard K. Knuttgen, and David L. Costill. Seated from left to right, Philip D. Gollnick, James S. Skinner, and Charles M. Tipton. (Photograph is a copy from the collection of Charles M. Tipton.)

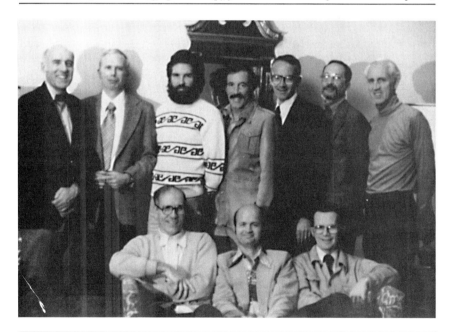

TABLE 12.2.
Exercise Physiology Subject Matter Areas Recommended in 1978 for Future Investigations[a]

Pharmacological Influences on Exercise Responses
Influence of Aging and Disease on Exercise Responses
Mechanisms Responsible for Membrane Changes with Exercise
Molecular Aspects of Muscular Responses to Exercise
Neuromuscular Aspects of Strength Development
Responses of the Immune System to Exercise
Responses of Connective Tissue to Exercise
Motor Control of the Recruitment of Muscle Fibers

[a] Material obtained from references [71] and [74], and originated by the individuals shown in Figure 12.4.

to be important professional matters that warrant discussion by exercise physiologists.

As suggested earlier, some ACSM members have advocated ASCM certification for individuals in clinical exercise physiology [69]. Although the 1996 ACSM Board of Trustees approved a membership recommendation to establish ". . . a specific designation for individuals who provide exercise services in a clinical setting: Clinical Exercise Physiologist . . . . " [1], the events preceding this designation created strife between the clinical and research-oriented physiologists within the organization; the latter group felt the category compromised the classical definition of a physiologist, regardless of his/her area of interest and expertise. One consequence of this disagreement has been an increase in the resolve of the advocates to have a different professional organization represent the interests of exercise physiologists.

In addition to the publication of journals, both APS and ASCM have an executive officer, schedule annual meetings, publish abstracts, encourage and support members to organize symposia, promote undergraduate and graduate student membership, establish "name" lectures, honor young and established investigators, recommend exercise physiologists for study sections and advisory boards, and have direct and indirect liaisons with health care and delivery policy makers in Washington, D.C. Moreover, both organizations have jointly sponsored events such as the "Integrative Biology of Exercise." Consequently, it is difficult to comprehend how a new organization of exercise physiologists would be superior to the ones currently representing their interests.

LEGACY OF THE HARVARD FATIGUE LABORATORY IN THE FUTURE OF EXERCISE PHYSIOLOGY

Chapman [21] was correct in labeling the Laboratory a "magnificent anomaly" because its stature has become enhanced, rather than diminished, with time. Contemporary exercise physiology textbooks continue to extol its accomplishments [15, 24, 51, 62], each semester many students are expected to recall its investigators, and yearly, ASCM members are reminded of its existence at the Dill Lecture or at the Dill Award given by the Southwest Regional Chapter. Combining the conditions of its creation, orientation, staffing, and the attraction of foreign scientists with the productivity of its investigators and the personal and professional influences of Dill, Keys, R.E. Johnson, Horvath, and Robinson, insures the fact that the Laboratory will always be a significant "landmark" for exercise physiologists. Moreover, its research accomplishments will be embellished with time and will be identified with exercise physiology even though its accomplishments are more related to applied physiology [27, 53]. According to Dill [27], Henderson in 1935 stated that the three objectives of the Laboratory were physiological, applied physiological, and sociological in nature.

The Laboratory should be remembered as an innovator that provided exercise physiology laboratory experiences for undergraduate students. Despite the fact the organizational structure did not allow credit hours to be given, many students had the opportunity to participate in research activities. Currently, many institutions incorporate this feature in their undergraduate programs, and this trend will undoubtedly increase in the next century. Since only two graduate students affiliated with the Laboratory graduated with Ph.D.s, no legacy in the academic preparation of doctoral candidates exists. However, the rigor the Laboratory followed in its methodology and the standards it established in the collection and presentation of their results are attributes that are relevant for any era, irrespective of its date.

Although the Laboratory did not leave a legacy related to cellular investigations, it will be necessary for most graduate programs preparing exercise physiologists to address the physiological and health care issues of the future, and to incorporate more didactic instruction in molecular biology and cellular processes, either from "home" departments or from traditional basic science units. For this later situation to become a reality, many exercise science or kinesiology administrators must be willing to collaborate by providing resources and faculty lines. Because of the costs and problems in redirecting traditional departments to have a molecular emphasis, as found at the University of Illinois, it is likely only a few will follow the Chicago model. Lastly, because of the changes in orientation and the name changes in the last 2 decades, the graduate preparation of exercise physiologists by departments of physical education in the next century will become a "thing of the past."

The post-doctoral training and experiences the Laboratory provided for the numerous scientists from the United States and abroad was a unique achievement and one that has become a universal expectation and requirement for biological scientists. Surprisingly, post-doctoral experience was not a universal stipulation in the recruitment notices for Ph.D. positions distributed by departments of exercise science, physical education, or kinesiology between 1989 and 1994 (Tipton, unpublished SW-ACSM Dill Lecture in 1994). However, this situation is rapidly becoming an exception for positions that specify exercise physiologists, and will become even more so after the turn of the century. During these past 50 years, individuals in the United States, such as Buskirk, Gollnick, Holloszy, Horvath, Mitchell, and Wasserman, to name a few, established impressive laboratories that emulated the Laboratory in providing post-doctoral training for countless individuals. Hopefully, this practice will continue in the future. In Europe, the laboratory of Saltin is one of many that have been established. The legacy established for human investigations, collaborative and interdisciplinary research, and field studies [21, 44] has been repeatedly demonstrated by others since the days of closure, and will be practiced by the researchers of the future.

Dill was active in both APS and ACSM, and served as president of each organization during his lifetime. He published his findings in their journals, endorsed the ACSM certification programs, and probably would have supported the recognition of the clinical exercise physiologist category because he knew this category would be important to individuals addressing the health care and delivery needs of the future. On the other hand, having known Dill since 1961, it is the author's opinion that Dill would not have endorsed the concept that the interest and concerns of exercise physiologists can best be served by a new and single professional organization.

SUMMARY

The relationships between the discipline of exercise physiology and the activities of the Harvard Fatigue Laboratory were examined. Even though 5 decades have elapsed since the Laboratory's closure, its existence, leaders, and accomplishments continue to be revered by exercise physiologists. The Laboratory was unique because it was the first research facility of its type and because no single exercise physiology laboratory in the United States since 1947 has been able to attract the stature of the national and international investigators that conducted the interdisciplinary research published by the Laboratory. Despite the inference from its name, the Laboratory's purpose was not to advance the discipline of exercise physiology; rather, it was to advance our understanding and interactions of applied physiology, physiology, and sociology [27]. Consequently, its contributions to the critical mass of exercise physiology literature were limited [21, 44, 53] even though many of the publications were seminal in nature. As documented by the Horvaths, the closure resulted in the establishment of many different research laboratories by former Laboratory staff members and associates (R.E. Johnson at Illinois, Horvath at Santa Barbara, and Dill at Nevada);

however, their impact on exercise physiology was delayed because Keys and Robinson had left for Minnesota and Indiana, respectively, well in advance of closing.

Unfortunately, the administrative structure and organization of the Laboratory was not conducive to the training of Ph.D. candidates with an interest in exercise physiology. Consequently, only two individuals graduated during its existence. Since departments of physiology or biology had limited faculty or interest in preparing students for such a future before and after closure, departments of physical education with specialization graduate programs in exercise physiology assumed this responsibility, which was facilitated by post-World War II funding that supported mass education, graduate training, health related research, and facility development. Today, the majority of the leaders in exercise physiology are the "products" of the specialization movement [71].

Although undergraduates were encouraged to participate in the research activities, the talented faculty of the Laboratory did not offer formal courses in exercise physiology. Thus, the development of an academic discipline in exercise physiology was left to institutions that required a science-oriented curriculum in their undergraduate and graduate degree programs in physical education, exercise science, or kinesiology.

The emergence of exercise physiology as a discipline in the United States was enhanced by the publications of the *Journal of Applied Physiology* in 1948 and by *Medicine and Science in Sports* in 1969. These were peer-reviewed journals that were interested in publishing research studies on exercise topics. Two other reasons contributed to its development. The first was the creation of an Applied Physiology Study Section at the National Institute of Health in 1964, whose purpose was to evaluate grant proposals in subject matter areas intrinsic to exercise physiology [71], while the second reason was the formation of the American College of Sports Medicine in 1954. ACSM was an important impetus for the establishment of the discipline because it had an organizational structure that encouraged exercise physiologists to join, provided opportunities for members to present at regional and national meetings, and would publish their findings. Although the American Physiological Society had been established more than a 100 years ago, only a limited number of its members were interested and active in exercise physiology at the time of the Laboratory's closure or at the beginning of the specialization era (1963). However, in 1977, APS created a membership section that included exercise physiology in its title. Currently, both APS and ACSM are effectively representing the professional interests of exercise physiologists.

While the future of exercise physiology is difficult to predict, it will undoubtedly contain an orientation in molecular biology that will include recent advances in computer utilization and imaging technology. It is also anticipated that more investigators with the attributes and abilities of Dill,

R.E. Johnson, Robinson, Horvath, Keys, and Taylor will emerge, and that more laboratories will be available to provide postdoctoral training for the "best and the brightest," while having the expertise to attract Nobel Prize caliber scientists to conduct collaborative research. Hopefully, all laboratory research or field studies will be conducted with the rigor and attention to detail that characterized the "Dill era." Finally, it is expected that more undergraduates will have had research experiences in exercise physiology. When any or all of these expectations occur, we will know that the legacy of the Harvard Fatigue Laboratory has continued.

REFERENCES

1. Action Items, ACSM Board of Trustees. *Sports Med. Bull.* 31: 6–7, 1996
2. Adolph, E.F. Physiology in North America, Section 1: purposes and methods of the study. *Fed. Proc.* 5: 408–416, 1946.
3. American Physiological Society. *History of the American Physiological Society: Semicentennial 1887-1937.* Baltimore, MD: American Physiological Society, 1938, pp. 179–189.
4. Anonymous. Foreword. *J. Appl. Physiol.* 1:1, 1948.
5. Abstract (McCurdy). Physical training as a profession. *Am. Phys. Ed. Rev.* 6: 311–312, 1901.
6. Astrand, P.O., and K. Rodahl. *Textbook of Work Physiology.* New York: McGraw-Hill Book Company, 1970, pp. 1–633.
7. Bainbridge, F.A. *The Physiology of Muscular Exercise.* London: Longmans, Green and Company. 1919, pp. 1–214.
8. Bergstrom, J. Muscle electrolytes in man. *Scan. J. Clin. Lab.* Invest. 14(Suppl. 68):1–110, 1962.
9. Bergstrom, J., and E. Hultman. Muscle glycogen synthesis after exercise: an enhancing factor localized to the muscle cells in man. *Nature.* 210:309–310, 1966.
10. Berryman, J.W. *Out of Many, One: A History of the American College of Sports Medicine.* Champaign, IL: Human Kinetics Publishers, 1995, pp. 316–333.
11. Bock, A.V., and D.B. Dill. *The Physiology of Muscular Exercise By the late F.A. Bainbridge. 3rd Edition.* London: Longmans, Green and Company. 1931, pp. 1–267.
12. Booth, F.W. Perspectives on molecular and cellular exercise physiology. *J. Appl. Physiol.* 65:1461–1471, 1988.
13. Booth, F.W. Application of molecular biology in exercise physiology. *Exerc. Sport Sci. Rev.* 17:1–27, 1989.
14. Brooks, G.A. 40 years of progress: Basic exercise physiology. *40th Anniversary Lectures.* Indianapolis, IN: American College of Sports Medicine, 1994, pp. 15–42.
15. Brooks, G.A., T.D. Fahey, and T.P. White. *Exercise Physiology: Human Bioenergetics and its Applications. 2nd ed.* Mountain View, CA: Mayfield Publishing Company, 1996, pp. 1–727.
16. Brouha, L., W.B. Cannon, and D.B. Dill. The heart rate of the sympathectomized dog in rest and exercise. *J. Physiol. (London)* 87:345–349, 1936.
17. Buskirk, E.R. From Harvard to Minnesota: keys to our history. *Exer. Sport Sci. Rev.* 20:1–26, 1992.
18. Buskirk, E.R. Exercise physiology, Part 1: early history in the United States. J.D. Massengale and R.A. Swanson (eds.). *The History of Exercise and Sport Science.* Champaign, IL: Human Kinetics Publishers, 1997, pp. 367–397, 428–431.
19. Byford, W.H. On the physiology of exercise. *Am. J. Med. Sci.* 30:32–42, 1855.
20. Chapman, C.B. Introduction. *Circ. Res.* 20(Suppl. I):I–1, 1967.
21. Chapman, C.B. The long reach of Harvard's Fatigue Laboratory, 1926-1947. *Perspect. Biol. Med.* 34:17–33, 1990.
22. Conant, J.B. *The Education of American Teachers.* New York: McGraw-Hill Book Company, 1963, pp. 1–275.

23. Costill, D.L. Applied Exercise Physiology. *40th Anniversary Lectures.* Indianapolis, IN: American College of Sports Medicine, 1994, pp. 69–80.
24. Costill, D.C., and J.H. Wilmore. *Physiology of Sport and Exercise.* Champaign, IL: Human Kinetics Publishers, 1994, pp. 1–533.
25. Dawson, P.M. *The Physiology of Physical Education.* Baltimore, MD: Williams and Wilkins Company, 1935, pp. 1–925.
26. Dill, D.B. *Life, Heat, and Altitude: Physiological Effects of Hot Climates and Great Heights.* Cambridge, MA: Harvard University Press, 1938, pp. 1–211.
27. Dill, D.B. Harvard Fatigue Laboratory: its development, contributions, and demise. *Circ. Res.* 1967, 20(Suppl. I):I161–I167.
28. Fenn, W.O. *History of the American Physiological Society: The Third Quarter Century, 1937-1962.* Washington, D.C.: The American Physiological Society, 1963, pp. 75, 92–112, 159–177.
29. Flint, A. *A Textbook of Human Physiology, 4th edition.* New York: D. Appleton and Company, 1896, pp. 1–850.
30. Flint, A. Jr. *On the Source of Muscular Power.* New York: D. Appleton and Company, 1878, pp. 1–104.
31. Folk, E.G., Jr. *Personal communication to CMT,* May 2, 1997.
32. Fye, W.B. *The Development of American Physiology.* Baltimore, MD: The John Hopkins University Press, 1987, pp. 1–295.
33. Geison, G.L. International relations and domestic elites in American physiology, 1900–1940. G.L. Geison (ed.). *Physiology in the American Context 1850-1940.* Bethesda, MD: American Physiological Society, 1987, pp. 115–154.
34. Gould, A.G., and J.A. Dye. *Exercise and its Physiology.* New York: A.S. Barnes and Company, 1932, pp. 1–434.
35. Guidelines for Graded Exercise Testing and Exercise Prescription. Philadelphia: Lea and Febiger, 1975, pp. 1–114.
36. Hartwell, E.M. On the physiology of exercise. *Boston Med. Surg. J.* 116:297–301, 1887.
37. Hellerstein, H.K., E.Z. Hirsch, R. Alder, et al. (eds.). *Exercise Testing and Exercise Training in Coronary Heart Disease.* New York: Academic Press, 1972, pp. 129–169.
38. Henderson, L.J. *Blood: A study in General Physiology.* New Haven, CN: Yale University Press, 1928, pp. 1–397.
39. Henderson, L.J. *Pareto's General Sociology: A Physiologist's Interpretation.* Cambridge, MA:- Harvard University Press, 1937, pp. 1–119.
40. Henderson, L.J. *On the Social System.* Chicago, IL: The University of Chicago Press, 1970, pp. 1–260.
41. Henry, F.M. Physical education: an academic discipline. *JHPER.* 35:32–33, 69, 1964.
42. Herxheimer, H. *The Principles of Medicine in Sport for Physicians and Students.* Berlin: George Thieme, (translated from German by W.W. Tuttle and G. C. Knowlton) 1933, pp. 1–299.
43. Horvath, S.M. *Personal communication to CMT.* May 1, 1997.
44. Horvath S.M., and E.C. Horvath. *The Harvard Fatigue Laboratory: Its History and Contributions.* Englewood Cliffs, NJ: Prentice-Hall, 1973, pp. 1–182.
45. Johnson, W.R. (ed.). *Science and Medicine of Exercise and Sport.* New York: Harper and Brothers Publishers, 1960, pp. 1–725.
46. Keys, A. *Forward. Physiology of Work Capacity and Fatigue.* E. Simonson (ed.). Springfield, IL: C.C. Thomas, 1971, pp. vii–ix.
47. Kolb, G. *Physiology of Sport. 2nd edition.* London: Krohne and Sesemann, 1893, pp. 1–184.
48. Kroll, W.P. *Graduate Study and Research in Physical Education.* Champaign, IL: Human Kinetics Publishers, 1982, pp. 1–342.
49. Lagrange, F. *Physiology of Bodily Exercise.* New York: D. Appleton and Company, 1890. pp. 1–395.
50. Maclaren, A. *Training in Theory and Practice.* London: Macmillian and Company, 1866, pp. 1–202.

51. McArdle, W.D., F.I. Katch, and V.L. Katch. *Exercise Physiology: Energy, Nutrition and Human Performance.* Baltimore, MD: Williams and Wilkins, 1996, pp. xiii–xliii.

52. McCurdy, J.H. *The Physiology of Exercise.* New York: Lea and Febiger, 1924, pp. 1–237.

53. McFarland, R, H. Russell, and L. Loring. *The Fatigue Laboratory, Harvard University, Bibliography 1921-1960.* Cambridge, MA: Mimeographic document from the Harvard Medical Library, pp. 1–38.

54. Morehouse, L.E., and A.T. Miller, Jr. *Physiology of Exercise.* St. Louis: C.V. Mosby Company, 1948, pp. 1–353.

55. Oscai, L. B. *Personal communication to CMT.* May 2, 1997.

56. Pappenheimer, R. S., Jr. *Physical Activity and Health. 40th Anniversary Lectures.* Indianapolis, IN: American College of Sports Medicine, 1994, pp. 93–109.

57. Park, R.J. The rise and demise of Harvard's B.S. program in anatomy, physiology, and physical training: a case of conflicts of interest and scarce resources. *Res. Q. Exer. Sports.* 63:246–260, 1992.

58. Rajor, J.E., and P.S. Brassie. Trends in the changing titles of departments of physical education in the United States. C.B. Corbin and H.M. Eckert (eds.). *The Academy Papers: The Evolving Undergraduate Major.* Champaign, IL: Human Kinetics Publishers, 1990, pp. 82–90.

59. Reed, C.I. Collateral maturation of physiology (1870-1910). *Physiologist* 5:300–307, 1962.

60. Reed, C.I. Physiology after the Civil War. *Physiologist* 5:90–96, 1962.

61. Richards, D.W. Lawrence Joseph Henderson. *Physiologist* 1:32–37, 1958.

62. Robergs, R.A., and S.O. Roberts. *Exercise Physiology: Exercise, Performance, and Clinical Applications.* St. Louis, MO: Mosby, 1997, pp. 1–801.

63. Schneider, E.C. *Physiology of Muscular Exercise.* Philadelphia, PA: W.B. Saunders Company, 1933, pp. 1–382.

64. Schneider, E.C., and P.V. Karpovich. *Physiology of Muscular Exercise. 3rd Edition.* Philadelphia, PA: W.B. Saunders Company, 1948, pp. 1–333.

65. Shephard, R.J. Putting medicine back into ACSM. *ACSM News.* 9:6–7, 1974.

66. Steinhaus, A.H. Studies in the physiology of exercise: I. Exercise and basal metabolism in dogs. *Am. J. Physiol.* 83:653–677, 1928.

67. Steinhaus, A.H. Chronic effects of exercise. *Physiol. Revs.* 13:103–147, 1933.

68. Steinhaus, A.H., L.A. Hoyt, and H.A. Rice. Studies in the physiology of exercise. X. The effects of running and swimming on the organ weight of growing dogs. *Am. J. Physiol.* 99: 512–520, 1932.

69. Strong, M. ACSM Certification Specialist. *Personal communication to CMT.* September 4, 1997.

70. Thomas, J.R. The body of knowledge: a common core. C.C. Corbin and H.M. Eckert (eds.). *The Academy Papers. The Evolving Undergraduate Major.* Champaign, IL: Human Kinetics Publishers, 1990, pp. 5–12.

71. Tipton, C.M. Exercise physiology, part II: a contemporary historical perspective. J.D. Massengale and R.A. Swanson (eds.). *The History of Exercise and Sport Science.* Champaign, IL: Human Kinetics Publishers, 1997, pp. 396–428, 431–438.

72. Tipton, C.M., J. Berryman, and W.P. Kroll. George Wells Fitz of Harvard: a forgotten advocate of exercise physiology. *FASEB J.*11:A53, 1997. (Abstract).

73. Wegner, N.K. Physical Activity in Primary and Secondary Prevention of Heart Disease. *40th Anniversary Lectures.* Indianapolis, IN: American College of Sports Medicine, 1994, pp. 43–54.

74. Wilmore, J.H. The challenge of change for physical education in 1980s: physiological view. M.G. Scott (ed.). *The Academy Papers, Issues and Challenges: A Kaleidoscope of Change.* Washington, D.C.: The American Academy of Physical Education, 1979, pp. 27–32.

75. Zeigler, E.F. Past, present, and future developments of physical education and sport. M.G. Scott (ed.). *The Academy Papers, Issues and Challenges: A Kaleidoscope of Change.* Washington, D.C.: The American Academy of Physical Education, 1979, pp. 9-19.

13
Physical Activity Epidemiology Applied to Children and Adolescents

CARL J. CASPERSEN, PH.D., M.P.H.
PATRICIA A. NIXON, PH.D.
ROBERT H. DuRANT, PH.D.

In 1996, the U.S. Department of Health and Human Services released the first Surgeon General's report on physical activity and health [186]. This report offered scientific evidence in support of the beneficial effects of regular physical activity on reduced mortality from all causes—from diseases such as cardiovascular diseases, non-insulin-dependent diabetes mellitus, and colon cancer, and from conditions such as obesity and high blood pressure. The value of this report to the public health community is considerable. But that value is diminished by the fact that the report did not address physical activity for child and adolescent populations.

Considerable efforts have been made in the areas of basic, clinical, and epidemiologic research to establish the beneficial influence of regular physical activity on health among child and adolescent populations. However, epidemiologic research is different from basic or clinical research. The latter two forms of research establish the biological and clinical basis for the health effects that physical activity can produce in the development and progression of chronic diseases and conditions that plague public health. Epidemiologic research, on the other hand, is particularly important to public health efforts because it must integrate its results with similar results from basic and clinical research in order to establish the relevance and applicability of its findings on a population basis [35]. This chapter is designed to introduce the practice and potential of physical activity epidemiology as applied to child and adolescent populations to both nonepidemiologists who are interested in the topic and to epidemiologists who have not focused on physical activity behaviors. The chapter begins with a brief discussion of what physical activity epidemiology involves and a description of health-related dimensions of physical activity. We then highlight how epidemiologists measure physical activity, review approaches being used for surveillance of physical activity among U.S. children and adolescents, offer prevalence estimates of some selected patterns of physical activity, provide examples of epidemiologic research in the area of physical activity among youth, and discuss the evidence of a potential beneficial association between physical activity and selected disease risks and health conditions. Finally, we present some current directions for the study of factors that help determine physical activity levels among children and adolescents, and some population-based efforts for the promotion of lifelong physical activity as a means of enhancing public health.

WHAT IS PHYSICAL ACTIVITY EPIDEMIOLOGY?

Physical activity epidemiology is applied to a behavior that can be linked to conditions and outcomes associated with health [32]. To understand this more fully, we first provide definitions that distinguish physical activity from exercise and physical fitness, and thereafter offer a definition of epidemiology.

Physical activity has been previously defined as "any bodily movement produced by skeletal muscles that results in caloric expenditure" [39]. At the same time, exercise is considered to be a subcategory of physical activity that is "planned, structured, and repetitive, and results in the improvement or maintenance of one or more facets of physical fitness." Physical fitness is not a behavior, but is more akin to a state or condition. Physical fitness has been defined as "something that people possess or achieve such as aerobic power, muscular endurance, muscular strength, body composition, and flexibility." Other attributes include agility, balance, coordination, reaction time, speed, and power [39].

Last [108] defined epidemiology as "the study of the distribution and determinants of health-related states and events in populations, and the application of this study to the control of health problems." Epidemiology involves: (1) defining a health problem and estimating its prevalence within particular populations; (2) identifying the factors that cause a health problem and the modes by which the factors are transmitted; (3) establishing the scientific basis for preventive activities or the allocation of resources; and (4) evaluating the effectiveness of preventive or therapeutic measures. Unlike basic or clinical research, which uses relatively small samples, epidemiology is interested in large, representative samples that will generalize to the public at large. By using large samples that have ample statistical power, epidemiologists are able to adjust for all the variables known to influence an association under investigation, and in so doing, establish the unique contribution of one factor (e.g., physical inactivity) to a suspected outcome of interest (e.g., the incidence of coronary heart disease) [32].

Caspersen [32] defined physical activity epidemiology as "a subspecialty of epidemiology that is concerned with (a) the association between physical activity behaviors and disease or other health outcomes, (b) the distribution and determinants of physical activity behaviors within given populations, and (c) the association between physical activity and other behaviors. The physical activity epidemiologist applies the results of descriptive and analytic research to the prevention and control of diseases and conditions within populations.'' Caspersen [32] asserted that physical activity measurement is a major part of physical activity epidemiology that, when not carefully understood and considered, can limit the researcher's ability to detect significant associations of physical activity with outcomes, determinants, and other behaviors. To provide a basis by which to understand the findings presented later in the chapter, we will first review measurement issues.

ISSUES IN MEASURING PHYSICAL ACTIVITY AMONG CHILDREN AND ADOLESCENTS

Physical activity epidemiologists must select the best measure of physical activity to effectively study a specific disease [32]. To make the best selection, it helps to consider which health-related dimension of physical activity one needs to address, along with its underlying mechanism of effect. Caspersen [32, 39] postulated that there are at least five health-related dimensions of physical activity that can be linked to specific diseases, conditions, and health outcomes—caloric expenditure, aerobic intensity, weight-bearing, muscular strength, and flexibility. Caloric expenditure, for example, is linked to diseases such as coronary heart disease, diabetes mellitus, and conditions such as obesity. Muscular strength and flexibility relate most to physical functioning (or disability), especially among older adult populations [35], and weight-bearing relates most to diseases such as osteoporosis (whose roots begin in childhood and adolescence [14]. Each dimension may exert its effect on specific diseases or conditions via different mechanisms [32]. Some mechanisms, such as the total rate or amount of caloric expenditure, are more physiological in nature. Other mechanisms, such as the force generated by skeletal muscles to produce strength, are more physical [32]. Knowing which health-related dimension of physical activity is measured and its underlying mechanism of effect is central to understanding disease-specific associations found in a specific population of interest.

Epidemiologists typically use surveys to measure physical activity among adult populations, children aged 10 yrs and older, and adolescents [17, 32, 99]. Surveys have several advantages over other methods: (1) they have acceptable accuracy in terms of reliability and validity; (2) they are relatively inexpensive; (3) they are convenient for study participants; and (4) they do not affect participants' behavior during measurement [107, 123]. Because most physical activity of children younger than 10 yrs of age is neither planned nor structured, surveys have limited use. Instead, studies of younger children can measure total caloric expenditure using the doubly-labeled water technique [79] or perhaps by using heart rate monitors [65, 77, 89, 106, 167], and can measure body movement by activity monitors [98, 157, 199] or direct observation [16, 60, 96, 120, 139]. Unfortunately, each of these objective measures of physical activity share several disadvantages; not only do they lack low cost and practicality required in epidemiologic studies seeking large, representative samples, they also (with the exception of certain direct observation procedures) do not identify specific types of physical activity being performed. Regardless, objective physical activity measures are still very useful as validation criteria to which physical activity surveys can be compared [99].

Two types of physical activity surveys are used—activity diaries [26] and self-administered or interviewer-administered activity questionnaires [1, 7, 26, 29, 50, 89, 158, 163]. The activity questionnaire can include a single question about usual activity [6, 78] or ask participants to recall activity during a day [89, 158], a week [158], a year [1], or even a lifetime [103]. Since shorter time frames are easier for children and adolescents to recall, surveys that use short time frames show greater evidence of reliability and validity than surveys that require long-term recall. However, short periods of recall may not reflect usual behavior [99]. Results of heart rate monitoring, a precise and objective measure, provide evidence of the potential for misclassification that could arise from the use of short time frames of measurement. For example, DuRant et al. [57] found that 16 days of physical activity would have to be observed to reliably estimate the average activity of 3-, 4-, and 5-yr-olds. In addition, surveys or other measurement procedures that use short time frames also cannot capture seasonal differences in physical activity [57].

It is not practical to use surveys as an accurate measure of the total caloric expenditure of a population because of the number and combination of physical activities that would have to be assessed. The need to assess basal metabolic rate presents an additional complexity. Nonetheless, researchers often try to overcome this limitation by assessing physical activities that require a caloric expenditure well above that needed to accomplish tasks of daily living or simple moving around [35]. For example, one survey might assess a variety of sports activities, household cleaning, vigorous conditioning exercises, strengthening exercise, stretching exercise, and transportation-related behaviors, such as walking or bicycling, for 30 minutes [92]. One could then approximate a measure of total caloric expenditure by tallying total time spent, or by calculating a kilocalorie index from common physical activities reported in a survey. Either of these calculations can then be used to rank children and adolescents on a scale of least active to most active [32]. Since most children and adolescents are not engaged in work for pay, physical activity surveys of these populations have not fully or fruitfully assessed occupational physical activity [41].

The limitations of physical activity surveys for children younger than 10 yrs of age make their use in physical activity surveillance problematic. Moreover, while objective procedures, such as activity monitoring, are being used more and more in epidemiologic and experimental studies among this population, there is, nonetheless, considerable uncertainty as to what precisely the units actually measure as well as how to standardize the instrument placement [99]. Because of these limitations, surveillance efforts undertaken as input to decision makers must rely on physical activity surveys among older children and adolescents to guide policy development or to promote meaningful increases in physical activity levels for individuals or groups.

PHYSICAL ACTIVITY SURVEILLANCE IN THE UNITED STATES

A central function in physical activity epidemiology is surveillance [37], which includes: (1) monitoring the prevalence and incidence of chronic diseases, conditions, and health events that can be influenced by physical activity; (2) assessing the prevalence of and changes in physical activity patterns; and (3) determining the prevalence of behavioral determinants of physical activity [32]. Epidemiologists often use data from different surveillance systems in the form of ecological comparisons to generate hypotheses or draw inferences. Surveillance data are also used to develop promotional efforts, to allocate limited resources, and to develop policies. Physical activity epidemiologists are not able to monitor as many diseases in child and adolescent populations as in adult populations since mortal and morbid outcomes are fortunately rare among children and adolescents [40, 128]. However, outcomes such as obesity levels, lipid levels, injuries, etc. are useful for monitoring purposes [37]. Moreover, surveillance in child and adolescent populations relies heavily on monitoring the total amounts of all activities, the prevalence or time spent in a specific physical activity, or the combinations of frequency, duration, and intensity of individual or group activities. Inherent in such formulations is the assumption that one will estimate either undesirable amounts (e.g., risk factor orientation) or desirable amounts (e.g., preventive orientation) of physical activity that are presumably linked to health outcomes. Information may be broken down by age, race/ethnicity, income status, or other sociodemographic variables [40].

In the U.S., four surveillance systems provide information on physical activity among children and adolescents (Table 13.1): (1) The National Health Interview Survey-Health Promotion Disease Prevention Supplement (NHIS-HPDP), which interviewed older adolescents aged 18–21 in 1990, 1991, and 1995; (2) the Behavioral Risk Factor Surveillance System (BRFSS), a monthly survey including adolescents ages 18–21 conducted by state health departments in a joint effort with the Centers for Disease Control and Prevention (CDC) in 1991 and in even-numbered years beginning in 1992; (3) the National Health Interview Survey-Youth Risk Behavior Survey (NHIS-YRBS), which interviewed children and adolescents aged 12–21 in 1992; (4) and the Youth Risk Behavior Survey (YRBS) which interviews students in grades 9–12 (roughly aged 14–19) in nationally representative

TABLE 13.1
Characteristics of Data Systems for Physical Activity Surveillance Among Children and Adolescents, United States, 1990–1997

Name of Survey	Survey Years	Months[a] Covered	Age of Sample	Survey Method[b]	Recall Period	Items in Survey	Method of Probing	Nature[c] and Detail of Survey Data
National Health Interview Survey– Health Promotion Disease Prevention Supplment	1990 1991 1992 1993 1994 1995	JFMAMJJASOND JFMAMJJASOND JFMAMJJASOND	18–21+	PI	past 2 wks	22	list specific	F/I/T/D
Behavioral Risk Factor Surveillance System	1990 1991 1992 1993 1994 1995 1996	JFMAMJJASOND JFMAMJJASOND JFMAMJJASOND JFMAMJJASOND JFMAMJJASOND	18–21+	TI	past mo	10	open-ended	F/I/T/D
National Health Interview Survey– Youth Risk Behavior Survey	1992	JFMAMJJASOND	12–21	PI	past wk	11	close-ended	F by I and/or D
Youth Risk Behavior Survey	1991 1992 1993 1994 1995 1996 1997	MAM MAM MAM MAM	14–19[d]	SAQ	past wk	11	close-ended	F by I and/or D

[a] JFMAMJJASOND = January, February, March, April, May, June, July, August, September, October, November, December.
[b] PI = personal interview; SAQ = self-administered questionnaire; TI = telephone interview.
[c] F = frequency; I = intensity; T = type; D = duration.
[d] Grades 9–12.

schools in the spring of odd-numbered years. Although the Third National Health and Nutrition Examination Survey has physical activity data for the years 1988 through 1994 [129], it has yet to be used as part of ongoing physical activity surveillance for children and adolescents.

Each of the above data systems uses a short-term recall of the frequency, and often the duration and intensity, of listed activities or as part of an open-ended solicitation (Table 13.1). Hence, each system is somewhat unique, in part, because there is currently no uniform method of assessing physical activity [37]. Each system has its own wording for questions, style and season of survey administration, sampling frame, sample size, technique, survey response rate, and so on [37]. However, while their methods of assessment differ, their physical activity summary scores were all designed to monitor selected behaviors as part of physical activity objectives for the year 2000 [185] (Table 13.2). Each objective is linked specifically to health-related physical activity dimensions of caloric expenditure, aerobic intensity, flexibility, and muscle strength [33]. In addition, while neither the reliability nor the validity of the four sets of survey questions has been demonstrated extensively among children and adolescents, the methodologies are well-described in the Surgeon General's Report on physical activity and health [186]; copies of the surveys and sample computations are available as well [143].

NHIS-HPDP

The HPDP supplement exists as part of the NHIS data collection effort that the National Center for Health Statistics conducted in 1990 through 1995 [133]. The NHIS typically selects a probability sample of the civilian, noninstitutionalized population of the U.S. aged 18 yrs or older [130, 131, 133] for in-home interviews. For the HPDP supplement, persons were randomly selected from each family that had been interviewed for the NHIS in 1990, 1991, and 1995. Although the overall sampling frame oversampled blacks, the final sample was poststratified by the age, sex, and racial distribution of the U.S. population for each survey year and weighted to provide national estimates. The overall response rate for the NHIS ranged between 83–88%.

Respondents to the HPDP interview indicated whether they had engaged in any of 22 exercises, sports, or physically active hobbies in the previous 2 wks [132], with open-ended solicitations that allowed respondents to report information on two other activities. For each activity, respondents provided the frequency, duration, and self-perceived physical effort associated with participation (none, small, moderate, or large increases in heart rate or breathing) [34, 38]. Then, based upon the perceived physical effort, an intensity code was assigned to the specific level of activity participation (only a single intensity code was used for golf, calisthenics or general exercise, swimming or water exercises, skating, and skiing). A computerized scoring system [34, 38] was used to group respondents according to four activity

TABLE 13.2
Health-Related Dimensions of Physical Activity with Possible Mechanism of Effect, Diseases or Conditions Affected, and Applicable Year 2000 Objectives

Physical Activity Dimension	Possible Mechanism	Diseases or Conditions Affected[a]	Year 2000 Objective
Caloric expenditure	Energy utilization	CHD, NIDDM, obesity, cancer	Objective 1.3: Increase to at least 30 percent the proportion of people aged 6 and older who engage regularly, preferably daily, in light to moderate physical activity for at least 30 minutes per day.
Aerobic intensity	Enhanced cardiac function	CHD, NIDDM, cancer	Objective 1.4: Increase to at least 20 percent the proportion of people aged 18 and older and to at least 75 percent the proportion of children and adolescents aged 6 through 17 who engage in vigorous physical activity that promotes the development and maintenance of cardiorespiratory fitness 3 or more days per week for 20 or more minutes per occasion.
Flexibility	Range of motion	Physical disability	Objective 1.6: Increase to at least 40 percent the proportion of people aged 6 and older who regularly perform physical activities that enhance and maintain muscular strength, muscular endurance, and flexibility.
Muscular strength	Muscle force generation	Physical disability	Object 1.6: Same as above
Weight-bearing	Gravitational force	Osteoporosis	n/a

[a] CHD = coronary heart disease; NIDDM = noninsulin-dependent diabetes mellitus; n/a = not applicable.

patterns: (1) physically inactive (no leisure-time physical activity); (2) irregularly active (activity performed < 3 times per wk, < 20 min per occasion, or both); (3) regularly active, not intensive (≥ 3 times per wk, ≥ 20 min per occasion, and < 50% of maximal cardiorespiratory capacity); and (4) regularly active, intensive (≥ 3 times per week, ≥ 20 minutes per occasion, ≥ 50 percent of maximal cardiorespiratory capacity, and rhythmically contracting large muscle groups). The first activity pattern estimates the year 2000 objective to reduce the percentage of Americans who report no leisure-time physical activity (objective 1.5), while the 4th pattern estimates the objective to increase regular, vigorous exercise (objective 1.4) [33, 185]. Respondents who perform 30 min of physical activity 5 times per wk provide an estimate of regular, sustained light-to-moderate physical activity (objective 1.3).

BRFSS

The BRFSS conducts monthly, year-round telephone interviews of older adolescents and adults aged 18 yrs and older, sampled by random-digit dialing [43, 46, 72, 194]. For 1990–1996, the total sample sizes for all participating states exceeded 100,000, and state-specific response rates ranged between 60–70%. Trained interviewers first ask respondents, "During the past month, did you participate in any physical activities or exercises such as running, calisthenics, golf, gardening, or walking for exercise?" Then, the interviewers question respondents about the frequency and duration of their two most common physical activities [36]. Using a computerized scoring system also used to analyze the NHIS-HPDP, this information, along with the activities' intensities and whether the activities involved the rhythmic contraction of large muscle groups, can classify how physically active the respondents were [34, 36, 38]. This system also calculates the percentage of each respondent's estimated maximal cardiorespiratory capacity [91] and calculates an intensity code using the velocity associated with running, jogging, walking, or swimming (see also Caspersen, C.J., and K.E.Powell. A computerized scoring method for the physical activity questions of the Behavioral Risk Factor Surveillance System. An unpublished technical monograph, 1986). With this procedure, the BRFSS can also estimate the prevalence of year 2000 objectives 1.3–1.5.

NHIS-YRBS

The 1992 NHIS-YRBS gathered information about risk behaviors among young people aged 18–21 yrs [44, 131]. Using the NHIS national probability sample of households, the NHIS-YRBS conducted a follow-back survey between April 1992 and April 1993, that oversampled youth not attending school. A total of 10,645 young people completed the interview, with an overall response rate of 74%.

The survey was administered via portable cassette players equipped with earphones, and respondents marked their answers on standardized answer sheets. This methodology was designed to ensure confidentiality of responses and to help those who would have difficulty answering a written questionnaire. Questions probed for the frequency of vigorous physical activity (e.g., exercise or take part in sports that made you sweat and breathe hard, such as basketball, jogging, fast dancing, swimming laps, tennis, fast bicycling, or other aerobic activities in the previous 7 days). Using the same time frame of recall, respondents were also asked how often they had engaged in 10 groups of activities: (1) stretching exercises, such as toe touching, knee bending, or leg stretching; (2) exercises to strengthen or tone muscles, such as pushups, sit-ups, or weight lifting; (3) house cleaning or yard work for ≥ 30 min at a time; (4) walking or bicycling for ≥ 30 min at a time; (5) baseball, softball, or Frisbee®; (6) basketball, football, or soccer; (7) roller skating, ice skating, skiing, or skateboarding; (8) running, jogging, or swimming for exercise; (9) tennis, racquetball, or squash; and (10) aerobics or dance.

To estimate the year 2000 objective for regular, sustained physical activity, the NHIS-YRBS, as well as the YRBS (see next section), used the combination of walking and bicycling the respondents said they performed 5 times per wk and 30 min per occasion in the previous week. Reports of no participation in either vigorous activity or walking or bicycling were used to estimate no reported leisure-time physical activity (objective 1.5) [186], although the concept of leisure time is a bit tenuous among young populations having large amounts of discretionary time [41]. Estimates of 3 days per wk of stretching and strength training are used to estimate year 2000 objective 1.6 (see Table 13.2) [185].

YRBS

The YRBS measures six categories of priority health-risk behaviors among adolescents, [100, 101] using national, state, and local school-based surveys of students in grades 9–12 in the spring of odd-numbered years [42, 45, 48].

The national YRBS uses a three-stage cluster sample design and includes students in public and private schools in all 50 states and the District of Columbia, with augmented sampling of black and Hispanic students. In 1995, North Carolina and Vermont conducted the YRBS in middle schools. Trained interviewers administer the questionnaire in the classroom, and students record their responses on sheets that later are scanned by computer for scoring. These procedures protect both student privacy and anonymity, and produce high response rates; school response rates range from 70–78%, student response rates range from 86–90%, and the overall response rates range from 60–70%. Between 10,000–16,000 students completed questionnaires between the years 1991–1995.

YRBS includes eight questions on physical activity [92]. The question on vigorous physical activity states, "On how many of the past 7 days did you exercise or participate in sports activities for at least 20 minutes that made you sweat and breathe hard, such as basketball, jogging, fast dancing, swimming laps, tennis, fast bicycling, or similar aerobic activities?'' This question is different from that used for the NHIS-YRBS since it asks respondents to base their answer on at least 20 min of vigorous exercise. Another question asks how many times respondents engaged in three specific activities in the previous 7 days: (1) walking or bicycling for at least 30 min at a time; (2) stretching exercises, such as toe touching, knee bending, or leg stretching; and (3) exercises to strengthen or tone the muscles, such as pushups, situps, or weight lifting. Respondents are asked two other questions: "In an average week when you are in school, on how many days do you go to physical education classes?" and "During an average physical education class, how many minutes do you spend actually exercising or playing sports?" These two questions are used to monitor the year 2000 objectives pertaining to physical education (PE) [33, 185]. Two questions can be used to monitor the influence of sport teams (outside of PE classes) on students' physical activity levels: "During the past 12 months, on how many sports teams run by your school did you play?" and "During the past 12 months, on how many sports teams run by organizations outside of your school did you play?"

Brenner et al. [29] has reported substantial reliability (using Kappa coefficients of percent agreement) for several YRBS questions: enrolled in PE class (91%), having exercised for more than 20 min per class period (75%), having played on school sport teams (69%), and having played on other sport teams (64%).

Examples From 1992 NHIS-YRBS for Selected Physical Activity Patterns

As implied previously, decision-makers can use surveillance data to guide the promotion of meaningful increases in physical activity patterns, which are known to vary by a variety of factors for individuals or groups of individuals. For example, the 1992 NHIS-YRBS revealed that physical activity patterns among children and adolescents vary substantially by sex, age, race/ethnicity, geographic region, the time of the survey, and household income [41, 186]. Twenty-nine percent of males surveyed reported walking or bicycling for 30 or more min, 5 or more days per wk—the year 2000 objective for regular, sustained activity—as compared to 24% of females. However, there were no statistically significant sex differences at any age from 12–21. Thirty-six percent of Hispanic males reported walking and bicycling, as compared with 28% percent of white, non-Hispanic males. The comparable figures for Hispanic females were 29% and 23%, respectively. The respective proportions for youth living in the West, Northeast, South, and Midwest were 31%, 29%, 25%, and 23%. Finally, 28% of youth reporting during September and October noted this pattern, as compared to 23% of youth reporting during January and February. Youth having a household income of $50,000 or more reported lower levels (albeit not statistically) of walking and bicycling as compared to other income groups.

1992 NHIS-YRBS also revealed that the proportion of youth reporting vigorous physical activity for 20 min or more, 3 or more days per wk—the year 2000 objective for regular, vigorous activity—also varied substantially according to sociodemographic and other factors [41, 186]. For example, 60% of males reported regular, vigorous activity, as compared to only 47% of females, although reported declines from ages 12 to 21 were less pronounced for males (from 71% to 42%) than for females (from 66% to 30%). A higher proportion of white, non-Hispanic females reported this pattern as compared to black, non-Hispanic or Hispanic females (42% each), while males of differing race/ethnicity status had similar rates. Rates of vigorous physical activity decreased from 60% for youth reporting household income of $50,000 or greater, to roughly 47% for household incomes of less than $10,000. Fifty-nine percent of youth reported vigorous activity during May through June, decreasing to 48% during November and December. Rates did not vary by geographic region.

From data such as the 1992 NHIS-HPDP, it is clear that physical activity promotional strategies for American children and adolescents should be cognizant of sociodemographic, geographic, and seasonal differences in physical activity patterns.

PHYSICAL ACTIVITY EPIDEMIOLOGIC RESEARCH

Research Designs

Two basic types of study designs are available to physical activity epidemiologists who wish to explore the association between physical activity and a specific disease or condition [32, 35]—an observational study design or an experimental design. Each has its strengths and weaknesses, as described below.

OBSERVATIONAL STUDIES. Physical activity epidemiologists can choose from four types of observational studies: (1) an ecologic study; (2) a cross-sectional study; (3) a case-control (or retrospective) study; or (4) a longitudinal study. In ecologic studies, epidemiologists examine data on a specific disease or condition from different sources or even complete surveillance systems to help generate hypotheses or draw inferences. This is often done by comparing a trend in the prevalence as revealed by one data set with the occurrence of a likely risk factor or determinant as revealed by a second data set. For example, an epidemiologist might compare the rate of increase of overweight with changes in physical activity over the same period. However, this approach has one serious limitation. If a factor such as dietary intake increases, the erroneous conclusion might be drawn that there is an association between the two variables being studied when, in fact, they share no relationship or only a limited one.

The cross-sectional study measures information about several potential risk factors and indices of health status concurrently in a population. Boreham et al. [25] used this methodology in their study of 12- and 15-yr-old male schoolchildren in Northern Ireland who reported sports participation based on extracurricular sports and other physical activity performed during a week. They found a significant association between an increasing score of total physical activity with lower systolic blood pressure. This finding prevailed after statistical adjustments for body size, sexual maturity, dietary intake, smoking, social class, and other potential confounding variables were made. The study design provided greater confidence, but not complete assurance, that the association was independent of the potential confounding influences. However, this design cannot identify a temporal or causal linkage between the suspected etiologic factor (physical activity) and the outcome (systolic blood pressure).

In case-control (or retrospective) study designs, individuals with and without a particular disease or condition are asked about their exposure to one or more risk factors prior to the diagnosis of the disease. When cases are found to have greater exposure to a suspected risk factor, one may begin to infer that the factor may have caused the disease. As children and adolescents often have problems recalling past events, especially physical activity [17], this design is not common among this population.

Finally, in longitudinal or prospective study designs, persons who do not have a particular disease or condition are followed over time to establish the presence or absence of risk factors that are measured at the beginning of the monitoring period. For example, in their 8-year longitudinal study of Danish adolescents, Andersen and Haraldsdottir [7] examined changes in the weekly time reported for sport and leisure activities relative to changes in percent of body fat measured via skinfolds. The main strength of this type of study—its long period of follow-up—is also one of its weaknesses, since such follow-up can be costly. Also contributing to the higher cost of longitudinal studies is their typically large sample size relative to the other observational study designs.

EXPERIMENTAL STUDIES. The most powerful epidemiologic study, like its basic or clinical research counterpart, is the experimental design. In this type of study, the epidemiologist attempts to eliminate or postpone the occurrence of a disease or condition by manipulating a risk factor. Although this design is the most powerful, it is also the most costly and the most time-consuming. First, the epidemiologist must identify a representative sample of persons without disease or condition for investigation. Then, each person in the sample must be randomly assigned to either a treatment (or intervention) group or a nontreatment (or control) group. The epidemiologist then follows the sample over time to establish either the proportion of each group that gets the disease or condition or the group that changes the most on a previously measured health-related parameter.

Hansen et al. [83] used an experimental design to study the relation between physical activity and blood pressure in a representative sample of more than 1500 Danish schoolchildren. They randomly allocated hypertensive and normotensive children to enhanced PE sessions performed 3 times per wk and found significant decreases in the systolic and diastolic blood pressure of both groups of children, as compared to a control group that followed their regular PE classes. Also using an experimental design, Sallis et al. [161] followed 4th grade students after randomly allocating four schools each to a traditional PE class (control group) or to a class that followed a special curriculum designed to enhance students' physical fitness and self-management skills in order to increase their in-school and out-of-school physical activity. In addition, students in the intervention group were randomly assigned to either a specialist-led class or a teacher-led class.

Some Findings of Physical Activity Epidemiologic Research

In the previous section, we briefly presented two basic types of study designs used in physical activity epidemiologic research. In this section, we focus closely on the findings of selected studies of physical activity among children and adolescents grouped (in sequence) into the following chronic disease risk factors or outcomes: (1) elevated serum lipids; (2) high blood pressure; (3) increased insulin; (4) obesity and overweight; (5) bone mineral density; and (6) unintentional injury. We also discuss findings of studies of determinants and interventions of physical activity among children and adolescents. Along with the narrative, we provide tables that focus on the study sample and some important sample characteristics that suggest its representativeness. Each table also includes study definitions or measures of physical activity (or determinant) exposure and outcomes of interest, the main findings, available dose-response information, and an indication of the statistical adjustments made to rule-out other explanatory or confounding factors. This information is provided to offer both insight into how the various study designs have been applied and a rudimentary view of the quality of the available epidemiologic data that may be used to infer health benefits of physical activity for children and adolescents.

SERUM LIPIDS. Cardiovascular diseases are the leading cause of death among adults in the U.S. [5, 170]. Cardiovascular disease risk factors develop early in life and tend to be maintained from year to year. Autopsy studies of children and adolescents reveal a relationship between both elevated lipid and lipoprotein levels as well as coronary artery plaques [136]. Although physical activity and exercise have been found to generally elicit positive changes in serum lipid and lipoprotein levels among adults, the experimental and epidemiologic evidence for a relationship among children and adolescents is less clear [7].

Two cross-sectional epidemiologic studies of older children and adolescents, by Perusse et al. [144] and by Tell and Vellar [181], reported an inverse relationship between physical activity and triglycerides [144, 181]. The first study also reported a positive correlation between physical activity and HDL-C [144] (Table 13.3). Physical activity was positively correlated with VO_2 max, which in turn was associated with lower total cholesterol and triglycerides and higher HDL-C/LDL-C and HDL-C/total cholesterol ratios [181]. Contradictory findings were found in a number of smaller studies that reported on the relationship between physical activity and lipids. Physical activity training studies have found higher HDL-C [11, 115, 137, 173, 188, 195] and HDL_2 [11] levels among trained adolescents as compared to untrained adolescents; however, no difference in total cholesterol was found. Trained individuals also had higher apolipoprotein levels than did untrained adolescents [115]. However, Armstrong and Simons-Morton [8] pointed out that these studies suffered from selection bias, such as small sample sizes and no control of training intensity, frequency, or duration of the training. Other studies have provided additional evidence that more active children and adolescents, as compared to sedentary youth, may have higher HDL-C [62, 63, 191, 192], lower ratios of total cholesterol/HDL-C and LDL-C/HDL-C [62, 63], and lower triglycerides [62, 63, 192]. Also, Craig et al. [50] found an inverse relationship between self-reported physical activity and LDL-C in preadolescent girls. By contrast, several other studies found no differences in serum lipids, lipoproteins, and apolipoproteins comparing active children with sedentary children [9, 116, 168], but these studies also had a number of methodologic shortcomings that limit the conclusions that can be drawn.

Several longitudinal studies suggest that there is a relationship between physical activity and serum lipids and lipoproteins in children and adolescents (Table 13.3). In a small sample (N = 123) of 3- and 4-yr-old white, black, and Hispanic children, DuRant et al. [59] observed physical activity and heart rates on 4 days over a yearlong period, every minute of each day for up to 12 hrs a day. They found that two indicators of physical activity were inversely associated with triglyceride levels at the one-year follow-up period, and that the slope of the exercise heart rate was associated with HDL_2. Although this small, nonrandom sample limits the ability to generalize from these findings, the methods used to measure physical activity greatly surpass those of all other studies reported to date.

In the Young Finns study, a 12-yr longitudinal investigation of 3-, 6-, 9-, 12-, 15-, and 18-yr-old children and adolescents, Porkka et al. [146] found that baseline exercise levels (defined as an index of physical activity from the product of intensity, duration, and monthly frequency of exercise) were inversely associated with triglyceride levels among males aged 12–18 yrs but not among their female counterparts. No effect of baseline exercise on lipid levels was found at the 12-yr follow-up among younger children. How-

TABLE 13.3.
Examples of Epidemiologic Studies of the Association Between Physical Activity and Serum Lipids and Lipoproteins Among Children and Adolescents

Study Design, Population, and Investigators	Response Rate, Completion Rate, and Final Response Rate[a]	Sex[b]	Age (Yrs)	Race[c]	Measurement of Physical Activity (PA)[d]	Measurement of Lipids and Lipoproteins[e]	Main Findings[f]	Dose Response[g]	Adjustments[h]
Cross-sectional									
French Canadian families, Perusse et al. (1989) [144]	RR = ? CR = ? FR = ?	484 M 419 F 903 T	14.5– 14.8 ± 3.3	903 W	3-day activity record of average number of 15-min periods in which subjects engaged in exercise activities; index of physical working capacity.	TOT-C, TRIG, HDL-C, LDL-C, HDL-C/ TOT-C	Standardized partial regression coefficients revealed that PA level was significantly correlated inversely with TRIG (B = −0.07) and positively with HDL-C (B = 0.10).	n/r	Age, gender, physical working capacity, body mass index, multiple skinfolds, caloric intake, alcohol intake, cigarette smoking.
Oslo Youth Study, Tell and Vellar (1988) [181]	RR = 81% CR = ? FR = ?	431 M 397 F 828 T	10– 15	828 W	Frequency of exercise ≥30 min resulting in being out of breath and sweating; VO₂max.	TOT-C, TRIG, HDL-C/ TOT-C	F: PA was significantly associated with lower mean TRIG and with higher VO$_2$max (r = 0.11). VO$_2$max associated with TOT-C (r = −0.10), TRIG (r = −0.09), and HDL-C/ TOT-C (r = 0.12).	Linear relation on a 5-point scale.	Tanner stage, BMI.
Longitudinal									
NHLBI Studies of Child Activity and Nutrition, DuRant et al. (1993) [59]	RR = ? CR = 65% FR = ?	59 M 64 F 123 T	3–4 to 4–5	44 W 50 B 29 H	Percentage of all day heart rates at 25% and 50% of resting level. Children's PA rating scale scored as percentage of min at level 3, 4, or 5; level 3, 4, 5 only; and levels 4 or 5 only. Slope of exercise heart rate.	TOT-C, TRIG, HDL$_1$-C, HDL$_2$-C, LDL-C, LDL-C/ HDL-C, TOT-C/ HDL-C	Significant correlation between mean PA at yr one and TRIG (r = −0.22) and percentage of PA at levels 3, 4, or 5 and TRIG (r = 0.18). Significant (correlation between slope of the exercise heart rate and HDL$_2$ (r = 0.21).	Linear relation between PA and lipids.	Sum of skin folds, height and gender. Average resting heart rate and waist to hip ratio.

Study		Sample	Age		PA Measure	Lipids	Results		Adjustments
Young Finns Study, Porkka et al. (1994) [146]	RR = 83% CR = 25% FR = 21%	414 M 469 F 883 T	3–18	883 W	Index of PA from the product of intensity, duration, and monthly frequency of exercise.	TOT-C, TRIG, HDL-C, LDL-C	Baseline PA levels were associated with 1992 lipid levels only for 12–18 yr-old males. Exercise explained 3% of variation in TRIG.	n/r	Baseline TRIG, subscapular skinfold, ratio of polyunsaturated to saturated fatty acids, daily smoking.
Adolescent and young adult women taking oral contraceptives, Linder et al. (1989) [111]	RR = ? CR = ? FR = ?	37 F	16–28	37 B	Frequency and number of mins 17 activities were performed over previous 2 wks. Aerobic PA defined as activities of ≥3 days/wk and ≥30 min/day at each month of follow-up.	TOT-C, TRIG, HDL-C, LDL-C, TOT-C/ HDL-C, LDL-C/ HDL-C	At 3 months, active subjects had significantly lower mean TOT-C and LDL-C (23–25 mg/dl) (independent of type of progestin) and significantly lower mean ratios (0.45–0.65) for TOT-C/HDL ratios than did nonactive subjects. PA moderated the negative effect of norgesterol on TOT-C/HDL-C and LDL-C/HDL-C.	n/r	Age, BMI, liver enzymes.
Experimental Boy Scouts, Linder, DuRant, Mahoney (1983) [112]	RR = ? CR = 78% FR = ?	50 M	11–17	50 W	Aerobic exercise 4 days/wk for 8 wks (3 days of run/walk at 80% of maximum heart rate for 25–30 min, 1 day of soccer or rugby for 1 hr)	TOT-C, TRIG, HDL-C, LDL-C, VLDL-C, LDL-C/ HDL-C, TOT-C/ HDL-C	No change in lipids despite increase in physical working capacity index (15.2%, p < 0.05).	n/a	n/a

(continued)

357

TABLE 13.3. *(continued)*

Study Design, Population, and Investigators	Response Rate, Completion Rate, and Final Response Rate[a]	Sex[b]	Age (Yrs)	Race[c]	Measurement of Physical Activity (PA)[d]	Measurement of Lipids and Lipoproteins[e]	Main Findings[f]	Dose Response[g]	Adjustments[h]
Middle school students, Rowland et al. (1996) [153]	RR = ? CR = 94% FR = ?	14 M 20 F 34 T	10– 12	32 W 2 B	Alternating 2-wk blocks of aerobic dance, step aerobics, running, and circuit activities 3 times/wk for 13 wks.	TOT-C, TRIG, HDL-C, LDL-C	No change in lipids despite increase in VO$_2$max (5.4%, p = 0.06).	n/a	n/a
CATCH study 3rd grade students, Webber et al., (1996) and Luepker et al. (1996) [113, 198]	RR = 60% CR = 79% FR = 48%	2645 M 2461 F 5106 T	Mean: 8.7 ± 0.5	2810 W 506 B 565 H 73 A 16 N 49 O	Behavioral intervention designed to increase PA and alter dieting behaviors	TOT-C on 40% of children, HDL-C, and apolipoprotein-B	No effect on lipids	n/a	n/a

[a] RR = response rate; CR = completion rate; FR = final response rate; n/r = not reported; CBD = cannot be determined.

[b] M = males; F = females; T = total.

[c] W = white; B = black; A = Asian; H = Hispanic/Latino; NA = Native American; O = other.

[d] VO$_2$max = estimated maximal oxygen consumption; n/a = not applicable.

[e] TOT-C = total serum cholesterol; HDL-C = high-density lipoprotein; LDL-C = low-density lipoprotein; VLDL-C = very low-density lipoprotein; TRIG = triglycerides.

[f] Multiple regression coefficients are not standardized or residualized except where indicated.

[g] n/r = not reported; n/a = not applicable.

[h] BMI = body mass index; n/a = not applicable.

ever, the investigators only used the measure of exercise levels from the baseline and did not analyze the measures of exercise at any of the four follow-up periods, thus creating a significant flaw in this study.

In a 3-mon longitudinal study nested within an experimental design that tested the effect of oral contraceptives containing two types of progestins on serum lipids, Linder et al. [111] (Table 13.3) found that active subjects—all of whom were black adolescents and young women—had lower total serum cholesterol and LDL-C than nonactive subjects, independent of the type of progestin in the oral contraceptive they were taking. Also, physical activity level moderated the negative effect that norgestrel had on the total cholesterol/HDL-C and LDL-C/HDL-C ratios. Nonactive subjects taking norgestrel had a significant increase in lipid ratios, whereas active subjects had no change.

Only one randomized experimental trial that tested the effect of exercise on serum lipids in children and adolescents has been conducted (Table 13.3). Linder et al. [112] tested the effect of an 8-wk aerobic exercise program on serum lipid levels among a small sample (N = 50) of white Boy Scouts. The boys' physical working capacity index was significantly higher following the exercise program, but no change was found in the boys' serum lipid levels. Rowland et al. [153] used a pretest-pretest-posttest design without a control group to test the effect of a 13-wk aerobic exercise program on serum lipids of 34 children aged 10–12 years. They found a 5.4% increase in VO_2 max following the exercise program but no change in lipid levels. Finally, the Child And Adolescent Trial for Cardiovascular Health (CATCH) used a quasi-experimental design, in which schools were the unit of randomization and students were the unit of analysis, to test two interventions on several outcomes [113, 198]. The interventions were designed to change physical activity and eating behaviors. Total cholesterol was measured on all 4019 children, and HDL-C and apolipoprotein-B were measured on 40% of the sample. The interventions were found to have no effect on serum lipids.

In summary, the epidemiologic studies to date are equivocal on the relationship between physical activity and the serum lipid and lipoprotein levels of children and adolescents. Nonetheless, that physical activity, exercise, and fitness, in various combinations, account for a small amount of the variability of lipid and lipoprotein levels of children and adolescents seems reasonable from the preponderance of evidence. Population-based, randomized controlled trials of both children and adolescents are required to establish if longer-term aerobic exercise, as well as other levels of physical activity, can have a beneficial effect on serum lipid, lipoprotein, and apolipoprotein levels. Moreover, such studies must control to ensure that confounders are not accounting for the relationships that are noted.

BLOOD PRESSURE. High blood pressure, or "hypertension," is a primary risk factor for cardiovascular morbidity and mortality. It is estimated that about 50 million Americans have high blood pressure [134], including 2.8 million children and adolescents aged 6–17 yrs [187]. Blacks have a higher prevalence of hypertension than whites, and there is some evidence that black children have higher blood pressure levels than white children [19]. The development of high blood pressure is believed to begin in childhood [85], and evidence suggests that elevated blood pressure tracks from adolescence into adulthood [109, 110].

The exact etiology of hypertension is unknown, but is attributed to both genetic and environmental factors [86]. Children with hypertensive parents are 2.5–5.0 times more likely to develop hypertension than children with normotensive parents [142, 169]. Obesity is also associated with elevated blood pressure [150], and the combination of parental history of hypertension and higher relative body weight increases the likelihood of developing hypertension later in life [140]. Environmental factors associated with high blood pressure include excessive sodium intake, weight gain, increased alcohol consumption, and physical inactivity [86]. As a consequence, intervention and prevention strategies aimed at children have targeted diet and exercise.

Of the 15 cross-sectional studies we reviewed, only five reported a significant inverse association between physical activity and either systolic blood pressure (SBP) [3, 25, 89, 90] or diastolic blood pressure (DBP) [3, 31, 90]. The majority found no such association [6, 10, 50, 88, 94, 119, 147, 148, 165, 181]. Several studies [25, 31, 90] reported both an inverse association and no association between physical activity and blood pressure depending on the sex and age of the study subjects. For example, Jenner et al. [90] found a significant inverse association between physical activity and SBP and DBP among females but not among males (Table 13.4). Boreham et al. [25] also reported a significant association between physical activity and SBP (but not DBP) among males. In the only study of black children, Bush et al. [31] found a significant difference between age groups. The researchers found physical activity to be a significant independent predictor of DBP among younger siblings aged 3–4 yrs but not older siblings aged 8–10 yrs. Despite the sex and age differences noted within these few studies, no consistent effects of sex or age was observed across all the studies. Another of the studies found SBP, but not DBP, to be lower in active males and females as compared to sedentary males and females [176]. However, the investigators apparently did not control for the higher body weight, triceps skinfold, or arm circumference of the sedentary children, all of which were significantly associated with blood pressure. Similarly, the potential effect of body weight was not considered in a study of children aged 3–6 yrs [97], in which a direct but weak (r = 0.15) association between physical activity and DBP was reported.

In general, the results of the cross-sectional studies we reviewed do not provide consistent evidence of an inverse relationship between physical activity and blood pressure. The inconsistent findings may be attributed to:

TABLE 13.4.
Examples of Epidemiologic Studies of the Association Between Physical Activity and Blood Pressure Among Children and Adolescents

Study Design, Population, and Investigators	Response Rate, Completion Rate, and Final Response Rate[a]	Sex[b]	Age (Yrs)	Race[c]	Measurement of Physical Activity (PA)	Measurement of Blood Pressure (BP)[d]	Main Findings[e]	Dose Response[f]	Adjustments[g]
Cross-sectional									
Australian schoolchildren, Jenner et al. (1992) [90]	RR = 64% CR = 78% FR = 50%	681 M 630 F 1311 T	11–12	n/r	Child's estimate of number of days/wk engaged in at least 1 hr of sport or out of school activity. School principal's estimate of total time spent in organized PA in school grouped above or below median of 150 min/wk of scheduled PA.	Oscillometric recorder (average of 3 readings).	Multiple regression between PA and blood pressure: M: PA not significantly related to SBP or DBP F: PA significantly related to SBP ($R^2 = 0.7\%$) and DBP ($R^2 = 2.7\%$).	F: Lowest category of days/wk of PA had highest DBP; equations imply that an increase in PA from 0 to 7 days would decrease SBP by 2.9 mm Hg.	Age, weight, height, BMI, sum of 4 skinfolds, waist-hip ratio, SES, outside temperature, fitness, energy intake, and respective quadratic terms.
Northern Irish schoolchildren, Boreham et al. (1997) [25]	RR = 78% CR = 100% FR = 78%	503 M 512 F 1990 T	12, 15	n/r	Recall of everyday PA coded by frequency, intensity, and duration (scored 1 to 100). Sports participation score based on number of extracurricular sports and other PA sessions/wk (scored 0 to 10).	Random-zero sphygmo-manometer (average of 2 measures), using Korotkoff sound I (SBP), sound IV (DBP) for 12-yr-olds, and sound V (DBP) for 15-yr-olds. At risk defined as DBP >95 mm Hg.	Standardized multiple regression coefficients between PA score and blood pressure: Results for 12 and 15-yr-olds by sex: M: Significant for SBP ($B = -0.14$); not significant for DBP; 20% difference in PA associated with 1.54-fold increase of being at risk. F: No significant effect.	n/r	Body size, sexual maturity, dietary intake, smoking, social class, school type.

(continued)

TABLE 13.4. *(continued)*

Study Design, Population, and Investigators	Response Rate, Completion Rate, and Final Response Rate[a]	Sex[b]	Age (Yrs)	Race[c]	Measurement of Physical Activity (PA)	Measurement of Blood Pressure (BP)[d]	Main Findings[e]	Dose Response[f]	Adjustments[g]
Longitudinal Danish schoolchildren, Andersen and Haraldsdottir, (1993) [7]	RR = 97% CR = 67% FR = 65%	88 M 115 F 203 T	15–19	n/r	Querstionnaire of sport and leisure activities recalled for past yr, expressed as hrs/wk of sport activity.	Mercury sphygmo-manometer (2 measures), using Korotkoff sound I (SBP) and IV (DBP).	PA change unrelated to changes in SBP or DBP.	n/a	n/a
Experimental Danish schoolchildren, Hansen et al., (1991) [83]	RR = 82% CR = 93%–100% FR = 76%–82%	66 M 64 F 132 T	9–11	n/r	Each child randomized to exercise group (extra 50 mins of physical education [PE], 3 times/wk for 8 mon) or control group (continued regular PE).	Random-zero sphygmo-manometer (1 measure), using Korotkoff sound I (SBP) and IV (DBP). Hypertensive defined as DBP ≥ 95 mm Hg; normotensive defined as DBP <95 mm Hg.	After 3 months no difference in SBP or DBP between groups. After 8 months hypertensive subjects had significantly decreased SBP (4.9 mm Hg) and DBP (3.8 mm Hg); normotensive subjects had significantly decreased SBP (6.5 mm Hg) and DBP (4.1 mm Hg) compared with control groups. SBP fell significantly more only for males in each group	n/r	Baseline weight, height, heart rate, and DBP.

Study		Demographics	Age	Intervention	BP measurement	Results		Covariates
CATCH study 3rd grade schoolchildren, Webber, et al. (1996), and Luepker et al. (1996) [113, 198]	RR = 60% CR = 79% FR = 48%	2645 M 2461 F 5106 T	Mean: 8.7 ± 0.5	2810 W 506 B 565 H 73 A 16 N 49 O	56 schools randomized to 2.5-yr program to increase to 40% time spent in moderate to vigorous PA in each PE class; 40 schools continued usual PE class.	Oscillometric automatic cuff (average of 3rd–5th readings).	No significant effect of PA intervention on BP for total group.	n/r	Age, height, BMI, and baseline BP.

[a] RR = response rate; CR = completion rate; FR = final response rate; n/r = not reported; CBD = cannot be determined.
[b] M = males; F = female.
[c] W = white; B = black; A = Asian; H = Hispanic/Latino; NA = Native American; O = other.
[d] SBP = systolic blood pressure; DBP = diastolic blood pressure.
[e] Multiple regression coefficients are not standardized or residualized except where indicated.
[f] n/r = not reported; n/a = not applicable.
[g] SES = Socioeconomic status; BMI = body mass index.

(1) differences in the measurement, type, and definition of physical activity; (2) differences in the measurement of blood pressure, including the use of different types of equipment, single vs multiple measures, and the IVth vs Vth Korotkoff sound to measure DBP; (3) differences in age, sex, body weight, and fat among the children studied; or (4) failure to control statistically for these differences.

In their 8-yr longitudinal study of Danish schoolchildren, Andersen and Haraldsdottir [7] found that both DBP and SBP tracked significantly in males and females, as reflected in correlation coefficients ranging from 0.38 to 0.54 (Table 13.4). In contrast, they found that physical activity estimated in mean hrs per wk of sports participation tracked significantly for males (r = 0.31) but not for females (r = 0.20) over the 8-yr period. Despite some evidence of tracking, the change from baseline to 8-yr follow-up in physical activity was not related to change in either SBP or DBP.

Four school-based, randomized experimental studies also yielded inconsistent findings. Two short-term intervention studies [66, 84] using more intense, aerobic physical activity reported no significant changes in SBP and DBP. However, the likelihood of finding significant blood pressure lowering in normotensive children—the control group—would be expected to be low. Similarly, Hansen et al. [83] found that 3 mon of increased physical activity (an extra 50 min of PE sessions, 3 times per wk) was insufficient to affect change in blood pressure. However, they also observed significant decreases in SBP and DBP after 8 mon of extra training in both normotensive and hypertensive children, as compared to children who continued the regular PE schedule. In contrast, the 2.5-yr CATCH intervention, which promoted an increase in moderate to vigorous activity to 40% of the PE class period, found no significant change in blood pressure for the overall group of 3rd grade children [113, 198].

These studies suggest that although short-term exercise intervention is not effective in lowering blood pressure among normotensive and hypertensive children, long-term exercise may lower blood pressure among hypertensive children and, perhaps, reduce the risk of developing high blood pressure among normotensive children. We suggest that future epidemiologic studies on the relation between physical activity and blood pressure meet the following criteria: (1) follow established guidelines for the standardized measurement of blood pressure [187]; (2) include black children, given the higher prevalence of hypertension in this race; (3) control for the potential effects of body weight and fat on blood pressure; and (4) examine the potential of a dose-response relationship between physical activity and blood pressure.

INSULIN. Circulating insulin has been found to be associated indirectly with the promotion of arteriosclerosis and cardiovascular diseases through its adverse effects on glucose, lipid metabolism, and blood pressure [205]. Yet, we could only identify two well-designed epidemiologic studies of physi-

cal activity or exercise on serum insulin, insulin resistance, or glucose tolerance among children or adolescents (Table 13.5). The Coronary Artery
Risk Development in Young Adults (CARDIA) epidemiologic study [117]
of 5115 18- to 30-yr olds found that logarithm-transformed insulin levels
were correlated with both heavy activity ($r = -0.14$) and treadmill duration
($r = -0.34$). These relationships weakened, but remained significant, after
adjusting for body mass index (BMI), age, race, and sex. In the Young Finns
Study [149], 1398 15-, 18-, 21-, and 24-yr-old males who engaged in one or
more physical activities per wk were found to have significantly lower serum
insulin levels than inactive males. No relation was found between this limited measure of physical activity and insulin in females. One limitation of
this study, however, is that only 39% of the subjects enrolled in the 1980
study were included in the 1986 analysis.

Most of the recommendations in the clinical medical literature on exercise and insulin appear to be based on experimental and cross-sectional
studies of adults. Although there are several studies on the effect of physical
activity and exercise on insulin, insulin resistance, and glucose tolerance
in children with either diabetes or obesity, these studies suffer from extremely small sample sizes or faulty designs. Thus, there is a need for cross-
sectional and longitudinal epidemiologic research on the relationship of
physical activity and serum insulin, insulin resistance, and glucose metabolism among children and adolescents who are healthy and among those
who have various forms of diabetes. Among both groups, population-based,
randomized controlled trials are needed on the effects of both longer-term
aerobic physical activity and less intensive physical activity on insulin levels.

OBESITY AND ADIPOSITY. Obesity and overweight are important public
health concerns because of their association with increased risk for hypertension, diabetes mellitus, coronary heart disease, osteoarthritis, lipid abnormalities, gall bladder disease, some cancers, and all-cause mortality
[145]. The public health concern extends to the pediatric population, in
which the prevalence of obesity has increased to nearly 22% [182]. Obesity
in children is significantly related to coronary risk factors, including higher
blood pressure and LDL-cholesterol and lower HDL-cholesterol [193, 197].
Obesity has been shown to track from childhood to adolescence to adulthood [203], and evidence suggests that obesity during adolescence is associated with chronic diseases that develop in adulthood, independent of adult
obesity [127].

Obesity and increased adiposity are attributed to an imbalance between
energy intake and energy expenditure. Because little evidence exists that
increased energy intake (or overeating) is a cause of obesity in children
[152, 178], research has focused on the role of energy expenditure, specifically physical activity, in the development of obesity and adiposity.

The findings of some cross-sectional studies suggest that obese children
and adolescents have lower levels of physical activity than their non-obese

TABLE 13.5.
Examples of Epidemiologic Studies of the Association Between Physical Activity and Serum Insulin Among Children and Adolescents

Study Design, Population, and Investigators	Response Rate, Completion Rate, and Final Response Rate[a]	Sex[b]	Age (Yrs)	Race[c]	Measurement of Physical Activity (PA)	Measurement of Insulin	Main Findings[d]	Dose Response[e]	Adjustments[f]
Cross-sectional Young Finns Study Raitakari et al. (1994) [148]	RR = n/r CR = n/r FR = CBD	640 M 758 F 1398 T	15, 18, 21, 24	1398 W	Participation in PA ≥ 1 time/wk.	Serum insulin	M: Significant regression coefficient of PA and insulin ($\beta = -1.53$) following adjustments for confounders. F: No significant association.	n/r	Use of butter, alcohol use, smoking, BMI, oral contraceptive use.

[a] RR = response rate; CR = completion rate; FR = final response rate; n/r = not reported; CBD = cannot be determined.
[b] M = males; F = females; T = total.
[c] W = white; B = black; A = Asian; H = Hispanic/Latino; NA = Native American; O = other.
[d] Multiple regression coefficients are not standardized or residualized except where indicated.
[e] n/r = not reported; n/a = not applicable.
[f] BMI = body mass index.

counterparts [30, 180], but the relationship between physical activity and adiposity in the general pediatric population is not clearly established. Many [3, 8, 119, 147, 165] but not all [126, 201] cross-sectional studies have reported no association between physical activity and BMI. Several studies [87, 179, 180] reported both a significant association and no association depending on the sex of subjects studied. The lack of a consistent relationship may be due to the fact that BMI, while easily measured, is more a measure of overweight than of adiposity and can reflect either higher lean body mass or higher fat mass. Further, because BMI is associated with both age and height in children and adolescents, this index may be a poor measure of relative body weight for this age group. Adiposity may be better assessed by skinfold measurements.

The results of studies comparing physical activity and skinfold measurements are also equivocal. Two studies [94, 180] reported an inverse association between physical activity and skinfold measurements, whereas three studies [3, 8, 178] reported no association. A number of studies reported mixed results depending on the age [25], sex [25, 90, 97, 179, 181], and race [138] of the study subjects. For example, Boreham et al. [25] found a significant inverse association between sports participation and percent body fat among girls aged 15 yrs but not girls aged 12 yrs, noting no association among boys of either age (Table 13.6). Furthermore, in their study of children aged 3–6 yrs, Klesges et al. [97] found a positive association ($r = 0.26$) between direct observation of physical activity and triceps skinfold thickness among girls, noting no association among boys. In general, we could detect no consistent effects of sex or age from the studies we reviewed. These disparate findings may arise from different methods of assessing overweight and adiposity (e.g., BMI and various skinfold sites) and physical activity (e.g., self-report questionnaire, heart rate monitors and motion sensors, and direct observation).

Two longitudinal studies of younger children aged 3–5 yrs yielded conflicting results. In the Framingham Children's Study [124], lower levels of physical activity (measured by Caltrac accelerometer) were associated with a significantly greater gain in subcutaneous fat (measured by triceps skinfold thickness) from preschool to 1st grade. In contrast, in a 1-yr longitudinal study of Texas children [59], the sum of seven skinfold measurements was not associated with physical activity level (measured by heart rate monitoring and direct observation), although a significant inverse correlation ($r = -0.21$) was found between mean activity level and waist/hip ratio (an index of fat patterning). Among adolescent populations, the relationship between physical activity and adiposity was more consistent. In an 8-yr follow-up study of Danish adolescents, Andersen and Haraldsdottir [7] found that change in physical activity was inversely related ($r = -0.35$) to change in percent body fat (estimated from skinfolds) in males but not females, while they noted no association with BMI for either sex (Table 13.6). Simi-

TABLE 13.6.
Examples of Epidemiologic Studies of the Association Between Physical Activity and Obesity and Adiposity Among Children and Adolescents

Study Design, Population, and Investigators	Response Rate, Completion Rate, and Final Response Rate[a]	Sex[b]	Age (Yrs)	Race[c]	Measurement of Physical Activity (PA)	Measurement of Obesity or Adiposity[d]	Main Findings[e]	Dose Response[f]	Adjustments[g]
Cross-sectional Finnish schoolchildren, Marti and Vartianen (1989) [119]	RR = n/r CR = 89% FR = CBD	565 M 577 F 1142 T	15	?	Questionnaire on leisure-time PA lasting ≥0.5 hr and causing out of breath and sweating, grouped as: 1) daily, 2) 2–3 times/wk, 3) once/wk, 4) 2–3 times/mo, 5) or less.	BMI	PA not related to BMI in M or F.	n/a	n/a
Northern Irish schoolchildren, Boreham et al. (1997) [25]	RR = 78% CR = 100% FR = 78%	503 M 512 F 1015 T	12, 15	?	Recall of everyday PA coded by frequency, intensity, and duration (scored 1 to 100). Sports participation score based on number of extracurricular sports and other PA sessions/wk (scored 0 to 10).	Weight, height, 4-site skinfolds used to determine percentage body fat; at risk defined as 20% for M and 30% for F.	M (aged 12 and 15 yrs): Standardized multiple regression coefficients for PA score not significantly related to percentage body fat. F (aged 12 yrs): No significant effect.	n/r	Body size, sexual maturity, dietary intake, smoking, social class, school type.

Longitudinal Danish schoolchildren, Andersen et al. (1994) [7]	RR = n/r CR = 64% FR = CBD	88 M 115 F 203 T	15– 19	?	Questionnaire on sport and leisure activities recalled for 1 yr; scored as mean hrs/wk in sport activity	Weight, height, suprapatellar, and abdominal skinfolds used to calculate percentage body fat.	F (aged 15 yrs): Significant standardized multiple regression coefficients between sports and percentage body fat (B = −0.10); sports PA difference of 20% associated with 2-fold increase of being at high risk. M: Change in PA inversely related to change in percentage body fat (r = −0.35) but not to change in BMI. F: Change in PA not related to change in percentage body fat or to change in BMI.	n/r	None

(continued)

TABLE 13.6. (continued)

Study Design, Population, and Investigators	Response Rate, Completion Rate, and Final Response Rate[a]	Sex[b]	Age (Yrs)	Race[c]	Measurement of Physical Activity (PA)	Measurement of Obesity or Adiposity[d]	Main Findings[e]	Dose Response[f]	Adjustments[g]
U.S. children and adolescents participating in NHES cycles II and III, Dietz and Gortmaker (1985) [52]	RR = n/r CR = 100% FR = CBD	2153 T	6–11 (cycle II) 12–17 (cycle III)	?	Hrs/day of TV watching, reading books or magazines, listening to radio, or playing sports, and time spent in leisure activities excluding sports and TV; stratified hrs/day of TV watching into 0–1, 1–2, 2–3, 3–4, 4–5, >5.	Triceps skinfold used to define obesity as ≥85th percentile and superobesity ≥95th percentile for same age and sex.	12–17 yr-olds who watched TV were significantly more obese and superobese than adolescents who watched less TV. Significant regression coefficients between cycle II TV watching and cycle III obesity (B = 0.008) and superobesity (B = 0.006).	Estimated regression coefficients indicated that for each added hr/day of TV, the percentage of obesity increased 1–3% and superobesity increased by 1–2%.	Dose response analyses adjusted for cycle II obesity or superobesity; season, region, and SES (e.g., population density; parental education, age, income, and number of children; birth order, race, condition restricting activity). Longitudinal analyses for cycle II obesity and SES.

Experimental

North Carolinian 3rd and 4th grade schoolchildren, Harrell et al. (1996) [84]	RR = n/r CR = 58% FR = CBD	616 M 658 F 1274 T	7–11 Mean: 8.9 ± 0.8	947 W 260 B 18 A 15 N 14 H 20 O	Schools randomized to an 8-wk intervention group (20 min of aerobic activities for 3 times/wk, plus classroom instruction on the importance of PA, food, and smoking to health) or a control group (regular health class instruction).	Weight, height, BMI, triceps, and subscapular skinfolds.	Sum of skinfolds decreased significantly in intervention compared with control group (mean change = −0.05). BMI did not change significantly.	n/r	Baseline values, sex, race, grade, and parental education.
CATCH study 3rd grade schoolchildren, Webber et al. (1996) and Luepker et al. (1996) [113, 198]	RR = 60% CR = 70% FR = 48%	4019 T	Mean: 8.7 ± 0.5	2819 W 506 B 565 H 73 A 16 N 49 O	56 schools randomized to 2.5-yr program to increase to 40% the time spent in moderate to vigorous PA in PE class; while 40 schools had usual PE class.	Weight, height, BMI, triceps, and subscapular skinfolds.	No difference in any measures between intervention and control groups.	n/r	Age, baseline value, site, sex, race and school random effect.

[a] RR = response rate; CR = completion rate; FR = final response rate; n/r = not reported; CBD = cannot be determined.

[b] M = males; F = females; T = total.

[c] W = white; B = black; A = Asian; H = Hispanic/Latino; NA = Native American; O = other.

[d] BMI = body mass index.

[e] Multiple regression coefficients are not standardized or residualized except where indicated.

[f] n/r = not reported; n/a = not applicable.

[g] SES = Socioeconomic status.

larly, lower skinfolds were observed in Finnish adolescents and young adults [149] who had consistently high physical activity scores on all three measurements over a 6-yr period, as compared to a sedentary group. In general, these studies provide evidence of a longitudinal inverse relationship between physical activity and adiposity.

The results of several studies suggest that the measure of physical inactivity may further elucidate the relationship between energy expenditure and obesity. In the National, Heart, Lung and Blood Institute's (NHLBI) Growth and Health Study [138] of 9- to 10-yr-old girls, television (TV) and video watching revealed significant direct associations between BMI and sum of skinfolds in both white girls and black girls, while a measure of physical activity revealed significant associations only in the black girls. These findings suggest that the measures of physical inactivity and activity are not merely reciprocals, and that the relationship of adiposity with these measures may be affected differentially by race.

An interrelationship between TV watching and obesity was also supported by data from two cycles of the National Health Examination Survey (NHES) which studied 6965 children aged 6–11 yrs between 1963 and 1965 (Cycle II), and 6671 adolescents aged 12–17 yrs between 1966 and 1970 (Cycle III). Dietz and Gortmaker [52] reported a significant association between TV watching and obesity and superobesity (defined as triceps skinfold > 85% and > 95% for same age and sex, respectively) in both groups (Table 13.6). From their analyses, the authors estimated that for each additional hr of TV watched per day, the prevalence of obesity and of superobesity increased by 1–3% and 1–2%, respectively.

Dietz and Gortmaker [52] also examined the relationship between TV watching and obesity longitudinally in a subsample of children (n = 2153) who participated in both NHES Cycle II and Cycle III (Table 13.6). Controlling for the prior obesity in Cycle II, these investigators found that TV watching in childhood (Cycle II) was positively associated with obesity and superobesity in adolescence (Cycle III). In contrast to these findings, TV watching was not associated with change in BMI or triceps skinfold in a sample of 279 6th and 7th grade girls that Robinson et al. [151] observed for 24 mon, or in BMI, sum of skinfolds, or waist/hip ratio in a sample of 191 3- to 4-yr-olds that DuRant and et al. [58] followed for 1 yr. The discrepancy between studies may be related to the methods used to assess TV watching. In the NHLBI [138] and NHES [52] studies, as well as in the study by Robinson et al. [151], TV watching was determined by the child's or parent's estimate of hrs of TV watched per day. In contrast, DuRant et al. [58] used direct observation for up to 4 days at 3-mon intervals for 1 yr to determine time spent watching TV. The results showed that TV watching was not related to body composition when multiple days of observation were used in the analysis. While direct observation provides a more accurate assessment of physically active and inactive behaviors than does self-report, this method would not be feasible in larger population-based studies. Nonetheless, the results of all of these studies emphasize the importance of measuring both physical activity and physical inactivity in the investigation of adiposity and obesity in children and adolescents.

Epstein et al. [68] critically reviewed the role of physical activity in the treatment of obesity in children and adolescents. In general, the results of nonepidemiologic randomized controlled intervention studies suggest that: (1) exercise alone is not an effective treatment for weight loss; (2) exercise in combination with dietary changes (reduced calorie or increased fiber intake) results in greater weight loss than dietary changes alone; (3) diet interventions and diet-plus-exercise interventions are equally effective in producing greater weight and body fat loss than no intervention; and (4) lifestyle exercise intervention may be more effective in producing long-term reductions in weight and percent overweight than either aerobic or calisthenics exercise intervention. In addition, Epstein et al. [69] provided evidence that an intervention aimed at decreasing sedentary behaviors, such as watching TV and videos and playing computer games, was more effective in reducing weight and body fat than was an intervention aimed at increasing physical activity. Moreover, these differences were maintained at a 1-yr follow-up.

Larger, randomized studies conducted in school settings have been limited to examining the effects of exercise intervention on adiposity, not obesity. In their short-term intervention studies, Harrell et al. [84] (Table 13.6) and Dwyer et al. [66] found that significantly greater decreases in skinfold measurements occurred in subjects who engaged in more intense aerobic activity, as compared to control subjects and nonaerobic exercise subjects, respectively. In stark contrast, the 2.5-year CATCH project [113, 198], which promoted an increase in moderate to vigorous activity to 40% of the PE class period, found no significant changes in indices of adiposity compared with control subjects.

Future epidemiologic studies on the association between physical activity and obesity or adiposity should: (1) target obese children and adolescents who are more likely to have coronary risk factors and an increased risk of developing chronic disease later in life; (2) follow the progression of risk factor relationships, particularly in obese children and adolescents; and (3) include interventions that promote increasing physical activity as well as decreasing physically inactive behaviors, such as TV and video watching.

BONE MINERAL DENSITY. With an aging population, bone mineral loss and osteoporosis are major public health concerns. An estimated 25 million Americans have osteoporosis, generating annual medical costs of about $13.8 billion [23, 135].

This discussion of the relation between physical activity and bone mineral density is restricted to studies that include larger samples that appear to be representative of the populations from which they were drawn. We could determine final response rates for only 3 of the 20 studies reviewed. Consequently, we could not judge the representativeness of these studies as a whole.

In general, some [70, 105, 155, 172, 183, 184] but not all [81, 172, 183] of the cross-sectional studies reported a significant positive association between physical activity and bone mineral density of the hip and forearm. Only a few studies [154, 155] found physical activity to be positively related to bone mineral density of the lumbar spine, while the majority of studies [24, 105, 155, 172, 183, 202] did not. An inverse correlation between physical activity and bone mineral density of the diaphyses of the second finger was found in girls and a positive correlation was found in boys [190]. Furthermore, in studies that stratified physical activity level, higher levels of bone mineral density were more often reported in groups with higher activity levels than in groups with lower levels [105, 172, 184], with some evidence of a dose-response relationship [184, 190]. We observed inconsistent findings within studies [105, 155, 172, 183, 184] depending on the sex and age of the subject, the bone site measured, and the adjustments made for potentially confounding variables. For example, Gunnes and Lehmann [82] found weight-bearing physical activity to be significantly associated to bone mineral density of the distal and ultradistal forearm among youth aged 11–17 yrs, but not among boys and girls aged 8–11 yrs (Table 13.7). However, the positive association that the investigators noted among the older children disappeared following adjustment for sex, weight, height, energy and nutrient intake, and exposure to daylight. Similarly, although Boot et al. [24] initially reported a significant correlation for physical activity with total and lumbar bone mineral density for males, those findings became nonsignificant following statistical adjustment for confounding variables. It is difficult to draw conclusions about the relationship between physical activity and bone mineral density from these studies since: (1) the study samples varied in age, sex, and pubertal status; (2) bone mineral density was measured using different equipment and at different bone sites, and was expressed in different units; (3) physical activity was measured and defined using different methods; and (4) not all studies adjusted for potentially confounding variables such as weight and pubertal status.

It is also unclear whether physical activity level during adolescence is associated with future bone mineral density. Two studies [71, 103] reported a significant association between physical activity assessed via long-term recall and bone mineral density of the forearm among adolescent females [71], but not among males in their twenties [71] or among post-menopausal women [103]. In the Amsterdam Growth and Health Longitudinal Study, in which physical activity level was measured prospectively six times from age 13–27 yrs and lumbar bone mineral density was measured at age 27, Welten et al. [200] found significant positive correlations between lumbar bone mineral density at age 27 and higher levels of weight-bearing activities

TABLE 13.7.
Examples of Epidemiologic Studies of the Association Between Physical Activity and Bone Mineral Density Among Children and Adolescents

Study Design, Population, and Investigators	Response Rate, Completion Rate, and Final Response Rate[a]	Sex[b]	Age (Yrs)	Race[c]	Measurement of Physical Activity (PA)	Measurement of BMC[d], BMD[d]	Main Findings[e]	Dose Response[f]	Adjustments
Cross-sectional									
Norwegian schoolchildren, Gunnes and Lehmann (1995) [81]	RR = n/r CR = 90% FR = CBD	495 T	8–17	W	Questionnaire on sports and leisure PA in 3 months; analysis restricted to weight-bearing PA in hrs/wk.	BMD (SPA[g]) of nondominant distal (BMD-D) and ultradistal (BMD-UD) forearm.	Simple regression: Weight-bearing PA significantly related to BMD-D and BMD-UD in 11- to 17-yr-olds, but not in 8- to 11-yr-olds. Multiple regression: Weight-bearing PA not a significant independent predictor of BMD-D or of BMD-UD.	n/r	Gender, weight, height, energy and nutrient intake, daylight exposure.
Rotterdam schoolchildren, Boot et. al. (1997) [24]	RR = n/r CR = 100% FR = CBD	205 M 295 F 500 T	4–20	444 W 21 B 35 A	Parent's or child's report of min/wk spent in PE class, organized sports, recreational activity, habitual walking and cycling.	BMD (DEXA[h]) of L2–L4 and total body; BMAD (apparent BMD) or L2–L4 (measured in only 43 children)	M: PA significantly correlated with L2–L4 and age-adjusted total body BMD. F: PA not related to BMD. Multiple regression: PA not associated with BMD or BMAD.	n/r	Age Multiple regression: Age, weight, height, Tanner stage, calcium intake.

(*continued*)

TABLE 13.7. *(continued)*

Study Design, Population, and Investigators	Response Rate, Completion Rate, and Final Response Rate[a]	Sex[b]	Age (Yrs)	Race[c]	Measurement of Physical Activity (PA)	Measurement of BMC[d], BMD[d]	Main Findings[e]	Dose Response[f]	Adjustments
Longitudinal Amsterdam children, Welten et al. (1994) [200]	RR = n/r CR = 59% FR = CBD	84 M 98 F 182 T	13– 27	?	Serial cross-check interview of weight-bearing activities >4 METS and >5 min duration over past 3 months; grouped into average weekly time spent in light (4–6 METS), medium heavy (7–10 METS), and heavy (>10 METS)	BMD (DEXA) of L2–L4 at age 27 yrs	Multiple regression: M: Significant coefficients between BMD at age 27 yrs and PA for 13–17 yr period (B = 0.178), and 13–27 yr period (B = 0.190), and 13–27 yr period (B = 0.158) (R^2 = 16–17%). F: Past and present PA not associated with BMD at 27 yrs.	n/r	Weight, sex, calcium intake, height.
Finnish schoolchildren, Kroger et al. (1993) [104]	RR = n/r CR = 100% FR = CBD	28 M 37 F 65 T	7– 20	?	Questionnaire categorized PA into 3 classes: little or no PA outside school, sports or PA ≥3 hrs/wk, and sports in arthletic clubs >5 hrs/wk.	BMC, bone width, and BMD (DEXA) of L2–L4, and femoral neck of left proximal femur.	No significant associations between PA class and BMD.	Trend reported for higher BMD among the most active group (no data provided)	Age, weight, height.

| Norwegian schoolchildren, Gunnes and Lehmann (1996) [82] | RR = n/r CR = 100% FR = CBD | 239 M 231 F 480 T | 8.2–16.5 | W | Questionnaire on sports and leisure PA in 3 months; analysis restricted to weight-bearing PA in hrs/wk (mean of baseline and yr 1 measure). | BMD (DEXA) of nondominant distal (BMD-D) and ultradistal (BMD-UD) forearm. | Simple regression: Mean weight-bearing PA significantly related to BMD-D ($r = 0.243$) and gain in BMD-UD in M but not F. Multiple regression: M: Significant coefficients between mean weight-bearing PA gain in BMD-D and BMD-UD in boys <11 yr ($B = 0.0002$) and of BMD-D in boys >11 yrs ($B = 0.0001$) F (<11 yrs): Significant coefficient between mean weight-bearing PA and gain in BMD-D. | n/r | Baseline weight and height; height gain; baseline BMD-D and BMD-UD; and energy, carbohydrate, fat, salt, niacin, and sodium intake. |

[a] RR = response rate; CR = completion rate; FR = final response rate; n/r = not reported; CBD = cannot be determined.
[b] M = males; F = females; T = total.
[c] W = white; B = black; A = Asian.
[d] BMC = bone mineral content; BMD = bone mineral density.
[e] Multiple regression coefficients are not standardized or residualized.
[f] n/r = not reported; n/a = not applicable.
[g] SPA = single photon absorptiometry.
[h] DEXA = dual energy X-ray absorptiometry.

in males, but not in females, at ages 13–17 yrs (R^2 = 0.16), 13–21 yrs (R^2 = 0.17), and the total period of 13–27 yrs (R^2 = 0.17) (Table 13.7). When physical activity was redefined by peak strain forces (based on ground reaction forces) in the same study sample, lumbar bone mineral density (at age 27) in both males and females was significantly related to peak strain physical activity over the total period of 13–27 yrs (R^2 = 0.25), although activity during the teenage years (13–17) accounted for a lower portion of the variance (R^2 = 0.08) in lumbar bone mineral density [80]. In an 11-yr longitudinal study [189] of physical activity in four cohorts of young Finns, the sum of physical activity over the 11-yr period correlated significantly with bone mineral density of the femoral neck in both males (r = 0.36) and females (r = 0.30) and with the lumbar spine in males (r = 0.29). Finally, two longitudinal studies that measured physical activity and bone mineral density at 1-yr follow-up yielded inconsistent findings. In their study of Finnish schoolchildren, Kroger et al. [104] reported no significant association between physical activity and bone mineral density of the lumbar spine or femoral neck. By contrast, in a study of Norwegian schoolchildren, Gunnes and Lehmann [82] found significant positive relationships between change in forearm bone mineral density and the average of weight-bearing physical activity over the year in both males and females less than 11 yrs of age and in males 11 yrs or older (Table 13.7). In general, these studies provide some evidence of a relationship between physical activity in childhood or adolescence and bone mineral density later in life. Future studies would benefit from the reporting of higher response rates (>80%), detailed reporting of physical activity exposure, consistent control for potentially confounding variables, such as weight, pubertal status, and calcium intake, and inclusion of nonwhite subjects.

Evidence of the modifiability of bone mineral density via exercise was demonstrated in a small, randomized controlled trial of 30 college women [174], who exhibited a 1% increase in lumbar bone mineral density after 8 mon of jogging or weight lifting. Additional evidence was found in a study of 268 Israeli infantry recruits. Margulies et al. [118] found that bone mineral content increased significantly by 8.3% in the right leg and 12.4% in the left leg among male recruits who had completed a 14-wk physical training program. In contrast, the investigators found significant increases of 9.4% for the left leg only among men who completed only part of the program as a result of an injury. To date, however, a population-based, randomized controlled trial to determine the effects of physical activity on bone mineral density in either children or adolescents has not been conducted. Well-designed experimental studies are warranted to determine: (1) if child or adolescent bone mineral density is modifiable via physical activity; (2) if a dose-response relationship or a minimal physical activity threshold exists for modifying bone mineral density; (3) if critical periods exist (such as puberty or growth spurts) during which the bone may be more or less influenced by physical activity; (4) if the effects of physical activity on bone mineral density might be sex, age, or bone-site specific; and finally, (5) if the modification of bone mineral density during adolescence via physical activity affects future bone health.

UNINTENTIONAL INJURY. Unintentional injury is a major cause of morbidity and mortality among children and adolescents [73]. A recent analysis of data from the 1988 National Health Interview Survey [21] estimated that 35.8% of all unintentional injury episodes among children aged 5–17 yrs are related to sports and recreational activities, with a recall-adjusted annual rate of 9.7 sports-related injuries per 100 children. This analysis also revealed that sports and recreational injuries resulted in 80,750 hospitalizations per year. In addition to the morbidity resulting from sports-related injury, such injuries may also lead to a decrease in physical activity. One study found that the main reason high school students gave for not completing a school-sponsored sport season was a sports-related injury requiring the student to stop playing [65].

The number and rate of injuries have been found to vary by age, sex, type of sport or activity, geographic location, and the context of participation. Elementary schoolchildren, for instance, were more likely to have playground-related injuries [28, 171] and twice as likely to have bicycle accidents not involving a motor vehicle [73] than older secondary school students, who were more likely to have injuries related to athletic pursuits [28, 171] and 20 times more likely to have bicycle accidents involving a motor vehicle [73]. The report of the NHIS data [21] revealed that sports and recreational injuries occurred more frequently among males than females (1.8:1), with the ratio (M:F) of injuries increasing to 2.4:1 among adolescents aged 14–17 yrs. Sex differences were also specific to the type of sport. In a study of Danish schoolchildren [175], boys had higher injury rates for soccer and skateboarding than did girls, who had higher injury rates for horseback riding, handball, and gymnastics. Another study [64] found that among sports participants, a higher percentage of female basketball players (33.3%) than male basketball players reported being injured; male baseball players, however, were more likely to be injured than were female softball players (19.4% vs 9.1%, respectively). The type of sport also affects the severity and body site of injury. Skateboarding, ice hockey, and skating account for head injuries, while soccer and gymnastics account for a larger proportion of lower extremity injuries [175].

Injury rates for individual sports or activities also varied by geographic location and the popularity of the sport in that region. In Massachusetts, for example, the largest proportion of sports injuries was attributed to football (19.9%) [73], whereas soccer injuries were more prevalent in Denmark [175].

Injury rates may also vary according to the physical context of participation or other factors associated with play. Sheps and Evans [171] reported sports-related injury rates of 0.10 and 0.35 per 100 student-yrs for elementary and secondary schoolchildren, respectively. For elementary schoolchildren, the highest injury rate (1.09 per 100 student-yrs) occurred on the playground (but not on equipment). For secondary school children, the highest injury rate (0.79 per 100 student-yrs) occurred off the playing field in sports-related areas (gym/pool/shower or dressing room). Also, Backx et al. [13] found that volleyball injuries were more prevalent during practice (6.7 per 1000 hrs of play), whereas the higher injury rate for basketball (23 per 1000 game-hrs) occurred during games.

The variability in injury rates observed among studies might be attributable to the different methodologies used to define and measure injury, accounting in part for the difficulty in comparing injury rates. In some studies, the measurement of injury was limited to injuries that required hospital or physician contact [2, 15, 21, 73, 175, 196]. Other studies relied on the report of the injured student [13], the student's parent [21], or a school nurse [28] or other member of the school or health department staff [171]. One study [65] relied on student self-report of injury that required medical care from a physician or caused an athlete to miss one or more games. Another study obtained data from an organized registry system [51], and still another obtained information from the response to a mailed questionnaire [22]. The definition of an injury also included injury that restricted sports activity [27, 75, 122] or resulted in the student missing PE class [13] or school for a day or more [13, 114]. Two studies only measured fractures [15, 22].

Another major limitation of many of these studies of unintentional injury is the failure to obtain reliable participation data [12], including the number of people engaged in specific sports or activities, as well as the level and precise position played by the sports participant. In fact, many of the sex and location differences in injury rates found by some studies may be attributable to different levels of participation in specific types of sports. For example, De Loës [51] used a registry of a Swiss organization, Youth and Sports, to examine the occurrence of acute injury in 32 sports from 1987 through 1989. She estimated that for each year, roughly 5000 or more injuries were recorded from 350,000 participants who engaged in 13.2 million hrs of sports activities. A comparison of injury rates (per 10,000 person-hrs) for 11 common sports revealed that males had a higher overall injury rate than did females (4.9 injuries vs 3.2 injuries). However, males had an almost 2.5-fold greater number of hrs of exposure to sports participation. When De Loës standardized her data by assuming equal hrs of exposure to each sport and equal total exposure for all sports participation, she found that the overall injury rate became equal for males and females (4.3 injuries).

At least one study offered evidence of a dose-response relationship along with an estimate of the burden associated with competitive athletics from a population-based vantage point. In their 3-yr injury surveillance study of 1245 adolescents, Aaron and LaPorte [2] reported an increasing injury risk for increasing team enrollment (0, 1, 2, 3+) in competitive athletics. To illustrate the extent of the burden imposed on males, the investigators estimated that 40 injuries would occur per 1000 adolescent males engaged in 175,500 hrs of competitive athletics, as compared to only 7 injuries per 1000 male adolescents spending an equivalent amount of time not engaged in such endeavors. This important distinction should be acknowledged, as these investigators noted that many researchers simply provide injury information for participants for a specific sport, and fail to examine rates of injury among persons who did not participate. When this occurs, a population-based relative risk of sports participation cannot be estimated.

Based on our review of epidemiologic studies of unintentional injuries, we suggest that future epidemiologic studies: (1) use standardized definitions and methods for assessing injury; (2) determine exposure time; (3) assess the total population at risk; (4) determine the unintentional injury rate in persons not exposed to sports or physical activity as a point of comparison; (5) examine the risk of injury during growth and development (e.g., during pubertal growth spurts); (6) assess the risks and benefits (both physiologically and monetarily) of participation in sports and other physical activities in the pediatric population; (7) examine the relationship of injury risk arising from specific types of sport by taking into account all forms of other exercise and physical activity participation; and (8) examine the efficacy of methods to decrease the risk of injury in children engaging in sports or recreational activities.

DETERMINANTS OF PHYSICAL ACTIVITY AND EXERCISE. The question of why children and adolescents engage in physical activity is an important one. Unfortunately, research in this area is scarce [160]. The handful of studies to date—either cross-sectional or longitudinal studies—have shown that a variety of personal, social, and physical environmental factors influence participation in physical activity [102, 125, 156, 162]. Because of the multidimensional aspects of these health behaviors, the predominant theoretical framework that has dominated the study of the determinants and promotion of physical activity has been social cognitive theory [61, 160]. In this theory, changes in physical activity are expected to be influenced by personal factors, environmental influences, and aspects of physical activity itself. A major part of this theory is the concept of physical activity or exercise self-efficacy—that is, a person's belief that he or she has the ability to perform physical activity. In this review, we discuss the epidemiologic research separately for children and adolescents because the determinants of physical activity vary by age.

The bulk of the research on children has focused on children aged 3–7 yrs. Research from two of the sites of NHLBI's SCAN project [18, 163] offer especially important insights on children's physical activity since the measurement of physical activity was based on direct observation over multiple hrs during the day over several days during the year. In their study at the San Diego project site, Sallis et al. [163] found ethnic and sex differences in the amount of physical activity that 4-yr-olds perform at home. The investigators also found that play rules, convenient play spaces, number of play spaces, and available time to play were predictive of the level of physical activity of the 4-yr-olds (Table 13.8). In a more recent analysis of these data, the same investigators [162] found that the selection of play spaces was influenced by whether the spaces were well-lit at night, by organized activities, by available supplies and drinking water, by distance from home (Mexican-American parents), by cost of admission, and by the child's friends also using the play spaces (among white parents). Level of physical activity was associated with observed requests by the child to engage in physical activity, time spent outdoors, and encouragement to play or exercise by child's friends, parents, or other adults [163].

In their analysis of the Galveston, Texas SCAN data, Baranowski et al. [18] found that male sex, being outside, and the month of the year accounted for 75% of the variance in the physical activity children aged 3- and 4-yrs, after adjusting for ethnicity and age. Using data from the same group of children, DuRant et al. [58] reported that several different indicators of observed television watching were inversely correlated with several different indices of physical activity (Table 13.8).

Moore et al. [125] used a Caltrac device to assess the physical activity of 100 children aged 4–7 yrs and their parents during two 5-day periods 6 mon apart. They then classified the children and their parents as either active or inactive, depending on whether counts per hr were above or below the median for age and sex groups. The investigators found that the activity level of the father was more strongly associated with the child's activity than was the mother's activity level. If both parents were active, children were 5.8 (95% confidence intervals, 1.9, 17.4) times more likely to be active.

In their study of older children residing in a Midwestern town, Stucky-Ropp and DeLorenzo [177] administered a physical activity questionnaire to 242 5th and 6th grade students and computed MET values for each child (Table 13.8). (One MET is the value of resting oxygen uptake relative to total body mass and is generally ascribed the value of 3.5 milliliters of oxygen per kilogram of body mass per minutes.) They investigated a model consisting of the child's enjoyment of physical activity and friend and family support of physical activity, and found that barriers to physical activity accounted for 13% of the variation in the males' level of physical activity. Among females, 12% of the variation in physical activity was accounted for by enjoyment, amount of exercise, equipment in home, family support, barriers, and parental modeling. The applicability of the results from this study is limited, however, since the sample was predominantly white and other sociodemographic variables were not controlled for.

TABLE 13.8.
Examples of Epidemiologic Studies of the Determinants of Physical Activity Among Children

Study Design, Population, and Investigators	Response Rate, Completion Rate, and Final Response Rate[a]	Sex[b]	Age (Yrs)	Race[c]	Measurement of Physical Activity (PA)	Main Findings[d]	Dose Response[e]	Adjustments[f]
Cross-sectional								
5th and 6th grade students, Stucky-Ropp and DeLorenzo (1993) [177]	RR = 82% CR = 85% FR = 70%	121 M 121 F 242 T	Mean: 11.2 ± 0.7	225 W 17 O	MET values from the Physical Activity Interview and Children's Physical Activity Questionnaire.	M: Child's enjoyment of PA ($R^2 = 0.09$), barriers to PA ($R^2 = 0.02$), and mother's report of family support ($R^2 = 0.01$) were significantly associated with PA. F: Child's enjoyment of PA ($R^2 = 0.06$), number of PA items in home ($R^2 = 0.02$), family support ($R^2 = 0.02$), barriers to PA ($R^2 = 0.01$), and parental modeling ($R^2 = 0.01$) were significantly associated with PA.	n/r	Gender
Longitudinal								
NHLBI Study of Children's Activity and Nutrition (SCAN) in San Diego, Calif., Sallis, et al. (1993) [163]	RR = 22% CR = 86% FR = 19%	351 T	Mean: 4.4 ± 0.5	150 W 201 H	Observed PA using Behaviors of Eating and Activity for Child Health Evaluation System. PA at home (kcal/kg/min) up to 4 days during the year.	Significantly greater PA for Anglo-Americans than for Mexican-Americans, and for boys than for girls. Fewer outdoor and indoor play rules, convenient play spaces, time in play spaces, and frequency of play spaces were significantly associated with PA. Requests for PA (r = 0.60), time outdoors (r = 0.74); prompts by parents (r = 0.30), other adults (r = 0.64), and other children (r = 0.44) were significantly associated with PA.	n/r	Demographic variables

(continued)

TABLE 13.8. *(continued)*

Study Design, Population, and Investigators	Response Rate, Completion Rate, and Final Response Rate[a]	Sex[b]	Age (Yrs)	Race[c]	Measurement of Physical Activity (PA)	Main Findings[d]	Dose Response[e]	Adjustments
NHLBI SCAN in Galveston, Tx., Baranowski et al. (1993), DuRant et al. (1994) [18, 58]	RR = n/r CR = 100% FR = CBD	90 M 101 F 191 T	3–4	68 W 79 B 44 H	Child Activity Rating Scale (CARS) measured every min up to 12 hrs/day from 1–4 days over 1 year.	A model including gender; month and location accounted for 75% of the variance in PA. Boys were more active than girls. Outside PA was significantly higher than inside PA, and was lower in the summer months. October–December boys' outside PA was higher than girls. Inside PA was lower during times of TV watching. Longest bout of TV watching was associated with percentage of time at CARS levels 3, 4, or 5 ($r = 0.27$), at CARS levels 4 or 5 ($r = 0.27$), and average CARS ($r = 0.24$). Similar relationships were found with percentage of min watching TV to total observed min.	n/r	Gender, ethnicity, age.
Framingham Children's Study, Moore et al. (1991) [125]	RR = 58% CR = 94% FR = 55%	63 M 37 F 100 T	4–7	?	Caltrac monitoring for 2 periods of 5-days 6 mon apart. Classified as active or inactive based on counts/hr above or below the median for age and for sex.	Children of active mothers were 2.0 times (95% CI = 0.9, 4.4) more likely to be active. Children of active fathers were 3.5 times (95% CI = 1.5, 8.3) more likely to be active, etc. If both parents were active, children were 5.8 times (1.9, 17.4) more likely to be active, with sons being 7.2 times (1.5, 35.5) more likely to be active.	n/r	Child's gender, parents' age, child's relative weight.

[a] RR = response rate; CR = completion rate; FR = final response rate; n/r = not reported; CBD = cannot be determined.
[b] M = males; F = females; T = total.
[c] W = white; B = black; A = Asian; H = Hispanic/Latino; NA = Native American; O = other.
[d] Multiple regression coefficients are not standardized or residualized except where indicated.
[e] n/r = not reported; n/a = not applicable.

Unlike some of the studies of children, none of the studies of the determinants of physical activity among adolescents are based on observed behaviors. Although two large studies were conducted among adolescents and adults in California [159] and Ontario [4], the analyses were not stratified by age. Therefore, we cannot draw any conclusions about the adolescents' behavior.

Zakarian et al. [204] conducted a cross-sectional study of a nonrandom sample of 9th and 11th grade students from a lower working-class community in California in which physical activity was based on three commonly used self-report measures (Table 13.9). They found that among males, physical activity outside school was significantly associated with lower school grade level, exercise self-efficacy, support by friends to exercise, beliefs in the benefits of exercise, and cigarette smoking. This model accounted for 16% of the variance in physical activity. Among females, 16% of the variation in physical activity outside school was accounted for by exercise self-efficacy, fewer perceived barriers to exercise, family support for exercise, lower school grade level, less dislike for PE, alcohol use, and a higher BMI. This study's strength is that the regression models contained up to 24 additional social, psychological, behavioral, and demographic variables whose significance was ruled-out. These models also accounted for over 20% of the variance in these students' overall vigorous exercise.

In a study of 150 Anglo students from a middle-class school district, Sallis et al. [166] administered the same instrument as Zakarian et al. [204]. The data was then combined for the working-class and middle-class samples. They found that boys reported a higher frequency of participation in vigorous exercise outside of school, total sports teams, PE classes and vigorous exercise in school when compared with girls. However, girls reported participating in a greater number of exercise lessons and classes than boys did. They found that there were ethnic and socioeconomic status (SES) differences in both the types of physical activities engaged in, and in the variables found to be associated with physical activity in the initial study by Zakarian et al. For example, high-SES Anglos were more likely to take activity lessons and participate in vigorous exercise during PE classes than were students from other ethnic groups, and black students were more likely to engage in dancing than were other students. A drawback of this study, however, is that SES was determined by the students' school, not by the demographic characteristics of each student.

Drewnowski et al. [54, 55] conducted a study of 3978 high school graduates attending a summer orientation session for the entering freshman class at the University of Michigan (Table 13.9). The students were asked how frequently they exercised for more than 1 hr per day for weight control. Among the women, higher SES was associated with the prevalence of dieting and exercise to lose weight. Among the men, there was no association with SES, although exercise was the preferred method to lose weight.

TABLE 13.9.
Examples of Epidemiologic Studies of the Determinants of Physical Activity Among Adolescents

Study Design, Population, and Investigators	Response Rate, Completion Rate, and Final Response Rate[a]	Sex[b]	Age (Yrs)	Race[c]	Measurement of Physical Activity (PA)[d]	Main Findings[e]	Dose Response[f]	Adjustments
Cross-sectional Lower working class 9th and 11th grade students, Zakarain et al. (1994) [204]	RR = 55% CR = 74% FR = 41%	807 M 827 F 1634 T	Mean: 15.88 ± 1.17	337 W 58 B 949 H 196 A 43 O	Frequency of PA outside of school for ≥20 min without stopping, which makes heart rate and breathing increase a large amount. Days of PE/wk. Days of vigorous exercise during PE/wk.	M: PA outside school was associated with lower school grade, exercise self-efficacy, friend support, benefits of exercise, and cigarette smoking. F: PA outside school was associated with self-efficacy, fewer perceived barriers, family support, lower school grade, less dislike for PE, alcohol use, and BMI.	n/r	Regression models were adjusted for 24 additional social, psychological, behavioral, and demographic variables.
Lower working class 9th and 11th grade students, and 150 Anglos from a middle-class school district, Zakarain et al. (1994) and Sallis, et al. (1996) [166, 204]	RR = n/r CR = 73% FR = CBD	1871 T	11–19	400 W 69 B 1126 H 225 A 51 ?	Same as above.	M: Significantly higher frequency of participation in total sports teams, PE classes, and vigorous exercise (40%) both in and outside school than females. F: Significantly more exercise lessons and classes than males. Race and SES differences in the types of PA performed and in the determinants of PA.	n/r	Race, sex, and SES.
College freshman, Drewnowski, Kurth, and Krahn (1994, 1995) [54, 55]	RR = 90% CR = 91% FR = 82%	2174 M 1804 F 3978 T	Mean: 17.7 ± 0.07	?	Frequency of exercise lasting >1 hr/day for purpose of weight control.	M: Exercise was the preferred method to lose weight. F: Higher SES was associated with increased prevalence of dieting and PA. Significantly greater weekly exercise for students whose parents had ≤ high school education (12.8%) compared with those whose parents had at least some college (25%).	n/r	None

Longitudinal 5th, 6th, and 8th grade students, Garcia, et al. (1995) [74]	RR = n/r CR = 72% FR = CBD	148 M 138 F 286 T	?	179 W 87 B	Child/Adolescent Exercise Log consisting of 16 items of PA frequency and duration. Index computed from metabolic cost of summed activities.	Only male gender, index of the benefits/barriers to exercise differential, and access to exercise facilities were associated with increased exercise ($R^2 = 0.193$) at 8–10 wks later. Significant multiple regression coefficients for gender ($B = 3.64$), beneficial barriers ($B = 1.27$), and access to facilities ($B = 0.60$).	n/r	Grade, race, self-esteem, perceived health status, previous exercise self-schema, self-efficacy, models, norms and social support, and sedentary time.
College students, Courneya and McAuley (1994) [49]	RR = n/r CR = 56% FR = 82%	81 M 89 F 170 T	Mean: 20.3 ± 2.15	?	Number of PA in the last 4 wks, min of PA/session, and perceived exertion using 15-point Borg scale.	Intention to exercise ($R^2 = 0.13$), exercise self-efficacy ($R^2 = 0.04$), and their interaction ($R^2 = 0.03$) were associated with exercise frequency 4 wks later. Intention to exercise ($R^2 = 0.21$), exercise self-efficacy ($R^2 = 0.03$), and their interaction ($R^2 = 0.11$) were associated with intensity of PA. Only intention to exercise was associated ($R^2 = 0.45$) with duration of PA.	n/r	Importance of exercise and Subjective Exercise Experience Scale.

[a] RR = response rate; CR = completion rate; FR = final response rate; n/r = not reported; CBD = cannot be determined.

[b] M = males; F = females; T = total.

[c] W = white; B = black; A = Asian; H = Hispanic/Latino; N = Native American; O = other.

[d] PE = physical education.

[e] Multiple regression coefficients are not standardized or residualized except where indicated; BMI = body mass index; SES = socioeconomic status.

[f] n/r = not reported; n/a = not applicable.

Garcia et al. [74] conducted a longitudinal study of a nonrandom sample of 286 5th, 6th, and 8th grade students from two schools (Table 13.9). Eight to 10 wks after completing a questionnaire on physical activity and exercise, students spent five morning class periods recording their previous day's exercise and physical activity using an exercise log. On Monday, students entered logs for Friday, Saturday, and Sunday. An index of the total metabolic cost of the activities was compiled from these data. The researchers found that a model consisting of male sex, a differential index of the benefits/barriers to exercise, and access to exercise facilities accounted for 19% of the variance in exercise level after adjusting for other variables and potential confounders.

Courneya and McAuley [49] conducted a 4-wk longitudinal study of the frequency, intensity, and duration of exercise among a nonrandom sample of 170 college students (Table 13.9). Physical activity was assessed using two self-report measures and a perceived effort scale at 2 and 4 wks after an initial survey. The researchers found that intention to exercise, exercise self-efficacy, and the interaction of the two accounted for 20% of the variation in exercise frequency and 33% of the variation in exercise intensity after adjusting for the importance of exercise and subjective exercise experience scales. Only intention to exercise ($R^2 = 0.45$) was associated with exercise duration.

The studies discussed here suggest that social, psychological, and attitudinal variables account for between 1/5 and 1/3 of the variation in adolescents' physical activity and exercise. Several other studies [20, 53, 76, 141] support this conclusion. Yet, most of the variation in adolescents' physical activity and exercise remains unaccounted for. Therefore, more prospective randomized epidemiologic studies that use valid and reliable measures of physical activity are needed to provide a complete picture of why adolescents engage in physical activity. This will help practitioners design and conduct more effective interventions to promote physical activity among children and adolescents.

INTERVENTIONS TO PROMOTE PHYSICAL ACTIVITY

Although the number of studies that have examined the effectiveness of interventions to promote increased physical activity and exercise among children and adolescents is limited, they nonetheless suggest that properly designed interventions can be effective in this population.

In a small study of two 5th grade classes (one intervention and one control), Duncan et al. [56] found that a 9-mon physical fitness program administered by a PE specialist resulted in a significant increase in the level of fitness of the intervention group at the end of the school year and at the end of the 3-mon summer recess (Table 13.10). A limitation of this study, however, is that the investigators did not assess and control for the out-of-school physical activities of students. In contrast, Sallis et al. [161] recently reported the findings from their well-designed study of 4th graders. They randomly assigned 12 elementary schools to the Sports, Play, and Active Recreation for Kids Study (SPARK) intervention taught by PE specialists, the SPARK intervention led by teachers, or a control condition of regular PE classes (Table 13.10). The SPARK intervention was designed to promote high levels of physical activity, teach movement skills, and be enjoyable. A typical SPARK lesson included 15 min of health-fitness activities and 15 min of skill-fitness activities. Ten health-related activity units included aerobic dance, aerobic games, walking, jogging, and jump rope. The investigators assessed several outcome variables, including self-reported physical activity outside school, Caltrac-monitored physical activity, cardiovascular endurance based on the time to complete a 1-mile run, the number of bent-knee sit-ups in 1 min, and the number of pull-ups the children could do. By the end of the 5th grade, specialist-led students participated in twice as much moderate-to-vigorous physical activity and expended twice as many calories during PE each wk as did control students. Teacher-led classes showed a lower level of improvement. The program did not have an effect on out-of-school physical activity. Girls in the specialist-led group reduced their time on the 1-mile run by 1 min (p = 0.03), with an effect size of 0.32. These girls also increased the number of sit-ups they could do in 1 min, with an effect size of 0.31. These differences were not significant among the boys.

Edmundsen et al. [67] recently reported findings from another intervention, the CATCH project of 7795 3rd grade students followed through the 5th grade (Table 13.10). They found that the intervention had a significant effect on exercise self-efficacy after the 3rd and 4th grades but not after the 5th grade. Although these investigators did not report the effect on out-of-school physical activity, exercise self-efficacy has been consistently found to be associated with increased physical activity among adolescents and young adults. McKenzie et al. [121] also evaluated CATCH PE intervention using a subset of these students (n = 5106). The program was designed to increase vigorous physical activity during PE by at least 90 min per wk, spread over 3 sessions. Children in the intervention schools engaged in vigorous physical activity during a higher percentage of the time than did those in control schools (51.9% vs 42.4%). Based on self-reports, children in the intervention schools spent more minutes breathing hard and had higher MET-weighted vigorous physical activity minutes than did control children.

Another intervention, the Class of 1989 [93] study, was a subcomponent of the Minnesota Heart Health Program (Table 13.10). In 1983, 2376 6th grade students were enrolled in the study and followed for 6 yrs. In addition to the regular interventions, additional aerobic PE classes and competitive

TABLE 13.10.
Examples of Experimental and Quasi-Experimental Studies of Interventions to Promote Physical Activity Among Children and Adolescents

Population, and Investigators	Response Rate, Completion Rate, and Final Response Rate[a]	Sex[b]	Age (Yrs)	Race[c]	Intervention[d]	Measurement of Outcome Variables	Main Findings[e]	Dose Response[f]	Adjustments
4th grade students, Sallis et al. (1997) [161]	RR = 75% (school) RR = 98% (student) CR = 60%–78.4% FR = CBD	815 M 723 F 1538 T	9.49–9.62	1261 W 30 B 62 H 185 A	SPARK study of enhanced PE was designed to increase health-fitness, skill-fitness, and self-management, and regular PA outside school. Schools were randomly assigned to PE specialist-led classes, teacher-led classes, or a control group.	Self-reported PA. Caltrac-monitored PA. Cardiovascular endurance (1 mile run). Muscular strength PA during PE (number of sit-ups in 1 minute).	M + F: Program increased PA during PE, but not outside school. F: Significant increases in the number of sit-ups and decreases in the 1 mile run time compared with control group.	n/r	n/a
3rd grade students, McKenzie et al. (1996) [121]	RR = 56% CR = 74% RR = 41%	2645 M 2461 F 5106 T	Mean: 8.76	3530 W 674 B 708 H 194 O	CATCH PE designed to increase vigorous PA during PE by at least 90 min/wk, over 3 sessions	Distance run in 9 min. Self-reports of PA converted to MET scores of moderate to vigorous PA during PE.	Compared with control subjects, children in intervention schools, engaged in more vigorous PE (51.9% versus 42.3%), spent more min breathing hard (58.6 versus 46.5), and had more MET-weighted vigorous PA min (339.5 versus 270.3)	n/r	n/a

Study	Response[a]	Sample[b]	Age/Grade	Race[c]	Intervention[d]	Measure	Results[e]		[f]
Class of 1989 study, Kelder, Perry, and Klepp (1993) [93]	RR = n/r (baseline) Yr: 1 CR = 88% 2 CR = 81% 3 CR = 70% 4 CR = 66% 5 CR = 59% 6 CR = 45% FR = CBD	?	Yr 1: 6th grade Yr 6: 12th grade	?	Additional aerobic PA classes and an exercise challenge in 8th grade and Slice of Life program in 10th grade.	Self-report of hrs/wk of exercise. Self-report of frequency of PA outside of school ≥3 times/wk and ≥20 min/occasion. Self-report of exercise intensity, combined into one PA score.	M: Intervention group exercised significantly more hrs in 7th and 11th grades. F: Intervention group exercised significantly more hrs in 7th–10th and in 12th grades. Intervention group had significantly higher PA scores in the 8th, 9th, and 11th grades.	n/r	n/a
10th grade students, Killen et al. (1988) [95]	RR = n/r CR = 78% FR = CBD	1447 T	14–16	998 W 29 B 93 H 190 A 4 N 4 PI 129 O	20 classroom sessions on PA, nutrition, cigarette smoking, stress, personal problems solving (there were 5 PA sessions)	Self-report of frequency and duration of 19 activities. Aerobic exercisers were students who performed ≥1 aerobic PA for ≥20 min non-stop for ≥3 times/wk.	M: Significantly increased aerobic exercise (12.8% to 17.4%) in the intervention group compared to a drop (13% to 11.4%) in the control group (p < 0.0001). F: Intervention group significantly increased aerobic exercise (13.6% to 19.6%) compared with no change (13.9%) in the control group (p < 0.0001).	n/r	n/a

[a] RR = response rate; CR = completion rate; FR = final response rate; n/r = not reported; CBD = cannot be determined.

[b] M = males; F = females; T = total.

[c] W = white; B = black; A = Asian; H = Hispanic/Latino; N = Native American; P = Pacific islander; O = other.

[d] PE = physical education; SPARK = Sports, Play, and Active Recreation for Kids Study; CATCH = Child and Adolescent Trial for Cardiovascular Health Study.

[e] Multiple regression coefficients are not standardized or residualized except where indicated.

[f] n/r = not reported; n/a = not applicable.

challenges to perform exercise outside school were introduced in the 8th grade. The Slice of Life Program, a peer-led curriculum designed to promote healthy eating and regular aerobic physical activity, was introduced in the 10th grade. An activity score and the number of hrs of exercise per wk were based on self-reports. Compared with controls, the overall intervention group exercised more hrs in the 7th and 11th grades. Females in the intervention group exercised more hrs in the 7th through 10th and 12th grades; they also had higher activity scores in the 8th, 9th, and 11th grades. These differences were not significant among the boys.

Finally, Killen et al. [95] evaluated a 20-session cardiovascular disease risk reduction intervention among 10th grade students in four high schools in two school districts (Table 13.10). Within each district, schools were randomly assigned to either an intervention group or control group, and students were the unit of analysis. Five of the 20 sessions were devoted to the promotion of increased physical activity. Each module provided the students with information on the effects of different health practices designed to increase the attractiveness of healthful lifestyles, cognitive and behavioral skills needed to change their personal behavior, skills for resisting social influences to adopt or readopt unhealthful habits, and specific practice skills to improve performance. At 2 mon after the completion of the 7-wk intervention, there were significant increases in the percentage of students who reported that they engaged in aerobic physical activities at least 3 times per wk for at least 20 min. The increases were similar for both boys and girls.

While limited in number, these studies have, nonetheless, helped to form the basis for public health recommendations for the promotion of physical activity among children and adolescents [47, 164].

SUMMARY AND CONCLUSIONS

Physical activity epidemiology is central to establishing the importance of physical activity to public health. However, epidemiologic research applied to children and adolescents is still in its infancy. For example, in the studies we reviewed, many instances could be found where samples were inadequately described or where response rates and completion rates suggest that the final sample may no longer be representative of the population of interest. Many studies also had incomplete statistical adjustment for confounding influences. The need for epidemiologic research was clearly demonstrated where initially beneficial findings were negated by such adjustment. Hence, physical activity epidemiologists can play a considerable role. Their research will be the basis for expanding policy and promotional efforts to educate children and adolescents on the benefits of physical activity and the skills needed to be active, thereby helping them to build a foundation for a lifetime of physical activity.

ACKNOWLEDGMENTS

The authors gratefully acknowledge the helpful advice that Dr. Matthew M. Zack provided in his review of the tables, and the very careful editorial review and suggestions made by Ms. Donna L. Brodsky and Dr. Rick Hull.

REFERENCES

1. Aaron, D.J., A.M. Kriska, S.R. Dearwater, et al. The epidemiology of leisure physical activity in an adolescent population. *Med. Sci. Sports Exerc.* 25:847–853, 1993.
2. Aaron D.J., R.E. LaPorte. Physical activity, adolescence, and health: an epidemiological perspective. *Exerc. Sports Sci. Rev.* 25:391–405, 1997.
3. Al-Hazzaa, H.M., M.A. Sulaiman, A.J. Al-Matar, and K.F. Al-Mobaireek. Cardiorespiratory fitness, physical activity patterns and coronary risk factors in preadolescent boys. *Int. J. Sports Med.* 15:267–272, 1994.
4. Allis, K.R. Predictors of inactivity: an analysis of the Ontario Health Survey. *Can. J. Pub. Health* 87:354–358, 1996.
5. American Heart Association. *1993 Heart and Stroke Facts Statistics.* Dallas, Texas, 1992, pp. 11.
6. Andersen, L.B. Blood pressure, physical fitness and physical activity in 17-year-old Danish adolescents. *J. Intern. Med.* 236:323–330, 1994.
7. Andersen, L.B., and J. Haraldsdottir. Tracking of cardiovascular disease risk factors including maximal oxygen uptake and physical activity from late teenage to adulthood: an 8-year follow-up study. *J. Intern. Med.* 234:309–315, 1993.
8. Armstrong, N., and B. Simons-Morton. Physical activity and blood lipids in adolescents. *Pediatr. Exerc. Sci.* 6:381–405, 1994.
9. Armstrong, N., J. Balding, P. Gentle, and B. Kirby. Estimation of coronary risk factors in British schoolchildren: a preliminary report. *Br. J. Sports Med.* 24:61–66, 1990.
10. Armstrong, N., J. Williams, J. Balding, P. Gentle, and B. Kirby. Cardiopulmonary fitness, physical activity patterns, and selected coronary risk factor variables in 11- to 16-year-olds. *Pediatr. Exerc. Sci.* 3:219–228, 1991.
11. Atomi, Y., Y. Kuroda, T. Asami, and T. Kawahara. HDL_2 cholesterol of children (10 to 12 years of age), related to VO_2max, body fat and sex. J. Rutenfranz, R. Mocellin, and F. Klimt (eds.). *Children and Exercise XII.* Champaign, IL: Human Kinetics, 1986, pp. 167–172.
12. Backx, F.J.G. Epidemiology of paediatric sports-related injuries. O. Bar-Or (ed.). *The Child and Adolescent Athlete.* Oxford (England): Blackwell Science, 1996, pp. 163–172.
13. Backx, F.J.G., W.B.M. Erich, A.B.A. Kemper, and A.L.M. Verbeek. Sports injuries in school-aged children. *Am. J. Sports Med.* 17:234–240, 1989.
14. Bailey, D.A. The role of physical activity in the regulation of bone mass during growth. O. Bar-Or (ed.). *The Child and Adolescent Athlete.* Oxford (England): Blackwell Science, 1996, pp. 138–152.
15. Bailey, D.A., J.H. Wedge, R.G. McCulloch, A.D. Martin, and S.C. Bernhardson. Epidemiology of fractures of the distal end of the radius in children as associated with growth. *J. Bone Joint Surg.* 71-A:1225–1230, 1989.
16. Bailey, R.C., J. Olson, S.L. Pepper, J. Porszasz, T.J. Barstow, and D.M. Cooper. The level and tempo of children's physical activities: an observational study. *Med. Sci. Sports Exerc.* 27:1033–1041, 1995.
17. Baranowski, T., C. Bouchard, O. Bar-Or, et al. Assessment, prevalence, and cardiovascular benefits of physical activity and fitness in youth. *Med. Sci. Sports Exerc.* 24:S237–S247, 1992.
18. Baranowski, T., W.O. Thompson, R.H. DuRant, J. Baranowski, and J. Puhl. Observations

on physical activity in physical locations: age, gender, ethnicity, and month effects. *Res. Q. Exer. Sport* 64:127–133, 1993.

19. Berenson, G.S., A.W. Voors, L.S. Webber, E.R. Dalferes, Jr., and D.W. Harsha. Racial difference of parameters associated with blood pressure levels in children: the Bogalusa Heart Study. *Metabolism* 28:1218–1228, 1979.

20. Biddle, S., and M. Goudas. Analysis of children's physical activity and its association with adult encouragement and social cognitive variables. *J. Sch. Health* 66:75–78, 1996.

21. Bijur, P.E., A. Trumble, Y. Harel, M.D. Overpeck, D. Jones, and P.C. Scheidt. Sports and recreation injuries in US children and adolescents. *Arch. Pediatr. Adolesc. Med.* 149: 1009–1016, 1995.

22. Blimkie, C.J.R., J. Lefevre, G.P. Beunen, R. Renson, J. Dequeker, and P. van Damme. Fractures, physical activity, and growth velocity in adolescent Belgian boys. *Med. Sci. Sports Exerc.* 25:801–808, 1993.

23. Bonjour, J.P., G. Theintz, F. Law, D. Slosman, and R. Rizzoli. Peak bone mass. *Osteoporos. Int.* 4(Supp. 1):S7–S13, 1994.

24. Boot, A.M., M.A.J. De Ridder, H.A.P. Pols, E.P. Krenning, and S.M.P.F. De Muinck Keizer-Schrama. Bone mineral density in children and adolescents: relation to puberty, calcium intake, and physical activity. *J. Clin. Endocrinol. Metab.* 82:57–62, 1997.

25. Boreham, C.A., J. Twisk, M.J. Savage, G.W. Cran, and J.J. Strain. Physical activity, sports participation, and risk factors in adolescents. *Med. Sci. Sports Exerc.* 29:788–793, 1997.

26. Bouchard, C., A. Tremblay, C. Leblanc, G. Lortie, R. Savard, and G. Theriault. A method to assess energy expenditure in children and adults. *Am. J. Clin. Nutr.* 37:461–467, 1983.

27. Boyce, W.T., and S. Sobolewski. Recurrent injuries in schoolchildren. *Am. J. Dis. Child.* 143:338-342, 1989.

28. Boyce, W.T., L.W. Sprunger, S. Sobolewski, and C. Schaefer. Epidemiology of injuries in a large, urban school district. *Pediatrics* 74:342–349, 1984.

29. Brener, N.D., J.L. Collins, L. Kann, C.W. Warren, and B.I. Williams. Reliability of the Youth Risk Behavior Survey questionnaire. *Am J. Epidemiol.* 141:575–580, 1995.

30. Bullen, B.A., R.B. Reed, and J. Mayer. Physical activity of obese and nonobese adolescent girls appraised by motion picture sampling. *Am. J. Clin. Nutr.* 14:211–223, 1964.

31. Bush, P.J., R.J. Iannotti, A.E. Zuckerman, R.W. O'Brien, and S.A. Smith. Cardiovascular disease risk factors. *Prev. Med.* 20:447–461, 1991.

32. Caspersen, C.J. Physical activity epidemiology: concepts, methods, and applications to exercise science. *Exerc. Sports Sci. Rev.* 17:423–473, 1989.

33. Caspersen, C.J. What are the lessons from the U.S. approach for setting targets. A.J. Killoran, P. Fentem, and C.J. Caspersen (eds.). *Moving On: International Perspectives on Promoting Physical Activity.* London: Health Education Authority, 1994, pp. 35–55.

34. Caspersen, C.J., G.M. Christenson, and R.A. Pollard. Status of the 1990 physical fitness and exercise objectives–evidence from NHIS 1985. *Public Health Rep.* 101:587–592, 1986.

35. Caspersen, C.J., A.M. Kriska, and S.R. Dearwater. Physical activity epidemiology as applied to elderly populations. *Clin. Rheumatol.* 8:7–27, 1994.

36. Caspersen, C.J., and R.K. Merritt. Physical activity trends among 26 states, 1986-1990. *Med. Sci. Sports Exerc.* 27:713–720, 1995.

37. Caspersen, C.J., R.K. Merritt, and T. Stephens. International physical activity patterns: a methodological perspective. R.K. Dishman (ed.). *Advances in Exercise Adherence.* Champaign: Human Kinetics, 1994, pp. 73–110.

38. Caspersen, C.J., R.A. Pollard, and S.O. Pratt. Scoring physical activity data with special consideration for elderly populations. Data for an Aging Population. *Proceedings of the 21st National Meeting of the Public Health Conference on Records and Statistics.* Hyattsville, Maryland: National Center for Health Statistics, 1987, pp. 30–34. DHHS Publication No. (PHS) 88-1214.

39. Caspersen, C.J., K.E. Powell, and G.M. Christenson. Physical activity, exercise and physical

fitness: definitions and distinctions for health-related research. *Public Health Rep.* 100: 126–130, 1985.

40. Caspersen, C.J., K.E. Powell, and R.K. Merritt. Measurement of health status and well being. Bouchard, C., R.J. Shephard, and T. Stephens (eds.). *Physical Activity, Fitness, and Health: International Proceedings and Consensus Statement.* Champaign, IL: Human Kinetics, pp. 180–202, 1994.

41. Caspersen, C.J., and M.M. Zack. The prevalence of physical inactivity in the United States. A. S. Leon (ed.). *Physical Activity and Cardiovascular Health: A National Consensus.* Champaign, IL: Human Kinetics, 1997, pp. 32–39.

42. Centers for Disease Control. *Youth Risk Behavior Survey, 1991.* Atlanta, GA: U.S. Department of Health and Human Services, Public Health Service, Centers for Disease Control, National Center for Chronic Disease Prevention and Health Promotion, 1991. National Technical Information Service Order No. PB94–500121.

43. Centers for Disease Control. *1992 BRFSS Summary Prevalence Report.* Atlanta, GA: U.S. Department of Health and Human Services, Public Health Service, Centers for Disease Control, National Center for Chronic Disease Prevention and Health Promotion, 1992.

44. Centers for Disease Control and Prevention. *National Health Interview Survey–Youth Risk Behavior Survey, 1992 machine readable data file and documentation.* Atlanta, GA: U.S. Department of Health and Human Services, Public Health Service, Centers for Disease Control and Prevention, National Center for Health Statistics, 1993.

45. Centers for Disease Control and Prevention. *Youth Risk Behavior Survey, 1993.* Atlanta, GA: U.S. Department of Health and Human Services, Public Health Service, Centers for Disease Control and Prevention, National Center for Chronic Disease Prevention and Health Promotion, 1993. National Technical Information Service Order No. PB95–503363.

46. Centers for Disease Control and Prevention. *1994 BRFSS Summary Prevalence Report.* Atlanta, GA: U.S. Department of Health and Human Services, Public Health Service, Centers for Disease Control and Prevention, National Center for Chronic Disease Prevention and Health Promotion, 1994.

47. Centers for Disease Control and Prevention. *Guidelines for school and community programs to promote lifelong physical activity among young people.* Atlanta, GA: U.S. Department of Health and Human Services, Public Health Service, Centers for Disease Control and Prevention, National Center for Chronic Disease Prevention and Health Promotion, MMWR 46(RR-6):1–36, 1997.

48. Centers for Disease Control and Prevention. *Youth Risk Behavior Survey, 1995.* Atlanta, GA: U.S. Department of Health and Human Services, Public Health Service, Centers for Disease Control and Prevention, National Center for Chronic Disease Prevention and Health Promotion, 1996. National Technical Information Service Order No. PB96–503123INC.

49. Courneya, K.S., and E. McAuley. Are there different determinants of frequency, intensity, and duration of physical activity? *Behav. Med.* 20:84–90, 1994.

50. Craig, S.B., L.G. Bandini, A.H. Lichtenstein, E.J. Schaefer, and W.H. Dietz. The impact of physical activity on lipids, lipoproteins, and blood pressure in preadolescent girls. *Pediatrics* 98(3 Part 1):389–395, 1996.

51. de Loës, M. Epidemiology of sports injuries in the Swiss organization "Youth and Sports" 1987-1989. *Int. J. Sports Med.* 16:134–138, 1995.

52. Dietz, W.H. Jr., and S.L. Gortmaker. Do we fatten our children at the television set? Obesity and television viewing in children and adolescents. *Pediatrics* 75:807–812, 1985.

53. Douthit, V.L. Psychological determinants of adolescent exercise adherence. *Adolescence* 29:711–722, 1994.

54. Drewnowski, A., C.L. Kurth, and D.D. Krahn. Body weight and dieting in adolescence: impact of socioeconomic status. *Int. J. Eat. Dis.* 16:61–65, 1994.

55. Drewnowski, A., C.L. Kurth, and D.D. Krahn. Effects of body image on dieting, exercise and anabolic steroid use in adolescent males. *Int. J. Eat. Dis.* 17:381–386, 1995.

56. Duncan, B., W.T. Boyce, R. Itami, and N. Puffenbarger. A controlled trial of a physical fitness program for fifth grade students. *J. Sch. Health.* 53:467–471, 1983.

57. DuRant, R.H., T. Baranowski, H. Davis, et al. Reliability and variability of heart rate monitoring in 3-, 4-, or 5-yr-old children. *Med. Sci. Sports Exerc.* 24:265–271, 1992.

58. DuRant, R.H., T. Baranowski, M. Johnson, and W.O. Thompson. The relationships among television watching, physical activity, and body composition of young children. *Pediatrics* 94:449–455, 1994.

59. DuRant, R.H., T. Baranowski, T. Rhodes, et al. Association among serum lipid and lipoprotein concentrations and physical activity, physical fitness, and body composition in young children. *J. Pediatr.* 133:185–192, 1993a.

60. DuRant, R. H., T. Baranowski, T. Rhodes, et al. Evaluation of the Children's Activity Rating Scale (CARS) in young children. *Med. Sci. Sports Exerc.* 25:1415–1421, 1993b.

61. DuRant, R.H., and A.C. Hergenroeder. Promotion of physical activity among adolescents by primary health care providers. *Pediatr. Exer. Sci.* 6:448–463, 1994.

62. DuRant, R.H., C.W. Linder, J.W. Harkness, and R.G. Gray. The relationship between physical activity and serum lipids and lipoproteins in black children and adolescents. *J Adolesc. Health Care* 4:55–60, 1983b.

63. DuRant, R.H., C.W. Linder, and O.M. Mahoney. Relationship between habitual activity and serum lipoprotein levels in white male adolescents. *J. Adolesc. Health Care* 4:235–240, 1983a.

64. DuRant, R.H., R.A. Pendergrast, J. Donner, C. Seymore, and C. Gaillard. Adolescents' attrition from school-sponsored sport. *Am. J. Dis. Child.* 145:1119–1123, 1991.

65. DuRant, R.H., R.A. Pendergrast, C. Seymore, C. Gaillard, and J. Donner. Findings from the preparticipation athletic examination and athletic injuries. *Am. J. Dis. Child.* 146: 85–91, 1992.

66. Dwyer, T., W.E. Coonan, D.R. Leitch, B.S. Hetzel, and R.A. Baghurst. An investigation of the effects of daily physical activity on the health of primary school students in South Australia. *Int. J. Epidemiol.* 12:308–313, 1983.

67. Edmundson, E., G.S. Parcel, H.A. Feldman, et al. The effects of the Child and Adolescent Trial for Cardiovascular Health upon psychosocial determinants of diet and physical activity behavior. *Prev. Med.* 25:442–454, 1996.

68. Epstein, L.H., K.J. Coleman, and M.D. Myers. Exercise in treating obesity in children and adolescents. *Med. Sci. Sports Exerc.* 28:428–435, 1996.

69. Epstein, L.H., A.M. Valoski, L.S. Vara, et al. Effects of decreasing sedentary behavior and increasing activity on weight changes in obese children. *Health Psychol.* 14:109–115, 1995.

70. Faulkner, R.A., C.S. Houston, D.A. Bailey, D.T. Drinkwater, H.A. McKay, and A.A. Wilkinson. Comparison of bone mineral content and bone mineral density between dominant and nondominant limbs in children 8–16 years of age. *Am. J. Hum. Biol.* 5:491–499, 1993.

71. Fehily, A.M., R.J. Coles, W.D. Evans, and P.C. Elwood. Factors affecting bone density in young adults. *Am. J. Clin. Nutr.* 56:579–586, 1992.

72. Frazier, E.L., A.L. Franks, and L.M. Sanderson. Behavioral risk factor data. *Using Chronic Disease Data: A Handbook For Public Health Practitioners.* Atlanta, GA: U.S. Department of Health and Human Services, Public Health Service, Centers for Disease Control, National Center for Chronic Disease Prevention and Health Promotion, 1992, Section 4–1, pp. 4–17.

73. Gallagher, S.S., K. Finison, B. Guyer, and S. Goodenough. The incidence of injuries among 87,000 Massachusetts children and adolescents: results of the 1980-1981 Statewide Childhood Injury Prevention Program Surveillance System. *Am. J. Publ. Health* 74: 1340–1347, 1984.

74. Garcia, A.W., M.A.N. Broda, M. Frenn, C. Covick, N.J. Pender, and D.L. Ronis. Gender

and developmental differences in exercise beliefs among youth and prediction of their exercise behavior. *J. Sch. Health* 65:213–219, 1995.

75. Garrick, J.G., and R.K. Requa. Injuries in high school sports. *Pediatrics* 61:465–469, 1978.

76. Gentle, P., R. Caves, N. Armstrong, J. Balding, and B. Kirby. High and low exercisers among 14- and 15-year-old children. *J. Pub. Health Med.* 16:186–194, 1994.

77. Gilliam, T.B., P.S. Freedson, D.L. Geenen, and B. Shahraray. Physical activity patterns determined by heart rate monitoring in 6–7 year old children. *Med. Sci. Sports Exerc.* 13:65–67, 1981.

78. Godin, G., and R.J. Shephard. Normative beliefs of school children concerning regular exercise. *J. Sch. Health* 54:443–445, 1984.

79. Goran, M.I., W.H. Carpenter, and E.T. Poehlman. Total energy expenditure in 4- to 6-yr-old children. *Am. J. Physiol.* 264:E706–E711, 1993.

80. Groothausen, J., H. Siemer, H.C.G. Kemper, J. Twisk, and D.C. Welten. Influence of peak strain on lumbar bone mineral density: an analysis of 15-year physical activity in young males and females. *Pediatr. Exerc. Sci.* 9:159–173, 1997.

81. Gunnes, M., and E.H. Lehmann. Dietary calcium, saturated fat, fiber and vitamin C as predictors of forearm cortical and trabecular bone mineral density in healthy children and adolescents. *Acta Paediatr.* 84:388–392, 1995.

82. Gunnes, M., and E.H. Lehmann. Physical activity and dietary constituents as predictors of forearm cortical trabecular bone gain in healthy children and adolescents: a prospective study. *Acta Paediatr.* 85:19–25, 1996.

83. Hansen, H.S., K. Froberg, N. Hyldebrandt, and J.R. Nielsen. A controlled study of eight months of physical training and reduction of blood pressure in children: the Odense Schoolchild Study. *B.M.J.* 303:682–685, 1991.

84. Harrell, J.S., R.G. McMurray, S.I. Bangdiwala, A.C. Frauman, S.A. Gansky, and C.B. Bradley. Effects of a school-based intervention to reduce cardiovascular disease risk factors in elementary-school children: the Cardiovascular Health in Children (CHIC) Study. *J. Pediatr.* 128:797–805, 1996.

85. Higgins, M.W., J.B. Keller, H.L. Metzner, et al. Studies of blood pressure in Tecumseh, Michigan: antecedents in childhood of high blood pressure in young adults. *Hypertension* 2:117–123, 1980.

86. Horan, M.J., and C. Lenfant. Epidemiology of blood pressure and predictors of hypertension. *Hypertension* 15(Suppl I):I20–I24, 1990.

87. Hovell, M.F., B. Kolody, and J.F. Sallis. Parent support, physical activity, and correlates of adiposity in nine year olds: an exploratory study. *J. Health Educ.* 27:126–129, 1996.

88. Janz, K.F., T.L. Burns, and L.T. Mahoney. Predictors of left ventricular mass and resting blood pressure in children: the Muscatine Study. *Med. Sci. Sports Exerc.* 27:818–825, 1995.

89. Janz, K.F., J.C. Golden, J.R. Hansen, and L.T. Mahoney. Heart rate monitoring of physical activity in children and adolescents: the Muscatine Study. *Pediatrics* 89:256–261, 1992.

90. Jenner, D.A., R. Vandongen, and L.J. Beilin. Relationships between blood pressure and measures of dietary energy intake, physical fitness, and physical activity in Australian children aged 11–12 years. *Epidemiol. Comm. Health* 46:108–113, 1992.

91. Jones, N.L., and E.J.M. Campbell. *Clinical Exercise Testing.* 2nd ed. Philadelphia: W.B. Saunders, 1982, p. 249.

92. Kann, L., W. Warren, J.L. Collins, J. Ross, B. Collins, and L.J. Kolbe. Results from the national school-based 1991 Youth Risk Behavior Survey and progress toward achieving related health objectives for the nation. *Public Health Rep.* 108(Suppl 1):47–67, 1993.

93. Kelder, S.H., C.L. Perry, and K.I. Klepp. Community-wide youth exercise promotion: long-term outcomes of the Minnesota Heart Health Program and the Class of 1989 Study. *J. Sch. Health* 63:218–223, 1993.

94. Kemper, H.C.G., J. Snel, R. Verschuur, and L. Storm-van Essen. Tracking of health and risk indicators of cardiovascular diseases from teenage to adult: Amsterdam Growth and Health Study. *Prev. Med.* 19:642–655, 1990.

95. Killen, J.D, M.J. Telch, T.N. Robinson, N. Maccoby, C.B. Taylor, and J.W. Farquhar. Cardiovascular disease risk reduction for tenth graders: a multiple-factor school-based approach. *J.A.M.A.* 260:1728–1733, 1988.

96. Klesges, R.C., T.J. Coates, L.M. Moldenhauer, B. Holzer, J. Gustavson, and J. Barnes. The FATS: an observational system for assessing physical activity in children and associated parent behavior. *Behav. Assessment* 6:333–345, 1984.

97. Klesges, R.C., C.K. Haddock, and L.H. Eck. A multimethod approach to the measurement of childhood physical activity and its relationship to blood pressure and body weight. *J. Pediatr.* 116:888–893, 1990.

98. Klesges, R.C., L.M. Klesges, A.M. Swenson, and A.M. Pheley. A validation of two motion sensors in the prediction of child and adult physical activity levels. *Am. J. Epidemiol.* 122: 400–410, 1985.

99. Kohl, H.W., J.E. Fulton, and C.J. Caspersen. Physical activity assessment among children and adolescents. *Prev. Med.* 1998 (in press).

100. Kolbe, L.J. An epidemiological surveillance system to monitor the prevalence of youth behaviors that most affect health. *Health Educ.* 21:44–48, 1990.

101. Kolbe, L.J., L. Kann, and J.L. Collins. Overview of the Youth Risk Behavior Surveillance System. *Public Health Rep.* 108(Suppl 1):2–10, 1993.

102. Kolody, B., and J.F. Sallis. A prospective study of ponderosity, body image, self-concept, and psychological variables in children. *Dev. Behav. Pediatr.* 16:1–5, 1995.

103. Kriska, A.M., R.B. Sandler, J.A. Cauley, R.E. LaPorte, D.L. Hom, and G. Pambianco. The assessment of historical physical activity and its relation to adult bone parameters. *Am. J. Epidemiol.* 127:1053–1063, 1988.

104. Kroger, H., A. Kotaniemi, L. Kroger, and E. Alhava. Development of bone mass and bone density of the spine and femoral neck: a prospective study of 65 children and adolescents. *Bone Miner.* 23:171–182, 1993.

105. Kroger, H., A. Kotaniemi, P. Vainio, and E. Alhava. Bone densitometry of the spine and femur in children by dual-energy x-ray absorptiometry. *Bone Miner.* 17:75–85, 1992.

106. Lansky, L.L., M.A. List, S.B. Lansky, M.E. Cohen, and L.F. Sinks. A validation of two motion sensors in the prediction of child and adult physical activity levels. *Am. J. Epidemiol.* 122:400–410, 1985.

107. LaPorte, R.E., H.J. Montoye, and C.J. Caspersen. Assessment of physical activity in epidemiologic research: problems and prospects. *Public Health Rep.* 100:131–146, 1985.

108. Last, J.M. *A Dictionary of Epidemiology. 3rd edition.* New York: Oxford University Press, 1995.

109. Lauer, R.M., T.L. Burns, L.T. Mahoney, and C.M. Tipton. Blood pressure in children. C.V. Gisolfi and D.R. Lamb (eds.). *Perspectives in Exercise Science and Sports Medicine: Vol. 2. Youth, Exercise, and Sport.* Indianapolis, IN: Benchmark Press, 1989, pp. 431–459.

110. Lieberman E. Hypertension in childhood and adolescence. N.M. Kaplan (ed.). *Clinical Hypertension.* Baltimore, MD: Williams and Wilkins. 1986, pp. 447–472.

111. Linder, C.W., R.H. DuRant, S. Jay, and N. Bryant-Pitts. The influence of oral contraceptives and habitual physical activity on serum lipids in black adolescents and young women. *J. Adolesc. Health Care* 10:275–282, 1989.

112. Linder, C.W., R.H. DuRant, and O.M. Mahoney. The effect of physical conditioning on serum lipids and lipoproteins in white male adolescents. *Med. Sci. Sports Exerc.* 15:232–236, 1983.

113. Luepker, R.V., C.L. Perry, S.M. McKinlay, et al. Outcomes of a field trial to improve children's dietary patterns and physical activity. *J.A.M.A.* 275:768–776, 1996.

114. Lysens, R.J., M.S. Ostyn, Y.V. Auweele, J. Lefevre, M. Vuylsteke, and L. Renson. The accident-prone and overuse-prone profiles of the young athlete. *Am. J. Sports Med.* 17: 612–619, 1989.

115. Macek, M., D. Bell, J. Rutenfranz, et al. A comparison of coronary risk factors in groups of trained and untrained adolescents. *Eur. J. Appl. Physiol.* 58:577–582, 1989.

116. Macek, M., J. Rutenfranz, K. Lange Anderson, et al. Favourable levels of cardiovascular health and risk indicators during childhood and adolescence. *Eur. J. Pediatr.* 144:360–367, 1985.

117. Manolio, T.A., P.J. Savage, G.L. Burke, et al. Association of fasting insulin with blood pressure and lipids in young adults: the CARDIA study. *Arteriosclerosis* 10:430–436, 1990.

118. Margulies, J.Y., A. Simkin, I. Leichter, et al. Effect of intense physical activity on the bone-mineral content in the lower limbs of young adults. *J. Bone Joint Surg.* 68-A: 1090–1093, 1986.

119. Marti, B., and E. Vartiainen. Relation between leisure time exercise and cardiovascular risk factors among 15-year-olds in eastern Finland. *J. Epidemiol. Comm. Health* 43:228–233, 1989.

120. McKenzie,T.L., J.F. Sallis, P.R. Nader, et al. BEACHES: an observational system for assessing children's eating and physical activity behaviors and associated events. *J. Appl. Behav. Anal.* 24:141–151, 1991.

121. McKenzie, T.L, P.R. Nader, P.K. Strikmiller, et al. School physical education: effect of the Child and Adolescent Trial for Cardiovascular Health. *Prev. Med.* 25:423–431, 1996.

122. McLain, L.G., and S. Reynolds. Sports injuries in a high school. *Pediatrics* 84:446–450, 1989.

123. Montoye, H.J., and H.L. Taylor. Measurement of physical activity in population studies: a review. *Hum. Biol.* 56:195–216, 1984.

124. Moore, L.L., U.S. Nguyen, K.J. Rothman, L.A. Cupples, and R.C. Ellison. Preschool physical activity level and change in body fatness in young children. *Am. J. Epidemiol.* 142: 982–988, 1995.

125. Moore, L.L., D.A. Lombardi, M.J. White, J.L. Campbell, S.A. Oliveria, and R.C. Ellison. Influence of parents' physical activity levels on activity levels of young children. *J. Pediatr.* 118:215–219, 1991.

126. Moussa, M.A.A., M.B. Skaik, S.B. Selwanes, O.Y. Yaghy, and S.A. Bin-Othman. Factors associated with obesity in school children. *Int. J. Obes.* 18:513–515, 1994.

127. Must, A., P.F. Jacques, G.E. Dallal, C.J. Bajema, and W.H. Dietz. Long-term morbidity and mortality of overweight adolescents. *N. Engl. J. Med.* 327:1350–1355, 1992.

128. National Center for Health Statistics. *Health, United States, 1995.* Hyattsville, MD: U.S. Department of Health and Human Services, Public Health Service, Centers for Disease Control and Prevention, National Center for Health Statistics, 1996. DHHS Publication No. (PHS) 96–1232.

129. National Center for Health Statistics. Plan and operation of the Third National Health and Nutrition Examination Survey, 1988-94. *Vital and Health Statistics, Series 1, No. 32.* Hyattsville, MD: U.S. Department of Health and Human Services, Public Health Service, Centers for Disease Control and Prevention, National Center for Health Statistics, 1994a. DHHS Publication No. (PHS)94–1308.

130. National Center for Health Statistics, P.F. Adams, and V. Benson. Current Estimates From the National Health Interview Survey, 1990. *Vital and Health Statistics, Series 10, No. 181.* Hyattsville, MD: U.S. Department of Health and Human Services, Public Health Service, Centers for Disease Control, National Center for Health Statistics, 1991. DHHS Publication No. (PHS)92–1509.

131. National Center for Health Statistics, Benson, V., and M.A. Marano. Current estimates from the National Health Interview Survey, 1992. *Vital and Health Statistics, Series 10, No. 189.* Hyattsville, MD: U.S. Department of Health and Human Services, Public Health Service, Centers for Disease Control and Prevention, National Center for Health Statistics, 1994b. DHHS Publication No. (PHS)94–1517.

132. National Center for Health Statistics, A.L. Piani, and C.A. Schoenborn. Health Promotion and Disease Prevention: United States, 1990. *Vital and Health Statistics, Series 10, No. 185.* Hyattsville, MD: U.S. Department of Health and Human Services, Public Health Service,

Centers for Disease Control and Prevention, National Center for Health Statistics, 1993. DHHS Publication No. (PHS)93–1513.

133. National Center for Health Statistics, and C.A. Schoenborn. Health Promotion and Disease Prevention: United States, 1985 *Vital and Health Statistics, Series 10, No. 163.* Hyattsville, MD:U.S. Department of Health and Human Services, Public Health Service, Centers for Disease Control, National Center for Health Statistics, 1988. DHHS Publication No. (PHS)88–1591.

134. National Institutes of Health. *The Fifth Report of the Joint National Committee on Detection, Evaluation, and Treatment of High Blood Pressure.* Bethesda, MD:National Institutes of Health, National Heart, Lung, and Blood Institute, 1993. NIH Publication No. 93-1088, pp. 1–48.

135. National Institutes of Health. National Institutes of Health Guide. *Prevention of osteoporosis, Volume 21, Number 21.* June 20, 1997.

136. Newman, W.P., W. Watigney, and G.S. Berenson. Autopsy studies of United States children and adolescents: relationships of risk factors to arteriosclerotic lesions. *Ann. N.Y. Acad. Sci.* 623:16–25, 1991.

137. Nizankowska-Blaz, T., and T. Abramowicz. Effects of intensive physical training on serum lipids and lipoproteins. *Acta Pediatr. Scand.* 72:357–359, 1983.

138. Obarzanek, E., G.B. Schreiber, P.B. Crawford, et al. Energy intake and physical activity in relation to indexes of body fat: the National Heart, Lung, and Blood Institute Growth and Health Study. *Am. J. Clin. Nutr.* 60:15–22, 1994.

139. O'Hara, N.V., T. Baranowksi, B.G. Simons-Morton, B.S. Wilson, and G.S. Parcel. Validity of the observation of children's physical activity. *Res. Q. Exerc. Sport* 60:42–47, 1989.

140. Paffenbarger, R.S., M.C. Thorne, and A.L. Wing. Chronic disease in former college students: VIII. Characteristics in youth predisposing to hypertension in later years. *Am. J. Epidemiol.* 88:24–32, 1968.

141. Page, R.M., and L.A. Tucker. Psychosocial discomfort and exercise frequency: an epidemiological study of adolescents. *Adolescence* 29:183–191, 1994.

142. Paul, O. Epidemiology of hypertension. J. Genest, E. Koiw, and O. Kutchel (eds.). *Hypertension: Physiopathology and Treatment.* New York:McGraw-Hill, 1977.

143. Pereira, M.A., S.J. FitzGerald, E.W. Gregg, et al. A collection of physical activity questionnaires for health-related research. *Med. Sci. Sports Exerc.* 29:S201–205, 1997.

144. Perusse, L., J.P. Despres, A. Tremblay, et al. Genetic and environmental determinants of serum lipid and lipoproteins in French Canadian families. *Arteriosclerosis* 9:308–318, 1989.

145. Pi-Sunyer, F.X. Health implications of obesity. *Am. J. Clin. Nutr.* 53:1595S–1603S, 1991.

146. Porkka K.V.K., J.S.A. Viikari, S. Taimela, M. Dahl, and H.K. Akerblom. Tracking and predictiveness of serum lipid and lipoprotein measurements in childhood: a 1-year follow-up. *Am. J. Epid.* 140:1096–1110, 1994.

147. Rabbia, F., F. Veglio, G. Pinna, et al. Cardiovascular risk factors in adolescence: prevalence and familial aggregation. *Prev. Med.* 23:809–815, 1994.

148. Raitakari, O.T., K.V.K. Porkka, L. Rasanen, and J.S.A. Viikari. Relations of life-style with lipids, blood pressure and insulin in adolescents and young adults: the Cardiovascular Risk in Young Finns Study. *Atherosclerosis* 111:237–246, 1994a.

149. Raitakari, O.T., K.V.K. Porkka, S. Taimela, R. Telama, L. Rasanen, and J.S.A. Viikari. Effects of persistent physical activity and inactivity on coronary risk factors in children and young adults. *Am. J. Epidemiol.* 140:195–205, 1994c.

150. Reisin, E., R. Abel, M. Modan, et al. Effect of weight loss without salt restriction on the reduction of blood pressure in overweight hypertensive patients. *N. Engl J. Med.* 298: 1–6, 1978.

151. Robinson, T.N., L.D. Hammer, J.D. Killen, et al. Does television viewing increase obesity and reduce physical activity? Cross-sectional and longitudinal analyses among adolescent girls. *Pediatrics* 91:273–280, 1993.

152. Rolland-Cachera, M.F., and F. Bellisle. No correlation between adiposity and food intake: why are working class children fatter? *Am. J. Clin. Nutr.* 44:779–787, 1986.

153. Rowland T.W., L. Martel, P. Vanderburgh, T. Manos, and N. Charkoudian. The influence of short-term aerobic training on blood lipids in healthy 10–12 year old children. *Int. J. Sports Med.* 17:487–492, 1996.

154. Rubin, K., V. Schirduan, P. Gendreau, M. Sarfarazi, R. Mendola, and G. Dalsky. Predictors of axial and peripheral bone mineral density in healthy children and adolescents, with special attention to the role of puberty. *J. Pediatr.* 123:868–870, 1993.

155. Ruiz, J.C., C. Mandel, and M. Garabedian. Influence of spontaneous calcium intake and physical exercise on the vertebral and femoral bone mineral density of children and adolescents. *J. Bone Miner. Res.* 10:675–682, 1995.

156. Sallis, J.F., C.C. Berry, S.L. Broyles, J.L. McKenzie, and P.R. Nader. Variability and tracking of physical activity over 2 yr in young children. *Med. Sci. Sports Exer.* 27:1042–1049, 1995.

157. Sallis, J.F., M.J. Buono, J.J. Roby, D. Carlson, and J.A. Nelson. The CALTRAC accelerometer as a physical activity monitor for school-age children. *Med. Sci. Sports Exerc.* 22:698–703, 1990.

158. Sallis, J.F., S.A. Condon, K.A. Goggin, J.J. Roby, B. Kolody, and J.E. Alcarez. The development of self-administered physical activity surveys for 4th grade students. *Res. Q. Exerc. Sport* 64:25–31, 1993a.

159. Sallis, J.F., W.L. Haskell, S.P. Fortmann, K.M. Vranizan, C.B. Taylor, and D.S. Soloman. Predictors of adoption and maintenance of physical activity in a community sample. *Prev. Med.* 15:331–341, 1986.

160. Sallis, J.F., and M.F. Hovell. Determinants of exercise behavior. J.O. Holloszy, and K.B. Pandolf (eds.). *Exercise and Sports Science Reviews.* Baltimore, MD: Williams and Wilkins, 1990, Vol. 18, pp. 307–330.

161. Sallis, J.F., T.L. McKenzie, J.E. Alcaraz, B. Kolody, N. Faucette, and M.F. Hovell. Effects of a 2-year education program (SPARK) on physical activity and fitness in elementary school students: SPARK. *Am. J. Pub. Health* 87:1328–1334, 1997.

162. Sallis, J.F., T.L. McKenzie, J.P. Elder, S.L. Broyles, and P.R. Nader. Factors parents use in selecting play spaces for young children. *Arch. Pediatr. Adolesc. Med.* 151:414–417, 1997.

163. Sallis, J.F., P.R. Nader, S.L. Broyles, et al. Correlates of physical activity at home in Mexican-American and Anglo-American preschool children. *Health Psych.* 12:390–398, 1993b.

164. Sallis J.F., and K. Patrick. Physical activity guidelines for adolescents: consensus statement. *Pediatr. Exerc. Sci.* 6:302–314, 1994.

165. Sallis, J.F., T.L. Patterson, M.J. Buono, and P.R. Nader. Relation of cardiovascular fitness and physical activity to cardiovascular disease risk factors in children and adults. *Am. J. Epidemiol.* 127:933–941, 1988.

166. Sallis, J.F., J.M. Zakarian, M.F. Hovell, and C.R. Hofstetter. Ethnic, socioeconomic, and sex differences in physical activity among adolescents. *J. Clin. Epidemiol.* 49:125–134, 1996.

167. Saris, W.H.M., P. Snel, J. Baecke, F. van Waesberghe, and R.A. Binkhorst. A portable miniature solid-state heart rate recorder for monitoring daily physical activity. *Biotelemetry* 4:131-140, 1977.

168. Schwane, J.A., and D.E. Cundiff. Relationships among cardiorespiratory fitness, regular physical activity and plasma lipids in young adults. *Metabolism* 28:771–776, 1979.

169. Schweitzer, M.D., F.R. Gearing, and G.A. Perara. Family studies of primary hypertension: their contributions to the understanding of genetic factors. J. Stamler, R. Stamler, and T.N. Pullman (eds.). *The Epidemiology of Hypertension.* New York: Grune and Stratton, 1964, pp. 28–38.

170. Shahar, E., A.R. Folsom, and R. Jackson. Effect of nonresponse on prevalence estimates for a referent population: insights from a population-based cohort study. Arteriosclerosis Risk in Communities (ARIC) Study Investigators. *Annals Epid.* 6:498–506, 1996.

171. Sheps, S.B., and G.D. Evans. Epidemiology of school injuries: a 2-year experience in a municipal health department. *Pediatrics* 79:69–75, 1987.

172. Slemenda, C.W., J.Z. Miller, S.L. Hui, T.K. Reister, and C.C. Johnston, Jr. Role of physical activity in the development of skeletal mass in children. *J. Bone Miner. Res.* 6:1227–1233, 1991.

173. Smith, B.W., W.P. Methrey, and A.W. Sparrow. Serum lipid and lipoprotein profiles in elite age group runners. M.R. Weiss, and D. Gould (eds.). *Sport for Children and Youth (1984 Olympic Scientific Congress Proceedings, Vol. 10.* Champaign, IL: Human Kinetics, 1986, pp. 269–273.

174. Snow-Harter, C., M.L. Bouxsein, B.T. Lewis, D.R. Carter, and R. Marcus. Effects of resistance and endurance exercise on bone mineral status of young women: a randomized exercise intervention trial. *J. Bone Miner. Res.* 7:761–769, 1992.

175. Sorensen, L., S.E. Larsen, and N.D. Rock. The epidemiology of sports injuries in school-aged children. *Scand. J. Med. Sci. Sports.* 6:281–286, 1996.

176. Strazzullo, P., F.P. Cappuccio, M. Trevisan, et al. Leisure time physical activity and blood pressure in schoolchildren. *Am. J. Epidemiol.* 127:726–733, 1988.

177. Stucky-Ropp, R.C., and T.M. DeLorenzo. Determinants of exercise in children. *Prev. Med.* 22:880–889, 1993.

178. Sunnegardh, J., L.E. Bratteby, U. Hagman, G. Samuelson, and S. Sjolin. Physical activity in relation to energy intake and body fat in 8- and 13-year-old children in Sweden. *Acta Paediatr. Scand.* 75:955–963, 1986.

179. Suter, E., and M.R. Hawes. Relationship of physical activity, body fat, diet, and blood lipid profile in youths 10–15 yr. *Med. Sci. Sports Exerc.* 25:748–754, 1993.

180. Taylor W., and T. Baranowski. Physical activity, cardiovascular fitness, and adiposity in children. *Res. Q. Exerc. Sport* 62:157–163, 1991.

181. Tell, G.S., and O.D. Vellar. Physical fitness, physical activity, and cardiovascular disease risk factors in adolescents: the Oslo Youth Study. *Prev. Med.* 17:12–24, 1988.

182. Troiano, R.P., K.M. Flegal, R.J. Kuczmarksi, S.M. Campbell, and C.L. Johnson. Overweight prevalence and trends for children and adolescents. The National Health and Nutrition Examination Surveys, 1963 to 1991. *Arch. Pediatr. Adolesc. Med.* 149:1085–1091, 1995.

183. Turner, J.G., N.L. Gilchrist, E.M. Ayling, A.J. Hassall, E.A. Hooke, and W.A. Sadler. Factors affecting bone mineral density in high school girls. *N.Z. Med. J.* 105:95–96, 1992.

184. Tylavsky, F.A., J.J.B. Anderson, R.V. Talmage, and T.N. Taft. Are calcium intakes and physical activity patterns during adolescence related to radial bone mass of white college-age females? *Osteopor. Int.* 2:232–240, 1992.

185. U.S. Department of Health and Human Services. *Healthy People 2000: National Health Promotion and Disease Prevention Objectives—Full Report, With Commentary.* Washington, DC: U.S. Department of Health and Human Services, Public Health Service, 1991. DHHS Publication No. (PHS)91–50212.

186. U.S. Department of Health and Human Services. *Physical Activity and Health: A Report of the Surgeon General.* Atlanta, GA: U.S. Department of Health and Human Services, Centers for Disease Control and Prevention, National Center for Chronic Disease Prevention and Health Promotion, 1996.

187. Update on the 1987 task force report on high blood pressure in children and adolescents: a working group report from the National High Blood Pressure Education Program. *Pediatrics* 98:649–658, 1996.

188. Valimaki, I., M.L. Hursti, L. Pihlakoski, and J. Viikari. Exercise performance and serum lipids in relation to physical activity. *Int. J. Sports Med.* 1:132–136, 1980.

189. Valimaki, M.J., M. Karkkainen, C. Lamberg-Allardt, et al. Exercise, smoking, and calcium intake during adolescence and early adulthood as determinants of peak bone mass. *B.M.J.* 309:230–235, 1994.

190. VandenBergh, M.F.Q., S.A. DeMan, J.C.M. Witteman, A. Hofman, W.T. Trouerbach, and D.E. Grobbee. Physical activity, calcium intake, and bone mineral content in children in The Netherlands. *J. Epidemiol. Comm. Health* 49:299–304, 1995.

191. Verschuur, R., H.C.G. Kemper, and C.W.M. Besseling. Habitual physical activity and health in 13 and 14-year-old teenagers. J. Ilmarinen and I. Valimaki (eds.). *Children and Sport.* New York: Springer-Verlag, 1984, pp. 155–161.

192. Viikari, J., I. Valimaki, R. Telama, et al. Atherosclerosis precursors in Finnish children: physical activity and plasma lipids in 13 and 12-year-old children. J. Ilmarinen and I. Valimaki (eds.). *Children and Sport.* New York: Springer-Verlag, 1984, pp. 231–240.

193. Voors, A.W., D.W. Harsha, L.S. Webber, B. Radhakrishnamurthy, S.R. Srinivasan, and G.S. Berenson. Clustering of anthropometric parameters, glucose tolerance, and serum lipids in children with high and low β- and pre-β-lipoproteins: Bogalusa Heart Study. *Atherosclerosis* 2:346–355, 1982.

194. Waksberg, J. Sampling methods for random digit dialing. *J. Am. Stat. Assoc.* 73:40–46, 1978.

195. Wanne, O., J. Viikari, and I. Valimaki. Physical performance and serum lipids in 14–16 year old trained, normally active and inactive children. J. Ilmarinen and I. Valimaki (eds.). *Children and Sport.* New York: Springer-Verlag, 1984, pp. 241–246.

196. Watkins, J., and P. Peabody. Sports injuries in children and adolescents treated at a sports injury clinic. *J. Sports Med. Phys. Fitness* 36:43–48, 1996.

197. Webber, L.S., D.S. Freedman, and J.L. Cresanta. Tracking of cardiovascular disease risk factor variables in school aged children. G.S. Berenson (ed.). *Causation of Cardiovascular Risk Factors in Children: Perspectives on Cardiovascular Risk in Early Life.* New York: Raven Press, 1986, pp. 42–64.

198. Webber, L.S., S.K. Osganian, H.A. Feldman, et al. Cardiovascular risk factors among children after a 2½-year intervention: the CATCH Study. *Prev. Med.* 25:432–441, 1996.

199. Welk, G.J., and C.B. Corbin. The validity of the Tritrac-R3D Activity Monitor for the assessment of physical activity in children. *Res. Q. Exerc. Sport* 66(3):202–209, 1995.

200. Welten, D.C., H.C.G. Kemper, G.B. Post, et al. Weight-bearing activity during youth is a more important factor for peak bone mass than calcium intake. *J. Bone Miner. Res.* 9: 1089–1096, 1994.

201. Wolf, A.M., S.L. Gortmaker, L. Cheung, et al. Activity, inactivity, and obesity: racial, ethnic, and age differences among schoolgirls. *Am. J. Public Health* 83:1625–1627, 1993.

202. Young, D., J.L. Hopper, C.A. Nowson, et al. Determinants of bone mass in 10- to 26-year-old females: a twin study. *J. Bone Miner. Res.* 10:558–567, 1995.

203. Zack, P.M., W.R. Harlan, P.E. Leaverton, and J. Cornoni-Huntley. A longitudinal study of body fatness in childhood and adolescence: the National Health Examination Survey. *J. Pediatr.* 95:126–130, 1979.

204. Zakarian, J.M., M.F. Hovell, C.R. Hofstetter, J.F. Sallis, and K.J. Keating. Correlates of vigorous exercise in a predominantly low SES and minority high school population. *Prev. Med.* 23:314–321, 1994.

205. Zavaroni, I., E. Dale'Aglio, E. Bonaora, O. Alpi, M. Passeri, and G. M. Reaven. Evidence that multiple risk factors for coronary artery disease exist in persons with abnormal glucose tolerance. *Am. J. Med.* 83:609–612, 1987.

Index

Page references followed by *t* or *f* indicate tables or figures, respectively.

Abdominal obesity, 70
in elderly, and aerobic
exercise and strength
training, 70–72
Acetylcarnitine, 22–23, 123
Acetyl-CoA
exercise and, 118–119,
299–300, 302
in fatty acid oxidation,
118–119, 122–124
phosphorylation, 124
regulation of, 21
in TCA cycle, 289*f*, 294,
299–300, 302,
307–308
Acetyl-CoA carboxylase
and 5′-amp-activated
protein kinase,
122–129, 124*f*
in fatty acid oxidation
regulation, 120,
122–129
inactivation, 125, 129
exercise intensity and,
127–128
isoforms of, 122
in malonyl-CoA synthesis,
120
in skeletal muscle,
122–123
phosphorylation, 120,
123–124, 124*f*, 125,
127
regulation, 122
in exercise or in
response to muscle
contraction, 125–127,
126*f*–127*f*
in liver, 123
in skeletal muscle,
123–128
Achilles' tendon, force, in
locomotion, 272–273,
273*f*
Acidosis, 239*t*, 291
ACSM. *See* American College
of Sports Medicine
Actin, 173–174, 180
Activity diaries, 344

Activity monitors, 343–344
Activity questionnaires, 344
Adenine nucleotide(s)
interaction with PCr and
glycogen metabolism,
4–6
as regulator of muscle
oxygen consumption
in contraction, 17–18
Adenosine diphosphate
in intense muscle
contraction, 2–4, 6,
9–10, 24
and muscle oxygen
consumption, 16–18,
23
and TCA cycle, 300
Adenosine diphosphate-
ribosylation, 169
Adenosine monophosphate
in ATP synthesis, 4–5
in fatty acid oxidation,
123, 125, 128–129
in glycogenolysis and
glycolysis regulation,
4–6
Adenosine monophosphate
deaminase, 6
activation in exercise, 299
ammonia production in,
292–293
Adenosine triphosphate
breakdown of, 293*f*
in fatty acid oxidation,
122, 124
in genetic translation,
168–169, 177, 180
hydrolysis, products of, 4
in protein degradation,
221–223, 229,
231–233, 238
repeated bouts of exercise
and, 13–16
store in skeletal muscle, 1
synthesis, in exercise,
1–30, 299–300
aerobic, 1, 6, 15–24
anaerobic, 1–24, 3*f*
in type I and type II

muscle fibers, 8–13,
11*f*
Adipose tissue, 191
lipoprotein lipase in, 191,
194–195, 210
and triglyceride
clearance, 207–210,
209*t*
Adiposity
in children and
adolescents, physical
activity and, 365–373,
368*t*–371*t*
development of, 365
Adolescent(s)
physical activity
epidemiology applied
to, 341–403
physical activity of
age and, 351–352
and blood pressure,
353–354, 359–364,
361*t*–363*t*
and bone mineral
density, 373–379,
375*t*–377*t*
determinants of, 381,
385–388, 386*t*–387*t*
geographic region and,
351–352
household income and,
351–352
and insulin, 364–365,
366*t*
interventions to
promote, 388–392,
390*t*–391*t*
measurement of,
343–345
and obesity and
adiposity, 365–373,
368*t*–371*t*
patterns in, 347–349,
351–352
race and, 351–352, 385
seasonal differences in,
351–352
and serum lipids,
354–359, 356*t*–358*t*

405

Adolescent(s) (*continued*)
  sex differences and,
    351–352, 355,
    360–367, 374–380,
    385–386, 389–392
  socioeconomic status
    and, 385
  surveillance, in United
    States, 345–352, 346*t*
  and unintentional
    injury, 379–381
  self-concept of, 149–150
  physical competence
    and, 154–155
Adolescent idiopathic
    scoliosis, 139
β-Adrenergic agonists, 239*t*
α-Adrenoreceptor, 175
Adulthood, self-concept in,
    150
Aerobic exercise
  in children and
    adolescents
    and blood pressure, 364
    interventions to
      promote, 389–392,
      391*t*
    and serum lipids,
      357*t*–358*t*, 359
  in elderly, 61–89
    and abdominal obesity,
      70–72
    and bone mineral
      density, 74–75
    and cardiovascular
      disease risk factors,
      62–73
    and cardiovascular
      fitness level, 62–64
    and fall prevention,
      75–76
    and hypertension,
      68–69
    and left ventricular
      hypertrophy, 69–70
    and lipoprotein-lipid
      profiles, 64–66
    and resting metabolic
      rate, 72–73
Aerobic intensity, 343, 347,
    348*t*
Aerobic metabolism,
    interaction with
    anaerobic metabolism
  in intense muscle
    contraction, 1–30
  repeated bouts of muscle
    contraction as model
    for studying, 13–16

Aging. *See also* Elderly
  and abdominal obesity, 70
  cardiovascular disease
    and, 61–62
  and cardiovascular fitness,
    62
  and health care costs, 61
  musculoskeletal health
    and, 61–62, 73–79
Alanine
  concentration gradient
    between muscle and
    blood, 291
  glucose and, 290*f*,
    294–295, 302
  muscle metabolism,
    288–296, 289*f*, 308
    in exercise, 299–302,
      306
    release, 289
      branched chain amino
        acids and, 288
      in exercise, 299, 302
      protein meal and, 296
    synthesis, 288, 290, 290*f*,
      308
      carbon and nitrogen
        sources for, 290*f*, 292,
        294–295, 308
    transport, 291
Alanine aminotransferase
    activity
  anaplerotic capacity, 306
  in exercise, 300–303, 301*f*,
    305–306, 308–309
  and TCA cycle, 300–303,
    301*f*, 305–306,
    308–309
Alcohol consumption, and
    hypertension, 360
American College of Sports
    Medicine, 326–327,
    331–333, 335–336
  certification, 330, 333
  D.B. Dill Lecture, 315,
    334
  membership categories,
    330
American Physiological
    Society, 324–326,
    331, 333, 335–336
Amino acid(s)
  aromatic, 291
  branched chain. *See*
    Branched chain
    amino acid(s)
  deamination, 292–293
    as alternative
      anaplerotic reaction,
      307–309
  forms of, 287

  free, 287
  in genetic translation,
    165–166, 168, 170,
    176
  muscle metabolism,
    287–314, 290*f*
    and blood glucose
      concentration,
      294–295, 302
    in exercise, 287–288,
      299–309
    protein meal and,
      295–296
    at rest, 287–298, 308
    schematic presentation
      of, 289*f*
    and TCA cycle,
      287–288, 289*f*, 294,
      299–309
  protein, 287
  in protein degradation,
    221, 225, 239*t*, 287
  in protein synthesis, 171,
    287
  transporters, 291–292
    System A (alanine), 291
    System ASC (alanine,
      serine and cysteine),
      291
    System L (leucine), 291
    System N (nitrogen)
      and N^m, 291
    System X⁻ (exchange),
      291–292
Amino acid biosynthesis,
    176
Aminoacyl-tRNA, 168–169,
    171
Aminolevulinic acid
    dehydratase, 235
Aminotransferase
    reaction(s), 292
  alanine, 300–303, 301*f*,
    305–306, 308–309
  branched chain amino
    acid, 288, 303–306
  in exercise, 300–306, 301*f*,
    308–309
  and TCA cycle, 300–306,
    301*f*, 308–309
Ammonia
  in alanine synthesis, 308
  from amino acid
    deamination, 307
  in ATP synthesis, 4
  branch amino acid
    supplementation and,
    305
  creatine supplementation
    and, 7–8

exercise and, 4, 7–8, 299, 301, 305, 307
and fatigue, 305
in glutamine synthesis, 288, 292–293, 308
and loss of motor coordination, 305
production, 292–293, 293*f*
transport, 297–298, 298*f*
urinary, 296
AMP. *See* Adenosine monophosphate
5′Amp-activated protein kinase (AMPK)
and acetyl-CoA carboxylase, 122–129, 124*f*
activation
in exercise, 125, 126*f*, 129
exercise intensity and, 127–128
in fatty acid oxidation regulation, 122–129
AMPK. *See* 5′amp-activated protein kinase (AMPK)
Amrinone, for sepsis, 176
Amsterdam Growth and Health Longitudinal Study, 374–378
β-Amyloid protein, 235
Anaerobic metabolism, interaction with aerobic metabolism
in intense muscle contraction, 1–30
repeated bouts of muscle contraction as model for studying, 13–16
Ankle(s)
energy stored and returned by, 274–275
in jogging, 271
muscle-tendon force at, 272
net muscle moments at, 268–271, 270*f*
in running, 269, 270*f*, 272, 274–275
in walking, 268
Ankle plantar flexion velocity, of elderly, improving, 76
Antigen presentation, 234
Antizyme, 233
Apolipoprotein, in children and adolescents, physical activity and, 355–359

Aponeurosis, 276
APS. *See* American Physiological Society
Aromatic amino acids, 291
Arteriosclerosis, 364
Asparagine, 288, 289*f*, 291, 307–308
Aspartate, 288, 289*f*, 291–292, 293*f*, 307–308
Astrand, P.O., 326
Atherogenesis, 194
Atherosclerosis, 191, 194
Atherothrombogenic syndrome, 70
Athletes, self-concept of, coaches and, 147–148
ATP. *See* Adenosine triphosphate
Atrophy
muscle
growth hormone and, 43
microgravity and, 242
myonuclei and satellite cells in, 50–51
protein degradation and, 241–242
and protein synthesis, 179–180
protein metabolism and, 219–220
Autocrine/paracrine function, of insulin-like growth factor-I, 34*f*, 34–35, 39*f*
and muscle adaptation, 44–46, 52*f*
Autophagy, lysosomal, 240
Avidin, 122

Bainbridge, F.A., 319
Balance, of elderly, improving, 76
Basal metabolic rate, 344
Baseball injury, 379
Baseline exercise, 355–359
Basic-fibroblast growth factor, 40
Basketball injury, 379–380
BCAA. *See* Branched chain amino acid(s)
Behavioral Risk Factor Surveillance System, 345, 346*t*, 349
bFGF. *See* Basic-fibroblast growth factor
Bicarbonate, in fatty acid oxidation, 122

Bicycle accidents, 379
Big Fish, Little Pond phenomenon, and self-concept, 148
Biomechanics of walking and running, 253–285
Biotin, 122
Blood fat-clearing factor, 191–192
Blood flow, 191
altered tissue due to physical activity, and triglyceride clearance, 210
and muscle ischemia, 100
and muscle oxygen consumption, 18–19
Blood pressure
of children and adolescents, physical activity and, 353–354, 359–364, 361*t*–363*t*
of elderly, 68
and aerobic exercise and strength training, 68–69
obesity and, 365
BMD. *See* Bone mineral density
Bock, A.V., 319, 326–327
Body Cathexis Scale, 141, 145
Body Esteem Scale, 142*t*, 145
Body fat
aerobic exercise and, 70–72
of children and adolescents, physical activity and, 353, 367
Body image, and self-concept, 137, 141, 145
Body weight, and self-concept, 149
Bohr effect, 16
Bone mineral density
in children and adolescents, physical activity and, 373–379, 375*t*–377*t*
in elderly, aerobic exercise and strength training and, 74–75
and hip fractures, 73–75
muscular strength and, 74–75
and osteoporosis, 73, 373

Booth, F.W., 329
Bouncing gait, 261, 265–267, 272, 274–275, 278
Branched chain amino acid(s), 239*t*
  in alanine synthesis, 292
  in glutamine synthesis, 292, 307
  in muscle, 288, 290
  protein meal and, 295–296
  release of alanine and glutamine and, 288
  supplementation, and performance, 304–305
  and TCA cycle, 303–307
  transport, 291
Branched chain amino acid α-keto acid dehydrogenase, 303–305
Branched chain aminotransferase activity, 288
  carbon drain of, and fatigue, 303–306
  and TCA cycle, 303–306
Branched chain α-keto acid, 288
BRFSS. *See* Behavioral Risk Factor Surveillance System
Bromo-deoxyuridine, 48, 49*f*
Brooks, G.A., 327–328
Buckle transducers, 272–273
Burns
  and amino acid metabolism, 291
  and protein degradation, 239*t*
Buskirk, Elsworth R., 328, 332*f*, 335

Calcium
  activation of muscle contraction by, 4
  in protein degradation, 222
  as regulator of muscle oxygen consumption in contraction, 16–17
  second-messenger signal, 170
  and TCA cycle, 300
Calcium-calmodulin dependent kinase, 179

Calcium-dependent neutral protease, 222
Calmodulin-dependent protein kinase III, 169
Caloric expenditure, 342–344, 347, 348*t*
Calpain system, of protein degradation, 222, 236
Calpastatin, 222
cAMP-dependent protein kinase, 50, 123
Cancer, 348*t*, 365
Carbohydrate(s)
  co-ingestion with branch amino acids, 305
  orally ingested, and TCA cycle, 306
  oxidation, 18, 117
Carbon, for alanine and glutamine synthesis, 290*f*, 292, 294
CARDIA, 365
Cardiac function, enhanced, 348*t*
Cardiac glycoside, 176
Cardiac muscle
  diabetes and, 175–176
  hypertrophy, 175
    thyroxine-induced, 178–179
  lipoprotein lipase and, 194, 196–197
  protein synthesis in, 172*t*
    modulation, 175, 177, 180
    translation and gene expression in, 182
    control of, 175, 177–179
    control points and mechanisms, 172*t*–173*t*
    elongation phase, 173*t*, 179
    initiation phase, 172*t*
    termination phase, 173*t*
Cardiovascular disease, 70, 354, 359, 364
  aging and, 61–62
  risk factors
    in elderly, aerobic exercise and strength training and, 62–73
    intervention in adolescence, 392
Cardiovascular fitness, in elderly, aerobic exercise and strength training and, 62–64

Carnitine, 21, 119, 123
Carnitine acetyltransferase reaction, 21
Carnitine palmitoyl-transferase
  in fatty acid oxidation, 118–122, 128–129
  inhibition, 118, 120–122
  liver, 120
  muscle, 120–122
Case-control studies, 352–353
Casein kinase II, 169, 176
CATCH. *See* Child and Adolescent Trial for Cardiovascular Health
Catecholamines, and lipoprotein lipase, 200, 206
Cathexis, 141
Cell phosphorylation state, 16–18, 20
Cellular redox state, 16
Center of mass mechanics, 254–267
  gait transitions, 261–263, 277
  ground reaction force
    for running, 254, 256*f*, 265
    for walking, 254, 255*f*, 264
  leg compression and, 264
  mechanical energy fluctuations, 254–261, 263–264
  similarities in diverse species, 253
Centers for Disease Control and Prevention, 345
Centripetal force, and gait transitions, 262
Chapman, C.B., 315, 323–324, 333–334
Child and Adolescent Trial for Cardiovascular Health
  blood pressure in, 363*t*, 364
  obesity in, 371*t*, 373
  physical activity intervention in, 389, 390*t*
  serum lipids in, 358*t*, 359
Children
  physical activity epidemiology applied to, 341–403

physical activity of
age and, 351–352
and blood pressure,
353–354, 359–364,
361*t*–363*t*
and bone mineral
density, 373–379,
375*t*–377*t*
determinants of,
381–384, 383*t*–384*t*
geographic region and,
351–352
household income and,
351–352
and insulin, 364–365,
366*t*
interventions to
promote, 388–392,
390*t*–391*t*
measurement of,
343–345
and obesity and
adiposity, 365–373,
368*t*–371*t*
parental modeling and,
382, 383*t*–384*t*
patterns in, 347–349,
351–352
race and, 351–352, 382,
383*t*
seasonal differences in,
351–352, 382, 384*t*
and serum lipids,
354–359, 356*t*–358*t*
sex differences and,
351–352, 355,
360–367, 374–380,
382, 389–392
surveillance, in United
States, 345–352, 346*t*
and unintentional
injury, 379–381
self-appraisals of, 147
self-concept of
body weight and, 149
development of,
147–148
exercise/sports and,
133, 147–149,
153–155
gender effects, 149–150
internal standards and,
149
measuring, 142*t*,
144–146
in preadolescence, 149
social comparisons and,
148

Cholesterol
in children and
adolescents, physical
activity and, 355–359,
356*t*–358*t*
in elderly, aerobic
exercise and strength
training and, 64–66
Chylomicronemia, 192
Citrate, in fatty acid
oxidation, 120,
122–125, 124*f*, 127*f*
Citrate lyase, 123
Citrate synthase reaction,
123
Citrate synthesis, 120
Citric acid cycle, and fatty
acid oxidation, 119
c-Jun, 225
CK reaction. *See* Creatine
kinase reaction
Class of 1989 study,
389–392, 391*t*
Clinical exercise
physiologists, 330,
333, 335
Coaches, and athletes' self-
concept, 147
Coenzyme-A derivatives of
fatty acids, 118
Competence
versus self-acceptance,
156*t*, 156–157
and self-concept/self-
esteem, 134, 144, 148,
154–155
Conant, J.B., 315
Conant Report (1963), 328
Congestive heart failure, 69
Conjugating enzymes,
223–225, 224*f*, 241
Conjugation, in protein
degradation,
223–225, 224*f*
Constant work rate exercise,
92
Contraceptives, oral, and
serum lipids, 357*t*,
359
Contraction(s), muscle
and acetyl-CoA
carboxylase
regulation, 125–127,
126*f*–127*f*
intense, interaction
between aerobic and
anaerobic metabolism
in, 1–30

isokinetic, fatigue and,
109–110
isometric, 11*f*, 274
oxygen consumption in,
regulators of, 16–20
protein and, 287
repeated bouts of, as
model for studying
interaction of
anaerobic and
aerobic metabolism,
13–16
voluntary static, and
fatigue
intermittent, 92, 93*f*
maximal, 92–110
sustained, 92
Coronary Artery Risk
Development in
Young Adults, 365
Coronary heart disease, 343,
348*t*, 365
Corticosteroid treatment,
and amino acid
metabolism, 291
Costill, David L., 327–328,
332*f*
CPT. *See* Carnitine
palmitoyl-transferase
Creatine, 3, 23
supplementation, and
exercise metabolism,
6–10, 8*f*–9*f*, 24
and type I muscle
fibers, 8
and type II muscle
fibers, 8
Creatine kinase, 23
Creatine kinase reaction,
2–3, 6, 8–9
Cross-bridges, 16, 19
Cross-sectional studies,
352–353
Cycle ergometry, 99–100,
110
for assessment of
hypobaric hypoxia,
109
and bone mineral density,
74
for cardiovascular fitness
assessment, 63–64
for dynamic exercise
assessment, 91
for exercise performance
assessment, 91–94,
104
test-retest variation in, 106

Cyclin-dependent kinases, 49
Cysteine, 291
Cytochrome *c* protein, 173–174, 181

Deadly quartet, 70
Denervation, 239*t*
Deoxyribonucleic aid, muscle, insulin-like growth factor-I and, 46, 48
Depression, in adolescence, 155
Development, cell, 32
Diabetes, 70, 343, 348*t*, 365
  in children, physical activity and, 365
  and lipoprotein lipase, 198
  protein synthesis and gene translation and, 175–179
Diaries, activity, 344
Diet
  and lipoprotein lipase, 196–198, 201
  and weight loss, 373
Differentiation, cell
  definition, 32
  insulin-like growth factor-I and, 40–41, 50, 51*f*
  of satellite cells, 50
Dihydrolipoyl dehydrogenase, 21
Dihydrolipoyl transacetylase, 21
Dill, David B., 319–320, 320*f*–321*f*, 324, 326–327, 334–335
D.B. Dill Lecture, 315, 334
Diphtheria toxin, 169
Disability, physical, 343, 348*t*
Discipline, academic, 316
Double support, in walking, 254
Doubly-labeled water technique, 343
Drosophila development, 241
Duty cycle, 13
Dynamic exercise
  electromyographic activity in, 101–102
  knee extension. *See* Knee extension exercise, dynamic
  muscle fatigue in, 91–116
  definitions, 92–93

point of exhaustion, 102–104
  power failure in, 110
Dynamic optimization, 276

Ecologic studies, 352–353
Edgerton, V. Reggie, 332*f*
Elderly
  aerobic exercise and strength training for, 61–89
  and abdominal obesity, 70–72
  and bone mineral density, 74–75
  and cardiovascular disease risk factors, 62–73
  and cardiovascular fitness level, 62–64
  and fall prevention, 75–76
  and glucose intolerance and insulin resistance, 66–68
  and hypertension, 68–69
  and left ventricular hypertrophy, 69–70
  and lipoprotein-lipid profiles, 64–66
  and muscle quality, 76–77
  and resting metabolic rate, 72–73
  cardiovascular disease in, 61–62
  demographics, 61
  flexibility in, 77–79
  growth hormone for, 41–42
  insulin-like growth factor-I for, 41–42
  musculoskeletal health of, 61–62, 73–79
  optimizing health in, 61–89
  physical self-concept of, 155
Electrical stimulation, in investigation of muscle metabolism and fatigue, 2, 3*f*, 11*f*, 11–12, 12*f*
Electromyographic activity
  in dynamic exercise, 101–102
  and fatigue, 92, 100–102

integrated, and MVCs, 101, 102*f*
  and muscle force development, 100–101
  in static contraction, 101
Electron transport chain, 16, 19
Elongation factors, in genetic translation, 167*f*, 169, 179, 181
Elongation of polypeptides, 168–170
EMG. *See* Electromyographic activity
Endoproteases, 221
Endurance time, assessment of, 92, 93*f*
Endurance training, and knee extension exercise, 105*f*, 106
Energy utilization, 348*t*
Epidemiology
  definition, 342
  physical activity. *See* Physical activity epidemiology
Epinephrine, 200
Estimation scale, and physical self-concept, 143–144
Estrogen, and lipoprotein lipase, 200–201
Euglycemia, 198–199, 201
Euphoria effects, and self-concept study, 139–140
Excitation, muscle
  diminished, and fatigue, 101–102
  and electromyographic activity, 100
Excitation-contraction coupling
  force production, inhibition of, 17
  inhibition of, 6, 19
Exercise. *See also* Aerobic exercise; Physical activity; Strength training
  aerobic and anaerobic metabolism in, 1–30
  amino acid metabolism in, 287–288, 299–309
  baseline, 355–359
  creatine supplementation and, 6–10, 8*f*

definition, 342
dynamic. *See* Dynamic
    exercise
for elderly, 61–89
fatty acid oxidation and,
    117–119, 121–122,
    125–129
lipoprotein lipase and,
    202–210
maximal, metabolic
    responses to, 2–16
performance
    branched amino acid
        supplementation and,
        304–305
    conventional
        approaches to
        studying, 91–100
    and protein metabolism,
        171–175, 308
    and self-concept/self-
        esteem, 133–134,
        147–149
    assessment, 136–147
    in hierarchical model,
        135*f*, 135–136
    self-enhancement and,
        152–154
    skill development and,
        151–152
self-efficacy, 381, 385,
    386*t*–387*t*, 388–389
and TCA cycle, 287–288,
    299–309
testing and prescription,
    330
and translation and gene
    expression, 171–175,
    202
and triglycerides, 65–66,
    204–210, 355,
    356*t*–358*f*
and weight loss, 373
Exercise and Self-Esteem
    Model, 135*f*,
    135–136, 152–153,
    156–157
Exercise leaders, 330
Exercise physiologists
    certification of, 330, 333
    clinical, 330, 333, 335
    definitions of, 316, 330
    preparation of, 328–330
Exercise physiology
    as academic discipline,
        316–317, 316*f*–317*f*
    emergence of, 317–319,
        325–326, 336

individuals contributing
    to, 320*f*–321*f*,
    320–322
education, 328–329, 336
history of, 317–319,
    324–327
Harvard Fatigue
    Laboratory and,
    315–316, 318–330,
    333–337
laboratory research in,
    318–319, 329, 334,
    336–337
molecular biology in,
    329–330, 334, 336
as profession, 317, 317*f*,
    330–333
subject matter investigated
    (1954–1994), 327*t*,
    327–328
subject matter
    recommended for
    further investigation
    (1978), 332–333, 333*t*
textbooks, 326–327
Exercise testing, 330
Exertion, perceived, ratings
    of, 92
Exhaustion, 92
    definition, 93
    in dynamic knee
        extension fatigue
        model, 97*f*–98*f*, 99,
        103–104
    versus muscle fatigue,
        92–93
    MVC force and, 93, 93*f*,
        97*f*
    point of
        in dynamic exercise,
            102–104
        in static exercise, 103
Exoproteases, 221
Experimental studies, in
    physical activity
    epidemiology,
    352–354
EXSEM. *See* Exercise and
    Self-Esteem Model
External free tendon, 276

FADH2, 119
Falls, preventing, aerobic
    exercise and strength
    training and, 75–76
Fasting. *See* Feeding and
    fasting

Fast-twitch muscle
    protein synthesis in,
        175–176, 179–180
    triglycerides in, 207
Fat. *See* Body fat
Fat free mass, aging and, 72
    aerobic exercise and
        strength training and,
        72–73
Fatigue, muscle
    amino acid metabolism
        and, 287–288,
        303–306, 309
    ATP and, 6, 14, 110
    branched chain amino
        acid supplementation
        and, 304–305
    conventional approaches
        to studying, 91–100
    definitions, 92–93
    and diminished muscle
        excitation, 101–102
    in dynamic exercise,
        91–116
    dynamic knee extension
        model of, 94–110,
        97*f*–98*f*
    in exercise intervention
        assessment, 104–107,
        105*f*
    in hypobaric hypoxia
        assessment, 104, 105*f*,
        107–109
    performance measures
        in, 104–106
    test-retest variation in,
        106–107, 107*f*
    electrical stimulation
        study of, 2
    and electromyographic
        activity, 92, 100–102
    versus exhaustion, 92–93
    in intermittent voluntary
        static contractions, 92
    schematic model for
        measuring, 93*f*
    ischemia and, 100
    in isokinetic contractions,
        109–110
    maximal voluntary static
        contraction force
        and, 92–110, 93*f*
    myoelectric manifestations
        of, 100–102
    point of exhaustion and,
        102–104
    in sustained voluntary
        static contractions, 92
    TCA cycle and, 287–288,
        303–306, 309

Fatty acid(s)
  availability of, 118
  lipoprotein lipase and,
      191, 194, 201, 206,
      210
  mobilization, 118*f*
      limit in, 305
  synthesis, 119–120, 123,
      207
  transport, 118–119, 191,
      194
  from triglycerides, 117,
      118*f*
Fatty acid oxidation,
      117–132, 118*f*, 302,
      309
  acetyl-CoA carboxylase
      and, 120, 122–129
  adenosine
      monophosphate and,
      123, 125, 128–129
  adenosine triphosphate
      and, 122, 124
  5′amp-activated protein
      kinase (AMPK) and,
      122–129
  carnitine palmitoyl-
      transferase system in,
      118–122, 128–129
  citrate and, 120, 122–125,
      124*f*, 127*f*
  in exercise, 117–119,
      121–122, 125–129
      trained versus non-
      trained subjects, 117
  in liver, 119–120, 123
  malonyl-CoA and,
      118–129
  possible rate-limiting sites
      of, 118–119
  rate at rest, 117
  regulation, 118–129
  sequence of events, 128*f*,
      128–129
  in skeletal muscle,
      117–129
      in exercise or fasting,
      121–122
Fatty acyl carnitine, 119
Fatty acyl-CoA, 118–119, 122
Faulkner, John A., 332*f*
Feeding and fasting
  and lipoprotein lipase,
      196–197
  and protein degradation,
      239*t*, 239–240
Femoral neck, bone mineral
      density in, 75,
      374–378, 376*t*

Femur, bone mineral
      density in, 376*t*
Fenn effect, 110
Ferritin protein expression,
      181
Fibroblast growth factor(s),
      48–49
Fibroblast growth factor type
      1 receptor, 50
Finger, diaphyses of, bone
      mineral density in,
      374
Fitness, physical, 342
Fitz, George W., 318
Flexibility, 77–79, 343, 347,
      348*t*
Flint, A., 319
Flint, A., Jr., 319, 324
Football injury, 379
Force transducers, 272–273
Forearm, bone mineral
      density in, 374–378,
      375*t*
Forward dynamic
      optimization, 276
Forward dynamic
      simulations, of
      muscle-tendon
      mechanics, 276–277
Fractures, 73–75
Framingham Children's
      Study, 367, 384*t*
Freud, Sigmund, 141
Froude number, 262
Fumarate, 300

Gait
  bouncing, 261, 265–267,
      272, 274–275, 278
  of elderly, improving, 76
Gait transitions, 261–263
  centripetal force/
      gravitational force
      ratio and, 262
  equine model of, 262, 277
  leg length and, 262
  metabolic energy costs
      and, 261–262
  rapid, 262–263
  speed and, 261–263, 277
Gall bladder disease, 365
GDP. *See* Guanosine 5′-
      diphosphate
Gene expression, in muscle,
      translational control
      of, 165–190
George Williams College,
      318
γ-Interferon, 234, 240–241
Glucagon, 123, 240

Glucocorticoids, and protein
      metabolism, 239*t*,
      239–240
Gluconeogenesis, 221, 290*f*,
      294–295, 302, 306
Glucose
  in amino acid metabolism,
      289*f*–290*f*, 294–295,
      302
  blood concentration,
      maintaining,
      294–295, 302
  fatty acid synthesis from,
      119–120, 123
  and lipoprotein lipase,
      198–199
  and malonyl-CoA,
      122–123
  and protein degradation,
      239*t*, 240
  in TCA cycle, 306
Glucose tolerance
  in children and
      adolescents, physical
      activity and, 364–365
  in elderly, aerobic
      exercise and strength
      training and, 66–68
Glucose-alanine cycle, 290*f*,
      294–295, 302
Glucose-1-phosphate, 4
Glucose-6-phosphate, 4
GLUT4, exercise and, 205
GLUT-4 transporter, 67
Glutamate
  in aminotransferase
      reactions, 292
  deamination, and TCA
      cycle, 307
  formation, 288
  and glutamine, 297–298,
      298*f*
  muscle metabolism, 288,
      289*f*, 290–292,
      295–298, 308
      in exercise, 299,
      301–302, 306
  protein meal and,
      295–296
  in splanchnic area, 295,
      297–298, 298*f*
  transport, 291–292
Glutamate dehydrogenase,
      301, 307
  ammonia production in,
      292–293
Glutaminase, 297
Glutamine
  concentration gradient
      between muscle and
      blood, 294

and gluconeogenesis, 290*f*, 294
muscle metabolism, 288–297, 289*f*, 308
physiological significance of, 296–297
release, 289, 291
  branched chain amino acids and, 288
  function of, 296–297
  protein meal and, 296
synthesis, 288, 290, 290*f*, 296
  as alternative anaplerotic reaction, 307–309
  ammonia for, 292–293
  carbon and nitrogen sources for, 290*f*, 292–294
  function of, 296–297
  rate in muscle, 293, 296
transport, 291
Glutamine synthase, 288
Glutamine-glutamate cycle, 297–298, 298*f*
Glycine, 291
Glycogen
in amino acid metabolism, 289*f*–290*f*, 294–295, 308
in ATP synthesis, 1–2, 4–6
in high intensity exercise, 305–306
interaction with adenine nucleotide and PCr, 4–6
in McArdle's disease, 305–308
repeated bouts of exercise and, 13
Glycogen depletion, in muscle, 287–288, 299, 302–305, 307–309
Glycogen phosphorylase, 4–6
deficiency, 305
Glycogenolysis
and ATP synthesis, 4–6, 11–13, 12*f*, 17, 19, 21, 24
definition, 4
in exercise, 4–6, 17, 21, 24
  in type I and type II muscle fibers, 11–13, 12*f*
inhibition of, 19
stimulators of, 4

Glycolysis, 21
in amino acid metabolism, 294, 301–302, 305–306
in ATP synthesis, 2, 3*f*, 4–6, 17
in exercise, 2, 3*f*, 4–6, 17, 301–302, 305–306
hepatic, 120
interaction with muscle oxygen consumption, 16
stimulation, 4, 19
Glycolytic enzymes, 300
Gollnick, Philip D., 328, 332*f*, 335
Gravitational force, 348*t*
Gravitational potential energy, 254–261, 259*f*–260*f*, 263, 278
Gravity, and gait transitions, 262
Ground reaction force
for running, 254, 256*f*, 265
for walking, 254, 255*f*, 264
Growth hormone
and insulin-like growth factor-I, 33–34, 34*f*, 34–35
and lipoprotein lipase, 201
treatment
  in animal models, 42–44
  in humans, 41–42
GTP. *See* Guanosine 5'-triphosphate
Guanosine 5'-diphosphate, 36
  in genetic translation, 167*f*, 168–170
Guanosine 5'-triphosphate, 36
  in genetic translation, 166, 167*f*, 168–170
Gut, glutamine-glutamate cycle in, 297
Gymnastics injury, 379

Handball injury, 379
Harter, Susan, 144
Harvard Fatigue Laboratory
closing of, 315
and establishment of new laboratories, 323–324, 335–336
factors in, 315

and transition to contemporary exercise physiology, 325–330
establishment of, 318
exercise physiology publications of, 322–323
individuals associated with, 320*f*–321*f*, 320–322
knowledge acquisition and integration at, 319–324
legacy of, 333–335, 337
methodology of, 322
name change, 315–316
preparation of future investigators, 324–325, 328, 336
purpose of, 319, 334–335
teaching activities of, 318–319, 336
Harvard University, 318, 324
Hawthorne effect, 139
HDL. *See* High-density lipoprotein
Head injury, 379
Health care costs, aging and, 61
Health/fitness directors, 330
Health/fitness instructors, 330
Heart. *See also* Cardiac muscle
pressure overload of, 175
Heart disease. *See also* Cardiovascular disease
coronary, 343, 348*t*, 365
Heart rate monitors, 343–344
Heat-shock proteins, 177, 180, 225, 235
Heme, 177
biosynthesis, 235
Henderson, L.J., 315, 320, 324, 334
Heparin, and lipoprotein lipase, 195, 197
Hexokinase II, 205
High-density lipoprotein
in children and adolescents, physical activity and, 355–359, 356*t*–358*t*
in elderly, aerobic exercise and strength training and, 64–66
obesity and, 365

Hind-limb suspension, 43, 50–51, 239*t*
Hip(s)
  bone mineral density of
    in children and adolescents, 374
    in postmenopausal women, 73–74
  muscle-tendon force at, 272
  net muscle moments at, 268–269, 270*f*
    in running, 269, 270*f*
    in walking, 268
Hip fracture(s)
  bone mineral density and, 73–75
  costs associated with, 73
  and functioning loss, 73
  risk
    for postmenopausal women, 73–75
    reducing, through exercise intervention, 74–75
Histidine, 291
Holloszy, John O., 332*f*, 335
Hormones. *See* Growth hormone; Thyroid hormone(s)
Horseback riding injury, 379
Horvath, Steven M., 320*f*–321*f*, 324, 328, 334–335
Hyperinsulinemia, 199, 201
Hypertension
  in children and adolescents, 359–360
    physical activity and, 354, 360–364, 362*t*
  development of, 360
  in elderly, 70
    aerobic exercise and strength training and, 68–69
  etiology of, 360
  obesity and, 365
  prevalence of, 359–360
  race and, 360
Hyperthyroidism, 175, 200
Hypertriglyceridemia, 192, 194, 199
Hypertrophy, cardiac, 175
  left ventricular, in elderly, 69–70
  thyroxine-induced, 178–179
Hypertrophy, skeletal muscle

insulin-like growth factor-I and, 33, 40, 44–46, 46*f*, 50, 51*f*–52*f*
  in animal models, 42–43
  myogenic aspects of, 47–53, 49*f*
  stimulated, 45–46
Hypobaric hypoxia, 104, 105*f*, 107–109
Hypothyroidism, 200
Hypoxanthine, creatine supplementation and, 7–8
Hypoxia, 19, 21–22. *See also* Hypobaric hypoxia

Ice hockey injury, 379
IGFBPs. *See* Insulin-like growth factor-I, binding proteins
IGF-I. *See* Insulin-like growth factor-I
IGF-II. *See* Insulin-like growth factor-II
IGFR1. *See* Insulin-like growth factor-I, receptors
Immortal cell lines, 32
IMP. *See* Inosine monophosphate
Indiana University, 315, 335
Infection, and protein degradation, 239*t*
Initiation factors, in genetic translation, 166–168, 167*f*, 175–178, 181
Injury, unintentional. *See also* Sports injury
  in children and adolescents, 379–381
Inosine monophosphate
  AMP deaminated to, 292
  in ATP synthesis, 4–5
  exercise and, 4–6, 299
  in glycogenolysis and glycolysis regulation, 4–6
  reamination, 292–293
Insulin
  and acetyl-CoA carboxylase, 123
  in children and adolescents, physical activity and, 364–365, 366*t*
  and genetic translation, 168, 170, 175, 177–178

and lipoprotein lipase, 197–200, 199*t*, 201, 206
and malonyl-CoA, 122–123
and protein degradation, 239*t*, 239–240
and protein synthesis, 168, 174–175, 178–179, 239
Insulin receptor, 35–37
Insulin receptor substrate, 36
Insulin resistance
  in children and adolescents, physical activity and, 364–365
  in elderly, 70
    aerobic exercise and strength training and, 66–68
Insulin resistance syndrome, 70
Insulin-like growth factor-I
  anabolic effects of, 40
  autocrine/paracrine function of, 34*f*, 34–35, 39*f*
  and muscle adaptation, 44–46, 52*f*
  binding proteins, 37–40, 39*f*
  circulating, increased
    in animal models, 42–44
    in humans, 41–42
  as component of GH control axis, 33–34, 34*f*
  expression, 34–35
  gene, structure of, 35
  and genetic translation, 178
  and muscle development, 33–34, 40–41
  and muscle hypertrophy, 33, 40, 42–46, 46*f*, 50, 51*f*–52*f*
  and muscle regeneration, 44–45
  receptors, 35–37
    knockout experiments, 35
    ligand interactions, 36–37
    structure, 35–36
  and satellite cells, 48–50, 51*f*
  signaling system, 35–40

components of, 39*f*
in skeletal muscle
adaptation, 31–60
somatomedin hypothesis
of, 33–34, 34*f*
system, components of,
34–40
systemic, and muscle,
41–44
thyroid hormones and,
51–53
tissue-specific regulation
of, 34–35, 37
Insulin-like growth factor-II,
38
receptors, 35–36
Interleukin-1 antagonist, for
sepsis, 176
Inverse dynamics, in muscle-
tendon mechanics,
272, 277–278
Inverse optimization, in
muscle-tendon force
measurement, 272
Inverted pendulum model,
of walking, 257*f*,
258–264, 278
Iron metabolism, 181
Iron responsive elements,
181
Ischemia, muscle, 100
Isocitrate, 300
Isocitrate dehydrogenase,
300
Isokinetic contraction(s),
fatigue and, 109–110
Isoleucine, 288, 289*f*, 303,
307–308
Isometric contractions, 11*f*,
274
Isopeptidase activity, in
protein degradation,
232–233
Isoproterenol, 200

Jogging, joint power and
work in, 271
Johns Hopkins University,
324–325
Johnson, Robert E.,
320*f*–321*f*, 334
Johnson, W.R., 326
Joint(s)
angular velocity, 269–271
dynamics, in locomotion,
267–271
kinematics
in calculating muscle-
tendon length
changes, 274

of elderly, improving,
76
net muscle moments at,
267–272, 270*f*
power and work, 269–271,
270*f*
Journal of Applied Physiology,
326, 331, 336

Karpovich, Peter V., 318,
327
Ketogenesis, 120, 123
α-Ketoglutarate, 288, 289*f*,
299–300, 302–303,
304*f*, 307
α-Ketoglutarate
dehydrogenase, 300
Keys, Ancel, 315, 323, 325,
334–336
Kidneys, gluconeogenesis in,
295
Kinematics
joint
in calculating muscle-
tendon length
changes, 274
improving in elderly, 76
walking, 268–269
Kinetic energy, for
locomotion, 257–261,
259*f*–260*f*, 261, 263,
278
Knee
coactivation of extensor
and flexor muscles,
272
in jogging, 271
muscle-tendon force at,
272
net muscle moments at,
268–272, 270*f*
in running, 269, 270*f*, 272
in walking, 268
Knee extension exercise,
dynamic
device, 95*f*, 95–96
fatigue model, 94–110,
98*f*
assessment procedure,
95*f*, 96–97
in exercise intervention
assessment, 104–107,
105*f*
in hypobaric hypoxia
assessment, 104, 105*f*,
107–109
performance measures
in, 104–106
schematic of, 97*f*

test-retest variation in,
106–107, 107*f*
point of exhaustion from,
103–104
relationship between
oxygen uptake and
work rate in, 99*f*,
99–100
Knuttgen, Howard K., 332*f*
Kolb, G., 326

Laboratory of Industrial
Physiology, 315–316.
See also Harvard
Fatigue Laboratory
Lactacystin, 236
Lactate
in amino acid
metabolism, 294
in ATP synthesis, 1–2, 5,
15, 20–21
and mitochondrial
respiration, 19
and muscle oxygen
consumption, 20–21
β-Lactone, 236
Lean body weight loss, and
knee extension
exercise, 104, 105*f*
Left ventricular
hypertrophy, in
elderly, aerobic
exercise and strength
training and, 69–70
Leg geometry, and walking,
264
Leg length
and running, 265
and walking, 262–264
Leg stiffness
and running, 265–267,
278
versus speed, 265, 266*f*
Leucine, 288, 289*f*, 308
in alanine and glutamine
synthesis, 292, 294
deamination, 307
and TCA cycle, 303, 304*f*,
307, 309
transamination, 303, 304*f*
transport, 291
Life adjustment, physical
self-concept and,
154–155
Ligaments, 267–268
Limb exchange, of amino
acids, 288–289
Limb girdle muscular
dystrophy, 222

Lipids, serum
  abnormalities, 365
  in children and
      adolescents, physical
      activity and, 354–359,
      356t–358t
  oral contraceptives and,
      357t, 359
Lipolysis, 118
Lipoprotein levels, in
      children and
      adolescents, physical
      activity and, 354–359,
      356t–358t
Lipoprotein lipase
  adipose, 191, 194–195,
      207–210, 209t
  catecholamines and, 200,
      206
  current understanding of,
      192–196
  degradation and
      clearance, 195–196
  diet and, 196–198, 201
  dietary changes and,
      197–198
  dysfunctional, 192
  estrogen and, 200–201
  fatty acids and, 191, 194,
      201, 206, 210
  feeding/fasting and,
      196–197
  gene, 192–194
  growth hormone and, 201
  history of blood fat-
      clearing factor,
      191–192
  hormones and, 198–201
  inactivation, 193–194
  insulin and, 197–200,
      199t, 201, 206
  mass, acute exercise and,
      202–205, 205f, 210
  messenger RNA, 192
      acute exercise and,
      202–204, 204f, 210
  species of, 193
  metabolism, 194–196
  in muscle, 191–218, 209t
      contractions and, 206
      exercise-induced,
          physiological
          relevance of, 206–210
      gene expression, 202,
          206, 210
      regulation by exercise,
          202–206
      resting, regulation of,
          196–201

overexpressed, 193–194
  physiological functions of,
      194
  production, 195
  protein structure, 193
  sepsis and, 201
  thyroid hormone and, 200
  tissue specific regulation,
      194, 210
  transgenic mouse lines,
      193–194
  and triglycerides,
      191–192, 194, 201,
      204–207
      altered body
          composition and, 210
      altered tissue blood
          flow due to physical
          activity and, 210
      clearance of, 207–210,
          209t
      eating and, 209
  weight (fat) loss and, 197
Lipoprotein-lipid profiles,
      abnormal, in elderly,
      70
  aerobic exercise and
      strength training and,
      64–66
Liver
  acetyl-CoA carboxylase in,
      123
  fatty acid oxidation in,
      119–120, 123
  gluconeogenesis in, 295,
      302
  glutamine-glutamate cycle
      in, 297–298
  malonyl-CoA in, 119–120
  protein degradation in,
      240
Loading, muscle, increased,
      31–60
Locomotion, 253–285. *See
      also* Jogging;
      Running; Walking
  behavioral models for,
      263–267, 278
  center of mass mechanics,
      254–267
  gait transitions, 261–263,
      277
  joint dynamics in,
      267–271
  joint power and work in,
      269–271, 270f
  mechanical energy
      fluctuations in,
      254–261, 263–264

metabolic energy costs of,
      260–262, 276–277
  muscle-tendon mechanics
      in, 253, 271–278
      electromyographic
          activity in, 275f
      force, 271–273, 275f
      forward dynamic
          simulations of,
          276–277
      inverse dynamics
          approach to, 277–278
      length changes,
          273–276, 275f
      net muscle moments in,
          267–272, 270f
      optimization criteria for,
          276–277
      performance goals of,
          277–278
      similarities in diverse
          species, 253
Longitudinal studies,
      352–353
Looking glass theory of self-
      concept, 147
Low-density lipoprotein
  in children and
      adolescents, physical
      activity and, 355–359,
      356t–358t
  in elderly, aerobic
      exercise and strength
      training and, 64–66
  obesity and, 365
Lumbar spine, bone mineral
      density in, 75,
      374–378
Lysosomal mechanisms, of
      protein degradation,
      221–222, 236

McArdle, W.D., 322
McArdle's disease, 305–308
McCurdy, J.H., 318
Macroautophagy, 221
Major histocompatibility
      complex, 234
Malate, 300
Malonyl-CoA
  carnitine palmitoyl-
      transferase inhibition
      by, 118, 120–122
  in fatty acid oxidation
      regulation, 118–129
  in fatty acid synthesis,
      119–120
  glucose and, 122–123
  insulin and, 122–123

significance in liver, 119–120
in skeletal muscle, 120–123
in exercise or fasting, 121–122, 125, 126*f*, 127–128
synthesis
by acetyl-CoA carboxylase, 120, 122–123
citrate and, 122–123
in skeletal muscle, 122–123
Mass effect, lactate production and, 21
MAT*α*2 regulator, 225
Maximal exercise, metabolic responses to, 2–16
Maximal voluntary static contraction force
exercise interventions and, 104–107, 105*f*
of exercising muscle, 98*f*, 98–99
and integrated electromyographic activity, 101–102, 102*f*
in muscle fatigue, 92–110, 93*f*
dynamic knee extension model of, 95*f*, 96–110, 97*f*–98*f*
at point of exhaustion, 103
of rested muscle, 93*f*, 97*f*–98*f*
and peak oxygen uptake, 100
Medicine and Science in Sports, 326, 331, 336
MET values, 382
Metabolic energy costs of locomotion, 260–262, 276–277
Metabolic rate, basal, 344
Metabolic syndrome, 70
Metabolism. *See* Aerobic metabolism; Anaerobic metabolism
7-Methyl-guanylate cap-binding, 167, 177
Microgravity
muscle atrophy and, 242
and protein degradation, 239*t*, 242
Minnesota Heart Health Program, 389–392

Mitochondria
density of, 19
function of, 6
respiration, 16, 18–19, 23
Mitogen(s), definition, 32
Mitogen-activated protein kinase, 36, 41, 168, 178
Mitogenesis, insulin-growth factor I and, 41
Molecular biology, and exercise physiology, 329–330, 334, 336
Morehouse, Lawrence E., 320*f*–321*f*, 325
Motion, range of, 348*t*. *See also* Locomotion
mRNA. *See* Ribonucleic acid, messenger
Muscle(s). *See also* Cardiac muscle; Skeletal muscle
atrophy of. *See* Atrophy, muscle
contraction of. *See* Contraction(s), muscle
fatigue of. *See* Fatigue, muscle
mass of
aging and, 66–67, 73
changes in, 33
oxygen consumption by. *See* Oxygen consumption
Muscle cell lines, definition, 32
Muscle moments, net, 267–272
at ankle, 268–271, 270*f*
at hip, 268–269, 270*f*
in jogging, 271
at knee, 268–272, 270*f*
in running, 269–272, 270*f*
in walking, 267–271
Muscle quality, in elderly, 76–77
Muscle wasting
glucocorticoids and, 239
sepsis and, 176
Muscle-tendon mechanics, in locomotion, 253, 271–278
electromyographic activity in, 275*f*
force, 271–273, 275*f*
forward dynamic simulations of, 276–277

inverse dynamics
approach to, 277–278
length changes, 273–276, 275*f*
partitioning into components, 274
Muscular dystrophy, limb girdle, 222
Muscular strength, 343, 347, 348*t*
and bone mineral density, 74–75
Musculoskeletal health, of elderly, 61–62, 73–79
MVC force. *See* Maximal voluntary static contraction force
Myoblasts, 45, 49
definition, 32–33
Myofibers
changes in, 33
formation, 32
insulin-like growth factor-I and, 34*f*, 45
in muscle hypertrophy, 33, 47
Myogenesis
definition, 32
insulin-like growth factor-I and, 33–34, 40–41, 44–45
and muscle atrophy, 50–51
and muscle hypertrophy, 33, 47–53
Myogenic regulatory factors, and insulin-like growth factor-I, 40–41
Myonuclei
and muscle atrophy, 50–51
and muscle hypertrophy, 47–48
Myosin heavy chain, 180–181
Myotubes, formation, 32, 40–41, 51

NAD$^+$-isocitrate dehydrogenase, 16
Na-K pump activity, aging and, 72
National Center for Health Statistics, 347
National Health Examination Survey, 370*t*, 372

National Health Interview Survey (1988), 379
National Health Interview Survey-Health Promotion Disease Prevention Supplement, 345, 346t, 347–349
National Health Interview Survey-Youth Risk Behavior Survey, 345, 346t, 349–350
examples, for selected physical activity patterns, 351–352
National Heart, Lung and Blood Institute Growth and Health Study, 372
Study of Child Activity and Nutrition, 356t, 381–382, 383t–384t
National Institute of Health, 326, 336
N-end rule proteins, 236
Nervous system, sympathetic, in elderly, 72
Neuromuscular function, of elderly, improving, 76
NHES. See National Health Examination Survey
NHIS-HPDP. See National Health Interview Survey-Health Promotion Disease Prevention Supplement
NHIS-YRBS. See National Health Interview Survey-Youth Risk Behavior Survey
Nicotinamide adenine dinucleotide, 2, 5, 16, 21–23, 119, 300
Nicotinamide adenine dinucleotide phosphate, 175–176
Nicotinamide adenine dinucleotide phosphate-dependent malic enzyme, 302
Nitrogen
for alanine and glutamine synthesis, 290f, 292–294
in amino acid metabolism, 289–290, 296
Nitrogen balance, 239–241

Nitrogen carriers, non-toxic, 288
Norepinephrine, 72, 200
Norgestrel, and serum lipids, 357t, 359
Normoxia, 21
assessment of, in knee extension exercise, 104, 107–109
Nutritional status, and protein synthesis, 175–176

Oberlin College, 318
Obesity, 343, 348t
in children and adolescents
physical activity and, 365–373, 368t–371t
physical inactivity and, 372–373
television watching and, 370t, 372–373
development of, 365
in elderly, aerobic exercise and strength training and, 70–72
and hypertension, 360
physical inactivity and, 370t
prevalence of, 365
Observational studies, 352–353
ODC. See Ornithine decarboxylase
Okadaic acid, 169–170
Older persons. See Elderly
Open reading frames (ORFs), 176
Oral contraceptives, and serum lipids, 357t, 359
Oral glucose tolerance test (OGTT), 67–68
Ornithine decarboxylase, degradation of, 233
Oslo Youth Study, 356t
Osteoarthritis, 365
Osteoporosis, 73
costs associated with, 73
weight-bearing and, 343, 348t
Outward Bound, and self-concept study, 139–140
Oxaloacetate, 123, 289f, 299–300, 303
2-Oxoglutarate, 23

Oxoglutarate dehydrogenase, 18
2-Oxoglutarate dehydrogenase, 16
Oxygen consumption, 23
interaction with glycolysis, 16
kinetics, 22
limits, in intense contraction, 18–19
maximum
in children and adolescents, physical activity and, 355
in elderly, 62, 72
aerobic exercise and strength training and, 62–63
regulation, 16–20
in the rest-to-steady-state transition period, 19–20
Oxygen partial pressure, at level of mitochondria (PO_{2mito}), 16, 19
Oxygen uptake
peak
assessment of, 92
MVC force and, 100
relationship with work rate, in dynamic knee extension exercise, 99f, 99–100

p53, 225
Palmitate oxidation, 117, 119
Palmitoyl-CoA, 124
Parental modeling, and physical activity, 382, 383t–384t
Passive walking machines, 264–265
PDC. See Pyruvate dehydrogenase complex
PEAS. See Physical Estimation and Attraction Scales
Peer status, 148
Pelvic rotation, and walking, 264
Pelvic tilt, and walking, 264
Pennsylvania State University, 328
meeting on exercise physiology (1978), 332f, 332–333, 333t
Peptide aldehydes, 236

Peptidyl-tRNA, 170
Perceived Competence Scale
  for Children, 144
PEST sequences, 225, 233
Phosphate, inorganic
  in ATP synthesis, 4
  in glycogenolysis
    regulation, 4–5
Phosphatidyl-inositol-3-
  kinase, 36, 40–41
Phosphocreatine, 23
  in ATP synthesis, 1–15, 3*f*,
    17–18, 21–22, 24
  creatine supplementation
    and, 6–10
  hydrolysis, products of, 4
  interaction with adenine
    nucleotide and
    glycogen metabolism,
    4–6
  and muscle oxygen
    consumption, 22
  repeated bouts of exercise
    and, 13–15, 15*f*
  synthesis, 3–4, 7, 14
  in type I and type II
    muscle fibers, 10–11,
    11*f*, 14–15, 15*f*
Phosphoenolpyruvate
  carboxykinase,
    reversal of, 302–303
Phosphofructokinase, 6
Phosphorylation
  oxidative, 16, 21
    in ATP synthesis, 1, 13,
      18, 24
  in phosphocreatine
    synthesis, 4
  regulation, 22–23
  substrate-level, in ATP
    synthesis, 1, 4, 6,
      17–18
Physical activity
  of children and
    adolescents
  age and, 351–352
  and blood pressure,
    353–354, 359–364,
    361*t*–363*t*
  and bone mineral
    density, 373–379,
    375*t*–377*t*
  determinants of,
    381–388, 383*t*–384*t*,
    386*t*–387*t*
  geographic region and,
    351–352
  household income and,
    351–352

and insulin, 364–365,
    366*t*
  interventions to
    promote, 388–392,
    390*t*–391*t*
  measurement of,
    343–345
  and obesity and
    adiposity, 365–373,
    368*t*–371*t*
  parental modeling and,
    382, 383*t*–384*t*
  patterns in, 347–349,
    351–352
  race and, 351–352, 382,
    383*t*, 385
  seasonal differences in,
    351–352, 382, 384*t*
  and serum lipids,
    354–359, 356*t*–358*t*
  sex differences and,
    351–352, 355,
    360–367, 374–380,
    382, 385–386,
    389–392
  socioeconomic status
    and, 385
  surveillance, in United
    States, 345–352, 346*t*
  and unintentional
    injury, 379–381
  definition, 342
  versus exercise and
    physical fitness, 342
  health-related dimensions
    of, 343, 347, 348*t*
  mechanisms of effect,
    343, 348*t*
  year 2000 objectives in,
    347, 348*t*, 349–351
Physical activity
  epidemiology
  applied to children and
    adolescents, 341–403
  case-control
    (retrospective)
    studies, 352–353
  cross-sectional studies,
    352–353
  definition, 342–343
  ecologic studies, 352–353
  experimental studies,
    352–354
  longitudinal studies,
    352–353
  measurement, 343–345
  observational studies,
    352–353

prospective studies, 353
  research designs, 352–354
  surveys, 343–345
Physical disability, 343, 348*t*
Physical Estimation and
  Attraction Scales, 143
Physical fitness, definition,
  342
Physical self-concept. *See*
  Self-concept, physical
Physical Self-Description
  Questionnaire, 137,
    143*t*, 147
Physical Self-Efficacy Scale,
  142*t*, 144
Physical Self-Perception
  Profile, 137, 143*t*,
    145–147, 152–153
Pi. *See* Phosphate, inorganic
PI31 protein inhibitor,
  234–235
Platelet-derived growth
  factors, 48
Play, 382
Playground-related injuries,
  379–380
Plurimetabolic syndrome, 70
Polyamine synthesis, 233
Polypeptides, genetic
  translation and,
    165–170, 175, 177,
    179
PO$_{2mito}$. *See* Oxygen partial
  pressure, at level of
  mitochondria
  (PO$_{2mito}$)
PPA, 146
Prescription, exercise, 330
Pressure overload, of heart,
  175
Primary cell structure,
  definition, 32
Progestin, and serum lipids,
  357*t*, 359
Program directors, 330
Proliferation, cell
  definition, 32
  insulin-like growth factor-I
    and, 40–41, 48, 50,
      51*f*
  in muscle development
    and adaptation,
      40–41, 47–50, 49*f*
  of satellite cells, 47–50
Prospective studies, 353
Protease(s), calcium-
  dependent, 222
Protease inhibitors, 228

Proteasome(s)
  archaebacterial, 226–228, 227*f*
  chymotrypsin-like activity of, 228
  crystal structures of, 226–229
  eukaryotic, 226–228, 227*f*
  inhibitors, 228, 234–235
  morphology of, 227
  peptidyl-glutamylpeptide hydrolyzing activity of, 228
  20S
    inhibitors, and protein degradation, 236–237
    as proteolytic core of 26S, 226–230, 231*f*
    regulators of, 229–235
    structure of, 227, 227*f*
  26S
    composition of, 226, 229–233, 231*f*
    degradation of non-ubiquitinated proteins, 233
    degradation of ubiquitinated proteins, 223–224, 226–233, 231*f*
    inhibitors, and protein degradation, 236–237
    proteolytic core of, 226–230, 231*f*
    regulatory complex of (PA700), 226, 229–233, 230*t*, 231*f*
    structure of, 226, 231*f*
    trypsin-like activity of, 228
    yeast, 227–229
Proteasome activator 28, 234
Proteasome activator 700, 226, 229–233, 230*t*, 231*f*
Protein(s)
  amino acids as, 287
  binding
    in genetic translation, 167–168
    to insulin-like growth factor-I, 37–40, 39*f*
    to iron responsive elements, 181
    to messenger RNA, 182, 196
  contractile, 287
  controlling levels of, 220–221
  long-lived, and protein degradation, 236

in muscle hypertrophy, 40
muscle-specific, and insulin-like growth factor-I, 40
selection for degradation, 221, 223–226, 224*f*
short-lived
  and cellular processes, 220
  and protein degradation, 236
in skeletal muscle, 287
total, in man's body, 287
ubiquitination of, 223–226, 224*f*
Protein deficiency, 239*t*
Protein degradation, 174, 219, 287, 308
  alteration of, 219
  and atrophy, 219–220, 241–242
  calpain system of, 222, 236
  conjugation in, 223–224, 224*f*
  glucocorticoids and, 239*t*, 239–240
  insulin and, 239*t*, 239–240
  lysosomal mechanisms of, 221–222, 236
  of non-ubiquitinated proteins, 233
  phosphorylation and, 225
  physiological importance and roles of, 220–221
  protein meal and, 295–296
  regulation of, 220
  sequences, 225–226
  in skeletal muscle, 219–221, 238–242
    physiological regulators of, 239*t*
  in steady-state conditions, 219
  and tissue growth, 219–220
  ubiquitin as marker for, 223–226, 224*f*
  ubiquitin-proteasome pathway of, 219–220, 222–252
    components of, 222–233, 231*f*, 238
    isopeptidase activity in, 232–233
    mutational analysis of, 235–236
    pharmacological intervention in, 243

physiological substrates of, 237, 237*t*
proteasome inhibitors and, 236–237
regulation by, 237–241
role of, 235–237
Protein expression, 174
  ferritin, 181
Protein synthesis, 287
  alteration of, 219
  and atrophy, 219–220
  initiation of, 166
  insulin and, 168, 174–175, 178–179, 239
  in muscle, 165, 219
    atrophy and, 179–180
    control points, 172*t*–173*t*, 175–182
    exercise and, 171–175, 308
    measuring rate of, 171
    modulation, 171–175
    nutritional status and, 175–176
  protein meal and, 295–296
  in steady-state conditions, 219
  and tissue growth, 219–220
Proteolysis. *See* Protein degradation
PSDQ. *See* Physical Self-Description Questionnaire
PSPP. *See* Physical Self-Perception Profile
Public health, 341–342, 392
Purine, biosynthesis of, 296
Purine nucleotide cycle, 292–293, 293*f*, 301, 307
Pyruvate, 4, 23
  in amino acid metabolism, 288, 289*f*, 294–295, 301–302, 305–306
  exercise and, 301–302, 305–306
Pyruvate carboxylase, 302
Pyruvate dehydrogenase, 16, 21, 300, 302
Pyruvate dehydrogenase complex
  and muscle oxygen consumption, 18
  as site for aerobic and anaerobic metabolism interaction, 20–24
Pyruvate dehydrogenase reaction, 123

Quadriceps
  composition, 10
  in dynamic knee
      extension exercise,
      94, 96
  ischemia, 100
Questionnaires, activity, 344

RAS protein, 36
Reaven syndrome, 70
Red blood cells, 16
Reflected appraisals, and
    self-concept, 147–148
Regeneration, muscle
  insulin-like growth factor-I
      and, 44–45
  satellite cells and, 47–48
Releasing factors, in genetic
    translation, 167*f*, 170
Reserpine, 200
Resistance training, for
    elderly, and insulin-
    like growth factor-I
    and growth hormone,
    41–42
Resting metabolic rate, in
    elderly, aerobic
    exercise and strength
    training and, 72–73
Rest-to-steady-state period,
    19–20, 22
Retrospective studies,
    352–353
Ribonucleic acid, messenger
  binding proteins, 182, 196
  exercise and, 174
  recognition and binding,
      167
    scanning model of, 167
  stability, 180–182, 196
  structure, 168
  synthesis, 196
  translation, 165–171, 167*f*,
      196
    in muscle, 171–182
Ribonucleic acid, ribosomal
  exercise and, 173
  in genetic translation, 166
  synthesis, 179
Ribonucleic acid, transfer
  formation, 168–169
  in genetic translation,
      166, 168–170
  in protein synthesis, 171
Ribonucleoprotein complex,
    167
Ribosome(s)
  in genetic translation,
      166, 170–171, 176,
      178, 181

synthesis, 180
Ribosome releasing factor,
    167*f*, 171
Riley, R.L., 325
Robergs, R.A., 327
Roberts, S.O., 327
Robinson, Sid, 315,
    320*f*–321*f*, 324, 334,
    336
Rodahl, K., 326
Rogerian counseling
    psychology, 147
Rolling egg mechanism, in
    walking, 258–259
rRNA. *See* Ribonucleic acid,
    ribosomal
Running
  Achilles' tendon force in,
      273
  behavioral models for,
      265–267
    in robots, 265–267
  biomechanics of, 253–285
  as bouncing gait, 261, 278
  energy storage and return
      in, 261, 274–275
  gravitational potential
      energy for, 257, 260*f*,
      261
  ground reaction force for,
      254, 256*f*, 265
  joint dynamics in,
      267–271
  joint power and work in,
      260–271, 270*f*
  kinetic energy for,
      257–258, 260*f*, 261
  leg length and, 265
  leg stiffness and, 265–267,
      278
    versus speed, 265, 266*f*
  mechanical energy
      fluctuations in,
      254–258, 261
  metabolic energy costs of,
      261–262
  net muscle moments in,
      269–272, 270*f*
  spring-mass model of,
      265, 278
  of single stance phase,
      258*f*
  speed in, 266*f*
  stick figure representation
      of, 258*f*
  surface stiffness and, 265
  transition from walking,
      261–263

Saccharomyces cerevisiae,
    234–236
Sarcopenia, 73
Satellite cells
  definition, 33
  differentiation, 50
  insulin-like growth factor-I
      and, 48–50, 51*f*
  in muscle adaptation,
      47–51
  in muscle atrophy, 50–51
  proliferation, 47–50
SCAN. *See* National Heart,
    Lung and Blood
    Institute, Study of
    Child Activity and
    Nutrition
Schneider, E.C., 327
SDQ. *See* Self-Description
    Questionnaire
SDQII. *See* Self-Description
    Questionnaire II
SDQIII. *See* Self-Description
    Questionnaire III
Self-acceptance, 134, 156*t*,
    156–157
Self-appraisals, 147
Self-concept, 133–164. *See
    also* Self-concept,
    physical
  academic, 133
  age and gender effects,
      149–151
    adolescence, 149–150
    adulthood, 150
    female scores, 150–151
    late adolescence-early
        adulthood, 150
    preadolescence, 149
  assessment items,
      136–138, 155–157
    relevance of, 136
    specificity/generality of,
        136–137, 137*t*
  Big Fish, Little Pond
      phenomenon and,
      148
  definition, 133–134
  hierarchical models of,
      135*f*, 135–136
  internal standards and,
      148–149
  longitudinal research in,
      139
  looking glass theory of,
      147
  reflected appraisals and,
      147–148

Self-concept (*continued*)
  scales, 136–147, 142*t*–143*t*
    component, advantages
      of, 138–141
    limitations of, 155–157
    narrow traits versus
      broad traits in,
      140–141
  and self-esteem, 134
  social, 133
  social comparisons and,
    147–148
  structure and
    measurement,
    133–138
Self-concept, physical, 133,
  139
  age and gender effects,
    149–151
  assessment items for,
    137–138
  competence and, 148,
    154–155, 156*t*,
    156–157
  development of, 147–149
  and life adjustment,
    154–155
  scales, 141–147, 142*t*–143*t*
    gender differences in,
      145
    social desirability and,
      140–141
  self-acceptance and, 156*t*,
    156–157
  self-enhancement and,
    152–154
  skill development and,
    151–152
Self-confidence, 133
Self-Description
  Questionnaire, 142*t*,
    144–146, 149
Self-Description
  Questionnaire II, 145,
    149–150
Self-Description
  Questionnaire III,
    139, 142*t*, 145–147,
    149
Self-efficacy, 138
  exercise, 381, 385,
    386*t*–387*t*, 388–389
  physical, 136
Self-enhancement, 134, 134*f*,
  152–154
Self-esteem. *See also* Self-
  concept

components of, 133
definition, 134
dimensions of, 134
exercise and, 134, 135*f*,
  135–136, 138–139,
  143–144
interactions with
  environment, 134,
  134*f*
and physical self-worth,
  135–136
and self-concept, 134
Self-identity, 147
Self-Liking/Self
  Competence Scale,
  156, 156*t*
Self-perception, 148
Self-Perception Profile for
  Children, 142*t*,
  144–155
Sepsis
  and amino acid
    metabolism, 291
  and genetic translation,
    176
  glutamine concentrations
    in, 296–297
  and lipoprotein lipase,
    201
  and muscle wasting, 176
  and triglycerides, 201
Serine, 291
Serum withdrawal, and
  lysosomal
  mechanisms of
  protein degradation,
  221–222
Shepherd, R.J., 331
Skateboarding injury, 379
Skating injury, 379
Skeletal muscle
  adaptation, 31, 33
    insulin-like growth
      factor-I and, 31–60
    satellite cells and,
      47–48
  aging and, 61–62, 73–79
  amino acid metabolism in,
    287–314, 290*f*
    in exercise, 287–288,
      299–309
    at rest, 287–298, 308
    schematic presentation
      of, 289*f*
  amino acids in, 287–288,
    308
  atrophy
    myonuclei and satellite
      cells in, 50–51

protein metabolism
  and, 179–180,
  219–220, 241–242
chronic stimulation of,
  174
development of, 33–34,
  40–41
energy, 1, 191, 207
fatty acid oxidation in,
  117–129
fiber types, 10
  metabolism, 8–13, 11*f*,
    13–15
hypertrophy
  insulin-like growth
    factor-I and, 33, 40,
    42–46, 46*f*, 50,
    51*f*–52*f*
  myogenic aspects of,
    47–53, 49*f*
lipoprotein lipase in,
  191–218
  exercise-induced,
    physiological
    relevance of, 206–210
  regulation at rest,
    196–201
  regulation by exercise,
    202–206
  and triglyceride
    clearance, 207–210,
    209*t*
malonyl-CoA in, and
  exercise or fasting,
  121–122, 125, 126*f*,
  127–128
oxygen consumption,
  regulators, in
  contraction, 16–20
protein degradation in,
  220–221, 238–240
  atrophy and, 219–220,
    241–242
  physiological regulators
    of, 239*t*
protein synthesis in, 165,
  219
  exercise and, 171–175,
    308
  measuring rate of, 171
  modulation, 171–182,
    172*t*–173*t*
  nutritional status and,
    175–176
proteins in, 287
regeneration
  insulin-like growth
    factor-I and, 44–45
  satellite cells in, 47–48

TCA cycle in, 287–288, 289f, 294, 299–309
thyroid hormones and, 51–53
translation and gene expression in, 165, 202
control of, 171–182
control points and mechanisms, 172t–173t, 175–182
elongation phase, 173t, 179–181
exercise and, 171–175, 206
initiation phase, 172t, 175–179
mechanical influence on, 181
termination phase, 173t, 179, 181–182
Skill development, self-concept/self-esteem and, 134, 134f, 151–152
Skinfold measurements, 367–373, 368t–371t
Skinner, James S., 332f
Slice of Life Program, 391t, 392
Slow-twitch muscle
microgravity and, 242
protein synthesis in, 175–176, 179–180
triglycerides in, 207
Soccer injury, 379
Social cognitive theory, and physical activity, 381
Social comparisons, and self-concept, 147–148
Sodium
and amino acid transporters, 291
and hypertension, 360
Softball injury, 379
Somatomedin C. *See* Insulin-like growth factor-I
Somatomedin hypothesis of insulin-like growth factor-I, 33–34, 34f
Sonomicrometry, 274, 275f
SPARK. *See* Sports, Play, and Active Recreation for Kids Study
Speed
for gait transitions, 261–263
equine model of, 262, 277

leg stiffness versus, 265, 266f
in spring-mass model of running, 266f
walking, optimum for energy transfer, 260–261
Splanchnic area, glutamine-glutamate cycle in, 295, 297–298, 298f
Sports injury, in children and adolescents, 379–381
activity type and, 379
age and, 379
geographic region and, 379–380
measurement of, 380
morbidity in, 379
participation data and, 380
physical participation context and, 379–380
population-based relative risk of, 380–381
sex differences in, 379–380
Sports, Play, and Active Recreation for Kids Study, 389, 390t
Springfield College, 318
Spring-mass model, of running, 258f, 265, 266f, 278
Starvation, protein synthesis and genetic translation and, 175–176
Static optimization, 272
Steinhaus, Arthur H., 318–319
Strain forces, peak, 378
Strength, aging and, 73
exercise intervention and, 76–77
Strength training
for elderly, 61–89
and abdominal obesity, 70–72
and bone mineral density, 74–75
and cardiovascular disease risk factors, 62–73
and cardiovascular fitness level, 62–64
and fall prevention, 75–76

and glucose intolerance and insulin resistance, 66–68
and hypertension, 68–69
and left ventricular hypertrophy, 69–70
and lipoprotein-lipid profiles, 64–66
and muscle quality, 76–77
and resting metabolic rate, 72–73
and knee extension exercise, 104–106, 105f
Striated muscle, translation and gene expression in, 165
Succinate, 300
Succinyl-CoA, 289f
Superobesity, 370t, 372
Support moment, in walking, 268
Surface stiffness, and running, 265
Surgeon General's report on physical activity and health (1996), 341, 347
Surveys, in physical activity epidemiology, 343–345
Swing limb, in walking, 264–265
Syndrome X, 70

Target force, 92–93, 93f, 103
Taylor, Henry L., 320f–321f, 323, 325
Television watching, by children and adolescents, 382
and obesity, 370t, 372–373
Tendons, 267–268, 271–278. *See also* Muscle-tendon mechanics, in locomotion
Tennessee Self-Concept Scale, 139, 144, 146, 154–156
Ternary complex, in genetic translation, 166–167, 175–177
Testing, exercise, 330
Tetrahydrolipstatin, 193
Texas Southwestern Medical School, 324

TGFβ. *See* Transforming growth factor-β
Thermoplasma acidophilum, 227
Third National Health and Nutrition Examination Survey, 347
Thyroid hormone(s)
and insulin-like growth factor-I, 51–53
and lipoprotein lipase, 200
and protein degradation, 239t
Thyroid response elements, 51
Tipton, Charles M., 328, 332f
Tolbutamide, 198
Transferrin receptor, 181
Transforming growth factor-β, 40, 50
Translation, genetic, 165–190
control of, 165, 171–182
control points and mechanisms, 172t–173t, 175–182
definition, 165
in muscle, 165, 171–182, 172t–173t
compartmentalization and localization, 182
sensitivity to metabolism, 182
phases of, 166
elongation, 166, 168–170, 173t, 179–181
initiation, 166–168, 172t, 175–179
termination, 166, 170–171, 173t, 179, 181–182
process of, 166–171
schematic representation of, 167f
terminology, 166
Trauma. *See also* Sports injury
and amino acid metabolism, 291
glutamine concentrations in, 296–297
TRE. *See* Thyroid response elements

Treadmill
for assessment of hypobaric hypoxia, 109
for cardiovascular fitness assessment, 62–64
for dynamic exercise assessment, 91
for exercise performance assessment, 91–94, 104
Tricarboxylic acid cycle
amino acid metabolism and, 287–288, 289f, 294, 299–309
anaplerosis
alanine aminotransferase reaction and, 300–303, 301f, 305–306, 308–309
amino acid deamination and, 307–309
branched chain aminotransferase reaction and, 303–306
in exercise, 287–288, 299–309
glutamine synthesis and, 307–309
for maximal rate of substrate oxidation, 305–306
role of orally ingested carbohydrate and blood glucose, 306
carbon drain on, and fatigue, 303–306, 304f, 309
multi-site modulation of, 300
and muscle oxygen consumption, 18
pyruvate dehydrogenase complex and, 21–23
substrate of, 299–300
Tricarboxylic acid cycle citrate synthase, 300
Triglycerides
in children and adolescents, 355, 356t–358t
clearance, 207–210, 209t
altered body composition and, 210

altered tissue blood flow due to physical activity and, 210
eating and, 209
in elderly, 65–66
exercise and, 65–66, 204–210, 355, 356t–358t
fatty acids from, 117, 118f
hydrolysis, 194
lipoprotein lipase and, 191–192, 194, 201, 204–210, 209t
sepsis and, 201
tRNA. *See* Ribonucleic acid, transfer
TSCS. *See* Tennessee Self-Concept Scale
Tubulin, 180
Tumor necrosis factor, 176
Tyrosine kinase activity, 35–36

Ubiquitin
activation, 223
as marker for protein degradation, 223–226, 224f
Ubiquitin-proteasome pathway, 219–220, 222–252
components of, 222–233, 231f, 238
proteasome activator 700, 226, 229–233, 230t, 231f
20S proteasome, 226–230, 227f, 231f
26S proteasome, 223–224, 226–233, 231f
ubiquitin, 223–226, 224f
isopeptidase activity in, 232–233
mutational analysis of, 235–236
pharmacological intervention in, 243
physiological substrates of, 237, 237t
proteasome inhibitors and, 236–237
regulation by, 237–241
role of, 235–237
Ubiquitin-protein ligase, 223
Ubiquitin-specific processing proteases (Ubps), 232

University of California at Los Angeles, 329
University of California at Santa Barbara, 323
University of Chicago, 324
University of Illinois, 323
University of Illinois (Chicago), 329–330, 334
University of Massachusetts, 328–329
University of Minnesota, 315, 323, 325, 336
University of Nevada, 323
University of Washington, 329
Unloading, muscle, 33, 50–51
  in animal models, 43
  protein degradation and, 241–242
Upstream open reading frames (uORFs), 176
Urea, 297–298, 298*f*

Valine, 288, 289*f*, 294, 303, 307–308
Velocity, movement, and muscle fatigue, 103–104, 110
VO_2. *See* Oxygen consumption
Volleyball injury, 380
VO_2max. *See* Oxygen consumption, maximum

Waist/hip ratio, 70–71, 372
Walking
  Achilles' tendon force in, 272–273, 273*f*
  behavioral models for, 263–265
  biomechanics of, 253–285

double support in, 254
energy transfer mechanism in, 258–261, 259*f*, 263–264
  optimum speed for, 260–261
gravitational potential energy for, 254–261, 259*f*, 263, 278
ground reaction force for, 254, 255*f*, 264
inverted pendulum model of, 258–264, 278
of single stance phase, 257*f*
joint dynamics in, 267–271
joint power and work in, 269–271
kinematics, 268–269
kinetic energy for, 257–261, 259*f*, 263, 278
leg geometry and, 264
leg length and, 262–264
mechanical energy fluctuations in, 254–261, 263–264
mechanics, in elderly, improving, 76
metabolic energy costs of, 260–262
net muscle moments in, 267–271
stick figure representation, 257*f*
support moment in, 268
transition to running, 261–263
Walking machines, passive, 264–265
Wasting. *See* Muscle wasting

Weight, and self-concept, 149
Weight gain, and hypertension, 360
Weight loss
  diet and, 373
  exercise and, 373
  and knee extension exercise, 104, 105*f*
  and lipoprotein lipase, 197
Weight-bearing activity, 343, 348*t*
  and bone mineral density, 374–378, 375*t*–377*t*
  and osteoporosis, 343
Weinberger Laboratory, 324
Wild-type cell, 32
Wilmore, Jack H., 332*f*
Women, postmenopausal
  bone mineral density of, 73–75
  hip fracture risk in, 73–75
  osteoporosis in, 73
Work rate
  peak, assessment of, 92
  relationship with oxygen uptake, in dynamic knee extension exercise, 99*f*, 99–100
Wrist, distal, bone mineral density in, 75
Wylie, Ruth, 141

Year 2000 objectives, in physical activity, 347, 348*t*, 349–351
Young Finns Study, 355–359, 357*t*, 365, 366*t*
Youth and Sports, 380
Youth Risk Behavior Survey, 345–347, 346*t*, 350–351